Advanced Surgical Facial Rejuvenation

Anthony Erian • Melvin A. Shiffman
(Editors)

Advanced Surgical Facial Rejuvenation

Art and Clinical Practice

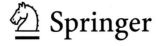

Editors
Anthony Erian, MD
Pear Tree Cottage
Cambridge Road
Wimpole 43
SG8 5QD Cambridge
United Kingdom
plasticsurgeon@anthonyerian.com

Melvin A. Shiffman, MD
17501 Chatham Drive
Tustin, California 92780-2302
USA
shiffmanmdjd@yahoo.com

ISBN 978-3-642-17837-5   e-ISBN 978-3-642-17838-2
DOI 10.1007/978-3-642-17838-2
Springer Heidelberg Dordrecht London New York

Library of Congress Control Number: 2011937179

© Springer-Verlag Berlin Heidelberg 2012

This work is subject to copyright. All rights are reserved, whether the whole or part of the material is concerned, specifically the rights of translation, reprinting, reuse of illustrations, recitation, broadcasting, reproduction on microfilm or in any other way, and storage in data banks. Duplication of this publication or parts thereof is permitted only under the provisions of the German Copyright Law of September 9, 1965, in its current version, and permission for use must always be obtained from Springer. Violations are liable to prosecution under the German Copyright Law.

The use of general descriptive names, registered names, trademarks, etc. in this publication does not imply, even in the absence of a specific statement, that such names are exempt from the relevant protective laws and regulations and therefore free for general use.

Product liability: The publishers cannot guarantee the accuracy of any information about dosage and application contained in this book. In every individual case the user must check such information by consulting the relevant literature.

Cover design: eStudioCalamar, Figueres/Berlin

Printed on acid-free paper

Springer is part of Springer Science+Business Media (www.springer.com)

Foreword

The trend of this last century is undoubtedly to look young and youthful for the longest time possible. I believe this is due to many factors. Certainly progress in medicine, precocious diagnosis of many diseases and new therapeutic protocols have contributed in increasing longevity but most of all never like in these last decades has the image of a person been so important. We have surely become a society of appearances.

This book will certainly help the young cosmetic surgeon to choose the best techniques in order to achieve excellent results. Another important aspect that comes out of this well-described book is that invasive surgery is not necessary all the times as we once used to believe. Today, traditional lifting is usually proposed in fewer patients than before. It is possible to achieve ameliorations with other, less-invasive techniques such as fat transfer and others. In this way the patient can have short postoperative recovery periods. We should learn to satisfy our patients with the less aggressive techniques possible. Theses combined techniques is the answer that this book can give to its readers. I think that we should really be grateful to Anthony Erian, Melvin Shiffman, and to the other authors for lending us their knowledge.

I would like to add a simple thought of mine to the reader of this book. Besides the technique chosen, the cosmetic surgeon should always keep in mind that he or she is not infallible. In no way does he or she have divine power, so humbleness should be his or her main character trait. Personal hypertrophic ego can lead to major mistakes! We should make our patients happy and try to help them find a better way of living with themselves. My advice is always not to promise your patients what they will not receive.

I would like to quote a beautiful thought of the author of the book *The Face* by Charles H. Willi, published in 1926: "The plastic surgeon is undoubtedly the greatest of all contemporary artists, he paints on living canvas and sculpts on human flesh contributing to the health and happiness and success of his patient."

Rome, Italy   Giorgio Fischer, M.D.

Preface

This book is the result of the hard work of many surgeons who wish to share with you their passion of facial aesthetic surgery. They are experts in their field and have agreed to share their knowledge and experience. The book covers comprehensive and "state-of-the-art" techniques in facial aesthetic surgery, and specific accounts and special techniques, both general and personal, are included.

The aim of this book is to give an up-to-date account of the latest in cosmetic facial surgery, as the trends and techniques seems to change with the times. We surgeons spend our lives learning and improving our techniques, honing and refining them. Both a beginner and an experienced surgeon will learn something from this text book.

A new trend of nonsurgical solutions has been added, as now facial rejuvenation encompasses both surgical and nonsurgical. It is acknowledged that anatomy is 90% of surgery, hence the inclusion of a detailed account relevant to facial rejuvenation.

This book has also stressed pre- and postoperative preparation to reduce complications and avoid litigation which is essential to our society nowadays.

Also, assessments and concepts of beauty have been added as it is difficult to have a basic parameter in this subjective industry.

I am very grateful to all the doctors who contributed with their time, knowledge, and dedication to make this book a special one.

I would like to refer to a facelift as surgical facial rejuvenation, as I feel the word "facelift" is confusing to both the patient and surgeon. It is also a misnomer. It is very difficult to divide the face into zones as all the anatomy is interlinked and interdependent.

In modern surgery today, one tends to combine more than one procedure, both surgical and nonsurgical, so it is more appropriate to name it Surgical Facial Rejuvenation.

I hope and believe that this book will be extremely useful to colleagues and students who want to know more about Facial Rejuvenation.

Cambridge, UK   Anthony Erian, M.D.

Contents

Part I Anatomy

1 Facial Anatomy 3
Peter M. Prendergast

2 Facial Proportions 15
Peter M. Prendergast

3 Danger Zones in Surgical Facial Rejuvenation 23
Peter M. Prendergast

4 Muscles Used in Facial Expression 31
Melvin A. Shiffman

**5 SMAFS (Superficial Musculoaponeurotic-Fatty System):
A Changed SMAS Concept; Anatomic Variants, Modes
of Handling, and Clinical Significance in Facelift Surgery** 35
Hassan Abbas Khawaja, Melvin A. Shiffman,
and Enrique Hernández-Pérez

Part II Anesthesia

**6 Anesthesia for Minimally Invasive Cosmetic Surgery
of the Head and Neck** 49
Gary Dean Bennett

7 Personal Method of Anesthesia in the Office 77
Stephen J. Gray

Part III Preoperative and Postoperative

8 Preoperative and Postoperative Plan 87
Anthony Erian and Ben Pocock

9 Facial Imaging 95
John Flynn

10	Skin Care and Adjuvant Techniques Pre and Post Facial Surgery..................................	107
	Anthony Erian and Clara Santos	

Part IV Psychological Aspects

11	What Is Human Beauty?..................................	117
	Pierre F. Fournier	

12	Body Dysmorphic Disorder..................................	123
	Melvin A. Shiffman	

Part V Techniques

13	Hair Transplantation..................................	129
	Paul C. Cotterill	

14	Ablative Laser Facial Resurfacing..................................	169
	P. Daniel Ward and Jessica H. Maxwell	

15	Photorejuvenation..................................	175
	Kenneth Beer and Rhoda S. Narins	

16	Superficial and Medium-Depth Chemical Peels..................	181
	Benjamin A. Bassichis	

17	Deep Phenol Chemical Peels..................................	193
	Michel Siegel and Benjamin A. Bassichis	

18	Chemical Blepharoplasty..................................	197
	Clara Santos	

19	Facial Implants..................................	205
	Benjamin A. Bassichis	

20	Injectable Facial Fillers..................................	211
	Donald W. Buck II, Murad Alam, and John Y.S. Kim	

21	Botulinum Toxin for Facial Rejuvenation..................................	219
	George J. Bitar, Daisi J. Choi, and Florencia Segura	

22	History of Fat Transfer..................................	231
	Melvin A. Shiffman	

23	Role of Fat Transfer in Facial Rejuvenation....................	233
	Anthony Erian	

24	**Cosmetic Surgical Rejuvenation of the Neck** 241
	L. Angelo Cuzalina and Colin E. Bailey

25	**Submental Liposuction** 267
	Mervyn Low

26	**Vaser UAL for the Heavy Face** 273
	Alberto Di Giuseppe and George Commons

27	**Suture Facelift Techniques** 279
	Peter M. Prendergast

28	**Bio-Lifting and Bio-Resurfacing** 315
	Pier Antonio Bacci

29	**Standard Facelifting** 329
	Shoib Allan Myint

30	**Suspension of the Retaining Ligaments and Platysma in Facelift: From "Fake-Lift" to "Facelift"** 335
	Keizo Fukuta

31	**Personal Technique of Facelifting in Office Under Sedation** 351
	Anthony Erian

32	**Design and Management of the Anterior Hairline Temporal Incision and Skin Take Out in the Vertical Facelift and Lateral Brow Lift Procedures** 363
	Mary E. Lester, Richard C. Hagerty, and J. Clayton Crantford

33	**Short-Scar Facelift with Extended SMAS/Platysma Dissection and Limited Skin Undermining** 373
	Hamid Massiha

34	**Extent of SMAS Advancement in Facelift with or without Zygomaticus Major Muscle Release** 379
	Henry A. Mentz III

35	**The Safe Facelift Using Bony Anatomic Landmarks to Elevate the SMAS** 397
	Bradon J. Wilhelmi and Yuron Hazani

36	**Anatomicohistologic Study of the Retaining Ligaments of the Face with Retaining Ligament Correction and SMAS Plication in Facelift** 405
	Ragip Ozdemir

37	**Vertical Temporal Lifting: A Short Preauricular–Pretrichal Scar**	425
	John Camblin	
38	**Deep Plane Face-lift: Integrating Safety and Reliability with Results**	437
	W. Gregory Chernoff	
39	**Subperiosteal Face-Lift**	445
	Lucas G. Patrocinio, Marcell M. Naves, Tomas G. Patrocinio, and Jose A. Patrocinio	
40	**Progression of Facelift Techniques Over the Years**	459
	W. Gregory Chernoff	
41	**Facial Contouring in the Postbariatric Surgery Patient**	463
	Anthony P. Sclafani and Vikas Mehta	
42	**Complications of Facelift Surgery**	471
	Melvin A. Shiffman	
43	**Forehead Lifting Approach and Techniques**	475
	Jaime Ramirez, Yhon Steve Amado, and Adriana Carolina Navarro	
44	**Endoscopic Forehead Lift**	495
	Jorge Espinosa and José Rafael Reyes	
45	**Minimally Invasive Ciliary-Frontoplasty Technique**	511
	German Guillermo Rojas Duarte	
46	**Treatment of Eyebrow Ptosis Through the Modified Technique of Castañares**	519
	Giovanni André Pires Viana and Giovanni Pires Viana	
47	**Endobrow Lift**	527
	Anthony Erian	
48	**Minimally Invasive Midface Lift**	541
	Enrique Andrade	
49	**Upper Eyelid Blepharoplasty**	547
	Amir M. Karam and Samuel M. Lam	
50	**Lower Eyelid Blepharoplasty**	555
	Amir M. Karam and Samuel M. Lam	

51	Upper Blepharoplasty of the Asian Eyelid	571
	Samuel M. Lam and Amir M. Karam	

52	Medial and Lateral Epicanthoplasty	577
	Dae Hwan Park	

53	Treatment of Tear Trough Deformity with Hyaluronic Acid Gel Filler	587
	Giovanni André Pires Viana	

54	Combined Technique in Otoplasty	595
	Marzia Salgarello	

55	Rhinoplasty	609
	Vladimir Kljajic and Slobodan Savovic	

56	Nonsurgical Rhinoplasty with Radiesse®	625
	George John Bitar, Olalesi Osunsade, and Anuradha Devabhaktuni	

57	Lip Enhancement: Personal Technique	641
	Anthony Erian	

58	Liposuction of the Neck: Technique and Pitfalls	647
	Anthony Erian	

59	Neck Lifting Variations	653
	Harry Mittelman and Joshua D. Rosenberg	

60	Exodermlift: Nonsurgical Facial Rejuvenation	671
	Clara Santos	

61	New Concepts of Makeup and Tattooing After Facial Rejuvenation Surgery	681
	Karen Betts	

Part VI   HIV Facial Lipodystrophy

62	Poly-L-Lactic Acid for the Treatment of HIV-Associated Facial Lipoatrophy	691
	Douglas R. Mest and Gail M. Humble	

63	Autologous Fat Transfer for HIV-Associated Facial Lipodystrophy	707
	Lisa Nelson and Kenneth J. Stewart	

64 **Comparison of Three Different Methods for Correction
of HIV-Associated Facial Lipodystrophy**.................. 723
Giovanni Guaraldi, Pier Luigi Bonucci, and Domenico De Fazio

Part VII Medical Legal

65 **Medical Malpractice Lawsuits: What Causes Them,
How to Prevent Them, and How to Deal with
Them When You Are the Defendant** 731
Ronald A. Fragen

Index 737

Part I

Anatomy

Facial Anatomy

Peter M. Prendergast

1.1 Introduction

Safe and effective surgical facial rejuvenation relies on a clear knowledge and understanding of facial anatomy. Techniques evolve and improve as the complex, layered architecture and soft tissue compartments of the face are discovered and delineated through imaging, staining techniques, and dissections both intraoperatively and in the research laboratory on cadavers [1]. To create a more youthful, natural-looking form, the surgeon endeavors to reverse some of the changes that occur due to aging. These include volumetric changes in soft tissue compartments, gravitational changes, and the attenuation of ligaments. Whether the plan of rejuvenation includes rhytidectomy, blepharoplasty, autologous fat transfer, implants, or endoscopic techniques, a sound knowledge of facial anatomy will increase the likelihood of success and reduce the incidence of undesirable results or complications.

This chapter describes the anatomy of the face in layers or planes, with some important structures or regions described separately, including the facial nerve, sensory nerves, and facial arteries. The facial skeleton forms the hard tissue of the face and provides important structural support and projection for the overlying soft tissues, as well as transmitting nerves through foramina and providing attachments for several mimetic muscles and muscles of mastication. Following a description of the hard tissue foundation, the soft tissues will be described, from superficial to deep, in the following order:

1. Superficial fat compartments
2. Superficial musculoaponeurotic system (SMAS)
3. Retaining ligaments
4. Mimetic muscles
5. Deep plane including the deep fat compartments

1.2 Facial Skeleton

Facial appearance is to a large extent determined by the convexities and concavities of the underlying facial bones (Fig. 1.1). The "high" cheekbones and strong chin associated with attractiveness are attributable to the convexities and projection provided by the zygomatic bone and mental protuberance of the mandible, respectively (Fig. 1.2). The facial skeleton consists of the frontal bone superiorly, the bones of the midface, and the mandible inferiorly. The midface is bounded superiorly by the zygomaticofrontal suture lines, inferiorly by the maxillary teeth, and posteriorly by the sphenoethmoid junction and the pterygoid plates. The bones of the midface include the maxillae, the zygomatic bones, palatine bones, nasal bones, the zygomatic processes of the temporal bones, the lacrimal bones, the ethmoid bones, and the turbinates. The facial skeleton contains four apertures: the two orbital apertures, the nasal aperture, and the oral aperture. The supraorbital foramen (or notch) and the frontal notch are found at the superior border of each orbit and transmit the supraorbital and supratrochlear nerves, respectively. The maxillary bones contribute to the nasal aperture, bridge of the nose, maxillary teeth, floor of the orbits, and cheekbones. The

P.M. Prendergast
Venus Medical, Heritage House,
Dundrum Office Park, Dundrum, Dublin 14, Ireland
e-mail: peter@venusmed.com

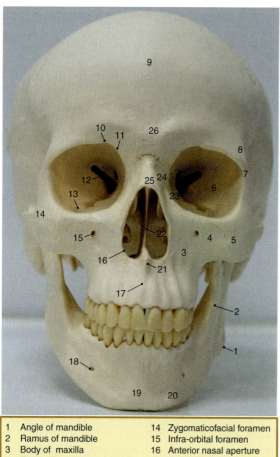

1	Angle of mandible	14	Zygomaticofacial foramen
2	Ramus of mandible	15	Infra-orbital foramen
3	Body of maxilla	16	Anterior nasal aperture
4	Zygomatic process of maxilla	17	Intermaxillary suture
5	Zygomatic bone	18	Mental foramen
6	Greater wing of sphenoid bone	19	Mental protuberance
7	Zygomaticofrontal suture	20	Body of mandible
8	Zygomatic process of frontal bone	21	Anterior nasal spine
9	Frontal bone	22	Nasal septum
10	Supra-orbital notch	23	Lacrimal bone
11	Frontal notch	24	Frontal process of maxilla
12	Superior orbital fissure	25	Nasal bone
13	Inferior orbital fissure	26	Glabella

Fig. 1.1 The facial skeleton

infraorbital foramen lies in the maxilla below the inferior orbital rim and transmits the infraorbital nerve. The zygomaticofacial foramen transmits the zygomaticofacial nerve inferolateral to the junction of the inferior and lateral orbital rim.

The mandible forms the lower part of the face. In the midline, the mental protuberance gives anterior projection to the overlying soft tissues. Laterally, the ramus of the mandible underlies the masseter muscle and continues superiorly to articulate with the cranium through the coronoid process and condylar process of the mandible.

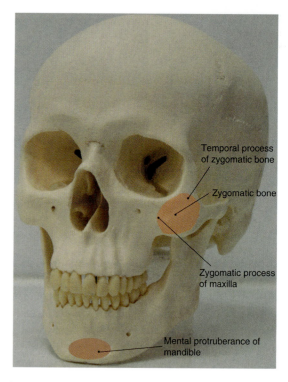

Fig. 1.2 Convexities of the facial skeleton

The mental nerve emerges from the mental foramen on the body of the mandible in line vertically with the infraorbital and supraorbital nerves.

As well as providing structural support, projection, and protection of sensory organs such as the eyes, the facial skeleton provides areas of attachment for the muscles of facial expression and the muscles of mastication (Fig. 1.3).

1.3 Superficial Fat Compartments

The pioneering work of Rohrich [2], using staining techniques and cadaver dissections, has revealed a number of distinct superficial fat compartments in the face. These compartments are separated from one another by delicate fascial tissue and septae that converge where adjacent compartments meet to form retaining ligaments. The superficial fat compartments of the face comprise the following: the nasolabial fat compartment, the medial, middle, and lateral temporal-cheek "malar" fat pads, the central, middle, and lateral temporal-cheek pads in the forehead, and the superior, inferior, and lateral orbital fat pads (Fig. 1.4). Nasolabial fat lies medial to the cheek fat pad

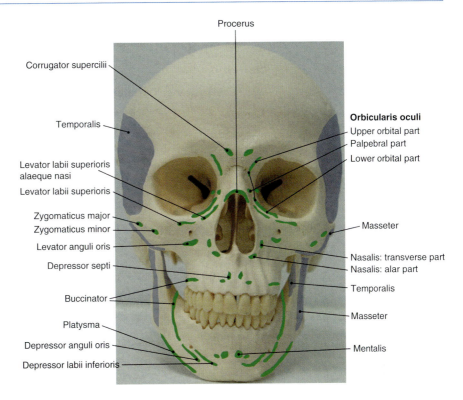

Fig. 1.3 Areas of muscle attachments to the facial skeleton

compartments and contributes to the overhang of the nasolabial fold. The orbicularis retaining ligament below the inferior orbital rim represents the superior border of the nasolabial fat compartment and the medial cheek compartment (Fig. 1.5). The middle cheek fat compartment lies between the medial and lateral temporal-cheek fat compartments and is bounded superiorly by a band of fascia termed the superior cheek septum. The borders of the middle cheek compartment, inferior, and lateral orbital fat pad compartments converge to form a tougher band of tissue called the zygomatic ligament [3]. The condensation of connective tissue at the borders of the medial and middle fat compartments correlates with the masseteric ligaments in the same location [4]. The lateral temporal-cheek fat pads span the entire face from the forehead to the cervical area. Its anterior boundary, the lateral cheek septum, is encountered during facelift procedures with medial dissection from the preauricular incision. In the forehead, its upper and lower boundaries are identifiable as the superior and inferior temporal septa. Medial to the lateral temporal-cheek fat compartment in the forehead, the middle forehead fat pad is bounded inferiorly by the orbicularis retaining ligament and medially by the central forehead fat compartment. Above and below the eyes, the superior

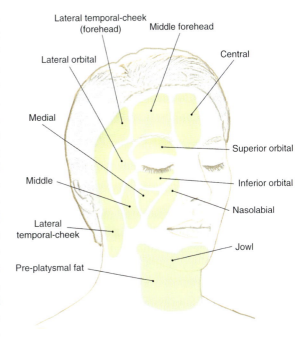

Fig. 1.4 The superficial fat compartments of the face

and inferior orbital fat compartments lie within the perimeter of the orbicularis retaining ligament. These periorbital fat pads are separated from one another medially and laterally by the medial and lateral canthi,

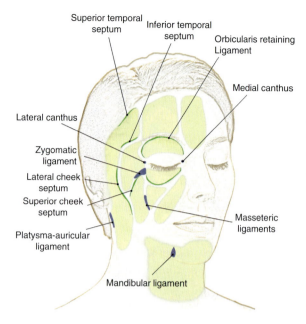

Fig. 1.5 Ligaments and septae between fat compartments of the face

respectively. The lateral orbital fat compartment is the third orbital fat pad and is bounded superiorly by the inferior temporal septum and inferiorly by the superior cheek septum. The zygomaticus major muscle attaches, through fibrous septae, to overlying superficial fat compartments along its length. In the lower third of the face, the jowl fat compartment adheres to the depressor anguli oris muscle and is bounded medially by the depressor labii and inferiorly by bands of the platysma muscle. Premental and preplatysmal fat abut the jowl fat compartment.

The compartmentalized anatomy of the superficial subcutaneous fat of the face has implications in the aging process. Volume loss appears to occur at different rates in different compartments, leading to irregularities in facial contour and loss of the seamless, smooth transitions between the convexities and concavities of the face associated with youthfulness and beauty.

1.4 Superficial Musculoaponeurotic System (SMAS)

In 1974, Mitz and Peyronie published their description of a fibrofatty superficial facial fascia they called the superficial musculoaponeurotic system (SMAS) [5]. This system or network of collagen fibers, elastic fibers, and fat cells connects the mimetic muscles to the overlying dermis and plays an important functional role in facial expression. The SMAS is central to most current facelift techniques where it is usually dissected, mobilized, and redraped. In simple terms, the SMAS can be considered as a sheet of tissue that extends from the neck (platysma) into the face (SMAS proper), temporal area (superficial temporal fascia), and medially beyond the temporal crest into the forehead (galea aponeurotica). However, the precise anatomy of the SMAS, regional variations, and even the existence of the SMAS are debated [6]. Ghassemi [7] describes two variations of SMAS architecture. Type I SMAS consists of a network of small fibrous septae that traverse perpendicularly between fat lobules to the dermis and deeply to the facial muscles or periosteum. This variation exists in the forehead, parotid, zygomatic, and infraorbital areas. Type II SMAS consists of a dense mesh of collagen, elastic, and muscle fibers and is found medial to the nasolabial fold, in the upper and lower lips. Although extremely thin, type II SMAS binds the facial muscles around the mouth to the overlying skin and has an important role in transmitting complex movements during animation. Over the parotid gland, the SMAS is relatively thick. Further medially, it thins considerably making it difficult to dissect. In the lower face, the SMAS covers the facial nerve branches as well as the sensory nerves. Dissection superficial to the SMAS in this region protects facial nerve branches [8]. Above the zygomatic arch, the SMAS exists as the superficial temporal fascia, which splits to enclose the temporal branch of the facial nerve and the intermediate temporal fat pad. Dissection in this area should proceed deep to the superficial temporal fascia, on the deep temporal fascia, to avoid nerve injury. Although considered as one "system" or plane, the surgeon should be mindful of the regional differences in SMAS anatomy from superior to inferior and lateral to medial.

1.5 Retaining Ligaments

True retaining ligaments are easily identifiable structures that connect the dermis to the underlying periosteum. False retaining ligaments are more diffuse condensations of fibrous tissue that connect superficial

1 Facial Anatomy

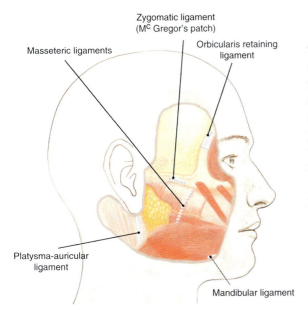

Fig. 1.6 The retaining ligaments of the face

1.6 Mimetic Muscles

The muscles of facial expression are thin, flat muscles that act either as sphincters of facial orifices, as dilators, or as elevators and depressors of the eyebrows and mouth. Frontalis, corrugator supercilii, depressor supercilii, procerus, and orbicularis oculi represent the periorbital facial muscles. The perioral muscles include the levator muscles, zygomaticus major and minor, risorius, orbicularis oris, depressor anguli oris, depressor labii, and mentalis. The nasal group includes compressor naris, dilator naris, and depressor septi. In the neck, the platysma muscle lies superficially and extends into the lower face (Fig. 1.7).

The frontalis represents the anterior belly of the occipitofrontalis muscle and is the main elevator of the brows. It arises from the epicranial aponeurosis and passes forward over the forehead to insert into fibers of the orbicularis oculi, corrugators, and dermis over the brows. Contraction raises the eyebrows and causes horizontal furrows over the forehead. Frontalis receives innervation from the temporal branch of the facial nerve.

The orbicularis oculi acts as a sphincter around the eye. It consists of three parts: the orbital, preseptal, and pretarsal parts. The orbital part arises from the nasal part of the frontal bone, the frontal process of the maxilla, and the anterior part of the medial canthal tendon. Its fibers pass in concentric loops around the orbit, well beyond the confines of the orbital rim. Contraction causes the eyes to squeeze closed forcefully. Superior fibers also depress the brow. Preseptal orbicularis oculi arises from the medial canthal tendon, passes over the fibrous orbital septum of the orbital rim, and inserts into the lateral palpebral raphe. The pretarsal portion, involved in blinking, overlies the tarsal plate of the eyelid and has similar origins and insertions to its preseptal counterpart. These muscles receive innervation from the temporal and zygomatic branches of the facial nerve.

The corrugator supercilii arises from the superomedial aspect of the orbital rim and passes upward and outward to insert into the dermis of the middle of the brow. From its origin deep to frontalis, two slips of muscle, one vertical and one transverse, pass through fibers of frontalis to reach the dermis. The superficial and deep branches of the supraorbital nerve are intimately related to corrugator supercilii at its origin and are prone to injury during resection of this muscle. Corrugator supercilii depresses the brow and pulls it medially, as in frowning.

and deep facial fasciae [9] (Fig. 1.6). The zygomatic ligament (McGregor's patch) is a true ligament that connects the inferior border of the zygomatic arch to the dermis and is found just posterior to the origin of the zygomaticus minor muscle [3]. Other true ligaments include the lateral orbital thickening on the superolateral orbital rim that arises as a thickening of the orbicularis retaining ligament, and the mandibular retaining ligament. The latter connects the periosteum of the mandible just medial to the origin of depressor anguli oris to the overlying dermis. This attachment gives rise to the labiomandibular fold just anterior to the jowl. The masseteric ligaments are false retaining ligaments that arise from the anterior border of masseter and insert into the SMAS and overlying dermis of the cheek. With aging, these ligaments attenuate, the SMAS over the masseter becomes ptotic, and this leads to the formation of jowls [10]. Below the lobule of the ear, the platysma-auricular ligament represents a condensation of fibrous tissue where the lateral temporal-cheek fat compartment meets the postauricular fat compartment. During facial rejuvenation procedures, true and false retaining ligaments are encountered and often released in order to mobilize and redrape tissue planes. Extra care should be taken when releasing ligaments as important facial nerve branches are intimately related to ligaments such as the zygomatic and mandibular retaining ligaments.

Fig. 1.7 The mimetic facial muscles

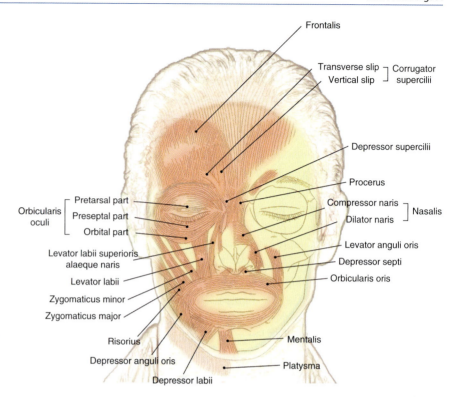

The depressor supercilii is a thin slip of muscle that is difficult to distinguish from the superomedial fibers of orbicularis oculi. It inserts into the medial brow and acts as a depressor.

The procerus arises from the nasal bone, passes superiorly, and insert into the dermis of the glabella between the brows. It depresses the lower forehead skin in the midline to create a horizontal crease at the bridge of the nose. Chemodenervation of procerus and corrugator supercilii to alleviate frown lines is one of the most common aesthetic indications for botulinum toxins. Procerus is sometimes debulked during endoscopic brow lift procedures to reduce the horizontal frown crease.

The zygomaticus major and minor are superficial muscles that originate from the body of the zygoma and pass downward to insert into the corner of the mouth and lateral aspect of the upper lip, respectively. They receive their nerve supply on their deep surface from the zygomatic and buccal branches of the facial nerve. Zygomaticus major and minor lift the corners of the mouth.

The levator labii lies deep to orbicularis oculi at its origin from the maxilla just above the infraorbital foramen. It passes downward to insert into the upper lip and orbicularis oris. A smaller slip of muscle medial to this, levator labii superioris alaeque nasi, originates from the frontal process of the maxilla and inserts into the nasal cartilage and upper lip. Both of these muscles are supplied from branches of the zygomatic and buccal branches of the facial nerve and elevate the upper lip.

The levator anguli oris arises deeply from the canine fossa of the maxilla below the infraorbital foramen and inserts into the upper lip. It is innervated on its superficial aspect by the zygomatic and buccal branches of the facial nerve and elevates the corner of the mouth.

The risorius is often underdeveloped and arises from a thickening of the platysma muscle over the lateral cheek, the parotidomasseteric fascia, or both. It inserts into the corner of the mouth and pulls the mouth corners laterally.

The orbicularis oris acts as a sphincter around the mouth and its fibers interlace with all of the other facial muscles that act on the mouth. The buccal and marginal mandibular branches of the facial nerve provide motor supply to orbicularis oris, which has various actions including pursing, dilation, and closure of the lips.

The depressor anguli oris arises from the periosteum of the mandible along the oblique line lateral to depressor labii inferioris. Its fibers converge on the modiolus with fibers of orbicularis oris, risorius, and sometimes levator anguli oris. It is supplied by the marginal mandibular branch of the facial nerve and depresses the mouth corners on contraction. Depressor labii inferioris arises from the oblique line of the mandible in front of the mental foramen, where fibers of depressor anguli oris cover it. It passes upward and medially to insert into the skin and mucosa of the lower lip and into fibers of orbicularis oris.

The mentalis arises from the incisive fossa of the mandible and descends to insert into the dermis of the chin. Contraction elevates and protrudes the lower lip and creates the characteristic "peach-pit" dimpling of the skin over the chin. Motor supply arises from the marginal mandibular nerve.

The nasalis consists of two parts: the transverse part (compressor naris) and the alar part (dilator naris). The compressor naris arises from the maxilla over the canine tooth and passes over the dorsum of the nose to interlace with fibers from the contralateral side. It compresses the nasal aperture. The dilator naris originates from the maxilla just below and medial to compressor naris and inserts into the alar cartilage of the nose. It dilates the nostrils during respiration. The depressor septi is a slip of muscle arising from the maxilla above the central incisor, deep to the mucous membrane of the upper lip. It inserts into the cartilaginous nasal septum and pulls the nose tip inferiorly. The nasalis and depressor septi receive innervation from the superior buccal branches of the facial nerve.

The platysma is a broad thin sheet of muscle that arises from the fascia of the muscles of the chest and shoulders and passes upward over the clavicles and neck toward the lower face. Fibers insert into the border of the mandible, perioral muscles, modiolus, and dermis of the cheek. Although variations exist [11], the platysma usually decussates with fibers from the other side 1–2 cm below the mandible. As part of aging, its medial fibers attenuate or thicken to create platysmal bands. Functionally, the platysma depresses the mandible during deep inspiration but is probably more important as a mimetic muscle to express horror or disgust. It is regarded as the inferior most extension of the SMAS and is innervated by the cervical branch of the facial nerve.

1.7 Deep Plane Including the Deep Fat Compartments

The superficial fat compartments described above lie above the muscles of facial expression in the subcutaneous plane. In the midface, the suborbicularis oculi fat and deep cheek fat represent deeper fat compartments that provide volume and shape to the face and act as gliding planes within which the muscles of facial expression can move freely. Suborbicularis oculi fat (SOOF) has two parts, medial and lateral [12]. The medial component extends along the inferior orbital rim from the medial limbus (sclerocorneal junction) to the lateral canthus and the lateral component from the lateral canthus to the temporal fat pad. Between the SOOF and the periosteum of the zygomatic process of maxilla there is a gliding space, the prezygomatic space [13]. This space is bounded superiorly by the orbicularis retaining ligament and inferiorly by the zygomatic retaining ligament (Fig. 1.8). The sublevator fat pad lies medial to the medial SOOF compartment and represents the most medial of the deep infraorbital fat pads. This fat pad is an extension of the buccal fat pad, behind levator labii superioris alaeque nasi and is continuous below and laterally with the melolabial and buccal extensions of the buccal fat pad

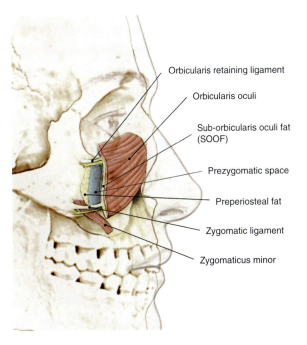

Fig. 1.8 The prezygomatic space

[1]. The buccal fat pad is an aesthetically important structure that sits on the posterolateral part of the maxilla superficial to the buccinator muscle and deep to the anterior part of masseter. Functionally, it facilitates a free gliding movement for the surrounding muscles of mastication [14]. As well as the medial extensions described above, it continues laterally as the pterygoid extension (Fig. 1.9). Buccal branches of the facial nerve and the parotid duct travel along its surface within the parotidomasseteric fascia after leaving the parotid gland.

The galea fat pad lies deep to frontalis in the forehead and extends superiorly for about 3 cm [15]. It envelops corrugator and procerus and aids gliding of these muscles during animation. The retroorbicularis oculi fat (ROOF) is part of the galea fat pad over the superolateral orbital rim from the middle of the rim to beyond the lateral part. It lies deep to the superolateral fibers of preseptal and orbital orbicularis oculi and contributes to the fullness (in youth) and heaviness (in senescence) of the lateral brow and lid.

With aging, the retaining ligaments under the eye attenuate. This, together with volume loss in the superficial and deep fat compartments, results in visible folds and grooves in the cheeks and under the eyes (Fig. 1.10).

The deep cervical fascia covering sternocleidomastoid in the neck continues upward to ensheath the parotid gland between the mandible and mastoid process. The layer of fascia covering the parotid gland and masseter, termed parotidomasseteric fascia, continues superiorly to insert into the inferior border of the zygomatic arch. In the temporal area, the corresponding fascia in the same plane is present as deep temporal fascia, which inserts into the superior border of the zygomatic arch. In the lower face, branches of

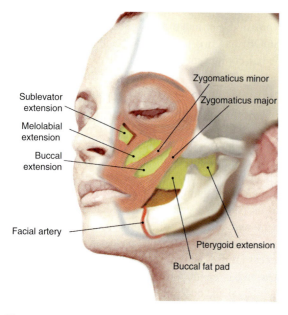

Fig. 1.9 The buccal fat pad and its extensions

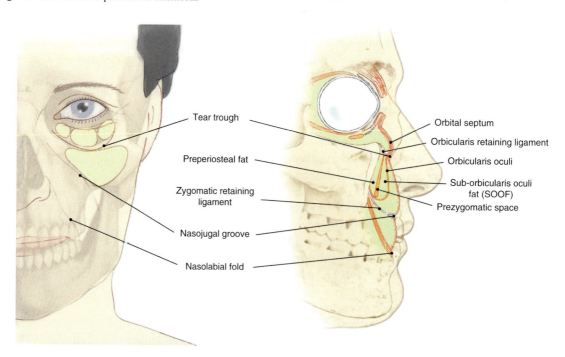

Fig. 1.10 Attenuated ligaments in the midface

the facial nerve lie underneath the deep fascia, whereas above the zygomatic arch and in the upper face, facial nerve branches lie superficial to the deep fascia and are susceptible to injury during superficial dissections.

1.8 Facial Nerve

The facial nerve (seventh cranial nerve) provides motor innervation to the muscles of facial expression. It begins in the face by emerging from the stylomastoid foramen 6–8 mm medial to the tympanomastoid suture of the skull. Before entering the substance of the parotid gland, the posterior auricular nerve and nerves to the posterior belly of digastric and stylohyoid branch from the main trunk. Within the parotid gland, the facial nerve divides into its main branches: temporal branch, zygomatic branch, buccal branch, marginal mandibular branch, and cervical branch (Fig. 1.11).

The temporal branch of the facial nerve leaves the superior border of the parotid gland as three or four rami. They cross the zygomatic arch between 0.8 and 3.5 cm anterior to the external acoustic meatus, and usually about 2.5 cm anterior to it. At the level of the zygomatic arch, the most anterior branch is always at least 2 cm posterior to the lateral orbital rim. The temporal branches pass in an envelope of superficial temporal fascia with the intermediate fat pad, superficial to the deep temporal fascia. The temporal branch enters frontalis about 2 cm above the brow, just below the anterior branch of the superficial temporal artery.

There are up to three zygomatic branches of the facial nerve. The upper branch passes above the eye to supply frontalis and orbicularis oculi. The lower branch always passes under the origin of zygomaticus major and supplies this muscle, other lip elevators and the lower orbicularis oculi. Smaller branches continue around the medial aspect of the eye to supply depressor supercilii and the superomedial orbicularis oculi.

The buccal branch exits the parotid and is tightly bound to the anterior surface of masseter within the parotidomasseteric fascia. It continues anteriorly over the buccal fat pad, below and parallel to the parotid duct, to supply the buccinators and muscles of the upper lip and nose. A second branch is occasionally present, but this travels superior to the parotid duct in its course anteriorly.

The marginal mandibular nerve exits the lower part of the parotid gland as one to three major branches. It usually runs above the inferior border of the mandible, but may drop up to 4 cm below it. About 2 cm posterior to the angle of the mouth, the nerve passes upward and more superficially to innervate the lip depressors. Although it remains deep to the platysma, it is vulnerable to injury during surgical procedures in the lower face at this location.

The cervical branch of the facial nerve passes into the neck at the level of the hyoid bone to innervate the platysma muscle.

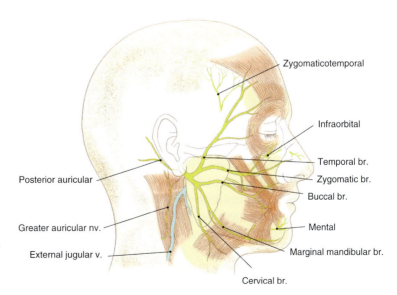

Fig. 1.11 The branches of the facial nerve. Note, the greater auricular, zygomaticotemporal, infraorbital, and mental nerves are sensory nerves

1.9 Sensory Nerves

The sensory innervation of the face is via the three divisions of the trigeminal nerve (fifth cranial nerve): ophthalmic nerve, maxillary nerve, and mandibular nerve. The ophthalmic nerve supplies the forehead, upper eyelid, and dorsum of the nose via the supraorbital, supratrochlear, infratrochlear, lacrimal, and external nasal nerves. The maxillary nerve supplies the lower eyelid, cheek, upper lip, ala of the nose, and part of the temple, through the infraorbital, zygomaticofacial, and zygomaticotemporal nerves. The maxillary nerve also supplies the maxillary teeth and nasal cavity via the alveolar nerves and pterygopalatine nerves, respectively. The mandibular nerve has motor and sensory fibers. Its branches include the inferior alveolar nerve, lingual nerve, buccal nerve, and auriculotemporal nerve. These supply the skin over the mandible, lower cheek, part of the temple and ear, the lower teeth, gingival mucosa, and the lower lip (Fig. 1.12). The greater auricular nerve, derived from the anterior primary rami of the second and third cervical nerves, supplies the skin over the angle of the mandible.

The supraorbital nerve emerges from the orbit at the supraorbital notch (or foramen) 2.3–2.7 cm from the midline in men and 2.2–2.5 cm from the midline in women [16]. It has superficial and deep branches that straddle the corrugator muscle. Sometimes these branches exit from separate foramina, the deep branch arising lateral to the superficial one. The deep branch usually runs superiorly between the galea and the periosteum of the forehead 0.5–1.5 cm medial to the superior temporal crest line. The supratrochlear nerve exits the orbit about 1 cm media to the supraorbital nerve and runs close to the periosteum under the corrugator and frontalis. Its several branches supply the skin over the medial eyelid and lower medial forehead. The infratrochlear nerve is a terminal branch of the nasociliary nerve that supplies a small area on the medial aspect of the upper eyelid and bridge of the nose. The external nasal nerve supplies the skin of the nose below the nasal bone, except for the skin over the external nares. The lacrimal nerve supplies the skin over the lateral part of the upper eyelid.

The infratrochlear nerve exits the orbit about 1 cm media to the supraorbital nerve and supplies the skin over the medial eyelid and bridge of the nose.

The infraorbital nerve is the largest cutaneous branch of the maxillary nerve. It enters the face through the infraorbital foramen 2.7–3 cm from the midline in men and 2.4–2.7 cm from the midline in women, about 7 and 6 mm inferior to the inferior orbital rim in men and women, respectively. The nerve appears from the foramen just below the origin of levator labii superioris. It supplies the lower eyelid, ala of the nose, and upper lip. The zygomaticofacial nerve arises from the zygomaticofacial foramen below and lateral to the orbital rim and supplies skin of the malar eminence. The zygomaticotemporal nerve emerges from its foramen on the deep surface of the zygomatic bone and supplies the anterior temple.

The mental nerve is a branch of the inferior alveolar nerve that exits the mental foramen in line vertically with the infraorbital foramen, between the apices of the premolar teeth. It is often visible and easily

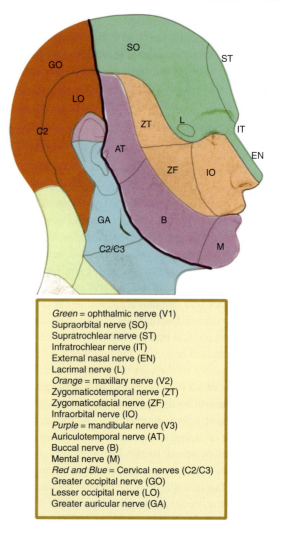

Fig. 1.12 Sensory innervation of the face

palpable through stretched oral mucosa. It supplies the skin over the lower lip and mandible. The buccal branch of the mandibular nerve supplies the buccal mucosa and skin of the cheek, and the lingual nerve provides sensory innervation to the anterior two-thirds of the tongue and the floor of the mouth. The auriculotemporal nerve emerges from behind the temporomandibular joint to supply the skin of the upper one-third of the ear, the external acoustic meatus, tympanic membrane, as well as the skin over the temporal region. Secretomotor fibers also pass via the auriculotemporal nerve to the parotid gland.

1.10 Arteries of the Face

The skin and soft tissue of the face receive their arterial supply from branches of the facial, maxillary, and superficial temporal arteries – all branches of the external carotid artery. The exception is a masklike area including the central forehead, eyelids, and upper part of the nose, which are supplied through the internal carotid system by the ophthalmic arteries (Fig. 1.13).

The facial artery arises from the external carotid and loops around the inferior and anterior borders of the mandible, just anterior to masseter. It pierces the masseteric fascia and ascends upward and medially toward the eye. It lies deep to the zygomaticus and risorius muscles but superficial to buccinator and levator anguli oris [17]. At the level of the mouth, the facial artery sends two labial arteries, inferior and superior, into the lips where they pass below orbicularis oris. The continuation of the facial artery near the medial canthus beside the nose is the angular artery.

The maxillary artery is a terminal branch of the external carotid with three main branches, mental, buccal, and infraorbital arteries. The mental artery is the terminal branch of the inferior alveolar artery that passes through the mental foramen to supply the chin and lower lip. The buccal artery crosses the buccinators to supply the cheek tissue. The infraorbital artery reaches the face through the infraorbital foramen and supplies the lower eyelid, cheek, and lateral nose. It anastomoses with branches of the transverse facial, ophthalmic, buccal, and facial arteries.

The superficial temporal artery is the terminal branch of the external carotid artery. In the substance of the parotid, just before reaching the zygomatic arch, it gives off the transverse facial artery which runs inferior and parallel to the arch and supplies the parotid, parotid duct, masseter, and skin of the lateral canthus. The superficial temporal artery crosses the zygomatic arch superficially within the superficial temporal fascia. Above the arch, it gives off a middle temporal artery that pierces the deep temporal fascia and supplies the temporalis muscle. Thereafter, about 2 cm above the zygomatic arch, the superficial temporal artery divides into anterior and posterior branches. The anterior branch supplies the forehead and forms anastomoses with the supraorbital and supratrochlear

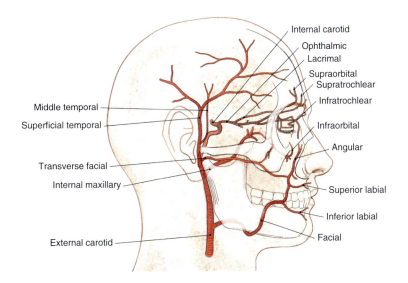

Fig. 1.13 Arterial supply to the face

vessels. The posterior part supplies the parietal scalp and periosteum.

The ophthalmic artery is a branch of the internal carotid system (Fig. 1.13). Its branches include the lacrimal, supraorbital, supratrochlear, infratrochlear, and external nasal arteries. There is significant communication between the external and internal carotid artery systems around the eye through several anastomoses. Inadvertent intra-arterial injection of fillers for soft tissue augmentation around the eye can lead to occlusion of the central retinal vessels and potentially blindness [18–20]. To avoid this complication, fillers should be injected in small volumes using a careful retrograde injection technique [21].

References

1. Gassner HG, Rafii A, Young A, Murakami C, Moe K, Larrabee WF. Surgical anatomy of the face. Implications for modern face-lift techniques. Arch Facial Plast Surg. 2008; 10(1):9–19.
2. Rohrich RJ, Pessa JE. The fat compartments of the face: anatomy and clinical implications for cosmetic surgery. Plast Reconstr Surg. 2007;119(7):2219–27.
3. Furnas DW. The retaining ligaments of the cheek. Plast Reconstr Surg. 1989;83(1):11–6.
4. Stuzin JM, Baker TJ, Gordon HL. The relationship of the superficial and deep facial fascias: relevance to rhytidectomy and aging. Plast Reconstr Surg. 1992;89(3):441–9.
5. Mitz V, Peyronie M. The superficial musculo-aponeurotic system in the parotid and cheek area. Plast Reconstr Surg. 1976;80(1):80–8.
6. Gardetto A, Dabernig J, Rainer C, Piegger J, Piza-Katzer H, Fritsch H. Does a superficial musculoaponeurotic system exist in the face and neck? An anatomical study by the tissue plastination technique. Plast Reconstr Surg. 2003;111(2): 664–72.
7. Ghassemi A, Prescher A, Riediger D, Axer H. Anatomy of the SMAS revisited. Aesthet Plast Surg. 2003;27(4): 258–64.
8. Wobig JL, Dailey RA. Facial anatomy. In: Wobig JL, Dailey RA, editors. Oculofacial plastic surgery. New York: Thieme; 2004. p. 5.
9. Jones BM, Grover R. Anatomical considerations. In: Jones BM, Grover R, editors. Facial rejuvenation surgery. Philadelphia: Mosby Elsevier; 2008. p. 18–22.
10. Mendelson BC, Freeman ME, Wu W, Huggins RJ. Surgical anatomy of the lower face: the premasseter space, the jowl, and the labiomandibular fold. Aesthet Plast Surg. 2008; 32(2):185–95.
11. Cardosa C. The anatomy of the platysma muscle. Plast Reconstr Surg. 1980;66(5):680–3.
12. Rohrich R, Arbique GM, Wong C, Brown S, Pessa JE. The anatomy of suborbicularis fat: implications for periorbital rejuvenation. Plast Reconstr Surg. 2009;124(3):946–51.
13. Mendelson BC, Muzaffar AR, Adams WP. Surgical anatomy of the midcheek and malar mounds. Plast Reconstr Surg. 2002;110(3):885–96.
14. Larrabee WF, Makielski KH, Henderson JL. Cheeks and neck. In: Larrabee WF, Makielski KH, Henderson JL, editors. Surgical anatomy of the face. Philadelphia: Lippincott Williams & Wilkins; 2004. p. 178.
15. Zide BM. ROOF and beyond (superolateral zone). In: Zide BM, editor. Surgical anatomy around the orbit. The system of zones. Philadelphia: Lippincott Williams & Wilkins; 2006. p. 57.
16. Zide BM. Supraorbital nerve. Nuances/dissections from above. In: Zide BM, editor. Surgical anatomy around the orbit. The system of zones. Philadelphia: Lippincott Williams & Wilkins; 2006. p. 77.
17. Berkovitz BKB, Moxham BJ. Head and neck anatomy. A clinical reference. Philadelphia: Taylor & Francis; 2002. p. 118.
18. Silva MT, Curi AL. Blindness and total ophthalmoplegia after aesthetic polymethylmethacrylate injection: case report. Arg Neuropsiquiatr. 2004;62(3B):873–4.
19. McCleve D, Goldstein JC. Blindness secondary to injections in the nose, mouth, and face: cause and prevention. Ear Nose Throat J. 1995;74(3):182–8.
20. Dreizen NG, Framm L. Sudden unilateral visual loss after autologous fat injection into the glabellar area. Am J Ophthalmol. 1989;107(1):85–7.
21. Coleman SR. Avoidance of arterial occlusion from injection of soft tissue fillers. Aesthet Surg J. 2002;22(6):555–7.

Facial Proportions

Peter M. Prendergast

2.1 Introduction

Although facial proportions, angles, and contours vary with age, sex, and race [1], it is worthwhile to consider aesthetic "ideals" when analyzing the face preoperatively and planning surgical rejuvenation. This chapter describes the surface markings of the face, soft-tissue cephalometric points for orientation, and commonly described facial planes and angles. Facial proportions, measurements, and angles that are deemed "ideal" are outlined to facilitate the surgeon with facial analysis and add a quantifiable dimension to perioperative assessment in surgical facial rejuvenation.

2.2 Surface Markings

The area anterior to the auricles, from the hairline superiorly to the chin inferiorly, represents the human face (Fig. 2.1). The forehead occupies the upper face, from the hairline to the eyebrows. Its contour, usually convex, is determined by the shape of the underlying frontal bone and distribution of subcutaneous and submuscular fat pads. There is a subtle prominence between the eyebrows called the glabella. Contraction of the procerus and corrugator muscles in this area results in hyperdynamic wrinkles. The eyebrows are positioned horizontally in males, overlying the supraorbital ridges.

P.M. Prendergast
Venus Medical, Heritage House,
Dundrum Office Park, Dundrum, Dublin 14, Ireland
e-mail: peter@venusmed.com

In females, the brows arch slightly from medial to lateral, with the highest part ideally in line vertically with the lateral limbus, or between the lateral limbus and lateral canthus.

In the midline, several soft-tissue cephalometric points are defined along the midsagittal plane from the glabella superiorly to the cervical point inferiorly (Fig. 2.2). These landmark points are used to describe facial proportions and angles. The external nose is pyramidal in shape with its base sitting over the nasal aperture of the skull. The root of the nose lies inferior to the glabella in the midline, over the frontonasal suture. The nose projects anteriorly and inferiorly from the nasion, or deepest part at the root, to the tip, or apex. The dorsum connects the nasion to the apex and is supported by immobile nasal bone superiorly and mobile cartilage inferiorly. The widest part of the nose consists of the alae, or nostrils, which lead into the nasal vestibule. Centrally, the columella connects the apex of the nose to the philtrum of the cutaneous upper lip. The junction of the red part of the lips with the skin is the vermillion border. Immediately adjacent to the vermillion border is the white roll, a tubelike structure that runs the length of the lip. In the midline, the top lip projects anteriorly as the tubercle. Below the lower lip, the labiomental groove passes between the lip and the chin. Between the alae of the nose and the lateral borders of the lip, the nasolabial groove or fold separates the upper lip from the cheek.

The soft tissue of the upper lateral cheek projects anteriorly over the zygomatic arch and represents a feature of beauty in most cultures. Anteriorly, the convexity of the cheek and smooth lid–cheek junction are attributable to the deep cheek fat compartments below the eye and deep to the cheek muscles. Further down and laterally, the buccal fat pad gives the cheek its roundness, especially in children.

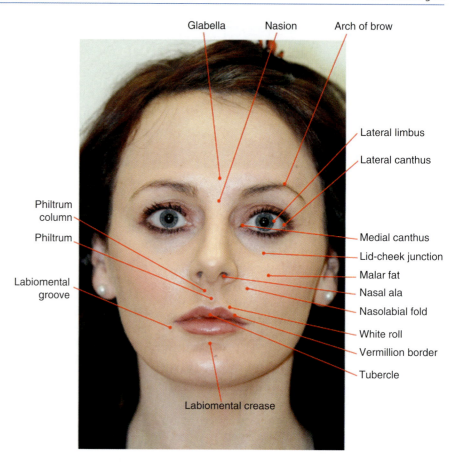

Fig. 2.1 Surface markings of the face

The inferior margin of the face runs from the menton in the midline at the chin, laterally along the inferior and lateral borders of the mandible, to the auricle. Jowl fat and laxity of platysma lead to ptosis and interrupt the definition of the jawline along this margin and are improved with lipoplasty and rhytidectomy.

2.3 Proportions

The face is divided into horizontal thirds (Fig. 2.3). The upper third extends from the hairline to the glabella, the middle third from the glabella to the subnasale, and the lower third from the subnasale to the menton. These facial thirds are rarely equal. In Caucasians, the middle third is often less than the upper third, and the middle and upper thirds are less than the lower third [2]. In East Asians, the middle third of the face is often greater than the upper third and equal to the lower third, and the upper third is less than the lower third [3]. The lower third is further divided into its own thirds, defining the upper lip, lower lip, and chin (Fig. 2.3). Anic-Milosevic et al. [4] compared the proportions of the lower facial third segments in males and females. The chin represented the largest segment and the lower lip height the smallest in both sexes. Although the vermilion height of upper and lower lips did not differ between men and women, the upper and lower lip heights were larger in males. In both genders, the upper vermilion height was smaller than the lower vermilion height. The height of the upper lip vermilion relative to the upper lip was significantly greater in females than in males. The width of the lips should be about 40% of the width of the lower face, and usually equal to the distance between the medial limbi. The width-to-height ratio of the face is typically 3:4, with an oval-shaped face being the aesthetic ideal.

The neoclassical canon of facial proportions divides the face vertically into fifths, with the width of each eye, the intercanthal distance, and the nasal width all

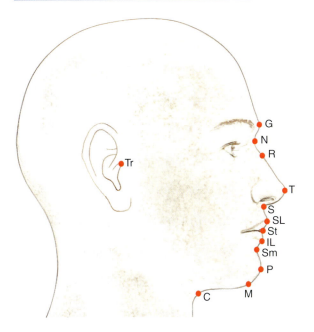

Fig. 2.2 Soft-tissue cephalometric points. The glabella (*G*) is the most prominent part in the midline between the brows. The nasion (*N*) lies at the root of the nose in the midline. The rhinion (*R*) is the junction of the bony and cartilaginous dorsum of the nose in the midline. The tip (*T*) is the most anterior part of the nose. The subnasale (*S*) is the junction of the columella and upper cutaneous lip. The superior labrum (*SL*) is the junction of the red and cutaneous parts of the lip at the vermilion border in the midline. The stomion (*St*) is the point where the lips meet in the midline. The inferior labrum (*IL*) is the point in the midline of the lower lip at the vermilion border. The supramentale (*Sm*) is midpoint of the labiomental crease between the lower lip and chin. The pogonion (*P*) is the most anterior point of the chin. The menton (*M*) is the most inferior point of the chin. The cervical point (*C*) is the point in the midline where the neck meets the submental area. The tragion (*Tr*) is the most superior point on the tragus

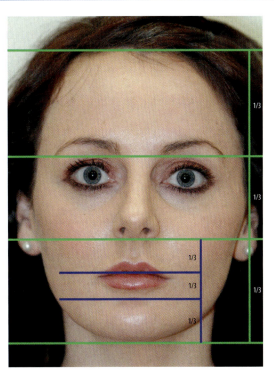

Fig. 2.3 Horizontal facial thirds. The upper third extends from the hairline to glabella, the middle third from glabella to subnasale, and lower third from subnasale to menton. The lower third is further divided into thirds: the upper third from subnasale to stomion, middle third from stomion to the labiomental crease, and the lower third from the labiomental crease to menton. These thirds define the upper lip, lower lip, and chin. Note that the thirds are not equal

measuring one-fifth (Fig. 2.4). However, studies using direct anthropometry and photogrammetric analyses in white and Asian subjects found variations in these proportions, with the width of the eyes and nasal widths often being either less than or greater than the intercanthal distance [2, 3, 5].

Crumley and Lancer describe appropriate projection of the nose and nasal tip [6]. A ratio of 5:4:3 should apply, respectively, to a line from the nasion to the nasal tip, a line from the nasion to the alar crease, and a perpendicular line joining the other two (Fig. 2.5). Nasal tip projection can be measured using other parameters. The Baum ratio is calculated by dividing the length of a line from the nasion to the nasal tip by the length of a perpendicular line from the nasal tip to a vertical line from the subnasale (Fig. 2.6). The Simons ratio also reflects nasal tip projection and is found by dividing the length from the subnasale to the nasal tip by the length from the subnasale to the superior labium (Fig. 2.7). According to Powell and Humphreys [7], the ideal Baum and Simons ratios for whites are 2.8:1 and 1, respectively. The rotation of the nose is described by the nasolabial angle: the angle formed between a line from the anterior columella and the subnasale and a line from the subnasale to the mucocutaneous border of the upper lip. According to Leach [8], this measurement is inaccurate as a representation of nasal rotation if the subject has a protruding maxilla or procumbent incisors. As such, a more accurate measurement is to use a line perpendicular to the Frankfurt horizontal plane in lieu of the subnasale to upper lip line (Fig. 2.8). The basal view of the nose can be divided into thirds with the ratio of the columella to the lobule about 2:1 (Fig. 2.9). Aesthetically,

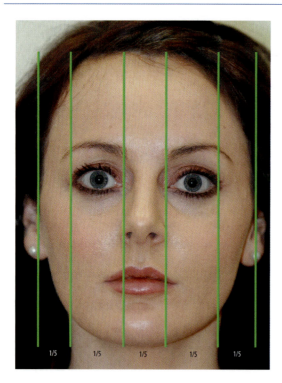

Fig. 2.4 Vertical fifths. The eye usually measures one-fifth the width of the face

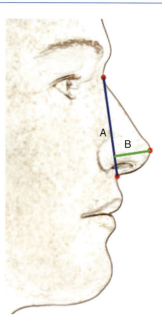

Fig. 2.6 The Baum ratio used to calculate nasal tip projection. The length of the nose (*a*) divided by a perpendicular line (*b*) from the nasal tip to the line from the nasion to subnasale gives the ratio

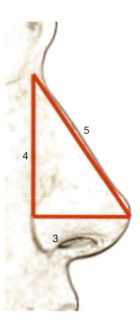

Fig. 2.5 Nasal proportions

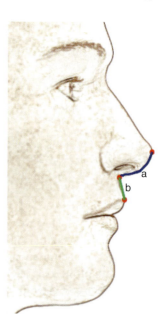

Fig. 2.7 The Simons ratio used to calculate nasal tip projection. A line from the subnasale along the anterior aspect of the columella to the nasal tip (*a*) divided by a line from the subnasale to the superior labium (*b*) gives the Simons ratio

a narrow nasal tip width, measured as a lobule to nasal base ratio, is preferred. Biller's study [9] showed a preference for a nasal tip width ratio of 0.35 in 30-year-old Asian women and 60-year-old white and Asian women, although a ratio of 0.45 was considered more attractive in 30-year-old white women. On basal view, the nasal apertures are usually oriented at an angle of 45–60° to the vertical, although racial variations exist (Fig. 2.10). Abdelkader et al. compared the length and

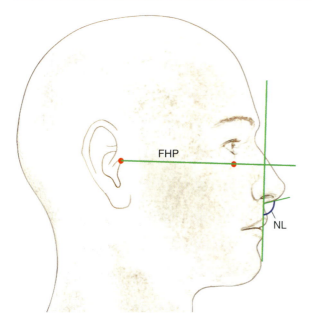

Fig. 2.8 Nasolabial angle. The Frankfurt horizontal plane (*FHP*) is found by drawing a line from the superior aspect of the external auditory canal to the most inferior point of the orbital rim. The nasolabial angle is formed between a line along the anterior part of the columella and a line perpendicular to the FHP

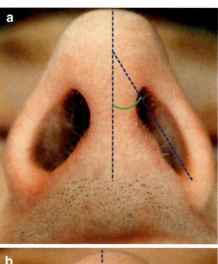

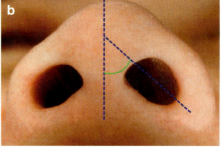

Fig. 2.10 Orientation of nasal apertures. (**a**) Caucasian nose showing an angle less than 45° and (**b**) Chinese nose showing an angle greater than 45°

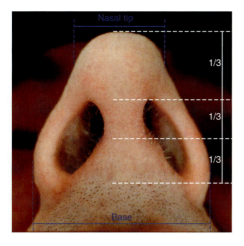

Fig. 2.9 Basal view of the nose. The lobule should represent approximately one-third (upper third) and the columella two-thirds (lower two-thirds) of the basal view. The width of the lobule (nasal tip) should be about 35–45% the width of the nasal base

width of the nasal aperture in men of three racial groups [10]. The nasal aperture was longer at maximum length in the Indian group compared to the Chinese and white groups. There was no significant difference between the length and width of the columella in all three racial groups.

2.4 The Golden Ratio

Beauty and facial attractiveness are easy to identify but difficult to quantify. Despite its subjective nature, we can attempt to define, measure, and explain the captivating phenomenon of beauty by describing it numerically and geometrically [11]. The measurement of aesthetically pleasing features, animate and inanimate, over at least the last two millennia, has produced an extraordinary finding. The same number, or ratio, appears so frequently as a measurement of beauty that it has almost become synonymous with beautiful and harmonious form. This number has been called the golden ratio.

The golden ratio, denoted by the symbol Φ (phi), is an irrational number of the order of 1.618033988. The ratio is obtained when a line $a+b$ is sectioned such that $a+b/a=a/b$ (Fig. 2.11). Although Indian mathematicians studied the golden ratio over 2,000 years ago, it first appeared in written documentation in Euclid's

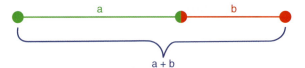

Fig. 2.11 The golden proportion. A line (a+b) is sectioned such that (a+b)/a = a/b = 1.618033988

elements about 300 B.C. [12]. The golden ratio, also known as the divine proportion, is considered by many to be the key to the mystery of aesthetics, attraction, and human beauty [13]. From the era of the ancient Greeks, through to the Renaissance, and the present day, mathematicians, scientists, architects, artists, and cosmetic surgeons have been intrigued by the ubiquitous nature of the divine proportion and its correlation with aesthetics. Ricketts showed that the proportions in a face generally perceived as being beautiful are intimately related to the golden ratio [14–17]. The width of the mouth is Φ times the width of the nose. The distance between the lateral canthi is Φ times the width of the mouth. The height of the face from pupils to chin is Φ times the height from the hairline to the pupils. Marquardt devised a mathematical model using Φ as the central measurement to map out facial proportions and aesthetically "ideal" shapes and sizes [18]. The result is a "Phi mask" that can be used as a tool to analyze facial beauty and determine its closeness to the aesthetically ideal golden proportion. Despite enthusiasm for the thesis that Φ is the Holy Grail in defining beauty and harmony of the human form, Holland [19] reminds us that several studies have not found a relationship between facial attractiveness and the golden ratio. Furthermore, Marquardt's mask does not represent the ideal female face but rather a masculinized face, with prominent supraorbital ridges, low eyebrows, high cheekbones, and a square jaw. These observations tell us that while the golden proportion is certainly a prominent and recurring theme in aesthetics, it should not be embraced as the only method by which we measure human beauty to the exclusion of other factors.

2.5 Planes and Angles

Powell and Humphreys [7] provide a detailed analysis of facial contours, proportions, and angles on profile (Fig. 2.12). These angles facilitate preoperative assessment and planning in facial rejuvenation. The ideal

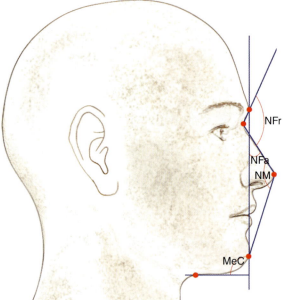

Fig. 2.12 Powell and Humphreys' aesthetic angles. A line from the glabella to pogonion creates the anterior facial plane. The angle formed by lines from the nasion to the glabella and from the nasion to the nasal tip is the nasofrontal angle (*NFr*). The nasomental angle (*NM*) lies between the line along the dorsum to the nasion, and a line drawn from the nasal tip to the pogonion. The nasofacial angle (*NFa*) is formed between the anterior facial plane and the line tangent to the dorsum of the nose. A line is drawn from the cervical point to the menton. This line intersects the anterior facial plane to create the mentocervical angle (*MeC*)

ranges in Caucasians are as follows: nasofrontal angle, 115–130°; nasofacial angle, 30–40°; nasomental angle, 120–130°; mentocervical angle, 80–95°. Racial variations include a wider nasofrontal angle in Chinese. The upper and lower lips are usually posterior to the nasomental line in Caucasians, but on or anterior to this line in individuals of African or Asian descent.

Peck and Peck [20] describe another orientation plane formed by a line from the tragion that bisects a line from the nasion to the pogonion (Fig. 2.13). The facial, maxillofacial, and nasomaxillary angles developed from these lines relate the upper lip to the chin and nasal tip and the nasion to the chin. In Caucasians, the mean facial angle as described by Peck and Peck is 102.5°, maxillofacial angle 5.9°, and nasomaxillary angle 106.1°. Holdaway's "H angle" [21] describes the degree of soft-tissue protrusion of the maxilla relative to the mandible and is ideally about 10° (Fig. 2.14). This angle can be manipulated by surgical intervention on the chin, by lip augmentation, or indeed by orthodontics.

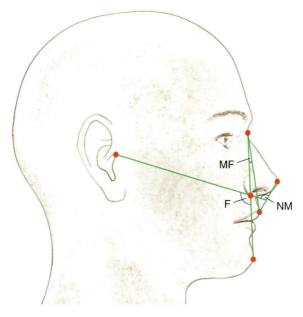

Fig. 2.13 Peck and Peck's aesthetic angles. A plane is developed by drawing a line from the tragion anteriorly to bisect a line from the nasion to pogonion. The angle created by the intersection of these two lines is the facial angle (*F*). A line dropped from the nasion to the superior labium creates the maxillofacial angle (*MF*) with the line from nasion to pogonion. The nasomaxillary angle (*NM*) relates the upper lip to the nasal tip and arises between a line from the tip to the superior labium and the orientation plane from the tragion

2.6 Conclusions

Patients often are specific in their request for facial rejuvenation procedures: nose reduction, nose tip elevation, lip enhancement, brow lift, or chin augmentation. Creating the aesthetic "ideal" relies less on site-specific reduction, augmentation, or straightening of facial features and more on a holistic approach, considering each feature as it relates to the rest of the face. The aesthetic surgeon should be mindful of average and ideal proportions and facial angles as they apply to the patient's race so that rejuvenation procedures can be performed with the goal in mind of achieving an attractive and harmonious appearance. Facial proportions and angles are easily determined in the office using photogrammetric analysis. With this information, the surgeon should educate the patient on the role of facial proportions in aesthetics, discuss the most appropriate measures, and tailor a plan to achieve the best results. Once there is an understanding of the importance of proportion in facial aesthetics, the proposed surgical plan is usually more acceptable, even if it deviates from the patient's initial requests.

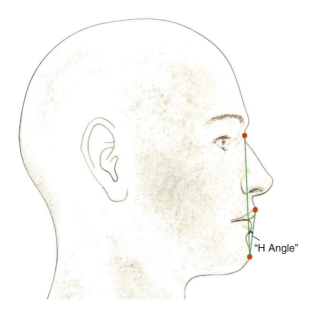

Fig. 2.14 Holdaway's "H angle." This angle is formed between a line from the nasion to pogonion and a line from the pogonion to the most anterior part of the upper lip. The angle is normally about 10°

References

1. Larrabee WF, Makielski KH, Henderson JL. Variations in facial anatomy with race, sex, and age. In: Larrabee WF, Makielski KH, Henderson JL, editors. Surgical anatomy of the face. Philadelphia: Lippincott Williams & Wilkins; 2004. p. 22–8.
2. Farkas LG, Hreczko TA, Kolar JC, Munro IR. Vertical and horizontal proportions of the face in young adult North American Caucasians: revision of neoclassical canons. Plast Reconstr Surg. 1985;75(3):328–38.
3. Sim RST, Smith JD, Chan ASY. Comparison of the aesthetic facial proportions of Southern Chinese and white women. Arch Facial Plast Surg. 2000;2(2):113–20.
4. Anic-Milosevic A, Mestrovic S, Prlic A, Slaj M. Proportions in the upper lip–lower lip–chin area of the lower face as determined by photogrammetric method. J Craniomaxillofac Surg. 2010;38(2):90–5.
5. Wang D, Qian G, Zhang M, Farkas LG. Differences in horizontal, neoclassical facial canons in Chinese (Han) and North American Caucasian populations. Aesthet Plast Surg. 1997;21(4):265–9.
6. Crumley RJ, Lanser M. Quantitative analysis of nasal tip projection. Laryngoscope. 1988;98(2):202–8.
7. Powell N, Humphreys B. Proportions of the aesthetic face. New York: Thieme-Stratton; 1984.

8. Leach J. Aesthetics and the Hispanic rhinoplasty. Laryngoscope. 2002;112(11):1903–16.
9. Biller JA, Kim DW. A contemporary assessment of facial aesthetic preferences. Arch Facial Plast Surg. 2009;11(2): 91–7.
10. Abdelkader M, Leong S, White PS. Aesthetic proportions of the nasal aperture in three different racial groups of men. Arch Facial Plast Surg. 2005;7(2):111–3.
11. Atiyeh BS, Hayek SN. Numeric expression of aesthetics and beauty. Aesthet Plast Surg. 2008;32(2):209–16.
12. Vegter F, Hage J. Clinical anthropometry and canons of the face in historical perspective. Plast Reconstr Surg. 2000; 106(5):1090–6.
13. Bashour M. History and current concepts in the analysis of facial attractiveness. Plast Reconstr Surg. 2006;118(3): 741–56.
14. Ricketts RM. Esthetics, environment, and the law of lip relation. Am J Orthod. 1968;54(4):272–89.
15. Ricketts RM. The biologic significance of the divine proportion and Fibonacci series. Am J Orthod. 1982;81(5): 351–70.
16. Ricketts RM. The golden divider. J Clin Orthod. 1981; 15(11):752–9.
17. Ricketts RM. Divine proportion in facial aesthetics. Clin Plast Surg. 1982;9(4):401–22.
18. Marquardt SR. Dr Stephen Marquardt and the golden decagon of human facial beauty. Interview with Dr Gottlieb. J Clin Orthod. 2002;36(6):317–8.
19. Holland E. Marquardt's phi mask: pitfalls of relying on fashion models and the golden ratio to describe a beautiful face. Aesthet Plast Surg. 2008;32(2):200–8.
20. Peck H, Peck S. A concept of facial esthetics. Angle Orthod. 1970;40(4):284–318.
21. Holdaway R. A soft tissue cephalometric analysis and its use in orthodontic treatment planning. Part II. Am J Orthod. 1984;85(4):279–93.

Danger Zones in Surgical Facial Rejuvenation

3

Peter M. Prendergast

3.1 Introduction

The increase in our knowledge of facial anatomy and the anatomy of aging has brought an evolution in techniques for aesthetic facial surgery [1]. More extensive procedures that access deeper planes and lift tissues in several vectors are favored over those that lift only subcutaneous tissue in a superolateral vector. These include extended sub-SMAS dissections, deep plane and composite rhytidectomies, and subperiosteal facelift techniques. Additionally, less invasive techniques such as the short scar facelift, minimal access cranial suspension (MACS) lift, and endoscopic brow lift have gained popularity because they provide effective rejuvenation and a relatively quick recovery. Since the first description of the superficial musculoaponeurotic system (SMAS) by Mitz and Peyronie in 1976 [2], the importance of addressing this layer for effective surgical rejuvenation has been realized. Dissecting, undermining, and redraping the SMAS provides a more natural and long-lasting rejuvenation compared to subcutaneous rhytidectomy alone. There are several regions, or danger zones, in the face where branches of the facial nerve lie immediately beneath the SMAS and are prone to injury if sharp dissection is performed in this plane. Nerve injuries can arise as a result of direct transection with sharp instruments, blunt trauma, traction, thermal injury from electrocautery, or inflammation. Facial nerve injuries can have serious sequelae such as brow ptosis, lid ptosis, lip weakness, and mouth asymmetries. Although most iatrogenic facial nerve palsies following aesthetic surgery are temporary, they can be distressing and may take months to fully recover. As such, preventing nerve injuries by careful planning, meticulous technique, and a sound knowledge of the precise location of important motor and sensory nerves in relation to the path of dissection is crucial.

This chapter outlines three main danger zones where facial nerve branches lie superficially and are susceptible to injury during commonly performed surgical rejuvenation techniques. The nerves associated with each zone are as follows:

Zone 1: Temporal branch of the facial nerve where it passes over the zygomatic arch and lies superficially within the superficial temporal fascia.

Zone 2: Zygomatic and buccal branches of the facial nerve where they emerge from the anterior aspect of the parotid and lie exposed during their course beneath a thin layer of SMAS.

Zone 3: Marginal mandibular branch of the facial nerve where it travels near the lower border of the mandible and passes superficially at its anterior part near the corner of the mouth.

In addition to the above motor nerves, four further danger zones are described that identify five sensory nerves. Although there are several other sensory nerves in the face, the ones highlighted here are regularly encountered during commonly performed surgical procedures, and are therefore more prone to injury. These procedures include coronal and endoscopic brow lift, subperiosteal midface lift, genioplasty, and SMAS-platysma rhytidectomy. The consequences of trauma to these sensory nerves, perhaps more than others, are more significant. Injury to the infraorbital or mental nerve can cause dysesthesias that impair

---

P.M. Prendergast
Venus Medical, Heritage House,
Dundrum Office Park, Dundrum, Dublin 14, Ireland
e-mail: peter@venusmed.com

speech and the ability to keep food in the mouth. The sensory nerves occupying these danger zones are:

Zone 4: The supraorbital and supratrochlear nerve trunks and the deep branch of the supraorbital nerve as it travels on the periosteum toward the frontoparietal scalp.

Zone 5: The infraorbital nerve where it emerges from its foramen on the anterior surface of the maxilla below the inferior orbital rim.

Zone 6: The mental nerve at the mental foramen below the root of the second mandibular premolar tooth on the lateral aspect of the chin.

Zone 7: The greater auricular nerve as it lies on the sternocleidomastoid muscle parallel to the external jugular vein and behind the posterior edge of the platysma.

3.2 Details of Zones

3.2.1 Zone 1

At the level of the zygomatic arch, the temporal branch of the facial nerve emerges from the substance of the parotid and passes over the bony arch toward the frontalis muscle between two slips of superficial temporal fascia. The nerve is prone to injury during its course superficially in this zone. The superficial temporal fascia is considered part of the superficial musculoaponeurotic system (SMAS) and splits at approximately the level of the hairline to envelop the intermediate fat pad, temporal branch of facial nerve, and frontal branch of superficial temporal artery. Although variations exist, the nerve always crosses the zygomatic arch between 0.8 and 3.5 cm anterior to the external auditory meatus (EAM), and not less than 2 cm posterior to the lateral orbital rim [3]. The temporal branch of facial nerve is usually described as having a consistent course from 0.5 cm below the tragus to 1.5 cm above the lateral brow [4]. However, soft tissue landmarks are not always reliable and should not be used as definite guides to the position of the nerve. More accurately, the nerve can be found 2.1–4 cm above the bony lateral canthus [3]. Therefore, this zone can be considered a triangle, with its base along the zygomatic arch from 0.8 to 3.5 cm anterior to the anterior border of EAM. A vertical line dropped from the superior part of the tragus represents the anterior border of EAM. A line is drawn from the anterior limit of the first line, superiorly to a point 4 cm above the bony lateral canthus, representing the anterior border of

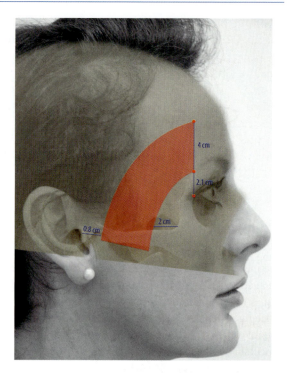

Fig. 3.1 Danger zone 1. This danger zone (*red*) extends from the inferior border of the zygomatic arch to a line above the bony lateral canthus. The zone curves anteriorly as shown from the lower line to the upper one. Within this zone, the temporal branch of the facial nerve is vulnerable to injury where it passes superficially in the superficial temporal fascia

this danger zone. A straight line connecting the first two lines completes the triangular danger zone (Fig. 3.1).

Dissecting immediately deep to the superficial temporal fascia above the zygomatic arch should be avoided. It is safe to dissect immediately below the dermis in the subcutaneous plane above the superficial temporal fascia [5], deep to the superficial temporal fascia along the deep temporal fascia [6], or under the deep temporal fascia. Injury to the temporal branch of the facial nerve results in weakness or paralysis of the ipsilateral frontalis muscle, leading to brow ptosis and smoothing of the forehead above the brow. Orbicularis oculi is usually spared since it also receives motor innervation from superior branches of the zygomatic branch of the facial nerve.

3.2.2 Zone 2

The zygomatic and buccal branches of the facial nerve emerge from the anterior border of the parotid invested in the parotidomasseteric fascia. There are up to three zygomatic branches and one or two buccal branches. The superior zygomatic branch passes over the orbit to innervate part of orbicularis oculi. Lower branches supply the lip elevators; one of the lower zygomatic branches always passes posterior to the origin of zygomaticus major on the body of the zygoma. The buccal nerve passes on the surface of the buccal fat pad below and parallel to the parotid duct and supplies the lip elevators, orbicularis oris, and nasalis. When a second buccal nerve is present, it passes above the parotid duct. The danger zone for these nerves lies anterior to the parotid and posterior to zygomaticus major and minor, where only the SMAS protects them (Fig. 3.2). The anterior border of parotid can be found by drawing a line from the most anterior inferior aspect of the temporal fossa to the masseteric tuberosity. Wilhelmi found that the most posterior part of the anterior border lies up to 2.5 mm posterior to this vector [7]. The upper lateral border of zygomaticus major is intimately related to the zygomatic branch of the facial nerve. The lateral border of zygomaticus major can be estimated to be 2.2–6.6 mm lateral and parallel to a line drawn from the mental protuberance to the most anterior inferior aspect of the temporal fossa [8]. The nerves, as well as parotid duct and facial vessels, are susceptible to injury during extended sub-SMAS dissections or composite rhytidectomy. Dissection should be performed only under direct vision in this zone. Signs of injury to the zygomatic and buccal branches of the facial nerve include weakness in forcefully closing the eyes, drooping of the ipsilateral upper lip and oral commissure, and significant asymmetry at rest and during animation [9, 10]. Since orbicularis oculi receives dual innervation from the temporal and zygomatic branches, complete iatrogenic paralysis of this muscle is rare following aesthetic surgery.

3.2.3 Zone 3

The marginal mandibular branch of the facial nerve emerges from the anterior aspect of the parotid as one to three main branches and runs along the mandible deep to the cervical fascia toward the lip depressors. The nerve usually runs along the inferior border of the mandible, but may drop up to 4 cm below it [11]. It starts its course deep to the cervical fascia, but pierces the fascia approximately halfway along the body of the mandible to lie just deep to the SMAS. Anteriorly, the nerve is prone to injury where the overlying SMAS becomes very thin and the nerve courses more superficially toward depressor anguli oris and depressor labii. About 2–3 cm posterior to the oral commissure, the nerve is most vulnerable where it crosses superficial to the anterior facial artery and vein. These vessels are also prone to injury during sub-SMAS dissections in this area. As such, this danger zone is defined by a circle with a radius of 2 cm with its center located 2 cm posterior to the oral commissure at the inferior border of the mandible (Fig. 3.3).

In this danger zone, the nerve can be injured during overzealous subcutaneous dissections from above or below when redraping the soft tissues over the mandible. Care should be taken to stay in the superficial subcutaneous plane in the jowl to avoid breaching the platysma where it exists only as a thin layer. Similarly, aggressive liposuction of the jowl should be avoided. Posteriorly, where the SMAS is more substantial, the nerve is

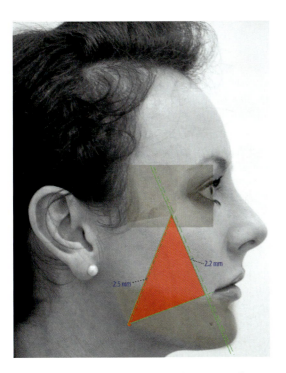

Fig. 3.2 Danger zone 2. The anterior continuous green line represents the most anterior position of the lateral border of zygomaticus major. The posterior continuous green line marks the most posterior part of the anterior border of the parotid gland. The borders of this triangular danger zone are formed in relation to these lines, with the base of the triangle running from the masseteric tuberosity at the angle of the mandible toward the oral commissure. The zygomatic and buccal branches of the facial nerve occupy this zone as they run on the buccal fat just underneath platysma

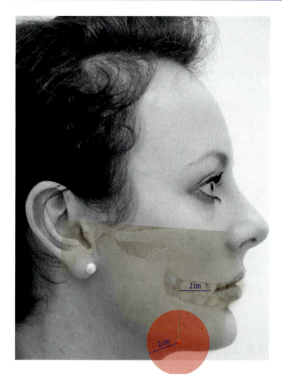

Fig. 3.3 Danger zone 3. The marginal mandibular nerve occupies this danger zone, represented by a circle centered on the inferior border of the mandible, 2 cm posterior to the oral commissure. The nerve courses superficially in this zone

susceptible to injury during composite rhytidectomy where the SMAS-platysma is mobilized over the anterior border of masseter. Dissection under direct vision and careful cautery of facial vein branches in this area are essential to preserve the nerve, especially where it crosses the facial vessels as they pass over the mandible. Injury to the marginal mandibular branch of the facial nerve results in elevation and protrusion of the lip on the ipsilateral side. The smile is asymmetric with an inability to show the lower teeth on the affected side. Abnormal lower lip elevation is also a sign of cervical branch injury due to weakness of platysma. However, since the mentalis receives innervation from the marginal mandibular nerve, the patient can still evert the lower lip if the marginal mandibular nerve has been spared [12].

3.2.4 Zone 4

This danger zone includes the supraorbital and supratrochlear nerves, branches of the ophthalmic division of the trigeminal nerve, and sensory nerves to the upper eyelid and forehead. The supraorbital nerve emerges from the supraorbital foramen or notch 2.3–2.7 cm from the midline in men and 2.2–2.5 cm from the midline in women [13]. The supratrochlear nerve appears from its foramen or notch about 1 cm medial to the supraorbital nerve. The supraorbital nerve has superficial and deep branches that straddle the corrugator muscle. Sometimes, the deep branch arises from its own foramen lateral to the superficial branch. These nerves are most commonly injured during coronal or endoscopic brow lift procedures where direct trauma or traction on the nerves leads to numbness or dysesthesias over the upper eyelid, dorsum of the nose, medial forehead, and scalp [14]. The deep branch of the supraorbital nerve runs superiorly between the galea and the periosteum 0.5–1.5 cm medial to the superior temporal crest line. Resection of the corrugator at its origin to alleviate glabellar frown lines is a frequent cause of injury to the supratrochlear nerve. To identify this danger zone, a circle of 3 cm diameter is centered on either the supraorbital foramen or notch if it is palpable, or a point along the superior orbital rim 2.5 cm from the midline. The danger zone is extended from the superolateral aspect of the circle along the superior temporal crest line and for 1.5 cm medially (Fig. 3.4). Any dissection or incision deep to the galea in the danger zone risks injury to the supraorbital nerve. Medially, fibers from the superficial branch of the supraorbital nerve and the supratrochlear nerves overlap so that injury to one of these nerves is not likely to result in significant sensory loss or disturbance.

3.2.5 Zone 5

This danger zone lies over the maxilla under the eye to include the infraorbital nerve. The nerve enters the face through the infraorbital foramen 2.5–3 cm from the midline, about 7 mm below the inferior orbital rim. The nerve appears from the foramen just below the origin of levator labii superioris. The infraorbital nerve is a branch of the maxillary division of the facial nerve and provides sensory innervation to the lower eyelid, cheek, side of the nose, and upper lip. The danger zone is a circular area centered on the foramen, with a diameter of 3 cm (Fig. 3.5). Deep dissections in this area, such as during an extended subperiosteal facelift, place the nerve at risk of injury. Subperiosteal dissections on the anterior maxilla can also injure the infraorbital vessels and the zygomatic branches of the facial nerve.

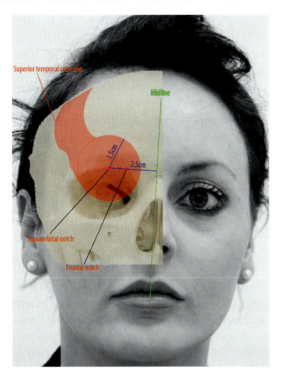

Fig. 3.4 Danger zone 4. A circle of 1.5 cm diameter is centered on a point 2.5 cm from the midline along the supraorbital ridge, or on the supraorbital foramen or notch if palpable. The danger zone extends from the superolateral part of the circle along the superior temporal crest lines and for 1.5 cm medial to it, where the deep branch of supraorbital nerve passes on the periosteum. This danger zone includes the supraorbital nerve, deep branch of supraorbital nerve, and supratrochlear nerve

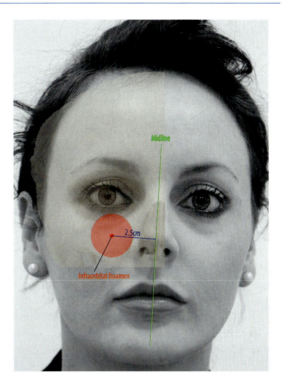

Fig. 3.5 Danger zone 5. This danger zone is circular, centered on the infraorbital foramen. The foramen is usually 2.5 cm from the midline, close to the midpupillary line. The infraorbital nerve can be damaged here during deep dissections over the maxilla

Direct visualization of these nerves and vessels using endoscopy may help prevent such injuries [15]. Trauma to the infraorbital nerve presents as numbness, dysesthesia, or hypesthesia of the skin it innervates.

3.2.6 Zone 6

The mental nerve is susceptible to injury during genioplasty either through a buccal or submental incision when the dissection is performed on the periosteum. The nerve arises roughly in line with the infraorbital and supraorbital nerves, emerging from the mental foramen below the lower second premolar tooth. A circle of 3 cm diameter centered on the mental foramen defines this danger zone (Fig. 3.6). Injury to the mental nerve can result in numbness of the lower lip, chin, and mucous membrane on the same side. Drooling can also occur due to sensory loss in this area.

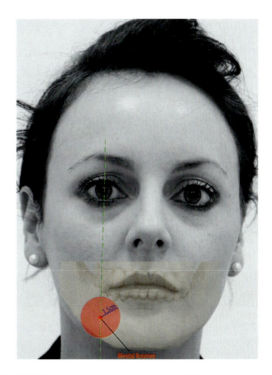

Fig. 3.6 Danger zone 6. A circular area of 3 cm diameter centered on the mental foramen defines this danger zone. Note that the foramen is approximately in the midpupillary line

3.2.7 Zone 7

The greater auricular nerve arises from the anterior primary rami of the second and third cervical nerves. It provides sensory innervation to the lower two-thirds of the auricle, the skin underneath the ear, and the posterior two-thirds of the jawline. The nerve pierces the deep cervical fascia at the posterior border of sternocleidomastoid and runs on the muscle, superficial and posterior to platysma toward the angle of the jaw. At a point 6.5 cm inferior to the external auditory canal, the nerve can be found halfway between the posterior and anterior borders of the sternocleidomastoid [16]. Below the ear it divides into anterior and posterior branches. This danger zone can be considered as an oblong, 2 cm wide and 6 cm long, with its center on a point 6.5 cm below the external auditory meatus oriented parallel to the external jugular vein (Fig. 3.7). The greater auricular nerve is prone to injury during neck dissections and suture plication of platysma to the mastoid fascia.

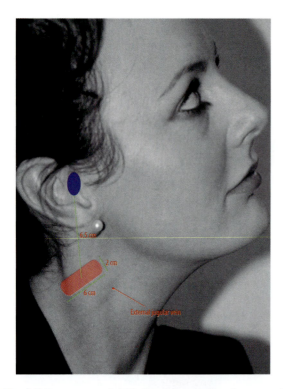

Fig. 3.7 Danger zone 7. This lies 6.5 cm below the external auditory meatus, in the middle of sternocleidomastoid, parallel to the external jugular vein. The greater auricular nerve is prone to injury as it passes through this danger zone behind the border of platysma

Great care should be taken as dissections proceed forward from the postauricular incision toward the nerve. It is identifiable about 1 cm posterior to the external jugular vein and runs parallel to it. The dissection in this zone should be in the subcutaneous plane, superficial to the nerve. When platysma is mobilized, it should be redraped over the nerve, and care should be taken not to compress or include the nerve or its branches in the suture. Injury to the greater auricular nerve may result in numbness, dysesthesia, or chronic hypesthesia in the skin of the inferior part of the ear, and skin anterior and inferior to this area.

3.3 Conclusions

No surgical procedure is without risks and potential complications. In the face, although there are several risks associated with surgery, such as infection, bleeding, and hematoma, the most serious complication is injury to one of the cranial nerves. Injury to one of the facial nerve branches, such as transection, traction, thermal injury, or blunt trauma, may present as weakness, asymmetry, or total paralysis of the brow, eye, lips, and mouth. There are several, well-defined areas or zones in the face where the important motor and sensory nerves have a predictable path. Mapping these danger zones out before surgical intervention, using bony landmarks where possible, helps orient the surgeon during dissections of the face and neck and may reduce the incidence of significant complications.

References

1. Adamson PA, Litner JA. Evolution of rhytidectomy techniques. Facial Plast Surg Clin North Am. 2005;13(3): 383–91.
2. Mitz V, Peyronie M. The superficial musculo-aponeurotic system (SMAS) in the parotid and cheek area. Plast Reconstr Surg. 1976;58(1):80–8.
3. Zide BM. The facial nerve–cranial nerve VII. In: Zide BM, editor. Surgical anatomy around the orbit. The system of zones. Philadelphia: Lippincott Williams & Wilkins; 2005. p. 19.
4. Pitanguy I, Ramos AS. The frontal branch of the facial nerve: the importance of its variation in face lifting. Plast Reconstr Surg. 1966;38(4):352–6.
5. Tellioglu AT, Hosaka Y. Temporoparietal fascia plication in rhytidectomy. Aesthet Plast Surg. 2006;30(2):175–80.

6. Toth BA, Daane SP. Subperiosteal midface lifting: a simplified approach. Ann Plast Surg. 2004;52(3):293–6.
7. Wilhelmi BJ, Mowlavi A, Neumeister MW. The safe face lift with bony anatomic landmarks to elevate the SMAS. Plast Reconstr Surg. 2003;111(5):1723–6.
8. Mowlavi A, Wilhelmi BJ. The extended SMAS facelift: identifying the lateral zygomaticus major muscle border using bony anatomic landmarks. Ann Plast Surg. 2004;52(4): 353–7.
9. Mendelson BC. Correction of the nasolabial fold: extended SMAS dissection with periosteal fixation. Plast Reconstr Surg. 1992;89(5):822–33.
10. Barton FE. Rhytidectomy and the nasolabial fold. Plast Reconstr Surg. 1992;90(4):601–7.
11. Dingman RO, Grabb WC. Surgical anatomy of the mandibular ramus of the facial nerve based on the dissection of 100 facial halves. Plast Reconstr Surg. 1962;29:266–72.
12. Daane SP, Owsley JQ. Incidence of cervical branch injury with "marginal mandibular nerve pseudo-paralysis" in patients undergoing face lift. Plast Reconstr Surg. 2003; 111(7):2414–8.
13. Zide BM. Supraorbital nerve: nuances/dissections from above. In: Zide BM, editor. Surgical anatomy around the orbit. The system of zones. Philadelphia: Lippincott Williams & Wilkins; 2005. p. 77.
14. Tabatabai N, Spinelli HM. Limited incision nonendoscopic brow lift. Plast Reconstr Surg. 2007;119(5):1563–70.
15. Williams JV. Transblepharoplasty endoscopic subperiosteal midface lift. Plast Reconstr Surg. 2002;110(7):1769–75.
16. McKinney P, Katrana DJ. Prevention of injury to the great auricular nerve during rhytidectomy. Plast Reconstr Surg. 1980;66(5):675–9.

Muscles Used in Facial Expression

Melvin A. Shiffman

4.1 Introduction

Facial expression is the mirror of our emotions. We express ourselves not only in words but in facial muscle contraction as well hand and body movement and body stature. Paralysis of facial muscles causes loss of expression of what we are trying to say or do. The face gives voice to what we are feeling.

The muscles used in human facial expression were reported by Duchenne de Boulogne in 1862 [1]. His research was through the use of electrophysiological analysis stimulating each of the facial muscles and correlating the muscles stimulated with facial expression and taking photographs of the results (Fig. 4.1).

Duchenne described a variety of neurologic and muscular disorders such as Duchenne–Aran motor neuron disease (1849) [2], Duchenne's pseudohypertrophic muscular dystrophy (1852) [3], and Duchenne–Erb palsy caused by upper brachial plexus injury during childbirth (1855) [4]. He was the first to use clinical photographs to illustrate neurological diseases (1862) [5].

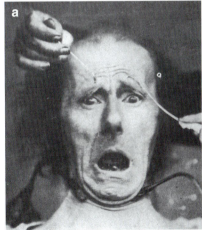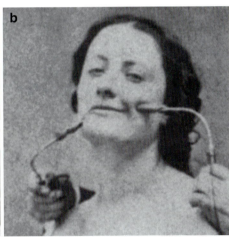

Fig. 4.1 Electrostimulation of muscles of the face by Duchenne. (**a**) Fear (**b**) Happy

M.A. Shiffman
17501 Chatham Drive,
Tustin, California 92780-2302, USA
e-mail: shiffmanmdjd@yahoo.com

Facial muscle contraction correlated to types of emotions [1]:

Isolated contraction of muscles	
Expression	Muscles involved
Attention, almost an expression of surprise or admiration	m. frontalis
Reflection	Superior part of m. orbicularis oculi, moderately contracted
Meditation, mental concentration	Superior part of m. orbicularis oculi, strongly contracted
Intentness of mind, somber thoughts, dissatisfaction	Superior part of m. orbicularis oculi, very strongly contracted
Pain	m. corrugator supercilii
Aggression, menace	m. procerus
Suffering, profound suffering with resignation	m. corrugator supercilii, moderate stimulus
Recollection, calling something to mind	Voluntary contraction of m. frontalis with upward gaze
Joy	m. zygomaticus major
False laughter	m. zygomaticus major

Combined contraction of muscles	
Weeping with hot tears	m. levator superiorus alaeque nasi plus palpebral part of m. orbicularis oculi
Moderate weeping	m. zygomaticus minor plus palpebral part of orbicularis oculi
Laughter	m. zygomaticus major plus palpebral part of m. orbicularis oculi
Irony, ironic laughter	m. buccinators plus m depressor labii inferioris
Sadness or despondency	m. depressor anguli oris plus flaring of the nostrils and downward gaze
Disdain or disgust	m. depressor anguli oris plus palpebral part of m. orbicularis oculi
Doubt	m. mentalis plus the outer fibers of m. orbicularis oris (either the inferior portion or the two portions at the same time) plus m. frontalis
Contempt or scorn	Palpebral part of m. orbicularis oculi plus m. depressor labii inferioris plus m. transversus plus m. levator labii superiorus alaeque nasi
Surprise	m. frontalis plus muscles lowering the mandible to a moderate degree
Astonishment	m. frontalis plus muscles lowering the mandible but stronger contraction of muscles
Stupefaction	m. frontalis plus muscles lowering the mandible but maximal contraction of muscles
Admiration, agreeable surprise	m. zygomaticus major plus m. frontalis plus lowering of the mandible with strong contraction of muscles
Fright	m. frontalis plus m. platysma
Terror	m. frontalis plus m. platysma and lowering of the mandible, maximally contracted
Terror, with pain or torture	m. corrugator supercilii plus m. platysma and muscles lowering the mandible
Anger	Superior part of m. orbicularis oculi plus m. masseter plus m. buccinators plus m. depressor labii inferiorus plus m. platysma
Carried away by ferocious anger	m. procerus plus platysma and muscles lowering the mandible, maximally contracted
Sad reflection	Superior part of m. orbicularis oculi plus m. depressor anguli oris
Agreeable reflection	Superior part of orbicularis oculi plus m. zygomaticus major
Ferocious joy	m. procerus plus zygomaticus major plus m. depressor labii inferiorus
Lasciviousness	m. transverus plus zygomaticus major
Sensual delirium	m. transverus plus zygomaticus major with gaze directed above and laterally, with spasm of the palpebral part of m. orbicularis oculi, the superior portion of which covers part of the iris
Ecstasy	m. zygomaticus major with gaze directed above and laterally, with spasm of the palpebral part of m. orbicularis oculi, the superior portion of which covers part of the iris
Great pain with tears and affliction	m. corrugator supercilii plus m. zygomaticus minor
Pain with despondency or despair	m. corrugator supercilii plus depressor anguli oris

4.2 Discussion

Surgery of the face is fraught with the danger of injury to motor nerves. Loss of facial nerve function is very distressing to patients. Surgeons should understand that not only can appearance be altered with motor nerve function loss but expression of emotions can also be altered. Perhaps in understanding what each facial muscle contributes to facial expression, the surgeon can understand the seriousness of the potential loss of any one of the muscles' function.

References

1. Duchenne de Boulogne GB. The mechanism of human facial expression. Paris: Jules Renouard, Libraire; 1862.
2. Duchenne de Boulogne GB. Recherches electro-physiologiques, pathologique et therapeutiques. Presented at the Academie des Sciences, Paris, 21 May 1849.
3. Duchenne de Boulogne GB. De la valeur de l'electricite dans traitement de maladies. Presented at the Societe Medico-Chiurgicale de Paris, 11 Mar and 6 Apr 1852.
4. Duchenne de Boulogne GB. De l'Electrisation Localisee, Paris, Chez J.-B. Bailliere; 1855.
5. Duchenne de Boulogne GB. Album des Photographies Pathologiques Complementaire du Livre Intitule de l'Electrisation Localisee. Paris, Bailliere et fils; 1862.

SMAFS (Superficial Musculoaponeurotic-Fatty System): A Changed SMAS Concept; Anatomic Variants, Modes of Handling, and Clinical Significance in Facelift Surgery

Hassan Abbas Khawaja, Melvin A. Shiffman, and Enrique Hernández-Pérez

5.1 Introduction

In the course of evolution, humans for the most part have lost the subdermal layer of muscles that covers the entire surface of many lower animals, and contracts around wounds, or contracts to flick off insects. Remnants of this musculocutaneous sheet exist in the skin as a fibrofatty layer. Because there are numerous connections via vertical fibrous septa, from the upper fibrofatty layer to the dermis of the skin and the fibrofatty-aponeurotic fascia encircles, envelopes, and interconnects the muscles of facial expression as a single unit, this interconnected system amplifies, transmits, and distributes mimetic muscular contractions, and translates them into a rich variety of complex facial expressions. Below the neck, only the Dartos muscle in the skin of the scrotum retains a muscular component. However, on the face and anterior neck, the superficial muscle layer has been retained, interposed between the skin and muscles of mastication. The purely muscular component consists of muscles of facial expression, whereas the fibrotic or aponeurotic component is referred to as the SMAS [1]. Somewhat confusingly, the fibrous portion of the SMAS, has also retained its designation as superficial fascia. Since its discovery, SMAS concept is not very clear cut, and confusion centers around its various components.

The SMAS consists of not only the fibro-aponeurotic part, but is a single unit "fibro-aponeurotic-fatty-fleshy system." The authors designate it as SMAFS (superficial musculoaponeurotic-fatty system). Therefore, SMAFS consists of a fibro-aponeurotic part, a superficial fatty layer, and superficial muscles of facial expression, as a single unit.

The lower subdivision of SMAFS, especially, is subject to considerable variations. Performing hundreds of facelifts over the last several years, we have seen variations such as thin and membranous SMAFS, thick and membranous SMAFS, thick and fibrous SMAFS, fibrofatty SMAFS, thick fleshy SMAFS, more fatty and less fibrous SMAFS, very fatty SMAFS, and patchy and broken down thin/thick SMAFS (which we call Island SMAFS). In addition, we have noticed attachment and regional variations; for example, not a very clear supra- and infrazygomatic divisions of SMAFS and discontinuity between the facial and neck SMAFS. Patchy/broken down SMAFS has been noticed by us either as a congenital anomaly or, apparently as a result of repeated Botox injections for obliterating the smile lines, lines around the cheek, nasolabial folds, and other facial/neck area lines. Broken down SMAFS has also been noticed as a result of repeated steroid injections into the face. Fatty SMAFS is noted in obese patients and those with well

---

H.A. Khawaja (✉)
Cosmetic Surgery & Skin Center, 53 A, Block B II,
Gulberg III, 54660 Lahore, Pakistan
e-mail: drhassan@nexlinx.net.pk, drhassan7@hotmail.com

M.A. Shiffman
17501 Chatham Drive,
Tustin, California 92780-2302, USA
e-mail: shiffmanmdjd@yahoo.com

E. Hernández-Pérez
Centro De Dermatologia Y Cirugia Cosmetica,
Villavicencio Plaza Suites 3-1, 3-2,
Paseo Escalón y 99 Av. Norte,
San Salvador, 01-177 El Salvador, C.A.
e-mail: drenrique@hernandezperez.com

developed and prominent cheeks. In thin patients, there may be fatty SMAFS as a result of repeated facial fat injections especially into the cheek region. There are considerable variations of anatomical landmarks especially frontal and marginal mandibular nerves in relation to the SMAFS.

The type, nature, and variations of SMAFS have an impact on the outcome of facelift surgery. Therefore, it is important for all surgeons, performing facelift surgery, to understand in detail the various types of SMAFS, and their variations, and plan the correct operative technique of debulking, plicating, lifting, and attaching the SMAFS to the bony periosteum, according to the nature and type of SMAFS present, in order to achieve good results. This is the aim of the following study.

5.2 Studies and Technique

The SMAFS (superficial musculoaponeurotic-fatty system) was studied in 800 facelift (Classical, Delta, S-lift, and Transcutaneous facelift) surgeries (661 females and 139 males) from August 1998 to March 2007, and the results of facelifts were analyzed according to the type of SMAFS. The age of the patients varied between 36 and 78 years. All patients were healthy, were not suffering from any physical or mental disability or illnesses. All female patients were nonpregnant and non-lactating. Seventy percent of the patients were of Fitzpatrick skin type III or IV and 30% of the patients were of skin type I or II. Preoperative SMAFS assessment was carried out in all cases. Facelifts in 70% of the patients were carried out as a result of sagging of skin and SMAFS, while in 30% of the cases, it was carried out to achieve a more youthful appearance in the face (for facial tightening). Faces of 75% of the patients were thin, while 25% of the patients had chubby (fatty) faces. A consent form was signed by all the patients. Pre- and postoperative photographs (after 1 month and 1 year) were taken in all cases. Intraopcrative gross SMAFS assessment was for thickness, thinness, consistency, continuity, nature, type of tissue present, mixed nature of the tissues present, density, tone, elasticity, rigidity, flaccidity, fattiness, fleshiness, breakage, and gaps in SMAFS (gross parameters), and were studied in detail.

In cases where the SMAFS was found to be thin, membranous, and flaccid, plication using Prolene 2/0 sutures, below the zygomatic arch, as in a Delta-lift or lifting and attaching to proximal zygoma, as in an S-lift, using vertical U and horizontal O sutures were carried out. In cases of classical lift, plication of SMAFS below the zygomatic arch was carried out using two Prolene sutures. In cases, where the SMAFS was found to be considerably fatty, as assessed preoperatively, closed liposuction using keel cobra tip or flat spatula cannula was carried out initially, in order to defat the SMAFS considerably; subsequently, lift was carried out as in a Classical, Delta, or S-lift. In cases of mild to moderately fatty SMAFS, defatting was carried out using open vacuum cleaner technique with a flat spatula cannula prior to Classical/Delta/S-lift. In cases where the SMAFS was found to be fleshy, thick, or rigid, relatively deeper and more SMAFS bites were taken and the SMAFS was attached to the periosteum of zygomatic arch. In cases where the SMAFS was found to be patchy, broken (Island SMAFS), or discontinuous, the aim was not to provide lift, but to restore continuity of SMAFS. In cases, where one or two discontinuous areas were present, the SMAFS was repaired and mild to moderate lift was provided while in other cases, SMAFS plication and lift was carried out after a year. In cases of mixed SMAFS, combination of liposuction, plication, and lifting were carried out according to the type of tissues present in the SMAFS. Bites of SMAFS were taken using curved needles with attached Prolene 2/0 through the superficial muscular part of SMAFS, in all cases, including thin and membranous SMAFS.

In cases where transcutaneous facelift (TCFL) was planned, preoperative SMAFS assessment with the thumb and index finger (Pinch Test) was carried out to assess density, tone, flaccidity, thickness, thinness, gaps, nature, tissue type, mixed patterns, and other palpable SMAFS parameters. In cases where the SMAFS was thin, membranous, and flaccid, superficial SMAFS bites, using the Khawaja-Hernandez (KH) needle, or the Keith needle and two to three sutures of Prolene 2/0, for lifting, were used. Where the SMAFS was thick, fatty, or fleshy, relatively deeper and more SMAFS bites were taken. More lift was provided in these cases. In all cases of TCFL, bites of SMAFS were taken through the superficial muscular layer and Prolene threads were attached to the thick temporal fascia or periosteum of the temporal bone.

5.3 Results

Results of intraoperative gross SMAFS variations showing various types of SMAFS are in Table 5.1. In cases of thin and membranous SMAFS, the density was decreased, tone was decreased, flaccidity was increased, elasticity was increased, and the SMAFS was soft and pliable. In these cases, the superficial fatty layer was practically nonexistent, and the fibro-aponeurotic and muscular layers were merged and in the form of a membrane. The muscle fibers were thin, long, stretched out, relatively atrophic, and membranous. In cases of thick and fatty SMAFS, consistency was somewhat harder, and it was more resistant, rigid, less elastic, more dense, and with increased tone. In these cases, superficial fatty layer was considerably increased. In cases of broken down (Island SMAFS), with gaps, very thin, and fragile SMAFS, elasticity was increased and tone and density were decreased considerably, while flaccidity was increased considerably. In these cases, the muscle layer was found to be considerably atrophic. In cases of fleshy SMAFS, tone, density, and thickness were increased, while elasticity was decreased. Superficial muscle layer was hypertrophic in these cases. In cases of mixed SMAFS, mixed characteristics were noted depending on the amount of tissue present in the SMAFS; for example, in cases of fibrofatty or fleshy-fatty SMAFS, tone, density, and thickness were increased, while elasticity was decreased. In case of fibrofatty SMAFS, fibro-aponeurotic and fatty layers were found to be thick, whereas, in case of fleshy-fatty SMAS, muscle layer was found to be hypertrophic, and fatty layer was considerably increased. In case of fibrous SMAFS, tone, thickness, rigidity, and density were increased, while elasticity and flaccidity were decreased. In these cases, fatty layer was nonexistent, while fibro-aponeurotic and muscular layers were found to be fibrotic, scarred, and hard.

Table 5.1 Gross SMAFS variations in a study of 800 facelifts

% Age	SMAFS type
57%	Membranous
23%	Fatty
12%	Mixed (membrano-fatty, fleshy-fatty etc.)
5%	Island (broken)
3%	Fleshy
2%	Fibrous

Table 5.2 Results of Classical, Delta, S-lift, and Transcutaneous facelifts according to SMAFS type

SMAFS type	Classical lift	Delta-lift	S-Lift	TCFL
Membranous (80%)	+++	+++	+++	++
Membranous (20%)	++	++	++	+
Fatty (60%)	++	++	++	−
Fatty (40%)	+	+	+	−
Fleshy	++	++	++	+
Mixed	+	+	+	+/−
Fibrous	−	−	−	−
Island	+	+	+	−

+++ (excellent), ++ (good), + (satisfactory), +/− (variable), and − (poor)

Results of Classical, Delta, and S-lift according to SMAFS type are in Table 5.2. In cases of membranous SMAFS, results of Classical/Delta/S-lift were considered as excellent (+++) in 80% of cases, and good (++) in 20% of cases (Figs. 5.1 and 5.2). In case of fatty SMAFS, after liposuction (closed/open), and after subsequent plication/lift, results were considered as good (++) in 60% of cases and as satisfactory (+) in 40% of cases. In cases of fleshy SMAFS, results of facelift were considered as good (++). In cases of mixed SMAFS, after liposuction (closed/open) and plication/lift, results were considered as satisfactory (+). In case of fibrous SMAFS, results were found to be poor (−). In case of transcutaneous facelift, results were good (++) in case of membranous SMAFS in 80% 0f the cases and satisfactory (+) in 20% of the cases. Results were found to be satisfactory (+) in case of fleshy SMAFS, variable (+/−) in case of mixed SMAFS, and poor (−) in cases of Island, fatty, and fibrous SMAFS.

5.4 Discussion

5.4.1 SMAS and SMAFS: Concept and Variations

The SMAS (superficial musculoaponeurotic system) described by Mitz and Peyronie in 1976 was an important landmark in surgical facial anatomy [1]. The SMAS concept was considered essential for a successful and

Fig. 5.1 (**a**) Preoperative patient with thin membranous SMAFS. (**b**) After modified S-lift with SMAFS plication and lift

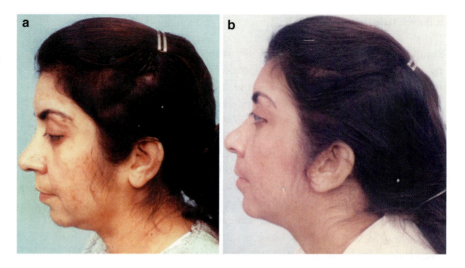

Fig. 5.2 (**a**) Fatty SMAFS. (**b**) Preoperative patient with thick moderately fatty SMAFS. (**c**) After modified temporal and retro-auricular lift with debulking, plication, lifting, and attachment of SMAFS to the temporal and mastoid bones

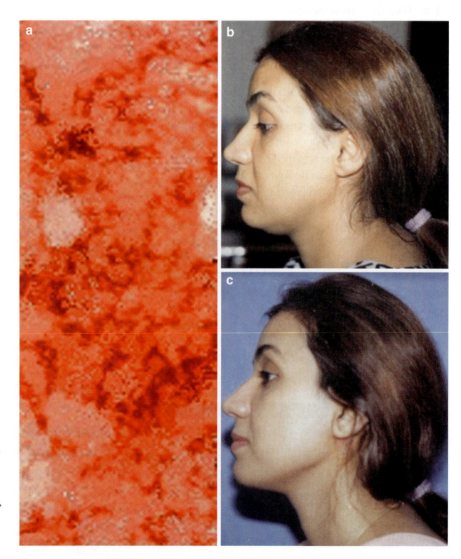

durable facelift. According to Mitz and Peyronie, SMAS is an extension of superficial cervical fascia into the face. It is continuous throughout the face and neck. Its thickness varies from region to region and from patient to patient. It is dense and thick over the parotid gland. Traced superiorly toward the zygomatic arch, it is termed temporoparietal fascia within the temporal region and galea within the scalp, both of which are substantial in terms of thickness [2]. As it is traced medially into the cheek, overlying the masseter and buccal fat pad, it becomes thinner and less distinct. In the malar region, it is quite thin and comprises the epimysium of the elevators of upper lip [3]. SMAS ensheathes the superficial mimetic muscles, platysma, zygomaticus major and minor, and risorius; fibrous septa connect the SMAS to the overlying dermis of skin. Therefore, mimetic muscles, SMAS, and skin function together as a single anatomical unit in producing facial movements. In view of the authors, however, the superficial mimetic muscles constitute a part of this system, which they call as SMAFS. The deeper layer of SMAS has no vertical fibrous connections. The deeper layer of cervical fascia continues into the face as the parotid-masseteric fascia. Some authors suggest that this layer is also part of SMAS. There appear to be two subdivisions of SMAS: (1) a suprazygomatic and (2) an infrazygomatic division. SMAS is attached firmly to the periosteum at the nuchal line posteriorly and at the mastoid process. Traced anteriorly, this attachment continues toward the zygomatic arch where it splits into two divisions: the upper division is attached below the eyebrow up to the dorsum of nose [4]; the lower subdivision descends downward at an angle of 45° to the lower lip margin. It is basically this lower subdivision which is clinically relevant in surgical facelifting [5]. The parotid fascia, risorius muscle, depressor anguli oris muscle, and platysma muscle can be pulled up together as one unit [6].

It appears that there are two major embryologically related subdivisions that interact at the buccal commissure. Those derived from the lower animal sphincter colli profundus muscle include the helmet-like muscles of skull, and mask-like muscles of the central face. The second division is related to the primitive platysma muscle, which in lower mammals consists of broad sheet of muscles covering the lower face and neck. In humans, it consists of platysma, risorius, depressor anguli oris, and the postauricular muscles, as well as the parotid fascia, which has lost its muscle fibers and has become fibrotic [7]. The components of the primitive platysma muscle lie in one plane. This plane, however, is not apparently continuous with the subgaleal plane of the forehead and scalp or with the lip elevators of the central face. Recognition of the disparate derivation of the two muscular systems makes it easier to understand why SMAFS is not continuous over the entire head and neck. However, embryological and acquired variations of SMAFS are somewhat more common than previously thought.

The platysma covers the upper parts of the pectoralis major and deltoideus, across the clavicle and mandible, joining the parotid fascia posteriorly, and enclosing the sternocleidomastoid attached to the mastoid process [8]. The SMAFS starts with the superficial fascia over the platysma (also embedded in platysma fibers), and extends over the mandible, to include the parotid fascia and the zygoma. The middle cervical fascia, invests the two layers of the infrahyoid muscles (has a superficial, middle, and deep sheath) and is attached to the hyoid bone and clavicle.

The frontal branch of facial nerve, unlike other nerve branches that lie deep to the deep facial fascia, is an anomaly. Once the frontal branch crosses the zygomatic arch, it travels underneath the temporoparietal fascia in the temporal region and then penetrates this layer peripherally to reach the deep surface of frontalis muscle. Therefore, if the temporoparietal fascia is violated during dissection, injury to this nerve can take place [9]. The area at greatest risk for damage to the temporal branch can be more easily demonstrated by drawing a line from the ear lobe to the lateral edge of the eyebrow and from the tragus to a point just above and behind the highest forehead crease. The temporal branches are at equal risk in the area defined by these lines, especially where they cross the zygomatic arch. At this point, the frontal nerve and its branches are especially vulnerable since they lie in the SMAFS just beneath its superficial fatty layer, and over the bony prominence [9]. The approximate path of the ramus to the frontalis muscle can be traced by drawing a line from 0.5 cm below the tragus to a point 1.5 cm above the lateral eyebrow. It is most vulnerable as it crosses the mid-zygomatic arch [9].

The S-lift procedure, in which the SMAFS is plicated, lifted, and attached to the periosteum of the zygomatic arch, can result in damage to the frontal nerve or its branches. Since the mid-zygomatic arch is the most vulnerable area, suturing of the SMAFS to the periosteum here should be avoided or one should proceed with extreme delicacy. Even suturing the SMAFS at the proximal zygomatic arch can result in nerve damage. In addition, pretragal pain and tension have been reported. If more knots are applied to the 2/0 Prolene sutures here, the knots can extrude through the skin. Damage to the temporal branch results in loss of function of the frontalis muscle, which derives its sole innervation from one solitary ramus that 85% of the time has no cross branches with the zygomatic nerve [9]. The forehead appears flat, the eyebrow falls to a lowered ptotic position, and there is inability to raise the eyebrow. There is no interference, however, with the eyelid closure. The upper part of orbicularis oculi and corrugator supercilii show little functional or cosmetic deficit. Single branching patterns are usual; however, as many as six or more branches have been traced crossing the zygomatic arch. It is probable that these variations account more commonly than previously thought. Therefore, in cases of multiple branching patterns, the S-lift procedure shows little functional or cosmetic deficit to the frontalis and other muscles of innervation by the frontal nerve. Despite the variety of branching patterns, these nerve fibers are nearly always medial and inferior to the frontal branch of the superficial temporal artery, which is easily palpated and serves a useful landmark in identifying the frontal nerve. The authors use the Delta-lift technique, in which the SMAFS is plicated well away from the frontal nerve/marginal mandibular nerves pathways, and therefore nerve injury practically never takes place. In case of S-lift, the authors attach Prolene to the proximal zygomatic arch. The authors have practically never seen damage to the frontal nerve using this technique.

The marginal mandibular nerve exits the parotid gland approximately 4 cm beneath the base of the earlobe near the angle of mandible. In 81% of patients, the nerve lies above the mandibular border. In 19% of cases, it lies inferior, although posterior to the facial vessels. The marginal mandibular nerve then crosses the facial vessels, and from this point anteriorly it runs superior to the mandibular border [10]. Where the facial artery and vein cross the mandibular border is a very useful landmark. The facial artery can be palpated just anterior to the angle of mandible along the anterior masseter border and serves as a quick method for localizing the marginal mandibular nerve [10]. Here, the nerve is superficial as it crosses over the facial vessels, and it is at this point that marginal mandibular nerve injury can take place [10]. It is very important to remember that as long as subcutaneous dissection remains superficial to SMAFS and platysma, motor nerve injury will be prevented [9, 10].

5.4.1.1 Sleep Lines

The underlying attachments of SMAFS become reflected superficially as skin folds, following certain chronic sleeping patterns. For example, sleep lines in the face become manifest as lines along the lower nasolabial fold and marionette areas, mid-cheek line, preauricular lines, arcus marginalis along the lower lid, nasal line along levator labii superioris, and as lines along the glabellar attachments. An oblique line appears across crow's feet, which reflects pressure on arcus marginalis attachment of SMAFS. These sleep lines become more prominent when compression is applied on tissues below these lines. Similarly, sleep line at the level of the levator labii superioris muscle from the SMAFS attachment becomes more prominent, when compression is applied on tissues toward the nose. Oblique fold across the marionette line reflects central condensation of SMAFS at the anterior mandibular ligament. Central cheek fold reflects the central condensation of SMAFS in the mid-cheek area. Skin folds may be created from SMAFS attachments from fibrous bands during the healing of scars.

5.4.1.2 Membranous SMAFS

This is the most common variant of SMAFS. Membranous SMAFS is usually thin, however, rarely, it is thick. In case of membranous SMAFS, adequate lift is achieved using three SMAFS sutures and plicating it below the zygomatic arch, as in a Classical/Delta-lift, or attaching it to the proximal periosteum of zygomatic arch, as in an S-lift using vertical U and horizontal O Prolene sutures. The lift is stable, and the results are longer lasting and usually excellent (Fig. 5.1) if the surgeon is an experienced rhytidectomist.

The results of Classical/Delta/S-lift are very satisfying when the SMAFS is thin and membranous as plication is easy and accurate and it is possible to lift the SMAFS considerably. SMAFS flaps have become obsolete in our hands now and are not created.

5.4.1.3 Fatty SMAFS

In case of Fatty SMAFS (Fig. 5.2), debulking of SMAFS via closed liposuction, using suction machine and either a keel cobra tip (3 mm diameter) or a flat spatula cannula should be carried out. However, if the SMAFS is mild to moderately fatty, an open vacuum cleaner technique of open liposuction should be followed using suction machine and a flat spatula cannula. Since, there will be a change in facial features if considerable debulking of SMAFS is done, this possibility should be discussed with the patient prior to surgery in order to prevent patient dissatisfaction. If the patient agrees to the thinning of face, surgery should be planned. After debulking of the SMAFS, plication and/or lift should be carried out as in a Classical/Delta or S-lift.

5.4.1.4 Flaccid SMAFS

When flaccidity of SMAFS is considerable, smaller SMAFS bites should be taken, and lifting and attaching it to the periosteum of zygoma using vertical U and horizontal O sutures, or tensing and plicating it below the zygoma using 2/3 Prolene sutures, should be considered.

5.4.1.5 Mixed SMAFS

A number of SMAFS variations can coexist in the form of mixed SMAFS, for example, fibrofatty SMAFS, thin and thick membranous SMAFS, fibro-membranous SMAFS, fleshy-fatty SMAFS, membranous-fatty SMAFS, membranous-fleshy SMAFS, fibro-fleshy SMAFS, and others. A number of technique variations can be planned according to the experience of the surgeon, and the type of tissues present in the SMAFS, for example; various combinations of closed/open liposuction, plication and lifting can be carried out in these cases.

5.4.1.6 Island SMAFS (Patchy/Discontinuous/ Broken Down SMAFS)

Island SMAFS is seen usually as a result of repeated Botox or steroid injections into the face. We have also seen Island SMAFS, as a congenital anomaly or as a result of repeated fat injections into the face, especially when sharp needles have been used for transfer and injections have been deeper. In these cases, SMAFS suturing should be considered primarily, and SMAFS repair should be carried out using 2/0 or 3/0 Prolene. Mild to moderate lift can be provided simultaneously if one or two discontinuous/patches exist. However, if the gaps in SMAFS are wide or discontinuity is more, only SMAFS repair should be carried out, and lifting should be deferred for several months to a year later.

5.4.1.7 Fleshy SMAFS

In case of fleshy SMAFS (Fig. 5.3), relatively deeper bites of SMAFS should be taken, three SMAFS sutures

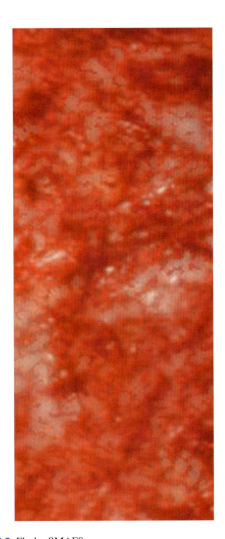

Fig. 5.3 Fleshy SMAFS

should be applied, and either plication as in a Delta/Classical lift or attachment to the periosteum of zygomatic bone as in an S-lift, should be done.

5.4.1.8 Fibrous SMAFS

In case of fibrous SMAFS, whether plication as in a Classical/Delta lift or attaching the SMAFS to the periosteum of the zygoma is carried out, results of facelifts are not so good.

5.4.1.9 SMAFS Sleep Lines Correction

SMAFS sleep lines can be corrected easily using either silk or Gore-Tex threads, using either a KH needle, or a conveniently sized Keith needle. Silk threads are suitable for persons of Asian descent or Hispanics, as in fair complexioned people, the black color of silk threads, reflects through the skin, especially, if these threads are inserted very superficially. The drawbacks of Gore-Tex threads are extrusion and infection. Other options are fat, collagen, Polymethol-Methacrylate, and Botox for these lines.

5.4.2 Clinical Significance of Attachment and Regional Variations of SMAFS in Facelift Surgery

Attachment and regional variations of SMAFS are in Tables 5.3 and 5.4.

Facelift results (Classical/Delta/S-lift) are excellent, when a clear cut supra- and infrazygomatic SMAFS exists [11, 12]. In open facelift surgery, Delta/S-lift/

Table 5.3 Attachment variations of SMAFS

Suprazygomatic and infrazygomatic SMAFS (usual)
Single unit (Unipolar) SMAFS
Discontinuous facial/neck SMAFS
Continuous/discontinuous suprazygomatic SMAFS
Continuous/discontinuous parotid/masseteric SMAFS
Thin and discontinuous central facial SMAFS (usual)
Thick and continuous central facial SMAFS (rare)

Table 5.4 Regional variations of SMAFS

Location	Variations
Infrazygomatic	Membranous, fatty, mixed, island, fleshy, fibrous (rare)
Suprazygomatic	Membranous, fleshy, fatty, mixed, island
Central face	Membranous, island, thick/continuous (rare)
Neck	Membranous, mixed, island, fatty, fleshy, fibrous (rare)

Classical lift and others, consideration should be paid to the entire SMAFS not only the fibro-aponeurotic part. It is important to take bites, plicate, lift, and attach not only the fibro-aponeurotic part but also the superficial muscular part of SMAFS [11, 12]. Only in this way, longer lasting and durable results of facelift will be achieved. If only superficial fibro-aponeurotic part is dissected and plicated/lifted, tissue sagging will reappear months after the procedure as the superficial fibrous part that is attached to the skin via fibrous septa will keep the skin lifted and the fibro-aponeurotic part, which ensheaths and encircles the superficial mimetic muscles will keep the muscles lifted. Over several months fascia lengthening takes place and muscles of facial expression that have not been plicated, droop. At the same time, it is also important, not to go deep into the muscles, otherwise, motor nerve injury will take place.

In the subperiosteal space, attachments are 1 cm above the orbital rim. Superomedial osteoperiosteal ligament is 13 mm from the midline and superolateral osteoperiosteal ligament is 23 mm from the midline [13]. Supraorbital nerve is lateral to the ligaments. At the orbital rim, inferomedial osteoperiosteal ligament is 12.6 mm from the midline. Supraorbital nerve is lateral to it. Release of the medially based ligaments results in easier lifting of the medial aspect of the eyebrow. The three subperiosteal ligaments extend into the subgaleal level. There is a broad ligament that extends across the lateral aspect of the supraorbital rim. Release of the lateral segment of the broad ligament results in easy elevation of the lateral portion of the eyebrow. Dissection between the medial retaining ligaments in the central tunnel provides exposure for treating the medial corrugator and procerus muscles in the glabellar area. The zygomatic ligament (McGregor's Patch) originates at or near the inferior border of the anterior zygomatic arch, and inserts into the skin [13]. The mandibular ligaments (Furnas Ligaments) originate from bone of mandible about 1 cm above the mandibular border [13]. It restrains anterior skin, preventing gravitational sagging. The platysma-auricular ligament is a condensation of the posterior border of platysma, often attached to the overlying skin [13]. Anterior-Platysma cutaneous ligaments are attachments of the anterior platysma to skin of the middle and anterior cheek [13]. These ligaments are closely associated with nearby vessels and facial nerve branches.

Results are better in case of single unit SMAFS, where no division exists. However, in these cases, if entire upper and lower SMAFS is not lifted, and only lower SMAFS is lifted like in Delta or S-lift, the upper sagging of SMAFS will become considerable, resulting in patient dissatisfaction. Plication of the condensed superficial parotid fascia and parotid fascia or attaching these fascias to the periosteum of zygomatic arch along with section of the platysma-auricular ligaments should be the aim in the lateral cheek area while performing facelift surgery. The authors do not recommend the subparotid fascia (masseteric fascia) plane for facelifting, going under the platysma muscle. The parotid gland is covered on its superior surface by the parotid fascia, which is a fibrotic degeneration of the primitive platysma muscle and is in direct continuity with platysma, risorius, and depressor anguli oris muscles. In the space between the parotid and masseteric fascia planes lie not only the parotid gland, but also Stenson's duct and emerging branches of the facial nerve; therefore, facial nerve injury can take place and parotid fistula can form if the surgeon works close to the masseteric fascia. When the SMAFS is thin and discontinuous, as in the central face, results of facelift are limiting here, for example, for the nasolabial folds, silk or Gore-Tex threads or other fillers like PMMA have to be used like in a Delta-lift to provide good results. However, rarely, when the SMAFS is continuous and thick in the central face, SMAFS plication results in obvious obliteration of nasolabial folds and fillers are not required in these cases. When the SMAFS is discontinuous or broken (Island SMAS) suprazygomatically, infrazygomatically, or in the neck, restoring continuity of SMAFS, rather than lifting should be the primary aim. When continuity of SMAFS has been restored, lifting should be planned at a subsequent stage, especially if gaps in SMAFS are more. The only exception to this rule is the central face, where discontinuous SMAFS is usual, and obliteration of nasolabial folds should be done with fillers, rather than achieving SMAFS continuity, otherwise, dissection will become very extensive, and branches of the facial nerve can get damaged, as the SMAFS is extremely thin here. Regional variations of SMAFS have an impact on the results of facelift surgery. However, generally, the surgeon should follow the general guidelines while dealing with regional SMAFS variations. The very fatty SMAFS assessed preoperatively should be defatted using suction machine and closed liposuction, using either a keel-cobra tip or a flat spatula cannula, in those regions. In cases of mild to moderately fatty SMAFS, defatting should be done using suction machine and a flat spatula cannula with an open vacuum cleaner technique. Deeper bites of SMAFS should be taken in case of fleshy SMAFS, more bites of SMAFS should be taken in case of membranous SMAFS, and continuity should be restored in case of Island (broken) SMAFS, in the SMAFS regions, where these variations are encountered; in all cases, including also thick, fibrous, flaccid and mixed.

Varieties, lifting and attaching either to the periosteum of zygomatic arch or plication should be considered, according to the skill and experience of the surgeon, and according to the type of SMAFS.

5.4.3 Importance of SMAFS Variations in Transcutaneous Facelifts, Mini-Invasive Lifts, and Thread Lifts

Transcutaneous facelift and thread lifts are blind procedures, where SMAFS assessment has to be done preoperatively and externally. Pinch test (lifting the SMAFS with the thumb and index finger) should be carried out over the face, neck, and temporal regions. Thickness, thinness, tone, density, elasticity, flaccidity, continuity, and other gross parameters should be assessed. In transcutaneous facelifting, where the SMAFS is thin and membranous, superficial SMAFS bites using the KH needle or a Keith needle, and two to three sutures for lifting and attaching the SMAFS to the thick temporal fascia or periosteum of the temporal bone provide a stable lift [14]. Where the SMAFS is thick, fatty, or fleshy, relatively deeper and more SMAFS bites should be taken, more lift should be provided and attachment should be to the periosteum of the temporal bone. Since there is discontinuity between the supra- and infrazygomatic SMAFS mostly, lifting the SMAFS infrazygomatically, and making Prolene 2/0 knots in the suprazygomatic SMAFS (thick temporal fascia) provides a stable lift in most of the cases. However, in cases of unipolar SMAFS (continuous supra- and infrazygomatic SMAFS), this attachment will result in certain sagging after a while, and the results of facelift will become poor. In these cases, attachment should be deep to the periosteum of temporal bone. If you are suspecting Island SMAFS on preoperative examination, TCFL can result in asymmetry of face. In these cases, restoring continuity of SMAFS, and mild/moderate lifting should be carried out via open technique and subsequent lift should be planned if considerable lift is required. The SMAS-Platysma facelift also aims at attaching the SMAS to the periosteum of mastoid bone, providing a stable lift [15].

A variety of thread lift procedures have also been advised to provide stability to the SMAFS; some use a feathering technique like the Sulamanidze threads for providing micro-stability and lift [16]; others aim at placing threads in the SMAFS providing a sort of micro-volume augmentation. Fournier [17] has developed a technique of cementing the threads with fat in the cheek areas, providing volume augmentation to SMAFS in the cheek areas. In any case, threads provide a very mild lift/stability to the SMAFS. The subperiosteal facelift of Hamra [18] was an intense procedure where undermining was carried deep to the SMAFS to the periosteum. It has been abandoned by most of the surgeons as a result of increased morbidity/complications. The argument was that in going deep to the bone and lifting the results were longer lasting. Some physicians are still using a somewhat modified technique for lifting the SMAFS, for example, for eyebrow lift, cheek lift, chin lift using blunt needles, going deep to the periosteum of bone and then coming back to the same point superficially taking SMAFS and dermis, using absorbable sutures. However, we believe that while performing these blind procedures, anatomical landmarks like the motor branches of facial nerve, should be taken into consideration to prevent motor nerve injury [19]. These procedures should only be performed by experienced surgeons and anatomical landmarks should be marked beforehand prior to needle insertion. In case of TCFL, and other suspension lifts, needle bites should be taken from the superficial muscular component of SMAFS, in order to provide a stable lift. In case of thread lifts, threads should be inserted into the superficial muscular component. The spikes of threads will go into the muscle fibers, thereby providing micro-lift. If the threads without spikes are used, whether they are inserted into the superficial muscular component, or into the fibro-aponeurotic component, threads will only provide a sort of volume augmentation in these cases.

5.5 Conclusions

The type, nature, and variations of SMAFS have an impact on the outcome of facelift surgery. Therefore, it is important for all surgeons performing facelift surgery to understand in detail the various types of SMAFS and their variations. They should be able to assess gross parameters of SMAFS by external manipulation and SMAFS examination and should be able to analyze various types of SMAFS preoperatively. They should be able to plan the correct operative technique of debulking, plicating, lifting, and attaching the SMAFS to the bony periosteum according to the nature and type of SMAFS present in order to achieve good results. Surgeons must undergo training programs from experienced rhytidectomists, before performing facelift surgery independently.

References

1. Mitz V, Peyronie M. The superficial musculoaponeurotic system (SMAS) in the parotid and cheek area. Plast Reconstr Surg. 1976;58(1):80–6.
2. Salasche SJ, Bernstein G. Surgical anatomy of the skin. 1st ed. Norwalk: Appleton & Lange; 1988. p. 89–97.
3. Pensler JM, Ward JW, Parry SW. The superficial musculoaponeurotic system in the upper lip. Plast Reconstr Surg. 1985;75(4):488–94.
4. Morales P, Castro R, Errea E, Nociti J. Suprazygomatic SMAS in rhytidectomy. Aesthetic Plast Surg. 1984;18(3):181–7.
5. Jost G, Lamouche G. SMAS in rhytidectomy. Aesthetic Plast Surg. 1982;6(2):69–74.
6. Jost G, Levet Y. Parotid fascia and face lifting: a critical evaluation of the SMAS concept. Plast Reconstr Surg. 1984;74(1):42–51.
7. Dzubow LM. A histologic pattern approach to the anatomy of the face. J Dermatol Surg Oncol. 1986;12(7):712–8.
8. de Castro CC. The anatomy of the platysma muscle. Plast Reconstr Surg. 1980;66(5):680–3.

9. Pitanguy I, Ramos AS. The frontal branch of the facial nerve: the importance of its variation in face lifting. Plast Reconstr Surg. 1966;38(4):352–6.
10. Moffat DA, Ramsden RT. The deformity produced by a palsy of the marginal mandibular branch of the facial nerve. J Laryngol Otol. 1977;91(5):401–6.
11. Khawaja HA, Hernandez-Perez E. The Delta-lift: a modification of S-lift for facial rejuvenation. Int J Cosmet Surg Aesthet Dermatol. 2002;4:309–15.
12. Saylan Z. The S-lift for facial rejuvenation. Int J Cosmet Surg. 1999;7:18–24.
13. Furnas DW. The retaining ligaments of the cheek. Plast Reconstr Surg. 1989;83(1):11–6.
14. Khawaja HA, Hernandez-Perez E. Transcutaneous face-lift. Dermatol Surg. 2005;31(4):453–7.
15. Serdev NP. Total ambulatory SMAS lift by hidden minimal incisions part 2: Lower SMAS-platysma face lift. Int J Cosmet Surg Aesthet Dermatol. 2002;4:285–92.
16. Sulamanidze MA, Shiffman MA. Facial lifting with aptos threads. Int J Cosmet Surg Aesthet Dermatol. 2001; 3: 275–81.
17. Fournier PF. Thread facelift. Meso-American Academy of Cosmetic Surgery meeting, San Salvador, May 2002.
18. Hamra ST. Subperiosteal face lift. Plast Reconstr Surg. 1995;96(2):493.
19. Baker DC, Conley J. Avoiding facial nerve injuries in rhytidectomy: anatomical variations and pitfalls. Plast Reconstr Surg. 1979;64(6):781–95.

Part II

Anesthesia

Anesthesia for Minimally Invasive Cosmetic Surgery of the Head and Neck

Gary Dean Bennett

6.1 Introduction

With progressive refinement of cosmetic and reconstructive surgical techniques, the development of less invasive surgical procedures, and the gradual demographic shift of the world's population toward the older age, the popularity of cosmetic and restorative treatments continues to increase. While more than 50% of all aesthetic surgeries are performed in the office [1], the majority of the newer noninvasive and minimally invasive cosmetic and restorative procedures are performed in the office setting. As a consequence of this shift toward less invasive procedures and greater office-based surgery, the surgeon has assumed a greater role in the selection and management of the anesthesia administered during the procedure.

Decisions relating to the preoperative evaluation, the selection of the anesthesia to be administered, the intraoperative monitoring, the postoperative pain management, and the discharge criteria, which were previously performed by the anesthesiologist or Certified Registered Nurse Anesthetist (CRNA), frequently become the responsibility of the surgeon. Evidence suggests that anesthesia-related deaths are significantly higher when the surgeon also administers the anesthesia [2]. Therefore, if the surgeon accepts the responsibility of the management of anesthesia, then it is incumbent on the surgeon to achieve an in-depth understanding of the concepts of anesthesia and to adhere to the same standards of care that are applied to the anesthesiologist or the CRNA [3]. The following chapter should serve as an introduction to understanding the standards-of-care relating to anesthesia for the cosmetic surgeon.

6.2 Surgical Facility

When deciding where to perform surgical procedures requiring anesthesia, the surgeon should be aware that studies demonstrate a threefold mortality in surgeries performed at the office-based setting compared to similar surgeries performed at other facilities such as free-standing surgical centers or hospitals [4]. Most states in the USA require that the surgical facility be accredited by one of the regulating agencies if general anesthesia or enough sedative medication is used which could potentially result in the loss of life-preserving protective reflexes [5, 6]. All operating rooms where anesthesia is administered must be equipped with the type of monitors required to fulfill monitoring standards established by the American Society of Anesthesiologists (ASA) [7], and resuscitative equipment and resuscitative medications [8, 9]. A transfer agreement should be established with a nearby hospital in the event of an unplanned admission. Preferably, the surgical facility should have convenient access to a laboratory in the event of a stat laboratory analysis. Essentially, office-based surgical facilities should comply with the same standard-of-care as accredited outpatient surgical centers and hospital-based outpatient surgery departments.

G.D. Bennett
Department of Anesthesiology, Chapman Medical Center,
2601 East Chapman Ave., Orange, CA 92869, USA
e-mail: dasseen@cox.net

Reprinted with permission of Springer

6.3 Ancillary Personnel

The facility or office must be staffed by individuals with the training and experience required to assist in the care of the patient [9, 10]. Use of qualified and experienced operating room personnel has been shown to improve operating room efficiency and reduce surgical morbidity [11, 12]. All personnel assisting in the operating room and recovery area should maintain Basic Life Support (BLS) Certification [13]. At least one health care provider in the facility must be certified to deliver advanced cardiac life support (ACLS) when anesthesia is administered [14]. The surgeon may prefer to enlist the assistance of an anesthesiologist or CRNA to provide intraoperative anesthesia and monitoring. If the surgeon elects to administer parenteral sedative or analgesic medication without the assistance of an anesthesiologist or CNRA, then a second licensed health care provider should be available to deliver the medications to the patient and monitor the patient throughout the perioperative period [15]. The use of untrained, unlicensed personnel to administer medication to the patient and monitor the patient is associated with an increased risk of anesthesia-related complications to the patient. The nurse who has been assigned to monitor the patient during the administration of sedative and analgesic medication should not be required to double as a circulating or scrub nurse [16]. Preferably, the surgeon who chooses to administer anesthesia should also be ACLS Certified.

6.4 Preoperative Evaluation

Despite the development of minimally invasive nonsurgical and surgical procedures, the importance of the preoperative anesthesia evaluation should not be minimized. An old adage within many anesthesia training programs is that while there may be minor surgical procedures, there is no such thing as a minor anesthetic. If the surgeon chooses to administer the anesthesia then he/she assumes the full responsibility of the preoperative assessment. Even if an anesthesiologist or CRNA is to be involved on the day of surgery, a carefully performed preoperative evaluation by the surgeon is instrumental in reducing potential delays or cancellations of surgery and improving the overall perioperative risk to the patient [17].

A comprehensive preoperative patient questionnaire is an invaluable tool to begin the initial assessment. Information contained in the history may determine the diagnosis of the medical condition in nearly 90% of patients [18]. Information requested by the questionnaire should include all current and prior medical conditions, prior surgeries and types of anesthesia received, adverse outcomes to previous anesthetics or other medications, eating disorders, prior or current use of antiobesity medications, current use of homeopathic or herbal supplements, and prior family history of severe reactions to anesthetics such as malignant hyperthermia. A complete review of systems, including questions about the presence of chest pain, shortness of breath, loss of consciousness, spontaneous bleeding or bruising, spontaneous weight loss, fever, or fatigue is crucial in identifying previously undiagnosed, untreated medical conditions, which could impact the outcome of anesthesia and surgery. Obtaining a family history of sudden, unsuspected illness or death is also important in identifying patients with potentially undiagnosed medical conditions.

A routine physical examination may alert the surgeon to certain medical conditions such as undiagnosed or inadequately treated hypertension, cardiac arrhythmias, cardiac failure, or bronchial asthma, which could result in increased risk to the patient during the perioperative period. Preliminary assessment of the head and neck anatomy may be useful to predict possible challenges in the event of an endotracheal intubation even if general anesthesia is not planned. Preoperative history and physical examination has been shown to be superior to laboratory analysis in determining the clinical course of anesthesia and surgery [19–23].

For patients with complicated, unstable, or previously unrecognized medical conditions, a consultation by the appropriate medical specialist is indicated to determine if the patient's medical conditional is optimally managed, if the medical condition may cause a significant increased in the perioperative risk to the patient, and to assist with the perioperative medical management of the patient if required. Additional preoperative testing may be considered medically necessary by the consultant.

Guidelines for the judicious use of preoperative laboratory screening tests for healthy patients not taking medications are presented in Table 6.1. Additional preoperative tests, noted in Table 6.2, may be indicated for patients with prior medical conditions or risk factors for anesthesia and surgery.

Excessive or indiscriminately ordered preoperative laboratory testing for healthy patients not taking medications has limited value in predicting surgical or anesthesia-related morbidity and mortality [26–30].

6.4.1 Preoperative Risk Assessment

One critical goal of the preoperative evaluation is the determination of a patient's overall level of risk related to the administration of anesthesia. By first establishing a patient's level of risk, strategies to reduce the patient's exposure may be considered. Compelling evidence suggests that certain coexisting medical conditions significantly increase the risk for perioperative morbidity and mortality [15, 31]. The risk classification system developed by the ASA in 1984 (Table 6.3) [32] has become the most widely accepted method of preoperative risk assessment. The value of the ASA system in predicting which patients are at higher risk for morbidity [33] and mortality [34–36] has been confirmed by numerous studies. Goldman and Caldera [37] established a risk assessment index based on cardiac disease, which has also been demonstrated to be effective in predicting perioperative mortality [38, 39]. Physicians should incorporate one of the acceptable risk classification systems as an integral part of the preoperative evaluation.

The type of surgery plays a key role in the overall risk of morbidity and mortality to the patient. The consensus of multiple studies confirms that more invasive surgeries, surgeries with multiple combined procedures, surgeries of prolonged duration, and surgeries with significant blood loss increases the risk of

Table 6.1 Guidelines for preoperative testing in healthy patients (ASA 1-11)

Age	Test
12–40[a]	CBC
40–60	CBC, EKG
Greater than 60	CBC, BUN, glucose, ECG, CXR

[a]Pregnancy test for potentially childbearing females suggested
Source: Adapted from Roizen et al. [24]

Table 6.2 Common indications for additional risk-specific testing

Electrocardiogram

 History: Coronary artery disease, congestive heart failure, prior myocardial infarction, hypertension, hyperthyroidism, hypothyroidism, obesity, compulsive eating disorders, deep venous thrombosis, pulmonary embolism, smoking, chemotherapeutic agents, chemical dependency, chronic liver disease.

 Symptoms: Chest pain, shortness of breath, dizziness

 Signs: Abnormal heart rate or rhythm, hypertension, cyanosis, peripheral edema, wheezing, rales, rhonchi

Chest X-ray

 History: Bronchial asthma, congestive heart failure, chronic obstructive pulmonary disease, and pulmonary embolism

 Symptoms: Chest pain, shortness of breath, wheezing, unexplained weight loss, and hemoptysis

 Signs: Cyanosis, wheezes, rales, rhonchi, decreased breath sounds, peripheral edema, abnormal heart rate or rhythm

Electrolytes, glucose, liver function tests, BUN, creatinine

 History: Diabetes mellitus, chronic renal failure, chronic liver disease, adrenal insufficiency, hypothyroidism, hyperthyroidism, diuretic use, compulsive eating disorders, diarrhea

 Symptoms: Dizziness, generalized fatigue or weakness

 Signs: Abnormal heart rate or rhythm, peripheral edema, jaundice

Urinalysis

 History: Diabetes mellitus, chronic renal disease, and recent urinary tract infection

 Symptoms: Dysuria, urgency, frequency, and bloody urine

Source: Adapted from Roizen et al. [25]

Table 6.3 The American Society of Anesthesiologists' physical status classification

ASA Class I	A healthy patient without systemic medical or psychiatric illness
ASA Class II	A patient with mild, treated and stable systemic medical or psychiatric illness
ASA Class III	A patient with severe systemic disease that is not considered incapacitating
ASA Class IV	A patient with severe systemic, incapacitating and life-threatening disease not necessarily correctable by medication or surgery
ASA Class V	A patient considered moribund and not expected to live more than 24 h

perioperative complications [40–44]. However, even with more minor procedures involving sedation or anesthesia, the physician should not neglect the preoperative evaluation and risk assessment.

6.4.2 Anesthesia and Patients with Preexisting Disease

Surgeons who perform outpatient surgery, especially office-based surgery, and particularly those surgeons who choose to administer sedative or analgesic medication, must appreciate how preexisting medical conditions may increase the risk of anesthesia in the surgical patient. Furthermore, the surgeon should maintain a reasonable understanding of the basic evaluation and treatment of these medical conditions. The following sections contain an introduction to considerations of medical conditions which may have a significant impact on a patient during the course of anesthesia and surgery.

6.4.3 Cardiac Disease

The leading cause of perioperative anesthetic and surgical mortality is complications related to cardiac disease, including myocardial infarction and congestive heart failure [45, 46]. Fortunately, a careful preoperative history and physical can identify most patients with preoperative heart disease [23]. When assessing patients who are apparently asymptomatic for heart disease, but have risk factors for heart disease such as smoking, hypertension, diabetes mellitus, obesity, hyperlipidemia, or a family history of severe heart disease, the prudent physician should be aware that 80% of all episodes of myocardial ischemia are silent [47, 48]. Patients with known cardiac disease must be evaluated by the internist or the cardiologist to ensure the medical condition is optimally managed. Anesthesia and all except the most minor surgical procedures on patients with significant heart disease should preferentially be performed in a hospital setting.

Most studies have demonstrated a dramatically greater risk of reinfarction and death in patients undergoing surgery within 6 months after sustaining a myocardial infarction [49–51]. More recent studies suggest that if patients are monitored postoperatively in the hospital cardiac care unit with invasive hemodynamic monitoring, the rate of perioperative reinfarction and death is reduced [52, 53]. At this time, postponing all but the most minor elective cosmetic surgeries for at least 6 months after a myocardial infarction remains the most prudent decision.

The cardiac risk index established by Goldman et al. [37] has proven extremely helpful in identifying patients with intermediate risk for perioperative cardiac complication [38]. Patients should be referred to a cardiologist for preoperative evaluation if the risk index score is greater than 13. Dipyridamole thallium scanning and dobutamine or adenosine stress echocardiography can predict potential perioperative cardiac complication [54]. A simple but reliable screening tool to evaluate the patient's cardiac status is the patient's exercise tolerance. The patient's ability to increase the heart rate of 85% of the age-adjusted maximal rate reliably predicts perioperative cardiac morbidity [55].

No one anesthetic technique or medication has ever emerged as the preferential method to reduce the incidence of perioperative complication in patients with cardiac disease [56, 57]. Most anesthesiologists agree that perioperative cardiac complications can be reduced through scrupulous patient monitoring and avoiding respiratory and hemodynamic fluctuations.

6.4.4 Obesity

With over 55% of the population of the USA afflicted, obesity has attained epidemic proportions [58]. In fact, obesity has emerged as one of the most prevalent health concerns in the developing world. Assuredly, physicians who work with patients undergoing cosmetic surgery will routinely encounter patients with this preexisting medical condition. These physicians must be aware that obesity is associated with other risk factors such as diabetes mellitus, heart disease, hypertension, sleep apnea, and occult liver disease [59]. A thorough preoperative evaluation must rule out these added risk factors prior to elective cosmetic surgery.

The body mass index (BMI), which is determined by weight (kg) divided by height (m) squared, has become the standard method of quantifying the level of obesity. Patients with a BMI over 30 are considered obese, while a BMI over 35 indicates morbid obesity [60]. Morbidly obese patients (BMI greater than 35) undergoing major surgery or any surgery where a general anesthetic is planned, should preferentially be referred to a hospital with health-care providers experienced with the management of this high-risk group.

Airway control in morbidly obese patients may be particularly challenging due to anatomical abnormalities of the airway [61]. The combination of higher gastric volume, lower gastric pH, and increased frequency of esophageal reflux elevates the risk of dreaded pulmonary aspiration [62]. The morbidly obese patient may have severe restriction in pulmonary function [63], which is further compromised in the supine position [64]. Pulmonary function may dangerously deteriorate when heavy sedation or general anesthesia is administered to the morbidly obese patient [65]. Hypoxemia may develop precipitously in this patient population while receiving heavy sedation or general anesthesia anytime in the perioperative period. Respiratory impairment may persist for up to 4 days after surgery or anesthesia [66].

Premedication with metaclopramide, or other dopamine receptor antagonist, and ranitidine, or similar histamine type-2 receptor antagonist, should be administered the evening prior to and on the morning of surgery to reduce the risk of pulmonary aspiration pneumonitis [67]. Because of the increased risk of deep venous thrombosis (DVT) [68] and pulmonary embolism (PE) [69], prophylactic measures such as lower extremity pneumatic compression devices and early ambulation should be used.

Fatal cardiac arrhythmias, sudden congestive heart failure, and intractable hypotension has developed in patients receiving anesthesia who have previously taken appetite suppressant medications such as aminorex fumarate, dexfenfluramine (Redux), fenfluramine (Pondimin), and phentermine (Ionam, Adipex-P, Fastin, Oby-Cap, Obenix, Oby-trim, or Zantryl). Some authors advocate a cardiac evaluation with an echocardiogram to rule out valvular disease associated with these medications, and continuous wave Doppler imaging with color-flow examination for any patient who has previously taken any antiobesity medications. Sustained hypotension may not respond to ephedrine, a popular vasopressor. Phenylephrine is the treatment of choice for hypotension in this patient population [70].

6.4.5 Hypertension

Perioperative mortality is significantly increased in patients with untreated or poorly controlled hypertension [71, 72]. Satisfactory control of hypertension reduces the risk of mortality due to complications related to cardiovascular and cerebral vascular disease [73–75]. Most authors concur that preoperative stabilization of hypertension reduces perioperative cardiovascular complications such as ischemia [76–78]. Patients with undiagnosed or poorly controlled hypertension can easily be identified in the preoperative examination and referred to the family physician or internist for evaluation and treatment. Attributing severe hypertension to the patient's preoperative level of anxiety can be a deadly assumption. Considering that many effective medications are available for the treatment of hypertension, there is little defense for the physician who proceeds with surgery in a patient with uncontrolled hypertension.

Previously prescribed antihypertensive medications should be continued up to and including the morning of surgery. Abrupt withdrawal from these medications may result in dangerous rebound hypertension [79]. The only exception are the class of medications known as angiotensin-converting enzyme (ACE) inhibitors, which have been associated with hypotension during the induction of general anesthesia [80].

While mild to moderate perioperative hypertension may be a response to anxiety, an inadequate level of anesthesia, or poor pain control, these cases of hypertension are usually accompanied by other signs such as verbal complaints of pain during local anesthesia, patient movement during general anesthesia, tachycardia, or tachypnea. If the pain treatment, anxiolytics, and depth of anesthesia have been deemed appropriate, then initiating treatment of the blood pressure is indicated.

Beta-adrenergic receptor blocking agents, such as propranolol, judiciously administered intravenously in doses of 0.5 mg at 10-min intervals, is especially effective in treating perioperative hypertension, which is accompanied by tachycardia. Even small doses of beta-adrenergic blocking agents can reduce the incidence of cardiac ischemia [78]. Labetalol, an antihypertensive medication with combined alpha-adrenergic and beta-adrenergic receptor blocking properties, administered in 10 mg doses every 10 min, is also a safe and effective alternative for treating both hypertension and tachycardia [81].

For severe hypertension, hydralazine, a potent vasodilator may be useful in 2.5–5 mg doses intravenously at 15-min intervals. The effects of hydralazine may be delayed up to 20 min and sustained for hours. Hydralazine may cause tachycardia or hypotension, especially if the patient is hypovolemic [82].

6.4.6 Diabetes Mellitus

Patients with diabetes mellitus have a significantly increased rate of surgical morbidity and mortality compared to nondiabetic patients [83]. These complications are primarily related to the consequences of the end-organ disease such as cardiovascular disease, renal disease, and altered wound healing which is associated with diabetes mellitus [31, 84, 85]. The preoperative evaluation should identify diabetic patients with poor control as well as medical conditions associated with diabetes such as cardiovascular disease and renal insufficiency. The physician should keep in mind that diabetic patients have a greater incidence of silent myocardial ischemia [86].

The minimum preoperative analysis for the diabetic patient should include fasting blood sugar, glycosylated hemoglobin, electrolytes, BUN, creatinine, and EKG. If there are any concerns regarding the patient's medical stability, the patients should be referred to a diabetologist, cardiologist, nephrologist, or other indicated specialist. Patients with brittle diabetes or other severe medical conditions should preferentially undergo surgery in a hospital-based surgical unit.

The primary objective of the perioperative management of the stable diabetic patient is to avoid hypoglycemia. Although patients are usually NPO after midnight prior to surgery, a glass of clear juice may be taken up to 2 h prior to surgery to avoid hypoglycemia. To minimize the risk of perioperative hypoglycemia, patients should not take their usual dose of insulin or oral agents on the morning of surgery. Surgery of the diabetic patient should be scheduled as early as possible in the morning to further reduce the risk of perioperative hypoglycemia. After the patient arrives, a preoperative fasting glucose should be determined. An intravenous infusion of fluid containing 5% dextrose should be initiated and continued at 1–2 ml/kg/h until oral fluids are tolerated in the recovery room. Usually, one-half of the patient's scheduled dose of insulin is administered after the intravenous dextrose fluid infusion has begun [87].

At least one intraoperative glucose should be measured for surgeries greater than 2 h, especially if general anesthesia is used. A final glucose level should be checked just prior to discharge. Glucose levels above 200 may be effectively managed with a sliding scale of insulin [88].

Treatment regimen directed toward tighter control of the blood glucose, such as insulin infusions, do not necessarily improve perioperative outcome, and recent data indicates that the risk of hypoglycemia may be greater with these regimen [89, 90]. It is imperative that diabetic patients tolerate oral fluids without nausea or vomiting prior to discharge.

6.4.7 Pulmonary Disease

An estimated 4.5% of the population may suffer some form of reactive airway disease which may influence perioperative pulmonary function [91]. These medical conditions include a recent upper airway infection, bronchial asthma, chronic bronchitis, chronic obstructive airway disease, and a history of smoking. A thorough evaluation of the patient's pulmonary function is indicated if any of these medical conditions are identified in the preoperative history. A careful history should help to separate these patients into low- and high-risk groups. The degree of preoperative respiratory dyspnea correlates closely with postoperative mortality [92]. Using a simple grading scale, the patients preoperative pulmonary function can be estimated (Table 6.4). Patients with level 2 dyspnea or greater should be referred to a pulmonologist for more

Table 6.4 Grade of dyspnea while walking

Level	Clinical response
0	No dyspnea
1	Dyspnea with fast walking only
2	Dyspnea with one or two blocks walking
3	Dyspnea with mild exertion (walking around the house)
4	Dyspnea at rest

Source: Adapted from Boushy et al. [92]

complete evaluation and possibly further medical stabilization. Patients with level 3 and 4 dyspnea are not suitable patients for outpatient surgery. The benefits of elective surgery in these patients should be carefully weighed against the increased risk.

Since upper airway infection may affect pulmonary function for up to 5 weeks [93], major surgery requiring general endotracheal anesthesia should be postponed, especially if the patient suffers residual symptoms such as fevers, chills, coughing, and sputum production, until the patient is completely asymptomatic.

Multiple studies have confirmed that patients who smoke more than one pack of cigarettes daily have a higher risk of perioperative respiratory complications compared to nonsmokers. However, cessation of smoking immediately prior to surgery may not improve the patient's outcome.

In fact, the risk of perioperative complications may actually increase if smoking is abruptly discontinued immediately prior to surgery. Cessation of smoking for a full 8 weeks may be required to successfully reduce the risk of perioperative pulmonary complications [94]. If the preoperative physical examination reveals respiratory wheezing, reversible bronchospasm should be optimally treated prior to surgery, even if this treatment requires that the surgery be delayed. Therapeutic agents include inhaled or systemic selective beta-adrenergic receptor type-2 agonist (albuterol) as a sole agent or in combination with anticholinergic (ipratropium) and locally active corticosteroid (beclomethasone diproponate) medications [95]. Continuing the patient's usual asthmatic medications up to the time of surgery [96], combined with postoperative use of incentive spirometry [97], effectively reduces postoperative pulmonary complications.

With regard to medically stabilized pulmonary disease, there are no conclusive, prospective, randomized studies to indicate which anesthesia technique or medication results in improved patient outcome.

6.4.8 Obstructive Sleep Apnea

The National Commission on Sleep Disorders Research estimates that 18 million Americans suffer with obstructive sleep apnea (OSA). Unfortunately, the majority of patients with sleep apnea remain undiagnosed [98]. The incidence of OSA increases among obese patients [99]. Since the target population for many cosmetic surgical procedures includes patients with morbid obesity, concern about the diagnosis and safe treatment of patients with OSA becomes even more relevant.

OSA is a result of a combination of excessive pharyngeal adipose tissue and inadequate pharyngeal soft tissue support [100]. During episodes of sleep apnea, patients may suffer significant and sustained hypoxemia. As a result of the pathophysiology of OSA, patients develop left and right ventricular hypertrophy [101]. Consequently, patients have a higher risk of ventricular dysarrhythmias and myocardial infarction [102].

Most medications used during anesthesia, including sedatives such as diazepam and midazolam; hypnotics such as propofol; and analgesics such as fentanyl, meperidine, and morphine, increase the risk for airway obstruction and respiratory depression in patients with OSA [103]. Death may occur suddenly and silently in patients with inadequate monitoring [104]. A combination of anatomical abnormalities makes airway management, including mask ventilation and endotracheal intubation, especially challenging in obese patients with OSA [105]. Perioperative monitoring, including visual observation, must be especially vigilant to avoid perioperative respiratory arrest in patients with OSA.

For patients with severe OSA, particularly those with additional coexisting medical conditions such as cardiac or pulmonary disease, surgery requiring sedation, analgesic, or general anesthesia, performed on an outpatient basis is not appropriate. For these high-risk patients, monitoring should continue in the intensive care unit until the patient no longer requires parenteral analgesics. If technically feasible, local or regional anesthesia may be preferable in patients with severe OSA. Postoperatively, patients with any history of OSA should not be discharged if they appear lethargic or somulent or there is evidence of even mild hypoxemia [106].

During the preoperative evaluation of the obese patient, a presumptive diagnosis of OSA may be made if the patient has a history of loud snoring, long pauses of breathing during sleep, as reported by the spouse, or daytime somnolence [107]. If OSA is suspected, patients should be referred for a sleep study to evaluate the severity of the condition.

6.4.9 Malignant Hyperthermia Susceptibility

Patients with susceptibility to malignant hyperthermia (MH) can be successfully managed on an outpatient basis if they are closely monitored postoperatively for at least 4 h [108]. Triggering agents include volatile inhalation agents such as halothane, enflurane, desflurane, isoflurane, and sevoflurane. Even trace amounts of these agents lingering in an anesthesia machine or breathing circuit may precipitate a MH crisis. Succinylcholine and chlorpromazine are other commonly used medications, which are known triggers of MH. However, many non-triggering medications may be safely used for local anesthesia, sedation-analgesia, postoperative pain control, and even, general anesthesia [109]. Nevertheless, anesthesia for patients suspected to have MH susceptibility should not be performed at an office-based setting. Standardized protocol to manage MH (available from the Malignant Hyperthermia Association of the United States, MHAUS) and supplies of dantrolene and cold intravenous fluids should be available for all patients.

Preferably, patients with MH susceptibility should be referred to an anesthesiologist for prior consultation. Intravenous dantrolene [110] and iced intravenous fluids are still the preferred treatment. MHAUS may be contacted at 800-98MHAUS and the MH hotline is 800-MH-HYPER.

6.5 Selections and Delivery of Anesthesia

Anesthesia may be divided into four broad categories, local anesthesia, and local anesthesia combined with sedation, regional anesthesia, and general anesthesia. The ultimate decision to select the type of anesthesia depends on the type and extent of the surgery planned, the patient's underlying health condition, and the psychological disposition of the patient. For example, a limited procedure in a calm, healthy patient could certainly be performed using strictly local anesthesia without sedation. As the scope of the surgery broadens, or the patient's anxiety level increases, the local anesthesia may be supplemented with oral or parenteral analgesic or anxiolytic medication. As the complexity of the surgery increases, general anesthesia may be the most appropriate choice.

6.5.1 Local Anesthesia

A variety of local anesthetics are available for infiltrative anesthesia. The selection of the local anesthetic depends on the duration of anesthesia required and the volume of anesthetic needed. The traditionally accepted, pharmacological profiles of common anesthetics used for infiltrative anesthesia for adults are summarized in Table 6.5 [111].

The maximum doses may vary widely depending on the type of tissue injected [112], the rate of administration [113], the age, underlying health, and body habitus of the patient [114], the degree of competitive protein binding [115], and possible cytochrome inhibition of concomitantly administered medications [116]. The maximum tolerable limits of local anesthetics have been redefined with the development of the tumescent anesthetic technique [117]. Lidocaine doses up to 35 mg/kg were found to be safe, if administered in conjunction with dilute epinephrine during liposuction [118]. With the tumescent technique, peak plasma

Table 6.5 Clinical pharmacology of common local anesthetics for infiltrative anesthesia

Agent	Without epinephrine					With epinephrine			
	Concentration (%)	Duration of action (min)	Maximum dose			Duration of action (min)	Maximum dose		
			mg/kg	Total mg	Total ml		mg/kg	Total mg	Total ml
Lidocaine	1.0	30–60	4	300	30	120	7	500	50
Mepivacaine	1.0	45–90	4	300	30	120	7	500	50
Etidocaine	0.5	120–180	4	300	60	180	5.5	400	80
Bupivacaine	0.25	120–240	2.5	185	75	180	3	225	90
Ropivacaine	0.2	120–360	2.7	200	80	120–360	2.7	200	80

Source: Adapted from Covino and Wildsmith [111]

levels occur 6–24 h after administration [118, 119]. More recently, doses up to 55 mg/kg have been found to be within the therapeutic safety margin [120]. However, recent guidelines by the American Academy of Cosmetic Surgery recommend a maximum dose of 45–50 mg/kg [14].

Certainly, significant toxicity has been associated with high doses of lidocaine as a result of tumescent anesthesia during liposuction [121]. The systemic toxicity of local anesthetic has been directly related to the serum concentration by many authors [113, 118–122]. Early signs of toxicity, usually occurring at serum levels of about 3–4 µg/ml for lidocaine, include circumoral numbness and lightheadedness, and tinnitus. As the serum concentration increases toward 8 µg/ml, tachycardia, tachypnea, confusion, disorientation, visual disturbance, muscular twitching, and cardiac depression may occur. At still higher serum levels above 8 µg/ml, unconsciousness and seizures may ensue. Complete cardiorespiratory arrest may occur between 10 and 20 µg/ml [113, 122]. However, the toxicity of lidocaine may not always correlate exactly with the plasma level of lidocaine presumably because of the variable extent of protein binding in each patient and the presence of active metabolites [113] and other factors already discussed including the age, ethnicity, health, and body habitus of the patient, and additional medications.

Ropivacaine, a long lasting local anesthetic has less cardiovascular toxicity than bupivacaine and may be a safer alternative to bupivacaine if a local anesthetic of longer duration is required [122, 123]. The cardiovascular toxicity of bupivacaine and etidocaine is much greater than lidocaine [122–124]. While bupivacaine toxicity has been associated with sustained ventricular tachycardia and sudden profound cardiovascular collapse [125, 126], the incidence of ventricular dysarrhythmias has not been as widely acknowledged with lidocaine or mepivacaine toxicity. In fact, ventricular tachycardia of fibrillation was not observed despite the use of supraconvulsant doses of intravenous doses of lidocaine, etidocaine, or mepivacaine in the animal model [123].

Indeed, during administration of infiltrative lidocaine anesthesia, rapid anesthetic injection into a highly vascular area or accidental intravascular injection leading to a sudden toxic level of anesthetic resulting in sudden onset of seizures or even cardiac arrest or cardiovascular collapse has been documented [127, 128]. One particularly disconcerting case presented by Christie [129] confirms the fatal consequence of a lidocaine injection of 200 mg in a healthy patient. Seizure and death occurred following a relatively low dose of lidocaine and a serum level of only 0.4 mg/100 ml or 4 µg/ml. A second patient suffered cardiac arrest with a blood level of 0.58 mg/100 ml or 5.8 µg/ml [129]. Although continued postmortem metabolism may artificially reduce serum lidocaine levels, the reported serum levels associated with mortality in these patients were well below the 8–20 µg/ml considered necessary to cause seizures, myocardial depression, and cardiorespiratory arrest. The 4 µg/ml level reported by Christie is uncomfortably close to the maximum serum levels reported by Ostad et al. [120] of 3.4 and 3.6 µg/ml following tumescent lidocaine doses of 51.3 and 76.7 mg/kg, respectively. Similar near toxic levels were reported in individual patients receiving about 35 mg/kg of lidocaine by Samdal et al. [130]. Pitman [131] reported that toxic manifestations occurred 8 h postoperatively after a total dose of 48.8 mg/kg which resulted from a 12-h plasma lidocaine level of 3.7 µg/kg. Ostad et al. [120] conclude that because of the poor correlation of lidocaine doses with the plasma lidocaine levels, an extrapolation of the maximum safe dose of lidocaine for liposuction cannot be determined. Given the devastating consequences of toxicity due to local anesthetics, physicians must exercise extreme caution when administering these medications.

Patients who report previous allergies to anesthetics may present a challenge to surgeons performing liposuction. Although local anesthetics of the aminoester class such as procaine are associated with allergic reactions, true allergic phenomena to local anesthetics of the aminoamide class, such as lidocaine, are extremely rare [132, 133]. Allergic reactions may occur to the preservative in the multidose vials. Tachycardia and generalized flushing may occur with rapid absorption of the epinephrine contained in some standard local anesthetic preparations. The development of vasovagal reactions after injections of any kind may cause hypotension, bradycardia, diaphoresis, pallor, nausea, and loss of consciousness. These adverse reactions may be misinterpreted by the patient and even the physician as allergic reactions [132]. A careful history from the patient describing the apparent reaction usually clarifies the cause. If there is still concern about the possibility of true allergy to local anesthetic, then the patient should be referred to an allergist for skin testing [133].

In the event of a seizure following a toxic dose of local anesthetic, proper airway management and maintaining oxygenation is critical. Seizure activity may be aborted with intravenous diazepam (10–20 mg), midazolam (5–10 mg), or thiopental (100–200 mg). Although the ventricular arrhythmias associated with bupivacaine toxicity are notoriously intractable [125, 126], treatment is still possible using large doses of atropine, epinephrine, and bretylium [134, 135]. Some studies indicate that lidocaine should not be used during the resuscitation of a patient from bupivacaine toxicity [136]. Pain associated with local anesthetic administration is due to pH of the solution and the may be reduced by the addition of 1 meq of sodium bicarbonate to 10 ml of anesthetic [137].

Topical anesthetics in a phospholipid base have become more popular as a technique for administering local anesthetics. Application of these topical agents may provide limited anesthesia over specific areas such as the face for minor procedures including limited laser resurfacing. EMLA (eutectic mixture of local anesthetics), a combination of lidocaine and prilocaine, was the first commercially available preparation. The topical anesthetic preparation must be applied under an occlusive dressing at least 60 min prior to the procedure to develop adequate local anesthesia [138]. Even after 60 min the anesthesia may not be complete and the patient may still experience significant discomfort. Many physicians prefer to use their own customized formula, which they obtain from a compounding pharmacy. However, these compounded formulas are not monitored by the FDA and compounding pharmacies may vary in the quality control standards. Some of the formulas may contain up to 40% local anesthetics in various combinations. This type of preparation could deliver up to 400 mg/g of ointment to the patient. The application of 30 g of a compounded formula containing a total of 20% local anesthetic over a wide area with subsequent occlusive dressing could expose the patient to 6,000 mg of local anesthetic. Studies have demonstrated that systemic absorption of local anesthetic after application of topical local anesthetic is limited to less than 5% [139, 140]. Even with limited systemic absorption, the development of toxic blood levels of local anesthetic, with the ensuing catastrophic results, would not be hard to envision if a large quantity of a concentrated compounded anesthetic ointment were applied under an occlusive dressing. There has been at least one case report of death after application of a compounded local anesthetic ointment while preparing for cosmetic surgery [141]. Physicians who prescribe compounded topical local anesthetics to patients prior to surgery should reevaluate the concentration of these medications as well as the total dose of medication that may be delivered to the patient. Frequently, the patient is given the topical anesthetic to be applied at home prior to arrival to the office or surgical center.

6.5.2 Sedative-Analgesic Medication (SAM)

Most minimally invasive procedures may be performed with a combination of local anesthesia and supplemental sedative-analgesic medication (SAM) administered orally (p.o.), intramuscularly (i.m.), or intravenously (i.v.). The goals of administering supplemental medications are to reduce anxiety (anxiolytics), the level of consciousness (sedation), unanticipated pain (analgesia), and, in some cases, to eliminate recall of the surgery (amnesia).

Sedation may be defined as the reduction of the level of consciousness usually resulting from pharmacological interventions. The level of sedation may be further divided into four broad categories, minimal sedation, moderate sedation, deep sedation (also referred to as conscious sedation), and general anesthesia. During minimal sedation patients may respond normally to verbal commands but have impaired cognitive function and coordination. Life-preserving protective reflexes (LPPRs), ventilatory, and cardiovascular functions are generally maintained during minimal sedation. During moderate sedation, while the level consciousness is depressed, the patient should respond in a purposeful manner to soft verbal commands. LPPRs, ventilation, and cardiovascular function are generally maintained in most patients. During deep sedation, the patient becomes difficult to arouse and may respond purposely only with loud verbal or painful tactile stimulation. During deep sedation the patient has a probability of loss of LPPRs and a depression of ventilatory function. Cardiovascular function is usually maintained. Finally, during general anesthesia, there is complete loss of consciousness and the patient is not arousable by any means. There is a high likelihood of loss of LPPRs and suppression of ventilatory and cardiac function under general anesthesia [142].

Life-preserving protective reflexes (LPPRs) may be defined as the involuntary physical and physiological responses that maintain the patient's life which, if interrupted, result in inevitable and catastrophic physiological consequences. The most obvious examples of LPPRs are the ability to maintain an open airway, swallowing, coughing, gagging, and spontaneous breathing. Some involuntary physical movements such as head turning or attempts to assume an erect posture may be considered LPPRs if these reflex actions occur in an attempt to improve airway patency such as expelling oropharyngeal contents. The myriad of homeostatic mechanisms to maintain blood pressure, heart function, and body temperature may even be considered LPPRs. When patient enters deep sedation, and the level of consciousness is depressed to the point that the patient is not able to respond purposefully to verbal commands or physical stimulation, there is a significant probability of loss of LPPRs. Ultimately, as total loss of consciousness occurs under general anesthesia and the patient no longer responds to verbal command or painful stimuli, the patient most likely looses the LPPRs [142].

In actual practice, the delineation between the levels of sedation becomes challenging at best. The loss of consciousness occurs as a continuum. With each incremental change in the level of consciousness, the likelihood of loss of LPPRs increases. The level of consciousness may vary from moment to moment, depending on the level of surgical stimulation. Since the definition of conscious sedation is vague, current ASA guidelines consider the term sedation-analgesia a more relevant term than conscious sedation [15]. The term sedative-analgesic medication (SAM) has been adopted by some facilities. Monitored anesthesia care (MAC) has been generally defined as the medical management of patients receiving local anesthesia during surgery with or without the use of supplemental medications. MAC usually refers to services provided by the anesthesiologist or the CRNA. The term "local standby" is no longer used because it mischaracterizes the purpose and activity of the anesthesiologist or CRNA.

Surgical procedures performed using a combination of local anesthetic and SAM usually have a shorter recovery time than similar procedures performed under regional or general anesthesia [143]. Using local anesthesia alone, without the benefit of supplemental medication is associated with a greater risk of cardiovascular and hemodynamic perturbations such as tachycardia, arrhythmias, and hypertension particularly in patients with preexisting cardiac disease or hypertension [144]. Patients usually prefer sedation while undergoing surgery with local anesthetics [145]. While the addition of sedatives and analgesics during surgery using local anesthesia seems to have some advantages, use of SAM during local anesthesia is certainly not free of risk. A study by the Federated Ambulatory Surgical Association concluded that local anesthesia, with supplemental medications, was associated with more than twice the number of complications than with local anesthesia alone. Furthermore, local anesthesia with SAM was associated with greater risks than general anesthesia [146]. Significant respiratory depression as determined by the development of hypoxemia, hypercarbia, and respiratory acidosis has been documented in patients after receiving even minimal doses of medications. This respiratory depression persists even in the recovery period [147, 148].

One explanation for the frequency of complications in patients receiving SAM is the wide variability of patients' responses to these medications. Up to 20-fold differences in the dose requirements for some medications such as diazepam, and up to fivefold variation for some narcotics such as fentanyl have been documented in some patients [149, 150]. Even small doses of fentanyl as low as 2 μg/kg, considered by many physicians as subclinical, produce respiratory depression for more than 1 h in some patients [151]. Combinations of even small doses of sedatives, such as midazolam, and narcotics, such as fentanyl, may act synergistically (effects greater than an additive effect) in producing adverse side effects such as respiratory depression and hemodynamic instability [152]. The clearance of many medications may vary depending on the amount and duration of administration, a phenomenon known as context-sensitive half-life. The net result is increased sensitivity and duration of action to medication for longer surgical cases [153]. Because of these variations and interactions, predicting any given patient's dose-response is a daunting task. Patients appearing awake and responsive may, in an instant, slip into unintended levels of deep sedation with greater potential of loss of LPPRs. Careful titration of these medications to the desired effect combined with vigilant monitoring are the critical elements in avoiding complications associated with the use of SAM. Klein acknowledges that most of the complications attributed to midazolam and narcotic combinations occurred as a result of inadequate monitoring [154]. Supplemental medication may be administered via multiple routes including oral, nasal, transmucosal, transcutaneous, intravenous, intramuscular, and rectal. While intermittent bolus has been the traditional method to administer medication, continuous infusion and patient controlled delivery result in comparable safety and patient satisfaction [155, 156].

Benzodiazepines such as diazepam, midazolam, and lorezepam remain popular for sedation and anxiolytics. Patients and physicians especially appreciate the potent amnestic effects of this class of medications, especially midazolam (using midazolam "means never having to say you're sorry") The disadvantages of diazepam include the higher incidence of pain on intravenous administration, the possibility of phlebitis [157], and the prolonged half-life of up to 20–50 h. Moreover, diazepam has active metabolites, which may prolong the effects of the medication even into the postoperative recovery time [158]. Midazolam, however, is more rapidly metabolized, allowing for a quicker and more complete recovery for outpatient surgery [158]. Because the sedative, anxiolytic and amnestic effects of midazolam are more profound than other benzodiazepines and the recovery is more rapid, patient acceptance is usually higher [159]. Since lorezepam is less affected by medications altering cytochrome P459 metabolisim [160], it has been recommended as the sedative of choice of liposuctions, which require a large dose of lidocaine tumescent anesthesia [121]. The disadvantage of lorezepam is the slower onset of action and the 11–22 h elimination half-life making titration cumbersome and postoperative recovery prolonged [158].

Generally, physicians who use SAM titrate a combination of medications from different classes to tailor the medications to the desired level of sedation and analgesia for each patient. Use of prepackaged or premixed combinations of medications defeats the purpose of the selective control of each medication. Typically, sedatives such as the benzodiazepines are combined with narcotic analgesics such as fentanyl, meperidine, or morphine during local anesthesia to decrease pain associated with local anesthetic injection or unanticipated breakthrough pain. Fentanyl has the advantage of rapid onset and duration of action of less than 60 min. However, because of synergistic action with sedative agents, even doses of 25–50 μg can result in respiratory depression [161]. Other medications with sedative and hypnotic effects such as a barbiturate, ketamine, or propofol are often added. Adjunctive analgesics such as ketorolac may be administered for additional analgesic activity. As long as the patient is carefully monitored, several medications may be titrated together to achieve the effects required for the patient characteristics and the complexity of the surgery. Fixed combinations of medications are not advised [15].

More potent narcotic analgesics with rapid onset of action and even shorter duration of action than fentanyl, including sufentanil, alfentanil, and remifentanil, may be administered using intermittent boluses or continuous infusion in combination with other sedative or hypnotic agents. However, extreme caution and scrupulous monitoring is required when these potent narcotics are used because of the risk of respiratory arrest [162, 163]. Use of these medications should be restricted to the anesthesiologist or the CRNA. A major disadvantage of narcotic medication is the perioperative nausea and vomiting [164].

Many surgeons feel comfortable administering SAM to patients. Others prefer to use the services of an anesthesiologist or CNRA. Prudence dictates that for prolonged or complicated surgeries or for patients with significant risk factors, the participation of the anesthesiologist or CRNA during MAC anesthesia is preferable. Regardless of who administers the anesthetic medications, the monitoring must have the same level of vigilance.

Propofol, a member of the alkylphenol family, has demonstrated its versatility as a supplemental sedative-hypnotic agent for local anesthesia and of regional anesthesia. Propofol may be used alone or in combination with a variety of other medications. Rapid metabolism and clearance result in faster and more complete recovery with less postoperative hangover than other sedative-hypnotic medications such as midazolam and methohexital [143, 165]. The documented antiemetic properties of propofol yield added benefits of this medication [166]. The disadvantages of propofol include pain on intravenous injection and the lack of amnestic effect [167]. However, the addition of 3 ml of 2% lidocaine to 20 ml of propofol virtually eliminates the pain on injection with no added risk. If an amnestic response is desired, a small dose of a benzodiazepine, such as midazolam (5 mg i.v.), given in combination with propofol, provides the adequate amnesia. Rapid administration of propofol may be associated with significant hypotension, decreased cardiac output [168], and respiratory depression [169]. Continuous infusion with propofol results in a more rapid recovery than similar infusions with midazolam [170]. Patient-controlled sedation with propofol has also been shown to be safe and effective [171].

Barbiturate sedative-hypnotic agents such as thiopental and methohexital, while older, still play a role in many clinical settings. In particular, methohexital, with controlled boluses (10–20 mg i.v.) or limited infusions remains a safe and effective sedative-hypnotic alternative with rapid recovery. However, with prolonged administration, recovery from methohexital may be delayed compared to propofol [172].

Ketamine, a phencyclidine derivative, is a unique agent because of its combined sedative and analgesic effects and the absence of cardiovascular depression in healthy patients [173]. Because the CNS effects of ketamine result in a state similar to catatonia, the resulting anesthesia is often described as dissociative anesthesia. Although gag and cough reflexes are more predictably maintained with ketamine, emesis and pulmonary aspiration of gastric contents is still possible [174]. Unfortunately, a significant number of patients suffer distressing postoperative psychomimetic reactions [175]. While concomitant administration of benzodiazepines attenuates these reactions, the postoperative psychological sequelae limit the usefulness of ketamine for most elective outpatient surgeries.

Droperidol, a butyrophenone and a derivative of haloperidol, acts as a sedative, hypnotic, and antiemetic medication. Rather than causing global CNS depression like barbiturates, droperidol causes more specific CNS changes similar to phenothiazines. For this reason, the cataleptic state caused by droperidol is referred to as neuroleptic anesthesia [176]. Droperidol has been used effectively in combination with various narcotic medications. While droperidol has minimal effect on respiratory function if used as a single agent, when combined with narcotic medication, a predictable dose-dependent respiratory depression may be anticipated [177]. Psychomimetic reactions such as dysphoria or hallucinations are frequent, unpleasant side effects of droperidol. Benzodiazepines or narcotics reduce the incidence of these unpleasant side effects [178, 179]. Extrapyramidal reactions such as dyskinesias, torticollis, or oculogyric spasms may also occur, even with small doses of droperidol. Diphenhydramine usually reverses these complications [179]. Hypotension may occur as a consequence of droperidol's alpha-adrenergic receptor blocking characteristics. One rare complication of droperidol is the neurolept malignant syndrome (NMS) [180], a condition very similar to malignant hyperthermia, characterized by extreme temperature elevations and rhabdomyolysis. The treatment of NMS and malignant hyperthermia is essentially the same. While droperidol has been used for years without appreciable myocardial depression [178], a surprising announcement from the Federal Drug Administration warned of sudden cardiac death resulting after the administration of standard, clinically useful doses [181]. Unfortunately, this potential complication makes the routine use of this once very useful medication difficult to justify given the presence of other alternative medications.

Butorphanol, buprenorphine, and nalbuphine are three synthetically derived opiates which share the properties of being mixed agonist-antagonists at the opiate receptors. These medications are sometimes preferred as supplemental analgesics during local, regional, or general anesthesia, because they partially reverse the analgesic and respiratory depressant effects of other narcotics. While these medications result in respiratory depression at lower doses, a ceiling effect occurs at higher dose, thereby limiting the respiratory depression. Still, respiratory arrest is possible, especially if these medications are combined with other medications with respiratory depressant properties [182]. While the duration of action of Butarphanol is 2–3 h, nalbuphine has a duration of action of about 3–6 h and buprenorphan up to 10 h, making these medications less suitable for surgeries of shorter duration. Table 6.6 summarizes the recommended doses for SAM.

6.5.3 Regional Anesthesia

Many limited cosmetic procedures may be performed using regional anesthesia, which is blockade of one or more sensory nerves with local anesthesia. Even though patients receive regional anesthesia, additional sedative analgesic medications can be administered.

6.5.4 General Anesthesia

Although significant advances have been made in the administration of local anesthetics, sedative-analgesic

Table 6.6 Common medications and dosages used for sedative analgesia[a]

Medication	Bolus dose	Average adult dose	Continuous infusion rate (μg/kg/min)
Narcotic analgesics			
Alfentanil	5–7 μg/kg	30–50 μg	0.2–0.5
Fentanyl	0.3–0.7 μg/kg	25–50 μg	0.01
Meperidine	0.2 mg/kg	10–20 mg i.v., 50–100 mg i.m.	NA
Morphine	0.02 mg/kg	1–2 mg i.v., 5–10 mg i.m.	NA
Remifentanil	0.5–1.0 μg/kg	10–25 μg	0.025–0.05
Sufentanil	0.1–0.2 μg/kg	10 μg	0.001–0.002
Opiate agonist-antagonist analgesics			
Buprenorphene	4–6 μg/kg	0.3 mg	NA
Butorphanol	2–7 μg/kg	0.1–0.2 mg	NA
Nalbupnine	0.03–0.1 mg/kg	10 mg	NA
Sedative-hypnotics			
Diazepam	0.05–0.1 mg/kg	5–7.5 mg	NA
Methohexital	0.2–0.5 mg/kg	10–20 mg	10–50
Midazolam	30–75 μg/kg	2.5–5.0	0.25–0.5
Propofol	0.2–0.5 mg/kg	10–20 mg	10–50
Thiopental	0.5–1.0 mg/kg	25–50 mg	50–100
Dissociative anesthetics			
Ketamine	0.2–0.5 mg/kg	10–20 mg	10

[a]These doses may vary depending on age, gender, underlying health status, and other concomitantly administered medications
Source: Adapted from references [183–185]

medications, and regional anesthesia, the use of general anesthesia may still be the anesthesia technique of choice for many patients. General anesthesia is especially appropriate when working with patients suffering extreme anxiety, high tolerance to narcotic or sedative medications, or if the surgery is particularly complex. The goals of a general anesthetic are a smooth induction, a prompt recovery, and minimal side effects, such as nausea, vomiting, or sore throat. The inhalation anesthetic agents, halothane, isoflurane, and enflurane, have been widely popular because of the safety, reliability, and convenience of use. The newer inhalation agents, sevoflurane and desflurane, share similar properties with the added benefit of prompt emergence [186, 187]. Nitrous oxide, a longtime favorite anesthetic inhalation agent, may be associated with postoperative nausea and vomiting [188]. Patients receiving nitrous oxide also have a greater risk of perioperative hypoxemia.

The development of potent, short-acting sedative, opiates analgesics, and muscle relaxant medications has resulted in newer medication regimen that permits the use of intravenous agents exclusively. The same medications that have been discussed for SAM can also be used during general anesthesia as sole agents or in combination with the inhalation agents [189]. The anesthesiologist or CRNA should preferentially be responsible for the administration and monitoring of a general anesthesia.

Airway control is a key element in the management of the patient under general anesthesia. Maintaining a patent airway, ensuring adequate ventilation, and prevention of aspiration of gastric contents are the goals of successful airway management. For shorter cases, the airway may be supported by an oropharyngeal airway and gas mixtures delivered by an occlusive mask. For longer or more complex cases, or if additional facial surgery is planned requiring surgical field avoidance, then the airway may be secured using laryngeal mask anesthesia (LMA) or endotracheal intubation [190].

Orthognathic surgeries that require unrestricted access to the oral and lower facial regions often require nasotracheal intubation. Obviously, this procedure requires an anesthesiologist with extensive training and experience to avoid serious complications to the upper airway. Techniques that facilitate nasotracheal intubation are listed in Table 6.7. Preflexing the tip of the endotracheal tube immediately prior to intubation that facilitates the passage of the tube around the nasopharyngeal junction is one helpful technique. When these precautions are followed, complications related to nasotracheal intubation, such as perioperative nasopharyngeal bleeding, or nasopharyngeal trauma are extremely rare (unpublished data from The Center for Oral and Facial Reconstruction and Reconstruction and Ambulatory Services, Irvine, CA).

6.5.5 Preoperative Preparation

Generally, medications which may have been required to stabilize the patient's medical conditions, should be continued up to the time of surgery. Notable exceptions include anticoagulant medications, monoamine oxidase inhibitors (MAO) [191, 192], and possibly the angiotensin converting enzyme (ACE) inhibitor medications [80, 193]. It is generally accepted that MAO inhibitors, carboxazial (Marplan), deprenyl (Eldepryl), paragyline (Eutonyl), phenelzine (Nardil), tranylcypromine (Parnate), be discontinued 2–3 weeks prior to surgery, especially for elective cases, because of the interactions with narcotic medication, specifically hyperpyrexia, and certain vasopressor agents, specifically, ephedrine [191, 192]. Patients taking ACE inhibitors (captopril, enalapril, and lisinopril) may have a greater risk for hypotension during general anesthesia [80]. As previously discussed, diabetics may require a reduction in dosage of their medication. However, if the risks of discontinuing any of these medications outweigh the benefits of the proposed elective surgery, the patient and physician may decide to postpone, modify, or cancel the proposed surgery.

Previous requirements of complete preoperative fasting for 10–16 h are considered unnecessary by many anesthesiologists [194, 195]. More recent investigations have demonstrated that gastric volume may be less 2 h after oral intake of 8 oz of clear liquid than after more prolonged fasting [196]. Furthermore, prolonged fasting may increase the risk of hypoglycemia [197]. Many patients appreciate an 8 oz feeding of their favorite caffeinated elixir 2 h prior to surgery. Preoperative sedative medications may also be taken with a small amount of water or juice. Abstinence from solid food ingestion for 10–12 h prior to surgery is still recommended. Liquids taken prior to surgery must be clear [198], for example, coffee without cream or juice without pulp.

Healthy outpatients are no longer considered to be at higher risk for gastric acid aspiration and therefore, routine use of antacids, histamine type-2 (H2) antagonists, or gastrokinetic medications is not indicated. However, patients with marked obesity, hiatal hernia, or diabetes mellitus have higher risks for aspiration. These patients may benefit from selected prophylactic treatment [199]. Sodium citrate, an orally administered, non-particulate antacid, rapidly increases gastric pH. However, its unpleasant taste and short duration of action limits its usefulness in elective surgery [200]. Gastric volume and pH may be effectively reduced by H2 receptor antagonists. Cimetidine (300 mg p.o., 1–2 h prior to surgery) reduces gastric volume and pH. However, cimetidine is also a potent cytochrome oxidase inhibitor and may increase the risk of reactions to lidocaine during tumescent anesthesia [201]. Ranitidine (150–300 mg 90–120 min prior to surgery) [202], or famotidine (20 mg p.o. 60 min prior to surgery) are

Table 6.7 Techniques to facilitate nasotracheal intubation

Pretreating of the nasopharynx with vasoconstrictor (oxymetazoline 0.05%).
Nasotracheal tube one size smaller than the size normally used for orotracheal intubation.
Prewarming the endotracheal tube to 45°C
Progressively dilating the nasopharynx with lubricated rubber nasopharyngeal tubes after induction
Copious lubrication of the endotracheal tube with a dental anesthetic lubricant (with benzocaine 10%)
Preflexing the tip of the endotracheal tube just prior to intubation to negotiate the nasopharynx
Using curved intubating forceps to direct the endotracheal tube through the larynx

Presented at the Winter Medical Conference of Chapman Medical Center, 2005, Salt Lake City, UT

equally effective but have a better safety profile than cimetidine [203].

Omeprazole, which decreases gastric acid secretion by inhibiting the proton pump mechanism of the gastric mucosa, may prove to be a safe and effective alternative to the H2 receptor antagonists [203]. Metaclopramide (10–20 mg p.o. or i.v.), a gastrokinetic agent, which increases gastric motility and lower esophageal sphincter tone, may be effective in patients with reduced gastric motility, such as diabetics or patients receiving opiates. However, extrapyramidal side effects limit the routine use of the medication [164, 204].

Postoperative nausea and vomiting (PONV) remains one of the more vexing complications of anesthesia and surgery [205]. In fact, patients dread PONV more than any other complication, even post operative pain [206]. PONV is the most common postoperative complication [207, 208], and the common cause of postoperative patient dissatisfaction [209]. Strategies to reduce PONV should be incorporated into the preoperative planning stages especially in patients with previous histories of PONV. Use of prophylactic antiemetic medication has been shown to reduce the incidence of PONV [210]. Even though many patients do not suffer PONV in the recovery period after ambulatory anesthesia, greater than 35% of patients develop PONV after discharge [211].

Droperidol, 0.625–1.25 mg i.v., is an extremely cost-effective antiemetic [212]. However, troublesome side effects such as sedation, dysphoria, extrapyramidal reactions [179], and more recently, cardiac arrest have been described [181]. These complications may preclude the widespread use of droperidol altogether. The serotonin antagonists, ondansetron (4–8 mg i.v.), dolasetron (12.5 mg i.v.), and granisetron (1 mg i.v.) are among the most effective antiemetic medications available without sedative, dysphoric, or extrapyramidal sequelae [213–215]. The antiemetic effects of ondansetron may reduce PONV for up to 24 h postoperatively [216]. The Effects of ondansetron may be augmented by the addition of dexamethasone (4–8 mg) [217], or droperidol (1.25 mg i.v.) [218]. Despite the efficacy of the newer serotonin antagonists, cost remains a prohibitive factor in the routine prophylactic use of these medications, especially in the office setting.

Promethazine (12.5–25 mg p.o., p.r., or i.m.), and chlorpromazine (5–10 mg p.o., or i.m. and 25 mg p.r.), are two older phenothiazines, which are still used by many physicians as prophylaxis, especially in combination with narcotic analgesics. Once again, sedation and extrapyramidal effects may complicate the routine prophylactic use of these medications [164].

Preoperative atropine (0.4 mg i.m.), glycopyrrolate (0.2 mg i.m.), and scopolamine (0.2 mg i.m.), anticholinergic agents, once considered standard preoperative medication because of their vagolytic and antisialogic effects, are no longer popular because of side effects such as dry mouth, dizziness, tachycardia, and disorientation [219]. Transdermal scopolamine, applied 90 min prior to surgery, effectively reduces PONV. However, the incidence of dry mouth and drowsiness is high [220], and toxic psychosis is a rare complication [221]. Antihistamines, such as diphenhydramine (25–50 mg p.o., i.m., or i.v.), and hydroxyzine (50 mg p.o. or i.m.), may also be used to treat and prevent PONV with few side effects except for possible postoperative sedation [222].

The selection of anesthetic agents may also play a major role in PONV. The direct antiemetic actions of propofol have been clearly demonstrated [223]. Anesthetic regimen utilizing propofol, alone or in combination with other medications, are associated with significantly less PONV [224]. Although still controversial, nitrous oxide is considered by many authors, a prime suspect among possible causes of PONV [188, 225, 226]. Opiates are also considered culprits in the development of PONV and the delay of discharge after outpatient surgery [164, 227–229]. Adequate fluid hydration has been shown to reduce PONV [230].

One goal of preoperative preparation is to reduce patients' anxiety. Many simple, non-pharmacological techniques may be extremely effective in reassuring both patients and families, starting with a relaxed, friendly atmosphere and a professional, caring, and attentive office staff. With proper preoperative preparation, pharmacological interventions may not even be necessary. However, a variety of oral and parenteral anxiolytic-sedative medications are frequently called upon to provide a smooth transition to the operative room. Diazepam (5–10 mg p.o.), given 1–2 h preoperatively, is a very effective medication, which usually does not prolong recovery time [231]. Parenteral diazepam (5–10 mg i.v. or i.m.), may also be given immediately preoperatively. However, because of a long elimination half-life of 24–48 h, and active metabolites with elimination half-life of 50–120 h, caution must be exercised when using diazepam, especially in shorter cases, so that recovery is not delayed [232]. Pain and phlebitis with i.v. or i.m. administration reduces the popularity of diazepam [157].

Lorezepam (1–2 mg p.o. or s.l., 1–2 h preoperatively), is also an effective choice for sedation or anxiolytics. However, the prolonged duration of action may prolong recovery time after shorter cases [233]. Midazolam (5–7.5 mg i.m., 30 min preoperatively, or 2 mg i.v. minutes prior to surgery) is a more potent anxiolytic-sedative medication with more rapid onset and shorter elimination half-life, compared to diazepam [234]. Unfortunately, oral midazolam has unpredictable results and is not considered a useful alternative for preoperative medication [235]. Oral narcotics, such as oxycodone (5–10 mg p.o.), may help relieve the patient's intraoperative breakthrough pain during cases involving more limited liposuction with minimal potential perioperative sequelae. Parenteral opioids, such as morphine (5–10 mg i.m., or 1–2 mg i.v.), demerol (50–100 mg i.m., or 10–20 mg i.v.), fentanyl (10–20 μg i.v.), or sufentanil (1–2 ug i.v.), may produce sedation and euphoria and may decrease the requirements for other sedative medication. The level of anxiolytics and sedation is still greater with the benzodiazepines than with the opioids. Premedication with narcotics has been shown to have minimal effects on postoperative recovery time. However, opioid premedication may increase PONV [236, 237].

Antihistamine medications, such as hydroxyzine (50–100 mg i.m, or 50–100 mg p.o.), dimenhydrinate (50 mg p.o., i.m., or 25 mg i.v.), are still used safely in combination with other premedications, especially the opioids, to add sedation and to reduce nausea and pruritus. However, the anxiolytic and amnestic effects are not as potent as the benzodiazepines [238]. Barbiturates, such as secobarbital and pentobarbital, once a standard premedication, have largely been replaced by the benzodiazepines.

Postoperative pulmonary embolism (PE) is an unpredictable and devastating complication with an estimated incidence of 0.1–5%, depending on the type of surgical cases [239], and a mortality rate of about 15% [240]. Risk factors for thromboembolism include prior history or family history of DVT or PE, obesity, smoking, hypertension, use of oral contraceptives and hormone replacement therapy, and patients over 60 year of age [240]. Estimates for the incidence of postoperative DVT vary between 0.8% for outpatients undergoing herniorrhaphies [241], to up to 80% for patients undergoing total hip replacement [239]. Estimates of fatal PE also vary from 0.1% for patients undergoing general surgeries to up to 1–5% of patients undergoing major joint replacement [239]. The incidence of pulmonary embolism may be more common than reported. One study revealed that unsuspected PE may actually occur in up to 40% of patients with who develop DVT [242].

Most minimally invasive cosmetic surgeries, especially of the head and neck, under local anesthesia, with or without sedation, are considered low risk for DVT or PE. Prevention of DVT and PE should be considered an essential component of the perioperative management, especially for cases which may last more than 2 h, with a general anesthetic used or the patient has increased risk factors for DVT or PE. Although unfractionated heparin reduces the rate of fatal PE [243], many surgeons are reluctant to use this prophylaxis because of concerns of perioperative hemorrhage. The low molecular weight heparins, enoxaparin, dalteparin, ardeparin, and danaparoid, a heparinoid, are available for prophylactic indications. Graduated compression stockings and intermittent pneumatic lower extremity compression devices applied throughout the perioperative period until the patient has become ambulatory are considered very effective and safe alternatives in the prevention of postoperative DVT and PE [244, 245]. Even with prophylactic therapy, PE may still occur up to 30 days after surgery [246]. Physicians should be suspicious of PE if patients present postoperatively with dyspnea, chest pain, cough, hemoptysis, pleuritic pain, dizziness, syncope, tachycardia, cyanosis, shortness of breath, or wheezing [240].

6.5.6 Perioperative Monitoring

The adoption of standardized perioperative monitoring protocol has resulted in a quantum leap in perioperative patient safety. The standards for basic perioperative monitoring were approved by the ASA in 1986 and amended in 1995 [7]. These monitoring standards are now considered applicable to all types of anesthetics, including local with or without sedation, regional, or general anesthesia, regardless of the duration or complexity of the surgical procedure and regardless of whether the surgeon or anesthesiologist is responsible for the anesthesia. Vigilant and continuous monitoring and compulsive documentation facilitates early recognition of deleterious physiological events and trends, which, if not recognized promptly, could lead to irreversible pathological spirals, ultimately endangering a patient's life.

During the course of any anesthetic, the patient's oxygenation, ventilation, circulation, and temperature should be continuously evaluated. The concentration of the inspired oxygen must be measured by an oxygen analyzer. Assessment of the perioperative oxygenation of the patient using pulse oximetry, now considered mandatory in every case, has been a significant advancement in monitoring. This monitor is so critical to the safety of the patient, that it has earned the nick-name "the monitor of life." Evaluation of ventilation includes observation of skin color, chest wall motion, and frequent auscultation of breath sounds. During general anesthesia with or without mechanical ventilation, a disconnect alarm on the anesthesia circuit is crucial. Capnography, a measurement of respiratory end-tidal CO_2, is required, especially when the patient is under heavy sedation or general anesthesia. Capnography provides the first alert in the event of airway obstruction, hypoventilation, or accidental anesthesia circuit disconnect, even before the oxygen saturation has begun to fall. End-expiratory or inspiratory volatile gas monitoring is also extremely useful. All patients must have continuous monitoring of the electrocardiogram (ECG) and intermittent determination of blood pressure (BP), and heart rate (HR) at a minimum of 5-min intervals. Superficial or core body temperature should be monitored. Of course, all electronic monitors must have preset alarms limits to alert physicians prior to the development of critical changes.

While the availability of electronic monitoring equipment has improved perioperative safety, there is no substitute for visual monitoring by a qualified, experienced practitioner, usually a CRNA or an anesthesiologist. During surgeries using local with SAM, if a surgeon elects not to use a CRNA or an anesthesiologist, a separate, designated, certified individual must perform these monitoring functions. Visual observation of the patient's position is also important in order to avoid untoward outcomes such as peripheral nerve or ocular injuries.

Documentation of perioperative events, interventions, and observations must be contemporaneously performed and should include BP and HR every 5 min and oximetry, capnography, ECG pattern, and temperature at 15 min intervals. Intravenous fluids, medication dosages in mgs, patient position, and other intraoperative events must also be recorded. Documentation may alert the physician to unrecognized physiological trends that may require treatment. Preparation for subsequent anesthetics may require information contained in the patient's prior records, especially if the patient suffered an unsatisfactory outcome due to the anesthetic regimen that was used. Treatment of subsequent complications by other physicians may require information contained in the records, such as the types of medications used, blood loss, or fluid totals. Finally, compulsive documentation may help exonerate a physician in many medical-legal situations.

When local anesthesia with SAM is used, monitoring must include an assessment of the patient's level of consciousness as previously described. For patients under general anesthesia, the level of consciousness may be determined using the bispectral index (BIS), a measurement derived from computerized analysis of the electroencephalogram. When used with patients receiving general anesthesia, BIS improves control of the level of consciousness, rate of emergence and recovery, and cost-control of medication usage. Moreover, BIS monitoring may reduce the risk of intraoperative recall [247].

6.5.7 Fluid Replacement

Management of perioperative fluids probably generates more controversy than any other anesthesia-related topic. For minimally invasive treatments in healthy patients, fluid replacement is not a critical part of the procedure. In this patient population, the intravenous access serves merely as a conduit for the administration of medications. Generally, the typical, healthy, 60 kg patient requires about 100 ml of water/h to replace metabolic, sensible, and insensible water losses. After a 12-h period of fasting, a 60 kg patient may be expected to have a 1 l volume deficit on the morning of surgery. This deficit should be replaced over the first few hours of surgery. The patient's usual maintenance fluid needs may be met with a crystalloid solution such as lactated Ringer's solution.

Replacement fluids may be divided into crystalloid solutions, such as normal saline or balance salt solution, colloids, such as fresh frozen plasma, 5% albumin, plasma protein fraction, or hetastarch, and blood products containing red blood cells, such as packed red blood cells. Generally, balanced salt solutions may be used as standard fluid maintenance and to replace small amounts of blood loss. For every milliliter of blood loss, 3 ml of fluid replacement is usually required [248]. However, as larger volumes of blood are lost, attempts to replace these losses with crystalloid reduces the serum oncotic pressure, one of the main forces supporting intravascular volume. Subsequently, crystalloid rapidly moves into the extracellular space. Intravascular volume cannot be adequately sustained with further crystalloid infusion [249]. At this point, many authors suggest that a colloid solution may be more effective in maintaining intravascular volume and hemodynamic stability [250, 251]. Given the ongoing crystalloid-colloid controversy in the literature, the most practical approach to fluid management is a compromise. Crystalloid replacement should be used for estimated blood losses (EBL) less than 500 ml, while colloids, such as hetastarch may be used for EBLs greater than 500 ml. One milliliter of colloid should be used to replace 1 ml of EBL [248]. However, not all authors agree on the benefits of colloid resuscitation. Moss and Gould [252] concluded that isotonic crystalloid replacement, even for large EBLs, restores plasma volume as well as colloid replacement.

Transfusion of red blood cells is rarely a consideration during minimally invasive cosmetic surgeries. Healthy, normovolemic patients, with hemodynamic and physiologic stability, should tolerate hemoglobin levels down to 7.5 g/dl [253]. The decision to transfuse must be made after careful consideration of the benefits and risks of transfusion and not rely on one transfusion trigger. Transfusion is generally indicated when hemoglobin concentrations fall below 6 g/dl [254]. The management of fluids during more invasive cases such as large volume liposuction or abdominoplasty has been described in detail in other references [255].

6.5.8 Recovery and Discharge

The same intensive monitoring and treatment which occurs in the operating room must be continued in the recovery room under the care of a designated, licensed, and experienced person for as long as is necessary to ensure the stability and safety of the patient, regardless of whether the facility is a hospital, an outpatient surgical center, or a physician's office. During the initial stages of recovery, the patient should not be left alone while hospital or office personnel attend to other duties. Vigilant monitoring including visual observation, continuous oximetry, continuous ECG, and intermittent BP and temperature determinations must be continued. Because the patient is still vulnerable to airway obstruction and respiratory arrest in the recovery period, continuous visual observation is still the best method of monitoring for this complication. Supplemental oxygenation should be continued during the initial stages of recovery and continued until the patient is able to maintain an oxygen saturation above 90% on room air.

The most common postoperative complication is nausea and vomiting. The antiemetic medications previously discussed with the same consideration of potential risks may be used in the postoperative period. Ondansetron (4–8 mg i.v. or s.l.) and other serotonin antagonists are probably the safest and most effective antiemetics [213–217]. However, the cost of this medication is often prohibitive, especially in an office setting [218]. Postoperative surgical pain may be managed with judiciously titrated i.v. narcotic medication such as demerol (10–20 mg i.v. every 5–10 min), morphine (1–2 mg i.v. every 5–10 min), or butorphanol (0.1–0.2 mg i.v. every 10 min).

The number of complications that occur after discharge may be more than twice the complications occurring intraoperatively and during recovery combined [256]. Accredited ambulatory surgical center generally have established discharge criteria. While these criteria may vary, the common goal is to ensure the patient's level of consciousness and physiological stability. Table 6.8 is one example of discharge criteria which may be used.

Use of medication intended to reverse the effects of anesthesia should be used only in the event of suspected overdose of medications. Naloxone (0.1–0.2 mg i.v.), a pure opiate receptor antagonist, with a therapeutic half-life of less than 2 h, may be used to reverse the respiratory depressant effects of narcotic medications, such as morphine, demerol, fentanyl, and butorphanol. Because potential adverse effects of rapid opiate reversal of narcotics include severe pain, seizures, pulmonary edema, hypertension, congestive heart failure, and cardiac arrest [258], naloxone must

Table 6.8 Ambulatory discharge criteria

1	All life-preserving protective reflexes, that is, airway, cough, and gag must be returned to normal
2	The vital signs must be stable without orthostatic changes
3	There must be no evidence of hypoxemia 20 min after the discontinuation of supplemental oxygen
4	Patients must be oriented to person, place, time, and situation (times 4)
5	Nausea and vomiting must be controlled and patients should tolerate p.o. fluids
6	There must be no evidence of postoperative hemorrhage or expanding ecchymosis
7	Incisional pain should be reasonably controlled
8	The patient should be able to sit up without support and walk with assistance

Source: Modified from Mecca [257]

be administered by careful titration. Naloxone has no effect on the actions of medications, such as the benzodiazepines, the barbiturates, propofol, or ketamine.

Flumazenil (0.1–0.2 mg i.v.), a specific competitive antagonist of the benzodiazepines, such as diazepam, midazolam, lorezepam, may be used to reverse excessive or prolonged sedation and respiratory depression resulting from these medications [259]. The effective half-life of flumazenil is 1 h or less [260].

The effective half-lives of many narcotics exceed the half-life of naloxone. The benzodiazepines have effective half-lives greater than 2 h and, in the case of diazepam, up to 50 h. Many active metabolites unpredictably extend the putative effects of the narcotics and benzodiazepines. A major risk associated with the use of naloxone and flumazenil is the recurrence of the effects of the narcotic or benzodiazepine after 1–2 h. If the patient has already been discharged home after these effects recur, the patient may be at risk for oversedation or respiratory arrest [258, 261]. Therefore, routine use of reversal agents, without specific indication, prior to discharge is ill advised and should not be a routine practice in postoperative management. Patients should be monitored for at least 2 h prior to discharge if these reversal agents are administered [15].

Physostigmine (1.25 mg i.v.), a centrally acting anticholinesterase inhibitor, functions as a nonspecific reversal agent which may be used to counteract the agitation, sedation, and psychomotor effects caused by a variety of sedative, analgesic, and inhalation anesthetic agents [262, 263]. Neuromuscular blocking drugs, if required during general anesthesia, are usually reversed by the anesthesiologist or CRNA prior to emergence in the operating room with anticholinesterase inhibitors such as neostigmine or edrophonium. Occasionally, a second dose may be required when the patient is in the recovery room.

In the event of patients failing to regain consciousness during recovery, reversal agents should be administered. If no response occurs, the patient should be evaluated for other possible causes of unconsciousness, including hypoglycemia, hyperglycemia, cerebral vascular accidents, or cerebral hypoxia. If hemodynamic instability occurs in the recovery period, causes such as occult hemorrhage, hypovolemia, pulmonary edema, congestive heart failure, or myocardial infarction must be considered. Access to laboratory analysis to assist with the evaluation of the patient is crucial. Unfortunately, stat laboratory analysis is usually not available if the surgery is performed in an office-based setting.

The above text is meant to serve as an overview of the extremely complex subject of anesthesia. It is the intent of this chapter to serve as an introduction to the physician who participates in the perioperative management of patients and should not be considered a comprehensive presentation. The physician is encouraged to seek additional information on this broad topic through the other suggested readings. At least one authoritative text on anesthesia should be considered a mandatory addition to the physician's resources.

References

1. Courtiss EH, Goldwyn RM, Joffe JM, Hannenberg AH. Anesthetic practices in ambulatory aesthetic surgery. Plast Reconstr Surg. 1994;93(4):792–801.
2. Bechtoldt AA. Committee on anesthesia study. Anesthetic-related death: 1969–1976. N C Med J. 1981;42(4):253–9.
3. White PF, Smith I. Ambulatory anesthesia: past present and future. Int Anesthesiol Clin. 1994;32(3):1–16.
4. Morello DC, Colon GA, Fredricks S, Iverson RE, Singer R. Patient safety in accredited office surgical facilities. Plast Reconstr Surg. 1997;99(6):1496–500.
5. West Group, West's Annotated California Codes, Business and Professions Code. 3A Article 11.5, Section 2216
6. West Group, West's Annotated Codes, Health and Safety Code. 38B, Chapter 1.3, Section 1248.
7. American Society of Anesthesiologists (ASA). Standards for basic anesthetic monitoring. Approved by the House of Delegates on 21 Oct 1986 and last amended on 13 Oct 1993. Park Ridge: Directory of Members, American Society of Anesthesiologists (ASA); 1997. p. 394.

8. Guidelines for ambulatory surgical facilities last amended 1988. Park Ridge: Directory of Members, American Society of Anesthesiologists; 1995. pp. 386–7.
9. American Academy of Cosmetic Surgery. Guidelines for liposuction; 1995. pp. 2–6.
10. West Group, West's Annotated California Codes, Health and Safety Code. 38B, Chapter 1.3, Section 1248.15.
11. Press I. The last word. Hospital and Health Networks; 1994. p. 60.
12. Anderson & Associates. Best practices. Putting insight into practice. Dallas: Anderson & Associates; 1992.
13. Graham III DH, Duplechain G. Anesthesia in facial plastic surgery. In: Willett JM, editor. Facial plastic surgery. Stamford: Appleton & Lange; 1997. p. 5–26.
14. The American Academy of Cosmetic Surgery. 2000 guidelines for liposuction surgery. Am J Cosmet Surg. 2000;25: 31–7.
15. Practice guidelines for sedation and analgesia by non-anesthesiologists. A report by the American Society of Anesthesiologists Task Force on Sedation and Analgesia by Non-Anesthesiologists. Anesthesiology. 1996;84(2):459–71.
16. Mannino MJ. Anesthesia for male aesthetic surgery. Clin Plast Surg. 1991;18(4):863–75.
17. Jamison RN, Parris WC, Maxson WS. Psychological factors influencing recovery from outpatient surgery. Behav Res Ther. 1987;25(1):31–7.
18. Hampton JR, Harrison MJG, Mitchell JR, Pritchard JS, Seymour C. Relative contributions of history taking, physical examination, and laboratory investigation to diagnosis and management of medical outpatients. Br Med J. 1975;2(5969):486–9.
19. Delahunt B, Turnbull PRG. How cost-effective are routine preoperative investigations? N Z Med J. 1980;92(673): 431–2.
20. Apfelbaum JL. Preoperative evaluation, laboratory screening, and selection of adult surgical outpatients in the 1990s. Anesthesiol Rev. 1990;17:4–12.
21. Gibby GL, Gravenstein JS, Layone AJ, Jackson KI. How often does the preoperative interview change anesthetic management? (Abstract). Anesthesiology. 1992;77:A1134.
22. Sandler G. Costs of unnecessary tests. Br Med J. 1979; 2(6181):21–4.
23. Rabkin SW, Horne JM. Preoperative electrocardiography effect of new abnormalities on clinical decisions. Can Med Assoc J. 1983;128(2):146–7.
24. Roizen MF, Foss JF, Fischer SP. Preoperative evaluation. In: Miller RD, editor. Anesthesia. 5th ed. Philadelphia: Churchill Livingstone; 2000. p. 854–5.
25. Roizen MF, Fischer SP. Preoperative evaluation: adults and children. In: White PF, editor. Ambulatory anesthesia & surgery. Philadelphia: W.B. Saunders; 1997. p. 155–72.
26. Korvin CC, Pearce RH, Stanley J. Admissions screening: clinical benefits. Ann Intern Med. 1975;83(2):197–203.
27. Tape TG, Mushlin AI. The utility of routine chest radiographs. Ann Intern Med. 1986;104(5):663–70.
28. Turnbull JM, Buck C. The value of preoperative screening investigations in otherwise healthy individuals. Arch Intern Med. 1987;147(6):1101–5.
29. Kaplan EB, Sheiner LB, Boeckman AJ, Roizen MF, Beal SL, Cohen SN, et al. The usefulness of preoperative laboratory testing. JAMA. 1985;253(24):3576–81.
30. Bates DW, Boyle DL, Rittenberg E, Kuperman GJ, Ma'Luf N, Menkin V, et al. What proportion of common diagnostic test appear redundant? Am J Med. 1998;104(4):361–8.
31. Fowkes FGR, Lunn JN, Farrow SC, Robertson IB, Samuel P. Epidemiology in anaesthesia. III. Mortality risk in patients with coexisting disease. Br J Anaesth. 1982;54(8):819–25.
32. American Society of Anesthesiologists. New classification of physical status. Anesthesiology. 1963;24:111.
33. Gold BS, Kitz DS, Lecky JH, Neuhaus JM. Unanticipated admission to the hospital following ambulatory surgery. JAMA. 1989;262(21):3008–10.
34. Tiret L, Desmonts JM, Hatton F, Vourc'h G. Complications associated with anesthesia - a prospective study in France. Can Anaesth Soc J. 1986;33(3 Pt 1):336–44.
35. Pedersen T, Eliasen K, Hendricksen E. A prospective study of mortality associated with anesthesia and surgery: risk indicators of mortality in hospital. Acta Anaesthesiol Scand. 1990;34:76.
36. Vacanti CJ, VanHouten RJ, Hill RC. A statistical analysis of the relationship of physical status to postoperative mortality in 68,388 cases. Anesth Analg. 1970;49(4):564–6.
37. Goldman L, Caldera DL, Nussbaum SR, Southwick FS, Krogstad D, Murray B, et al. Multifactorial index of cardiac risk in noncardiac surgical procedures. N Engl J Med. 1977;297(16):845–50.
38. Goldman L, Caldera DL, Southwick FS, Nussbaum SR, Murray B, O'Malley TA, et al. Cardiac risk factors and complications in non-cardiac surgery. Medicine. 1978; 57(4):357–70.
39. Mangano DT, Browner WS, Hollenberg M, London MJ, Tubau JF, Tateo IM. Association of perioperative myocardial ischemia with cardiac morbidity and mortality in men undergoing non-cardiac surgery. N Engl J Med. 1990; 323(26):1781–8.
40. Krupski WC, Layug EL, Reilly LM, Rapp JH, Mangano DT. Comparison of cardiac morbidity between aortic and infrainguinal operations. Study of Perioperative Ischemia (SPI) Research Group. J Vasc Surg. 1992;15(2):354–63.
41. L'Italien GJ, Cambria RP, Cutler BS, Leppo JA, Paul SD, Brewster DC, et al. Comparative early and late cardiac morbidity among patients requiring different vascular surgery procedures. J Vasc Surg. 1995;21(6):935–44.
42. Detsky AS, Abram HB, Mclaughlin JR, Drucker DJ, Sasson Z, Johnston N, et al. Predicting cardiac complication in patients undergoing non-cardiac surgery. J Gen Intern Med. 1986;1(4):211–9.
43. Rose SD, Corman LC, Mason DT. Cardiac risk factors in patients undergoing noncardiac surgery. Med Clin North Am. 1979;63(6):1271–88.
44. Pasternak LR. Screening patients: strategies and studies. In: McGoldrick KE, editor. Ambulatory anesthesiology, a problem-oriented approach. Baltimore: Williams & Wilkins; 1995. p. 10.
45. Buck N, Devlin HB, Lunn JN. Report of confidential inquiry into perioperative deaths: Nuffield Provincial Hospitals Trust. London: King's Fund Publishing House; 1987.
46. Lunn JN, Devlin HB. Lessons from the confidential inquiry into perioperative death in three NHS regions. Lancet. 1987;2(8572):1384–6.
47. McCann RL, Clements FM. Silent myocardial ischemia in patients undergoing peripheral vascular surgery: incidence

and association with preoperative cardiac morbidity and mortality. J Vasc Surg. 1989;9(4):583–7.
48. Deanfield JE, Maseri A, Selwyn AP, Ribeiro P, Chierchia S, Krikler S, et al. Myocardial ischaemia during daily life in patients with stable angina: its relation to symptoms and heart rate changes. Lancet. 1983;2(8353):753–8.
49. Tarhan S, Moffitt EA, Taylor WF, Giuliani ER. Myocardial infarction after general anesthesia. JAMA. 1972;220(11): 1451–4.
50. Sapala JA, Ponka JL, Duvernoy WF. Operative and nonoperative risks in the cardiac patient. J Am Geriatr Soc. 1975;23(12):529–34.
51. Steen PA, Tinker JH, Tarhan S. Myocardial reinfarction after anesthesia and surgery. JAMA. 1978;239(24):2566.
52. Rao TLK, Jacobs KH, El-Etr AA. Reinfarction following anesthesia in patients with myocardial infarction. Anesthesiology. 1983;59(6):499–505.
53. Shah KB, Kleinman BS, Sami H, Patel J, Rao TL. Reevaluation of perioperative myocardial infarction in patients with prior myocardial infarction undergoing non-cardiac operations. Anesth Analg. 1990;71(3):231–5.
54. Mantha S, Roizen MF, Barnard J, Thisted RA, Ellis JE, Foss J. Relative effectiveness of preoperative noninvasive cardiac evaluation test on predicting adverse cardiac outcome following vascular surgery: a metaanalysis. Anesth Analg. 1994;79(3):422–33.
55. McPhail N, Calvin JE, Shariatmader A, Barber GG, Scobie TK. The use of preoperative exercise testing to predict cardiac complication after arterial reconstruction. J Vasc Surg. 1988;7(1):60–8.
56. Christopherson R, Beattie L, Frank SM, Norris EJ, Meinert CL, Gottlieb SO, et al. Perioperative morbidity in patients randomized to epidural or general anesthesia for lower extremity vascular surgery. Perioperative Ischemia Randomized Anesthesia Trial Study Group. Anesthesiology. 1993;79(3):422–34.
57. Slogoff S, Keats AS. Randomized trial of primary anesthetic agents on outcome of coronary artery bypass operations. Anesthesiology. 1989;70(2):179–88.
58. Abraham S, Johnson CL. Prevalence of severe obesity in adults in the United States. Am J Clin Nutr. 1980;33(2 Suppl):364–9.
59. Anderson T, Gluud C. Liver morphology in morbid obesity: a literature study. Int J Obes. 1984;8(2):97–106.
60. Fauci AS, Braunwald E, Isselbacher KJ, Wilson JD, Martin JB, Kaspper DL, et al. Harrison's principles of internal medicine. 14th ed. New York: McGraw-Hill; 1998. p. 454–5.
61. Lee JJ, Larson RH, Buckley JJ, Roberts RS. Airway maintenance in the morbidly obese. Anesthesiol Rev. 1980; 71:33–6.
62. Vaughan RW, Bauer S, Wise L. Volume and pH of gastric juice in obese patients. Anesthesiology. 1975;43(6):686–9.
63. Ray CS, Sue DY, Bray G, Hansen JE, Wasserman K. Effects of obesity on respiratory function. Am Rev Respir Dis. 1983;128(3):501–6.
64. Paul DR, Hoyt JL, Boutros AR. Cardiovascular and respiratory changes in response to change of posture in the very obese. Anesthesiology. 1976;45(1):73–8.
65. Drummond GB, Park GR. Arterial oxygen saturation before intubation of the trachea: an assessment of oxygenation techniques. Br J Anaesth. 1984;56(9):987–93.
66. Vaughn RW, Englehardt RC, Wise L. Postoperative hypoxemia in obese patients. Ann Surg. 1974;180(6):877–82.
67. Manchikanti L, Roush JR, Colliver JA. Effect of preanesthetic ranitidine and metaclopromide on gastric contents in morbidly obese patients. Anesth Analg. 1986;65(2): 195–9.
68. Rakoczi I, Chamone D, Collen D, Verstraete M. Prediction of postoperative leg-vein thrombosis in gynaecological patients. Lancet. 1978;1(8062):509–10.
69. Snell AM. The relation of obesity to fatal post operative pulmonary embolism. Arch Surg. 1927;15:237–44.
70. Shiffman MA. Anesthesia risks in patients who have had antiobesity medication. Am J Cosmet Surg. 1998;15:3–4.
71. Smithwick RH, Thompson JE. Splanchnicectomy for essential hypertension; results in 1,266 cases. JAMA. 1953; 152(6):1501–4.
72. Brown BR. Anesthesia and essential hypertension. In: Hershey SG, editor. ASA refresher courses in anesthesiology, vol. 7. Philadelphia: JB Lippincott; 1979. p. 47.
73. Veterans' Administration Cooperative Study Group on Antihypertensive Agents. Effects of treatment on morbidity in hypertension. II. Results in patients with diastolic blood pressure averaging 90 through 114 Hg. JAMA. 1970;213(7): 1143–52.
74. The effect of treatment on mortality in "mild" hypertension: results of the hypertension detection and follow-up program. N Engl J Med. 1982;307(16):976–80.
75. Kannel WB. Blood pressure as a cardiovascular risk factor. Prevention and treatment. JAMA. 1996;275(20):1571–6.
76. Prys-Roberts C, Meloche R, Foex P. Studies of anesthesia in relation to hypertension. I. Cardiovascular responses of treated and untreated patients. Br J Anaesth. 1971;43(2): 122–37.
77. Bedford RF, Feinstein B. Hospital admission blood pressure: a predictor for hypertension following endotracheal intubation. Anesth Analg. 1980;59(5):367–70.
78. Stone JG, Foex P, Sear JW, Johnson LL, Khambatta HJ, Triner L. Myocardial ischemia in untreated hypertension patients: effect of a single small oral dose of a beta-adrenergic blocking agent. Anesthesiology. 1988;68(4): 495–500.
79. Katz JD, Cronau LH, Barash PG. Postoperative hypertension: a hazard of abrupt cessation on antihypertensive medication in preoperative period. Am Heart J. 1976;92(1): 79–80.
80. Coriat P, Richer C, Douraki T, Gomez C, Hendricks K, Giudicelli JF, et al. Influence of chronic angiotensin-converting enzyme inhibition in anesthetic induction. Anesthesiology. 1994;81(2):299–307.
81. Leslie JB, Kalayjian RW, Sirgo MA, Plachetka JR, Watkins WD. Intravenous labetolol for treatment of postoperative hypertension. Anesthesiology. 1987;67(3):413–6.
82. O'Malley K, Segal JL, Israili ZH, Boles M, McNay JL, Dayton PG. Duration of hydralazine action in hypertension. Clin Pharmacol Ther. 1975;18(5 Pt 1):581–6.
83. Walsh DB, Eckhauser FE, Ramsburgh SR, Burney RB. Risk associated with diabetes mellitus in patients undergoing gall-bladder surgery. Surgery. 1982;91(3):254–7.
84. Hjortrup A, Rasmussen BF, Kehlet H. Morbidity in diabetic and non-diabetic patients after major vascular surgery. Br Med J. 1983;287(6399):1107–8.

85. Burgos LG, Ebert TJ, Asiddao C, Turner LA, Pattison CZ, Wang-Cheng R, et al. Increased intraoperative cardiovascular morbidity in diabetics with autonomic neuropathy. Anesthesiology. 1989;70(4):591–7.
86. Hirsch IB, McGill JB, Cryer PE, White PF. Perioperative management of surgical patients with diabetes mellitus. Anesthesiology. 1991;74(2):346–59.
87. Roizen M. Anesthetic implications of concurrent disease. In: Miller RD, editor. Anesthesia. 5th ed. Philadelphia: Churchill Livingstone; 2000. p. 909.
88. Walts LF, Miller J, Davidson MD, Brown J. Perioperative management of diabetes mellitus. Anesthesiology. 1981; 55(2):104–9.
89. Malling B, Knudsen L, Christiansen BA, Schurzek BA, Hermansen K. Insulin treatment in non-insulin dependent diabetic patients undergoing minor surgery. Diabetes Nutr Metab. 1989;2:125–31.
90. Hirsch IB, White PF. Management of surgical patients with insulin dependent diabetes mellitus. Anesthesiol Rev. 1994; 21:53–9.
91. Weiss KB, Wagner DK. Changing patterns of asthma mortality. Identifying target populations at high risk. JAMA. 1990;264(13):1683–7.
92. Boushy SF, Billing DM, North LB, Helgason AH. Clinical course related to preoperative pulmonary function in patients with bronchogenic carcinoma. Chest. 1971;59(4): 383–91.
93. Hall WJ, Douglas RG, Hyde RW, Roth FK, Cross AS, Speers DM. Pulmonary mechanics after uncomplicated influenza A infections. Am Rev Respir Dis. 1976;113(2): 141–8.
94. Warner MA, Offord KP, Warner ME, Lennon RL, Conover MA, Jansson-Schumacher U. Role of preoperative cessation of smoking and other factors in postoperative pulmonary complication: a clinical prospective study of coronary artery bypass patients. Mayo Clin Proc. 1989;64(6): 609–14.
95. Homer CJ. Asthma disease management. N Engl J Med. 1997;337(20):1461–3.
96. Stein M, Cassara EL. Preoperative pulmonary evaluation and therapy for surgical patients. JAMA. 1970;211(5): 787–90.
97. Bartlett RH, Brennan ML, Gazzaniga AB, Hansen EL. Studies on the pathogenesis and prevention of postoperative pulmonary complication. Surg Gynecol Obstet. 1973; 137(6):925–33.
98. National Commission on Sleep Disorders Research. Wake up America. A national sleep alert. Washington, DC: GPO; 1993.
99. Barsh CI. The origin of pharyngeal obstruction during sleep. Sleep Breath. 1999;31:17–21.
100. Shelton KE, Gay SB, Woodson H, Gay S, Suratt PM. Pharyngeal fat in obstructive sleep apnea. Am Rev Respir Dis. 1993;148(2):462–6.
101. Berman EJ, DiBenedetto RJ, Causey DE, Mims T, Conneff M, Goodman LS, et al. Right ventricular hypertrophy detected in echocardiography in newly diagnosed obstructive sleep apnea. Chest. 1991;100(2):347–50.
102. Orr WC. Sleep apnea, hypoxemia, and cardiac arrhythmias. Chest. 1986;89(1):1–2.
103. Chung F, Crago RR. Sleep apnea syndrome and analgesia. Can Anaesth Soc J. 1982;29(5):439–45.
104. Ostermeier AM, Roizen MF, Hautekappe M, Klock PA, Klafta JM. Three sudden postoperative respiratory arrests associated with epidural opioids in patients with sleep apnea. Anesth Analg. 1997;85(2):452–60.
105. Benumof JL. Obstructive sleep apnea in the adult obese patient: implications for airway management. J Clin Anesth. 2001;13(2):144–56.
106. Strollo Jr PJ, Rogers RM. Obstructive sleep apnea. N Engl J Med. 1996;334(2):99–104.
107. Wilson K, Stooks RA, Mulroony TF, Johnson IJ, Guilleminault C, Huang Z. The snoring spectrum: acoustic assessment of snoring sound intensity in 1,139 individuals undergoing polysomnography. Chest. 1999;115(3): 762–70.
108. Yentis SM, Levine MF, Hartley EJ. Should all children with suspected or confirmed malignant hyperthermia susceptibility be admitted after surgery? A 10-year review. Anesth Analg. 1992;75(3):345–50.
109. Gronert GA, Antognini JF, Pessah IN. Malignant hyperthermia. In: Miller RD, editor. Anesthesia. 5th ed. Philadelphia: Churchill Livingstone; 2000. p. 1047–8.
110. Kolb ME, Horne ML, Martz R. Dantrolene in human malignant hyperthermia: a multicenter study. Anesthesiology. 1982;56(4):254–62.
111. Covino BG, Wildsmith JAW. Clinical pharmacology of local anesthetics. In: Cousins MJ, Bridenbaugh DL, editors. Neural blockade in clinical anesthesia and management of pain. 3rd ed. Philadelphia: Lippincott Raven; 1998. p. 98.
112. Braid DP, Scott DB. The systemic absorption of local anesthetic drugs. Br J Anaesth. 1965;37:394–404.
113. Moore DC, Bridenbaugh DL, Thompson GE, Balfour RI, Horton WG. Factors determining doses of amide-type anesthetic drugs. Anesthesiology. 1977;47(3):263–8.
114. Nation R, Triggs F, Selig M. Lignocaine kinetics in cardiac and aged subjects. Br J Clin Pharmacol. 1977;4(4):439–48.
115. Meister F. Possible association between tumescent technique and life-threatening pulmonary edema. Clin Plast Surg. 1996;23:642–5.
116. Shiffman M. Medications potentially causing lidocaine toxicity. Am J Cosmet Surg. 1998;15:227–8.
117. Klein JA. The tumescent technique of liposuction surgery. Am J Cosmet Surg. 1987;4:263–76.
118. Klein JA. Tumescent technique for regional anesthesia permits lidocaine doses 35 mg/kg for liposuction. J Dermatol Surg Oncol. 1990;16(3):248–63.
119. Klein JA. Pharmacokinetic of tumescent lidocaine. In: Klein JA, editor. Tumescent technique: tumescent anesthesia and microcannular liposuction. St Louis: Mosby; 2000. p. 141–61.
120. Ostad A, Kageyama N, Moy RL. Tumescent anesthesia with a lidocaine dose of 55 mg/kg is safe for liposuction. Dermatol Surg. 1996;22(11):921–7.
121. Klein JA, Kassarjdian N. Lidocaine toxicity with tumescent liposuction. Dermatol Surg. 1997;23(12):1169–74.
122. Corvino BG, Wildsmith JAW. Clinical pharmacology of local anesthetic agents. In: Cousins MJ, Bridenbaugh DL, editors. Neural blockade in clinical anesthesia and management of pain. 3rd ed. Philadelphia: Lippincott Raven; 1998. p. 107–8.
123. Feldman HS, Arthur GR, Covino BG. Comparative systemic toxicity of convulsant and supraconvulsant doses of

123. intravenous ropivacaine, bupivacaine and lidocaine in the conscious dog. Anesth Analg. 1989;69(6):794–801.
124. Morishma HO, Peterson H, Finster M. Is bupivacaine more cardiotoxic than lidocaine? Anesthesiology. 1983;59:A409.
125. Albright GA. Cardiac arrest following regional anesthesia with etidocaine or bupivacaine. Anesthesiology. 1979;51(4):285–7.
126. Rosen M, Thigpen J, Shnider SM, Foutz SE, Levinson G, Koike M. Bupivacaine-induced cardiotoxicity in hypoxic and acidotic sheep. Anesth Analg. 1985;64(11):1089–96.
127. Sunshine I, Fike WW. Value of thin-layer chromatography in two fatal cases of intoxication due to lidocaine and mepivacaine. N Engl J Med. 1964;271:487–90.
128. Yukioka H, Hayashi M, Fujimori M. Lidocaine intoxication during general anesthesia (letter). Anesth Analg. 1990;71(2):207–8.
129. Christie JL. Fatal consequences of local anesthesia: report of five cases and a review of the literature. J Forensic Sci. 1976;21:671–9.
130. Samdal F, Amland PF, Bugge JF. Plasma lidocaine levels during suction-assisted lipectomy using large doses of dilute lidocaine with epinephrine. Plast Reconstr Surg. 1994;93(6):1217–23.
131. Pitman GH. Tumescent technique for local anesthesia improves safety in large-volume liposuction (Discussion). Plast Reconstr Surg. 1993;92:1099–100.
132. Fisher MM, Graham R. Adverse responses to local anesthetics. Anaesth Intensive Care. 1984;12(4):325–7.
133. Aldrete J, Johnson DA. Evaluation of intracutaneous testing for investigation of allergy to local anesthetic agents. Anesth Analg. 1970;49(1):173–83.
134. Kaster GW, Martin ST. Successful resuscitation after massive intravenous bupivacaine overdose in the hypoxic dog. Anesthesiology. 1984;61:A206.
135. Feldman H, Arthur G, Pitkanen M, Hudley R, Doucette AM, Covino BG. Treatment of acute systemic toxicity after the rapid intravenous injection of ropivacaine, bupivacaine, and lidocaine in the conscious dog. Anesth Analg. 1991;73(4):373–84.
136. Kasten GW, Martin ST. Bupivacaine cardiovascular toxicity: comparison of treatment with bretylium and lidocaine. Anesth Analg. 1985;64(9):911–6.
137. McKay W, Morris R, Mushlin P. Sodium bicarbonate attenuates pain on skin infiltration with lidocaine, with or without epinephrine. Anesth Analg. 1987;66(6):572–4.
138. Buckley MM, Benfield P. Eutectic lidocaine/prilocaine cream: a review of the topical anesthetic/analgesic efficacy of a eutectic mixture of local anesthetics (EMLA). Drugs. 1993;46(1):126–51.
139. Gammaitoni AR, Davis MW. Pharmacokinetics and tolerablitly of lidocaine patch 5% with extended dosing. Ann Pharmacother. 2002;36(2):236–40.
140. Endo Pharmaceuticals. Lidoderm. In: Physicians desk reference. 60th ed. Monyvale: Thompson PDR; 2006. p. 1107–8.
141. Young D. Student's death sparks concerns about compounded preparations. Am J Health Syst Pharm. 2005;62:450–4.
142. Holzman RS, Cullen DJ, Eichhorn JH, Phillip JH. Guidelines for sedation by nonanesthesilogists during diagnostic and therapeutic procedures. J Clin Anesth. 1994;6(4):265–76.
143. White PF, Negus JB. Sedative infusions during local and regional anesthesia: a comparison of midazolam and propoful. J Clin Anesth. 1991;3(1):32–9.
144. Rothfusz ER, Kitz DS, Andrews RW. O_2 sat, HR and MAP amoung patients receiving local anesthesia: how low/high do they go? Anesth Analg. 1988;67:S189.
145. Lundgren S, Rosenquist JB. Amnesia, pain experience, and patient satisfaction after sedation with intravenous diazepam. J Oral Maxillofac Surg. 1983;41(2):99–102.
146. Federated Ambulatory Surgical Association. FASA special study I. Alexandria: FASA; 1986.
147. McNabb TG, Goldwyn RM. Blood gas and hemodynamic effects of sedatives and analgisics when used as as suppliment to local anesthesia in plastic surgery. Plast Reconstr Surg. 1976;58(1):37–43.
148. Singer R, Thomas PE. Pulse oximeter in the ambulatory anesthetic surgical facility. Plast Reconstr Surg. 1988;82(1):111–4.
149. Giles HG, MacLeod SM, Wright JR, Sellers EM. Influence of age and previous use on diazepam dosing requirements for endoscopy. Can Med Assoc J. 1978;118(5):513–4.
150. Wynands JE, Wong P, Townsend G, Sprigge JS, Whalley DG. Narcotic requirements for intravenous ansthesia. Anesth Analg. 1984;63(2):101–5.
151. Kay B, Rolly G. Duration of action of analgesic suppliment to anesthesia. Acta Anaesthesiol Belg. 1977;28(1):25–32.
152. Bailey PL, Andriano KP, Pace NL. Small doses of fentanyl potentiate and prolong diazepam induced respiratory depression. Anesth Analg. 1984;63:183.
153. Reves JG. Benzodiazapines. In: Prys-Roberts C, Hugg CC, editors. Pharmacokinetics of anesthesia. Boston: Blackwell Scientific Publications; 1984.
154. Klein JA. Tumescent technique for local anesthesia improves safety in large-volume liposuction. Plast Reconstr Surg. 1993;92(6):1085–98.
155. Osborne GA, Rudkin GE, Curtis NJ, Vickers D, Craker AJ. Intraoperative patient-controlled sedation; comparison of patient-controlled propofol with anaesthetist-administered midazolam and fentanyl. Anesthesiology. 1991;46(7):553–6.
156. Zelcer J, White PF, Chester S, Paull JD, Molnar R. Intraoperative patient-controlled analgesia: an alternative to physician administration during outpatient monitored anesthesia care. Anesth Analg. 1992;75(1):41–4.
157. Hegarty JE, Dundee JW. Sequelae after intravenous injection of three benzodiazepines: diazepam, lorazepam, and flunitrazepam. Br Med J. 1977;2(6099):1384–5.
158. Greenblatt DJ, Shader RI, Dwoll M, Harmatz JS. Benzodiazepines: a summary of the pharmacokinetics. Br J Clin Pharmacol. 1981;11 Suppl 1:11S–6.
159. White PF, Vasconez CO, Mathes SA, Way WL, Wender LA. Comparison of midazolam and diazepam for sedation during plastic surgery. Plast Reconstr Surg. 1998;81(5):703–12.
160. Blitt CD. Clinical pharmacology of lorezepam. In: Brown BRJ, editor. New pharmacologic vista in anesthesia. Philadelphia: FA Davis; 1983. p. 135.
161. Rigg JR, Goldsmith CH. Recovery of ventilatory response to carbon dioxide after thiopentone, morphine and fentanyl in man. Can Anaesth Soc J. 1976;23(4):370–82.
162. White PF, Coe V, Shafer A, Sung ML. Comparison of alfentanil with fentanyl for outpatient anesthesia. Anesthesiology. 1986;64(1):99–106.

163. SaRego MM, Inagoki Y, White PF. Use of remifentanil during lithotripsy: intermittant boluses vs continuous infusion [abstract]. Anesth Analg. 1997;84:5541.
164. Watcha MR, White PF. Postoperative nausea and vomiting: its etiology, treatment and prevention. Anesthesiology. 1992;77(1):162–84.
165. Mackenzie N, Grant IS. Propofol (Diprovan) for continuous intravenous anaesthesia: a comparison with methohexitone. Postgrad Med J. 1985;61 Suppl 3:70–5.
166. McCollum JS, Milligan KR, Dundee JW. The antiemetic action of propofol. Anaesthesia. 1988;43(3):239–40.
167. Smith I, Monk TG, White PF, Ding Y. Propofol infusion during regional anesthesia: sedative, amnestic, anxiolytic properties. Anesth Analg. 1994;79(2):313–9.
168. Grounds RM, Twigley AJ, Carli F, Whitwam JG, Morgan M. The haemodynamic effects of thiopentone and propofol. Anaesthesiology. 1985;40(8):735–40.
169. Goodman NW, Black AM, Carter JA. Some ventilatory effects of propofol as sole anesthetic agent. Br J Anaesth. 1987;59(12):1497–503.
170. Fanard L, Van Steenberge A, Demeire X, van der Puyl F. Comparison between propofol and midazolam as sedative agents for surgery under regional anesthesia. Anaesthesia. 1988;43(Suppl):87–9.
171. Rudkin GE, Osborne GA, Finn BP, Jarvis DA, Vickers D. Intraoperative patient-controlled sedation: comparison of patient-controlled propofol with patient-controlled midazolam. Anesthesiology. 1992;47(5):376–81.
172. Meyers CJ, Eisig SB, Kraut RA. Comparison of propofol and methohexital for deep sedation. J Maxillofac Surg. 1994;52(5):448–52.
173. White PF, Way WL, Trevor AJ. Ketamine: its pharmacology and therapeutic uses. Anesthesiology. 1982;56(2):119–36.
174. Taylor PA, Towey RM. Depression of laryngeal reflexes during ketamine anesthesia. Br Med J. 1971;2(763): 688–9.
175. Garfield JM, Garfield FB, Stone JG, Hopkins D, Johns LA. A comparison of psychological responses to ketamine and thiopental, nitrous oxide, halothane anesthesia. Anesthesiology. 1972;36(4):329–38.
176. Corssen G, Reves JG, Stanley TH. Neuroleptanalgesia and neuroleptanesthesia. Intravenous anesthesia and analgesia. Philadelphia: Lea & Febig; 1988. p. 175.
177. Prys-Roberts C, Kelman GR. The influence of drugs used in neurolept analgesia on cardiovascular and ventilatory function. Br J Anaesth. 1967;39(2):134–45.
178. Edmonds-Seal J, Prys-Roberts C. Pharmacology of drugs used in neurolept analgesia. Anaesth Analg (Paris). 1959; 16:1022.
179. Melnick BM. Extrapyramidal reactions to low-dose droperidol. Anesthesiology. 1988;69(3):424–6.
180. Guze BH, Baxter Jr LR. Current concepts: neuroletic malignant syndrome. N Engl J Med. 1985;313(3):163–6.
181. FDA strengthens warnings for Droperidol. FDA Talk Paper, 12/5/01;T01-62.
182. Bailey PL, Egan TD, Stanlet TE. Intravenous opiod anesthetics. In: Miller RD, editor. Anesthesia. 5th ed. Philadelphia: Churchill Livingstone; 2000. p. 345–8.
183. Philip BK. Supplemental medication for ambulatory procedures under regional anesthesia. Anesth Analg. 1985;64(11): 1117–25.
184. Sa Rego MM, Watcha MF, White PF. The changing role of monitored anesthesia care in the ambulatory setting. Anesthesiology. 1997;85(5):1020–36.
185. Fragen RJ, editor. Drug infusions in anesthesiology. New York: Raven Press; 1991.
186. Naito Y, Tamai S, Shingu K, Fujimori R, Mori K. Comparison between sevoflurane and halothane for paediatric ambulatory anesthesia. Br J Anaesth. 1991;67(4):387–9.
187. Ghouri AF, Bodner M, White PF. Recovery profile following desflurane-nitrous oxide versus isoflurane-nitrous oxide in outpatients. Anesthesiology. 1991;74(3):419–24.
188. Bodman RI, Morton HJ, Thomas ET. Vomiting by outpatients after nitrous oxide anesthesia. Br Med J. 1960;5182: 1327–30.
189. Van Hemelrijck J, White PF. Intravenous anesthesia for day-care surgery. In: Kay B, editor. Total intravenous anesthesia. Amsterdam: Elsevier; 1991. p. 323–50.
190. Benumof JL. Laryngeal mask airway: indication and contraindications. Anesthesiology. 1992;77(5):843–6.
191. Campbell GD. Dangers of monoamine oxidase inhibitors. Br Med J. 1963;1:750.
192. Sjoqvist F. Psychotropic drugs, 2. Interaction between monoamine oxidase (MAO) inhibitors and other substances. Proc R Soc Med. 1965;58(11 Part 2):967–78.
193. Roizen M. Anesthetic implications of concurrent diseases. In: Miller RD, editor. Anesthesia. 5th ed. Philadelphia: Churchill Livingstone; 2000. p. 998.
194. Green CR, Pandit SK, Schork MA. Preoperative fasting time: is the traditional policy changing? Results of a national survey. Anesth Analg. 1996;83(1):123–8.
195. Schreiner MS, Nicolson SC. Pediatric ambulatory anesthesia: NPO before or after surgery? J Clin Anesth. 1995;7(7): 589–96.
196. Maltby JR, Sutherland AD, Sale JP, Schaffer EA. Preoperative oral fluids. Is a five-hour fast justified prior to elective surgery? Anesth Analg. 1986;65(11):1112–6.
197. Doze VA, White PF. Effects of fluid therapy on serum glucose in fasted outpatients. Anesthesiology. 1987;66(2): 223–6.
198. Kallar SK, Everett LL. Potential risks and preventative measures for pulmonary aspiration: new concepts in preoperative fasting guideline. Anesth Analg. 1993;77(1): 171–82.
199. Manchikanti L, Canella MG, Hohlbein LJ, Colliver JA. Assessment of effects of various modes of premedication on acid aspiration risk factors in outpatient surgery. Anesth Analg. 1987;66(1):81–4.
200. Morgan M. Control of gastric pH and volume. Br J Anaesth. 1984;56(1):47–57.
201. Manchikanti L, Kraus JW, Edds SP. Cimetidine and related drugs in anesthesia. Anesth Analg. 1982;61(7):595–608.
202. Manchikanti L, Colliver JA, Roush JR, Canella MG. Evaluation of ranitidine as an oral antacid in outpatient anesthesia. South Med J. 1985;78(7):818–22.
203. Boulay K, Blanloeil Y, Bourveau M, Gray G. Comparison of oral ranitidine(R), famotidine (F), and omeprazole (O) effects on gastric pH and volume in elective general surgery (Abstract). Anesthesiology. 1992;77:A431.
204. Diamond MJ, Keeri-Szanto M. Reduction of postoperative vomiting by preoperative administration of oral metaclopromide. Can Anaesth Soc J. 1980;27(1):36–9.

205. Kapur PA. The big 'little' problem (Editorial). Anesth Analg. 1991;73(3):243–5.
206. van Wijk MG, Smalhout B. Postoperative analysis of the patients' view of anesthesia in a Netherlands's teaching hospital. Anaesthesia. 1990;45(8):679–82.
207. Hines R, Barash PG, Watrous G, O'Connor T. Complications occurring in the post anesthesia care unit. Anesth Analg. 1992;74(4):503–9.
208. Green G, Jonsson L. Nausea: the most important factor determining length of stay after ambulatory anaesthesia. A comparison study of isoflurane and/or propofol techniques. Acta Anaesthesiol Scand. 1993;37(8):742–6.
209. Madej TH, Simpson KH. Comparison of the use of domperidone, droperidol, and metaclopramide on the prevention of nausea and vomiting following gynaecological surgery in day cases. Br J Anaesth. 1986;58(8):879–83.
210. White PF, Shafer A. Nausea and vomiting: causes and prophylaxis. Sem Anesth. 1987;6:300–8.
211. Carroll NV, Miederhoff P, Cox FM, Hirsch JD. Postoperative nausea and vomiting after discharge from outpatient surgery centers. Anesth Analg. 1995;80(5):903–9.
212. Tang J, Watcha MF, White PF. A comparison of costs and efficacy of ondansetron and droperidol as prophylactic antiemetic therapy for elective outpatient gynecologic procedures. Anesth Analg. 1996;83(2):304–13.
213. Alon E, Himmelseher S. Ondansetron in the treatment of postoperative vomiting: a randomized double-blind comparison with droperidol and metaclopromide (Abstract). Anesth Analg. 1993;79:A8.
214. Wilson AJ, Diemunsch P, Lindeque BG, Scheinin H, Helbo-Hansen HS, Kroeks MV, et al. Single-dose i.v. granisetron in the prevention of postoperative nausea and vomiting. Br J Anaesth. 1996;76(4):515–8.
215. Sung YF, Wetcher BV, Duncalf D, Joslyn AF. A double-blind placebo-controlled pilot study examining the effectiveness of intravenous ondansetron in the prevention of postoperative nausea and emesis. J Clin Anesth. 1993;5(1):22–9.
216. McKenzie R, Kovac A, O'Connor T, Duncalf D, Angel J, Gratz I, et al. Comparison of ondansetron versus placebo to prevent postoperative nausea and vomiting in women undergoing gynecological surgery. Anesthesiology. 1993;78(1):21–8.
217. McKenzie R, Tantisira B, Karambelkan DJ, Riley TJ, Abdelhady H. Comparison of ondansetron with ondansetron plus dexamethasone, 4 to 8 mg, in the prevention of postoperative nausea and vomiting. Anesth Analg. 1994;79(5):961–4.
218. McKenzie R, Uy NT, Riley TJ, Hamilton DL. Droperidol/ondansetron combination controls nausea and vomiting after tubal ligation. Anesth Analg. 1996;83(6):1218–22.
219. Shafer A. Preoperative medication: adults and children. In: White PF, editor. Ambulatory anesthesia and surgery. London: W.B. Saunders; 1997. p. 173.
220. Kotelko DM, Rottman RL, Wright WC, Stone JJ, Yamashiro AY, Rosenblatt RM. Transdermal scopolamine decreases nausea and vomiting following cesarean section in patients receiving epidural morphine. Anesthesiology. 1989;71(5):675–8.
221. Rodysill KJ, Warren JB. Transdermal scopolamine and toxic psychosis. Ann Intern Med. 1983;98(4):561.
222. Vener DF, Carr AS, Sikich N, Bissonette B, Lerman J. Dimenhydrinate decreases vomiting after stabismus surgery in children. Anesth Analg. 1996;82(4):728–31.
223. Borgeat A, Wilder-Smith OH, Saiah M, Rifat K. Subhypnotic doses of propofol possess direct antiemetic properties. Anesth Analg. 1992;74(4):539–41.
224. Raftery S, Sherry E. Total intravenous anaesthesia with propofol and alfentanil protects against nausea and vomiting. Can J Anaesth. 1992;39(1):37–40.
225. Felts JA, Poler SM, Spitznagel EL. Nitrous oxide, nausea and vomiting after outpatient gynecological surgery. J Clin Anesth. 1990;2(3):168–71.
226. Melnick BM, Johnson LJ. Effects of eliminating nitrous oxide in outpatient anesthesia. Anesthesiology. 1987;67(6):982–4.
227. Shafer A, White PF, Urquhart ML, Doze UA. Outpatient premedication: use of midazolam and opioid analgesics. Anesthesiology. 1989;71(4):495–501.
228. Meridy HW. Criteria for selection of ambulatory surgical patients and guidelines for anesthetic management: a retrospective study of 1553 cases. Anesth Analg. 1982; 61(11):921–6.
229. Janhumen L, Tommisto T. Postoperative vomiting after different modes of general anesthesia. Ann Chir Gynaecol. 1972;61:152.
230. Yogendran S, Asokumar B, Chang DC, Chung F. A prospective randomized double-blind study of the effects of intravenous fluid therapy on adverse outcomes on outpatient surgery. Anesth Analg. 1995;80(4):682–6.
231. Jakobsen H, Hertz JB, Johansen JR, Hansen A, Kolliker K. Premedication before day surgery. Br J Anaesth. 1985;57(3):300–5.
232. Baird ES, Hailey DM. Delayed recovery from a sedative: correlation of the plasma levels of diazepam with clinical effects after oral and intravenous administration. Br J Anaesth. 1972;44(8):803–8.
233. Gale GD, Galloon S, Porter WR. Sublingual lorazepam: a better premedication? Br J Anaesth. 1983;55(8):761–5.
234. Reinhart K, Dallinger-Stiller G, Dennhardt R, Heinnemeyer G, Eyrich K. Comparison of midazolam and diazepam and placebo i.m. as premedication for regional anesthesia. Br J Anaesth. 1985;57(3):294–9.
235. Raybould D, Bradshaw EG. Premedication for day case surgery. Anesthesiology. 1987;42(6):591–5.
236. Conner JT, Bellville JW, Katz RL. Meperidine and morphine as intravenous surgical premedicants. Can Anaesth Soc J. 1977;24(5):559–64.
237. Pandit SK, Kothary SP. Intravenous narcotics for premedication in outpatient anaesthesia. Acta Anaesthesiol Scand. 1989;33(5):353–8.
238. Wender RH, Conner JT, Bellville JW, Schehl D, Dorey F, Katz RL. Comparison of i.v. diazepam and hydroxyzine as surgical premedicants. Br J Anaesth. 1977;49(9):907–12.
239. Roisen MF. Anesthetic implications of concurrent disease. In: Miller R, editor. Anesthesia. 5th ed. Philadelphia: Churchill Livingstone; 2000. p. 959–60.
240. Goldhaber SZ. Pulmonary embolism. N Engl J Med. 1998;339(2):93–104.
241. Sandison AJP, Jones SE, Jones PA. A daycare modified Shouldice hernia repair follow-up. J One-day Surg. 1994;3:16–7.

242. Moser KM, Fedullo PF, LittleJohn JK, Crawford R. Frequent asymptomatic pulmonary embolism in patients with deep venous thrombosis. JAMA. 1994;271:223. [erratum] J Am Med Assoc 1994;271(24):1908.
243. Collins R, Scrimgeour A, Yusuf S, Peto R. Reduction in fatal pulmonary embolism and venous thrombosis by perioperative administration of subcutaneous heparin, an overview of results of randomized trials in general, orthopedic and urologic surgery. N Engl J Med. 1988;318(18): 1162–73.
244. Prevention of venous thrombosis and pulmonary embolism. NIH consensus conference. JAMA. 1986;256(6):744–9.
245. Gallus A, Raman K, Darby T. Venous thrombosis after elective hips replacement-the influence of preventative intermittent calf compression on surgical technique. Br J Surg. 1983;70(1):17–9.
246. Bergqvist D, Lindblad B. A 30-year survey of pulmonary embolism verified at autopsy: an analysis of 1274 surgical patients. Br J Surg. 1985;72(2):105–8.
247. Gan TJ, Glass PS, Windsor A, Payne F, Rosow C, Sebel P, et al. Bispectral index monitoring allows faster emergence and improved recovery from propofol, fentanyl and nitrous oxide anesthesia. Anesthesiology. 1997;87(4):808–15.
248. Tonnesen AS. Crystalloids and colloids. In: Miller R, editor. Anesthesia. 4th ed. New York: Churchill Livingstone; 1994. p. 1595–618.
249. Linko K, Makelainen A. Cardiorespiratory function after replacement of blood loss with hydroxyethyl starch 120, Dextran-70, and Ringer's lactate in pigs. Crit Care Med. 1989;17(10):1031–5.
250. Hankeln K, Radel C, Beez M, Laniewski P, Bohmert F. Comparison of hydroxyethyl starch and lactated Ringer's solution in hemodynamics and oxygen transport of critically ill patients in prospective cross over studies. Crit Care Med. 1989;17(2):133–5.
251. Dawidson I. Fluid resuscitation of shock: current controversies. Crit Care Med. 1989;17(10):1078–80.
252. Moss GS, Gould SA. Plasma expanders: an update. Am J Surg. 1988;155(3):425–34.
253. Leone BJ, Spahn DR. Anemia, hemodilution, and oxygen delivery. Anesth Analg. 1992;75(5):651–3.
254. American Society of Anesthesiologists Task Force on Blood Component Therapy. Practice guidelines for blood component therapy. Anesthesiology. 1996;84(3):732–47.
255. Bennett GD. Anesthesia for liposuction and abdominoplasty. In: Shiffman MA, Mirrafati S, editors. Aesthetic surgery of the abdominal wall. Berlin: Springer; 2005. p. 29–54.
256. Natof HE, Gold B, Kitz DS. Complications. In: Wetcher BV, editor. Anesthesia of ambulatory surgery. 2nd ed. Philadelphia: Lippincott; 1991. p. 374–474.
257. Mecca RS. Postoperative recovery. In: Borash PG, Cullen BF, Stoelting RK, editors. Clinical anesthesia. Philadelphia: J.B. Lippincott; 1992. p. 1517–8.
258. Bailey PL, Egar TD, Stanley TH. Intravenous opioid anesthetics. In: Miller RD, editor. Anesthesia. 5th ed. Philadelphia: Churchill Livingstone; 2000. p. 273–376.
259. Jensen S, Knudsen L, Kirkegaard L, Kruse A, Knudsen EB. Flumazenil used for antagonizing the central effects of midazolam and diazepam in outpatients. Acta Anaesthesiol Scand. 1989;33(1):26–8.
260. Klotz U. Drug interactions and clinical pharmacokinetics of flumazenil. Eur J Anaesthesiol. 1988;2:103–8.
261. McCloy RF. Reversal of conscious sedation by flumazenil: current status and future prospects. Acta Anaesthsiol Scand Suppl. 1995;108:35–42.
262. Bourke DL, Rosenberg M, Allen PD. Physostigmine: effectiveness as an antagonist of respiratory depression and psychomotor effects caused by morphine or diazepam. Anesthesiology. 1984;61(5):523–8.
263. Hill GE, Stanley TH, Slentker CR. Physostigmine reversal of postoperative somnolence. Can Anaesth Soc J. 1977; 24(6):707–11.

Recommended Reading

McGoldrick K, editor. Ambulatory anesthesiology. A problem-oriented approach. Baltimore: Williams & Wilkins; 1995.

Miller RD. Anesthesia. 5th ed. Philadelphia: Churchill Livingstone; 2000.

White PF, editor. Ambulatory anesthesia & surgery. Philadelphia: W.B. Saunders; 1997.

Personal Method of Anesthesia in the Office

Stephen J. Gray

7.1 Introduction

Multimodal anesthesia has been in the ascendency for some time. Chilvers [1] landmark paper gave this technique impetus by highlighting the merits of this approach as opposed to traditional epidural analgesia in colorectal surgery. This is old news! Office-based anesthetic practitioners have been using this approach, with opioid sparing if not outright exclusion, in spontaneously breathing patients since the late 1990s [2]. Emesis is the one outcome most feared by patients [3] and once again it has been the office-based practitioners who have redefined endpoints in this area.

7.2 Definition of Sedation

In 2002 the American Society of Anesthesiologists [4] assembled a Task Force and defined four specific levels of sedation/analgesia.

Minimal Sedation (Anxiolysis): A drug-induced state during which patients respond normally to verbal commands. Although cognitive function and coordination may be impaired, ventilatory and cardiovascular functions are unaffected.

Moderate Sedation/Analgesia (Conscious Sedation): A drug-induced depression of consciousness during which patients respond purposefully to verbal commands, either alone or accompanied by light tactile stimulation.

No interventions are required to maintain a patent airway and spontaneous ventilation is adequate. Cardiovascular function is usually maintained.

Deep Sedation/Analgesia: A drug-induced depression of consciousness during which patients cannot easily be aroused but respond purposefully following repeated or painful stimulation. The ability to independently maintain airway function may be impaired. Patients may require assistance in maintaining a patent airway and spontaneous ventilation may be inadequate. Cardiovascular function is usually maintained.

General Anesthesia: A drug-induced loss of consciousness during which patients are not arousable, even by painful stimulation. The ability to independently maintain ventilatory function is often impaired. Patients often require assistance in maintaining a patent airway and positive pressure ventilation may be required because of depressed spontaneous ventilation or drug-induced depression of neuromuscular function. Cardiovascular function may be impaired.

The Society rightly contends that sedation is a continuum and it is not always possible to gauge how a patient will respond. So where the intention was moderate sedation, it is always possible the patient may move into deep sedation and even general anesthesia. It behooves the practitioner to have the requisite skills to be able to rescue the situation. Undoubtedly, this has implications for personnel and facilities.

The situation in the UK is more polarized; deep sedation is regarded as general anesthesia. The demarcation being, moderate sedation can be given by non-anesthesiologists whereas deep sedation (general anesthesia) requires a physician trained in anesthesia.

The American Society of Anesthesiologists has recently examined Monitored Anesthesia Care (latest update September 2, 2008). The Society is emphatic that Monitored Anesthesia Care (MAC) is a physician-led

S.J. Gray
Papworth Hospital NHS Trust, Papworth Everard, Cambridge, CB23 3RE, UK
e-mail: sjgray@tiscali.co.uk

service facilitating the safe administration of a maximal depth of sedation/analgesia in excess of that provided by moderate sedation. The MAC provider must have the skills to convert to general anesthesia should the clinical need arise. The MAC provider has an extended role beyond that furnished by a practitioner of moderate sedation, namely, preoperative assessment, management concomitant medical problems, supervision of recovery, and pain relief.

7.3 Other Considerations

Sedation has inherent risks: hemodynamic instability [5], respiratory depression [6], and uncontrolled movements [7]. Elderly patients need less sedation [8] and are at greater risk of desaturation and cardiovascular lability [9]. Sedation can unmask obstructive sleep apnea [10].

7.4 Assessing Level of Sedation

The two most commonly used scales are Modified Wilson Sedation scale (Table 7.1) and Observer's Assessment of Alertness/Sedation (OAA/S) (Table 7.2).

Table 7.1 Modified Wilson sedation scale

Score	Description
1	Oriented, eyes may be closed but can respond to "Can you tell me your name?" "Can you tell me where you are right now?"
2	Drowsy, eyes may be closed, arousable only to command: "Please open your eyes?"
3	Arousable to mild physical stimulation (ear lobe tug)
4	Unarousable to mild physical stimulation

The latter, though more detailed, produces a more accurate record and has an impressive inter-rater agreement of 85–96% [11].

A plethora of Level of Consciousness (LOC) monitors have appeared since Bispectral Index (BIS Aspect Medical) was granted FDA approval in 1996. These include Entropy (Datex-Ohmeda, Finland), Patient State Index (Physiometrix), Cerebral State Monitor (Danmeter), and Narcotrend (Schiller Medical). Auditory evoked potentials have created interest, in particular the mid-latency signal, though it has been Bispectral Index (BIS) and Spectral Entropy that have found their way into clinical practice.

BIS takes power-spectral analysis (relationship between power and frequency over time) a step further by examining the phase relationships between component waves of different frequencies that make up the composite EEG. The monitor generates a dimensionless number on a continuous scale of 0–100, with "100" representing awake normal cortical electrical activity and "0" signifying cortical electrical silence. Surgical anesthesia is deemed to occur between 60 and 40 (Table 7.3).

BIS correlates well with the hypnotic state and anesthetic drug concentration [12–14]. BIS can shorten recovery times [15]. The Australian "B-aware" trial [16] recruited 2,463 patients and elegantly established that BIS-guided anesthesia reduces awareness by 82% in an at-risk adult surgical population. However, BIS does not predict movement in response to surgical stimulation, such responses often stem from the spinal cord.

Interestingly, adding nitrous oxide to an inhalational agent has little effect on BIS in the absence

Table 7.2 Observer's Assessment of Alertness/Sedation Scale (OAA/S)

Score	Sedation level	Responsiveness	Speech	Facial expression	Eyes
5	Alert	Responds readily to name	Normal	Normal	Clear no ptosis
4	Light	Lethargic	Mild slowing response to name	Mild relaxation	Glazed or mild ptosis
3	Moderate	Response only after name called loudly	Slurring or marked slowing	Mild relaxation	Glazed and marked ptosis
2	Deep	Responds after mild prodding or shaking	Few recognizable words	–	–
1	Deep sleep Unconscious	Does not respond to mild prodding or shaking	–	–	–

Table 7.3 BIS levels and levels of sedation/anesthesia

BIS	
100–85	Awake: capable of memory processing and explicit recall
85–75	Minimal sedation (anxiolysis)
75–70	Moderate ("conscious") sedation
70–60	Deep sedation
60–40	General anesthesia
<40	Over anesthetized

of surgical stimulation, but during surgery the antinociceptive influence leads to a decrease in BIS. Ketamine causes a dose-dependent activation of the EEG with subsequent increase in BIS values.

The concept of "entropy" has been applied to the EEG, as a way of quantifying its degree of order [17, 18]. One particular entropy concept, Shannon entropy, has been shown to correlate with anesthetic drug effect [19]. In essence, Shannon entropy measures the predictability of future amplitude values of the EEG based on amplitude values previously observed in the signal. Spectral entropy applies this Shannon entropy concept. Presently, the only commercially available entropy module (M-Entropy, Datex-Ohmeda, Finland) looks at two spectral entropy indicators: "state entropy" (SE) covering the dominant EEG frequency (0.8–32 Hz) and "response entropy" (RE) over the complete range of frequencies (0.8–47 Hz). The latter range includes both EEG and EMG components. The SE has a range (0–91) and RE (0–100) with lower numbers denoting a deeper level of anesthesia.

Vanluchene ALG et al. [20] compared BIS and spectral entropy in patients receiving a propofol infusion with or without remifentanil. BIS and spectral entropy accurately detected loss of consciousness to verbal command and decreased proportionately when remifentanil was used.

It is important to understand that BIS displays considerable variability within study populations, so making it difficult to identify sensitive and specific threshold values. Importantly, no BIS value predicts an individual threshold. Level of consciousness monitors is no substitute for vigilance, their true merit lies in their ability to enable the anesthetist to tailor the anesthetic to the individual.

7.5 Agents Used in Sedation

7.5.1 Propofol

A phenolic derivative (2,6 diisopropylphenol) is highly lipid soluble, a weak organic acid ($pK_a = 11$), and almost entirely unionized at $pH = 7.4$. It is close to being the ideal agent for sedation and possesses a very favorable pharmacokinetic profile, with fast induction and ability to rapidly change sedation level together with a prompt recovery. Propofol exerts its effects via the β subunit of the $GABA_A$ receptor as well as releasing the neuroinhibitory transmitter, glycine. Sedation and amnesia are dose related though the amnesic effect is not as powerful as midazolam [9, 21]. Anxiolysis is not dose related. Pain on injection can occur, especially if a small calibre vein is used. Propofol is a poor analgesic [6] but has valuable antiemetic properties [21]. Doses in excess of 200 mg/h can induce hypotension and bradycardia. In the office setting, this can be offset with the use of low dose ketamine [22].

7.5.2 Benzodiazepines

Midazolam is the favored benzodiazepine (BDZ). Midazolam is a clear solution with a $pH = 3.5$ but is unique in that its structure depends on the surrounding pH. With increasing pH, the diazepine ring closes becoming unionized and lipid soluble [23]. Midazolam has the highest clearance (6–10 ml/kg/min) of all the commonly used BDZ and has a reasonable onset/offset profile but considerably slower than propofol. Like other benzodiazepines, midazolam is an agonist at the BZD receptor site (interface between α,γ subunits on the $GABA_A$ receptor) and is a good sedative with excellent amnesic properties but no analgesic action [24]. Flumzenil is a specific antagonist, thereby providing a layer of safety, though it clears faster than midazolam and rebound sedation can occur.

7.5.3 Clonidine and Dexmedetomidine

These drugs are $α_2$ adrenoceptor agonists, possessing potent anxiolytic and sedative actions. These agents stimulate $α_2$ adrenoceptors in the lateral reticular nucleus, so reducing central sympathetic outflow and in the spinal cord promote opioid release thereby modulating the descending noradrenergic pathway involved in spinal nociceptive processing. Clonidine has a relatively slow onset/offset profile with a distribution half-life of 1.2 h and an elimination half-life of 14.6 h. So, if used orally, the dose must be given 30–60 min before surgery. Clonidine at high doses (5 µg/kg orally or 4 µg/kg intravenous) has analgesic properties, does not impair respiration or induce nausea/vomiting [25]. Cardiovascular instability is more common in the elderly.

Dexmedetomidine is up to eight times more potent than clonidine, has a faster onset/offset profile (elimination half-life 2 h), making it more readily titratable. It is much more expensive with concerns being raised regarding hemodynamic instability and associated nausea/vomiting [26].

Both agents impair thermoregulatory mechanisms and can decrease postoperative shivering.

7.5.4 Ketamine

Developed in the 1960s, ketamine, a phencyclidine derivative, is a racemic mixture of S(+) enantiomer, which is two to three times more potent than the R(−) enantiomer. The (S+) enantiomer causes less dysphoria and is the preferred preparation in Europe. S(+) also has a role moderating opioid-induced hyperalgesia. Ketamine is water soluble forming an acidic solution with pH = 3.5–5.5 and is known to act by inhibiting the NMDA receptor in a noncompetitive manner, producing dissociative anesthesia. EEG analysis depicts dissociation between thalamocortical and limbic systems. Outpatient anesthesia has provided the foundation for its resurgence with low dose (0.5–1.0 mg/kg) regimes providing weak sedation but excellent analgesia. Additionally, ketamine's stimulation of the sympathetic nervous system counters the hypotension and respiratory depression associated with propofol [22]. Dose-related nausea/vomiting can be troublesome. Sedative doses of propofol can allay the disturbing dysphorias/hallucinations.

7.5.5 Opioids

Despite techniques employing propofol, ketamine, and clonidine, the author's practice is not devoid of opioids.

From an office-based perspective, remifentanil has provided substantial interest. Remifentanil is a very potent, pure µ agonist with a time-independent context half time (duration of action determined by metabolism not distribution). The elimination half-life is 3–10 min, being metabolized by nonspecific plasma and tissue esterases. This contrasts with alfentanil, sufentanil, and fentanyl all having longer context sensitive half times. Notwithstanding its intense analgesic action, remifentanil is a poor anxiolytic and amnesic [27]. Hemodynamic instability does not seem to be a problem and probably due to its ultrashort duration of action, nausea/vomiting is less common. Perhaps its major drawback in the office setting is the profound respiratory depression this agent induces [28].

7.5.6 Acetaminophen

A para-aminophenol derivative, acetaminophen has no effect on cyclooxygenase in vitro and is a capable antipyretic and analgesic in mild to moderate pain. In Europe, the use of the intravenous preparation is ubiquitous. In an office-based practice, acetaminophen has secured a role through its opioid-sparing effect. Overdose can be fatal as it leads to exhaustion of hepatic glutathione reserves and possible liver failure.

7.5.7 Nonsteroidal Anti-inflammatory Drugs (NSAIDs)

NSAIDs inhibit the enzyme cyclooxygenase (COX). Cyclooxygenase exists as two isoenzymes. COX-1 (the constitutive form) mediates the synthesis of thromboxane, produces prostaglandins controlling renal blood flow, and is instrumental in forming the protective gastric mucosal barrier. Platelets generate thromboxane on exposure to collagen, adenosine, and adrenaline thereby encouraging hemostasis through vasoconstriction and platelet aggregation. COX-2 (the inducible form) is produced where there is tissue damage. It amplifies the inflammatory response yet paradoxically generates prostcyclin (PGI_2) in the vascular endothelium. Prostacyclin causes vasodilatation and inhibits platelet aggregation.

So inhibition of COX-2 may tip the thromboxane/prostacyclin balance in favor of vasoconstriction, platelet aggregation, and thromboembolism.

Amid reports of increased cardiac deaths many of the earlier COX-2 inhibitors have been withdrawn from the market. In the USA, celeoxib survives, whilst in Europe, parecoxib is available intravenously. Mounting concerns have placed a cloud over this whole class of drugs (Table 7.4).

7.5.8 Other Agents

Glycopyrrolate, used for its antisialogogue action, counters the increase in secretions accompanying ketamine usage. Dexamethasone has a dual role as an anti-inflammatory and antiemetic. Ondanestron a $5HT_3$ receptor antagonist, is a powerful antiemetic, and a crucial drug in any rescue strategy. Adrenoceptor agonists/antagonists (epinephrine, ephedrine, metaraminol, labetalol, esmolol) assist in maintaining cardiovascular stability. Rocuronium, a non-depolarizing muscle relaxant, when administered at 25% intubating dose, enables rectus muscle repair while the patient continues to breathe spontaneously.

7.6 Devices Used in the Delivery of Sedation

Currently, there is a difference as to how propofol is delivered between the USA and Europe. The USA predominantly uses manually controlled devices with or without a bolus facility whereas much of Europe has target-controlled infusion (TCI) devices. These TCI pumps deliver propofol in accordance with microprocessor-controlled algorithms, based on pharmacokinetic modeling, aimed at rapidly achieving and maintaining a constant drug concentration in the plasma or at the drug effect site [29]. Continuing research into effect site TCI demonstrates a faster onset and greater predictability of drug action, without adverse hemodynamic consequences [30].

Clinically, the distinction between the two infusion regimes blurs when propofol is titrated with a loss-of-consciousness monitor like BIS.

Table 7.4 Anesthetic agents

Class	Drug	Site of action	Main effect	Role
Sedative/hypnotic	Propofol	CNS β subunit $GABA_A$ Glycine release	Sedation/anesthesia	Principle sedative hypnotic
Benzodiazepines	Midazolam	CNS α/γ subunit $GABA_A$	Anxiolysis/sedation amnesia	Preop anxiolytic amnestic
$α_2$ agonists	Clonidine Dexmedetomodine	CNS/spinal cord $α_2$ adrenoceptors	Anxiolysis/sedation analgesia	Preop anxiolytic Intraop sedation analgesia sparing other agents
Dissociative agent	Ketamine	NMDA receptors	Dissociation/analgesia	Dissociation/analgesia
Opioids	Remifentanil/Fentanyl Alfentanil/Sufentanil	μ receptors	Systemic analgesia	Systemic analgesia
Para-aminophenol derivatives	Acetaminophen	CNS? inhibit prostaglandins via COX-3 (variant COX-1)	Analgesia	Pain relief mild/moderate
NSAIDs	COX inhibition Ketorolac, diclofenac Ibuprofen, naproxen	Cyclooxygenase (COX) inhibition	Analgesia	Pain relief mild/moderate
	COX-2 inhibitors Celecoxib, parecoxib			Analgesia Anti-inflammatory

7.7 Postoperative Nausea and Vomiting (PONV)

Macario's study [3] elegantly showed that fear of PONV is the primary concern of patients. The hallmark of a successful office-based practice resides in the combined efforts of the anesthesiologist and surgeon to eliminate this outcome. Friedberg [31] elegantly showed that using a non-opioid propofol/ketamine technique, the incidence of PONV can be an exceptional, 0.5%.

7.7.1 Risk Factors

A number of studies, including Apfel's [32], highlight the main risk factors: (1) female, (2) young, (3) non-smoker, (4) previous history of PONV and or motion sickness, (5) emetogenic procedure (gynecology, laparoscopic, strabismus, facial surgery, (6) duration 2 h or more, (7) opioid exposure, and (8) volatile anesthetic used.

The preoperative assessment, usually a phone call the day before surgery, is vital in determining the patient's relative risk of PONV and goes a long way to providing reassurance that this issue will be addressed.

Guided by the work of Scuderi and White [33], patients assessed as high risk may benefit by receiving multimodal antiemetic therapy. This focuses on the use of small doses of differing classes of antiemetics so as to target the emesis pathway at different points. Numerous cocktails abound but one which the author has found useful incorporates: droperidol (0.625 mg), dexamethasone 8 mg, given after induction, then granisteron (0.5–1.0 mg) at the conclusion of the procedure.

7.8 Techniques of Sedation

The author has tried all manners of drug combinations with propofol: midazolam, fentanyl, remifentanil, but settled on a simpler non-opioid propofol TCI/midazolam technique.

Deference to such luminaries as Friedberg et al. [34], who have mastered Propofol-Ketamine/BIS/Monitored Anesthetic Care, producing spectacular results, in particular PONV <1%.

In the resource constrained environment in which the author works, sadly, BIS is not readily available, so ketamine is not routinely used. Traditional teaching may question the use of BIS in spontaneously breathing patients, citing the prime validation for BIS coming from the at-risk paralyzed adult surgical population [16]. Infusing propofol by means of target-controlled plasma or effect site concentration counters the interindividual variability in the way propofol is hydrolyzed in the liver [35]. Admittedly, by not using BIS, the ability to distinguish movement as being spinal cord or brain generated is lost. Usually a further injection of local solves the problem; after all the guiding tenet of the whole technique is reliant upon the surgeon providing adequate local analgesia.

The author's reluctance to use ketamine without BIS resides in not knowing that a stable hypnotic level of propofol has been achieved. On the downside, ketamine's effect though relatively short lived, can produce significant cerebral excitation with a concomitant increase in blood pressure and bleeding. Often, this excitation can progress to agitation manifest by additional movement within the surgical field. Table 7.5 outlines the technique.

Table 7.5 Propofol target-controlled infusion (TCI) – Midazolam technique

Clonidine 200 mcg po, 30–60 min prior to surgery (defer if sys BP < 100 mmHg)
Anesthetic room • Monitoring: EKG, NIBP, SpO_2 • Intravenous line with appropriate non-return valve • Midazolam 2–3 mg, Glycopyrrolate 200 mcg • Supplemental oxygen: 2 l/min via nasal prongs
Operating room • Propofol TCI: start with plasma conc (C_p = 2.0 mcg/ml) stepwise increments of 0.5 mcg/ml till stable breathing pattern emerges • Before injection of local anesthesia: bolus = 1.0–1.5 mcg/ml expect some movement • Basal C_p = 2.5–3.5 mcg/ml
Prophylactic antibiotics, antiemetics (if high risk), Dexamethasone = 8 mg
Acetaminophen 1 g (intravenously 20 min before end procedure)
Levobupivacaine 0.25% to field (topical or via drains)

7.9 Conclusions

A successful office-based practice is reliant on Propofol Intravenous Anesthesia, avoidance of opioids, minimal airway intervention and enlightened use of local analgesia. Undoubtedly, level-of-consciousness monitoring provides further assurance, making the use of ketamine a more realistic proposition however, with vigilance and attention to detail, a simple and safe technique, as described does afford excellent outcomes for all concerned.

References

1. Chilvers CR, Nguyen MH, Robertson IK. Changing from epidural to multimodal analgesia for colorectal laparotomy: an audit. Anaesth Intensive Care. 2007;35(2):230–8.
2. Friedberg BL. Propofol-ketamine technique, dissociative anesthesia for office surgery: a five-year review of 1, 264 cases. Aesthetic Plast Surg. 1999;23(1):70–5.
3. Macario A, Weinger M, Carney K, Kim A. Which clinical anesthesia outcomes are important to avoid? The perspective of patients. Anesth Analg. 1999;89(3):652–8.
4. Practice Guidelines for Sedation and Analgesia by Non-Anesthesiologists. An updated report by the American Society of Anesthesiologists Task Force on Sedation and Analgesia by Non-anesthesiologists. Anesthesiology. 2002;96(4):1004–17.
5. Mingus ML, Monk TG, Gold MI, Jenkins W, Roland C. Remifentanil versus propofol as adjuncts to regional anaesthesia. J Clin Anesth. 1998;10(1):46–53.
6. Servin F, Desmonts JM, Watkins WD. Remifentanil as an analgesic adjunct in local/regional anaesthesia and in monitored anaesthesia care. Anesth Analg. 1999;89(4 Suppl): S28–32.
7. Martinez-Telleria A, Cano ME, Carlos R. Paradoxical reaction to midazolam after its use as a sedative in regional anaesthesia. Rev Esp Anestesiol Reanim. 1992;39(6): 379–80.
8. Schnider TW, Minto CF, Shafer SL, Gambus PL, Andresen C, Goodale DB, et al. The influence of age on propofol pharmacodynamics. Anesthesiology. 1999;90(6):1502–16.
9. Holas A, Kraft P, Marcovic M, Quehenberger F. Remifentanil, propofol or both for conscious sedation during eye surgery under regional anaesthesia. Eur J Anaesthesiol. 1999;16(11): 741–8.
10. Sharma VK, Galli W, Haber H, Pressman MR, Stevenson R, Meyer TJ, et al. Unexpected risks during administration of conscious sedation: previously undiagnosed obstructive sleep apnea. Ann Intern Med. 2003;139(8):707–8.
11. Chernik DA, Gillings D, Laine H, Hendler J, Silver JM, Davidson AB, et al. Validity and reliability of the observer's assessment of alertness/sedation scale: study with intravenous midazolam. J Clin Psychopharmacol. 1990;10(4):244–51.
12. Leslie K, Sessler DI, Schroeder M, Walters K. Propofol blood concentration and the bispectral index predicts suppression of learning during propofol/epidural anesthesia in volunteers. Anesth Analg. 1995;81(16):1269–74.
13. Liu J, Singh H, White PF. Electroencephalographic bispectral analysis predicts the depth of midazolam-induced sedation. Anesthesiology. 1996;84(1):64–9.
14. Liu J, Singh H, White PF. Electroencephalographic bispectral index correlates with intraoperative recall and depth of propofol-induced sedation. Anesth Analg. 1997;84(1): 185–9.
15. Gan TJ, Glass PS, Windsor A, Payne F, Rosow C, Sebel P, et al. Bispectral index monitoring allows faster emergence and improved recovery form propofol, alfentanil, and nitrous oxide anesthesia. Anesthesiology. 1997;87(4):808–15.
16. Myles PS, Leslie K, McNeil J, Forbes A, Chan MT. Bispectral index monitoring to prevent awareness during anaesthesia: the B-Aware randomised trial. Lancet. 2004;363(9423):1757–63.
17. Struys M, Verisichelen L, Mortier E, Ryckaert D, De Mey JC, de Deyne C, et al. Comparison of spontaneous frontal EMG, EEG power spectrum and bispectral index to monitor propofol effect and emergence. Acta Anaesthesiol Scand. 1998;42(6):628–36.
18. Bruhn J, Ropcke H, Hoeft A. Approximate entropy as an electroencephalographic measure of anesthetic drug effect during desflurane anesthesia. Anesthesiology. 2000;92(3): 715–26.
19. Bruhn J, Lehmann LE, Ropcke H, Bouillon TW, Hoeft A. Shannon entropy applied to the electoencephalographic effects of desflurane. Anesthesiology. 2001;95(1):30–5.
20. Vanluchene AL, Struys MM, Heyse BE, Mortier EP. Spectral entropy measurement of patient responsiveness during propofol and remifentanil comparison bispectral index. Br J Anaesth. 2004;93(5):645–54.
21. Smith I, Monk TG, White PF, Ding Y. Propofol infusion during regional anaesthesia: sedative, amnestic, and anxiolytic properties. Anesth Analg. 1994;79(2):313–9.
22. Frizelle HP, Duranteau J, Samii K. A comparison of propofol with a propofol-ketamine combination for sedation during spinal anaesthesia. Anesth Analg. 1997;84(6):1318–22.
23. Peck TE, Hill SA, Williams M. Pharmacology for anaesthesia and intensive care. 3rd ed. Cambridge: Cambridge University Press; 2008.
24. de Andres J, Bolinches R. Comparative study of propofol and midazolam for sedation in regional anaesthesia. Rev Esp Anestesiol Reanim. 1993;40(6):354–9.
25. Hall JE, Uhrich TD, Ebert TJ. Sedative, analgesic and cognitive effects of clonidine infusions in humans. Br J Anaesth. 2001;86(1):5–12.
26. Bhana N, Goa KL, McClellan KJ. Dexmedetomidine. Drugs. 2000;59(2):263–8.
27. Lauwers MH, Vanlersberghe C, Camu F. Comparison of remifentanil and propofol infusions for sedation during regional anaesthesia. Reg Anesth Pain Med. 1998;23(1): 64–70.
28. Murdoch JA, Hyde RA, Kenny GN. Target-controlled remifentanil in combination with propofol for spontaneously breathing day-case patients. Anaesthesia. 1999;54(11): 1028–31.
29. Shafer SL, Gregg KM. Algorithms to rapidly achieve and maintain stable drug concentrations at the site of drug effect with a computer-controlled infusion pump. J Pharmakinet Biopharm. 1992;20(2):147–69.
30. Struys MM, De Smet T, Depoorter B, Versichelen LF, Mortier EP, Deneve N, et al. Comparison of plasma

compartment versus two methods for effect compartment-controlled target-controlled infusion for propofol. Anesthesiology. 2000;92:399–406.
31. Friedberg BL. Propofol ketamine anesthesia for cosmetic surgery in the office suite. Anesthesia for outside the operating room. Int Anesthesiol Clin. 2003;41(2):39–50.
32. Apfel CC, Kortilla K, Abdalla M, Kerger H, Turan A, Vedder I, et al. A factorial trial of six interventions for the prevention of PONV. N Engl J Med. 2004;350:2441.
33. Scuderi P, James R, Harris L, Mims III GR. Multimodal antiemetic management prevents early postoperative vomiting after outpatient laparoscopy. Anesth Analg. 2000;91(6): 1408–14.
34. Freidberg BL. Anesthesia in cosmetic surgery. Cambridge: Cambridge University Press; 2007.
35. Court MH, Duan SX, Hesse LM, Venkatakrishnan K, Greenblatt DJ. Cytochrome P-450 2B6 is responsible for interindividual variability of propofol hydroxylation by the human liver. Anesthesiology. 2001;94(1):110–9.

Part III
Preoperative and Postoperative

Preoperative and Postoperative Plan

Anthony Erian and Ben Pocock

8.1 Plan for Facelift Surgery

1. Preoperative Assessment
   During the initial visit, a consultation form is created by the authors and is used to thoroughly address each point of the first encounter with our client (Table 8.1).

2. Assessment of the Degree of Suitability for Surgery
   Once the initial consultation has been performed, the patient's degree of suitability for surgery is assessed. Patients lie within one of three categories:
   (A) Not suitable
   (B) Suitable, once certain conditions have been met
   (C) Suitable

3. Assessment of the Biological Suitability for Surgery
   Various preoperative tests need to be performed in order that patients can safely undergo surgery. This list serves as an example of which tests may be requested preoperatively as each client will have different tests depending on their individual medical history [1–3].
   Baseline Study
   (A) Blood tests, such as kidney function, hemoglobin, and clotting factors
   (B) Urinalysis
   (C) Electrocardiogram
   (D) Report from general practitioner or family doctor

4. Analysis of Anatomy
   During this stage of the assessment, the patient's face is analyzed in detail, with the aid of photography. Particular note is made of deficiencies, asymmetries, and abnormalities such as scars. Preoperative photography is valuable in further defining this facial assessment, as well as being extremely useful for medicolegal purposes [4–6]. As well as the photographs, notes are made in the patient's chart on standard diagrams (Fig. 8.1).

5. Discussion of Surgery
   For those patients felt to be suitable for surgery, a full consultation is conducted and the patient is asked what exactly is bothering them with their face and after we agree in principle on the procedure, whether it is surgical or nonsurgical, the procedure is discussed in detail together with the possible complications and show them some examples of pre- and postoperative cases of similar age and deformity for them to get an idea of the likely outcome of surgery [7–10]. The mental state is assessed, as the authors consider patients not suitable if:
   (A) They have unrealistic expectations of surgery.
   (B) Suffer from any mental condition, whether it is depression or body dismorphophobia or a body image problem, they should be excluded from surgery.
   (C) Very aggressive patients who seem angry about something not related to the surgery.
   (D) The deformity is so minute and the patient magnifies its significance and its magnitude. Remember, a millimeter on the face is a mile on the brain in the thinking of those patients.
   (E) Patients with relationship difficulties and depression must not undergo surgery until they are stable.

A. Erian (✉) and B. Pocock
Pear Tree Cottage, Cambridge Road,
Wimpole 43, SG8 5QD Cambridge, United Kingdom
e-mail: plasticsurgeon@anthonyerian.com

Table 8.1 Consultation form for preoperative assessment

MR ERIAN
CONSULTATION REPORT

Consultation Date ....

Ref by ....

Tel. No ....

Patents Details:-

Forename/s ....

Surname ....

Address ....

Date of Birth ....

Sex ....

Tel. No ....

Patient's GP:-

Name ....

Address ....

....

....

Procedure/Interest..

History of Present Complaint............................

....

Previous Surgery and Medical Illness...............

Previous Mental Problems.................................

....

Family History:

Husband/Wife..

Children..

Work...

Social..

Family/Friends...

Patient's Hope & Expectations of Surgery ....

....

....

....

General History :-

Smoking .... Drinking ....

Pill ....

Drugs/Medications...

Allergies ....

Previous Anesthetic ....

(continued)

Table 8.1 (continued)

Examination and General Description...	
Specific Description of Relevant Areas	
....	
General Examination :	
BP ....H.S ....Pulse ....CVS	
Chest ....Abdomen	
My Opinion/Comments	
Patient is (A) Good Candidate	
(B) Suitable with Reservations	
(C) Poor Candidate and Surgery not indicated	
Operation Recommended :	
Clinic .... No. of Nights .... Type	
Anesthetic	
Date .... Time to Report .... Last	
Food/Liquid	
Special Instructions to Patient	
....	
Signature	
I agree to your contacting my GP and for him to provide you with details of my medical history.	
Signed	
Date	
I do not wish you to contact my GP	
Signed	
Date	

(F) Heavy smokers with long-term damage as a result of nicotine should be excluded and the surgeon should point out the increased risk of bleeding necrosis and infection [11].

(G) Patients with medical conditions that interfere with the anesthetics should be considered carefully and their medication should be reviewed by a physician prior to undergoing surgery [1, 3, 8].

(H) Patients with infectious diseases and sexually transmitted diseases are counseled carefully prior to surgery.

Careful examination is conducted in the presence of a chaperone to identify the clinical problems with the consent of the patient.

Further discussion is carried out. A copy of the consent is given to the patient and this is discussed in detail. During the 2 weeks before surgery which we consider the minimum time to allow clients to reflect on surgery, the patient has time to read this copy of the consent, so that any remaining questions may be answered before the form is signed. As well as discussing consent, the type of anesthesia, the dressings, and the likely postoperative course are discussed.

8.2 Facelift Preoperative Instructions

Before surgery, patients receive a copy of the preoperative instructions. This allows patients to have time to read this information at least 2 weeks before surgery, as well as giving them time to follow the instructions.

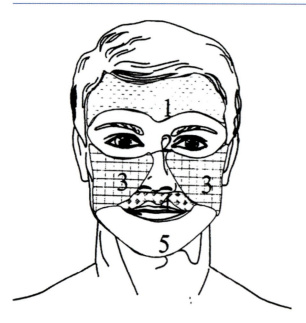

Fig. 8.1 Standard diagram for patient analysis. *1* – Brow, *2* – peri-orbital (eye area), *3* – cheek, *4* – upper lip, *5* – chin and jowl area

Along with this, patients also receive a copy of the postoperative instructions and the consent form, so that they may be fully informed and prepared for the operation.

The authors have found that preoperative instructions are best presented in the form of a list. This allows patients to more easily understand the instructions, as they are able to go through the list item by item. As patients have a copy of this at hand, they may even use the list to check off items as they have understood and completed them.

Preoperative Instructions

(A) Your facelift will be performed under twilight anesthesia (intravenous sedation and injection of local anesthetic solution into the tissues). You will not have general anesthesia, and the twilight technique will allow for a speedier recovery. Because you will not have general anesthesia, you will not have many of the side effects such as a sore throat or significant nausea and vomiting. Though you will not remember, the intravenous sedation allows you to obey commands during the operation, which is important, for example, in turning your head. Because the muscles are not completely paralyzed, the surgery is safer, since nerves can be tested and thereby are less likely to be injured. Due to the large amount of local anesthetic put into the tissues during the operation, there will be very little pain when waking up in the recovery room, and this also helps in a speedier recovery [1, 10, 12, 13].

(B) Please bring with you a pair of sunglasses, a headscarf, and/or a hat to wear upon discharge. This is for your comfort. In addition, plan to wear shirts that open at the front and do not require being pulled over your head [3, 14].

(C) Please do not wear any makeup, lotions, or creams on the day of your surgery. Wash your hair and face on the morning of the operation.

(D) Do not take aspirin or other medicines that may thin your blood, and thus lead to bleeding and bruising complications, for 1 week before your surgery. This includes vitamin E and other herbal/nonmedical preparations, as well as alcohol consumption, which can lead to excessive bruising and bleeding. Please ask the surgeon if you are unsure of what not to take. If you take medicines such as warfarin in order to thin your blood, please consult with the surgeon in order that this is managed properly [3, 15].

(E) Within the week before your operation, do not have you hair bleached, tinted, colored, or permed, as this may affect the skin on your scalp. You will be able to have your hair treated again 6 weeks after surgery, as fresh scars can be sensitive to chemicals used in treating hair.

(F) Do not have your hair cut before surgery. During surgery, your hair will not be cut, and will eventually cover the incisions of your operation. It may be better to have longer hair as this can cover up the scars. There will be postoperative instructions about when you will be able to wash your hair after the operation.

(G) Please write down any questions you may have thought about since the consultation and you will be able to ask these on the day of your operation.

(H) Please expect to stay in the hospital overnight and arrange for someone to pick you up the next day. You will not be able to drive, and a responsible adult will need to come pick you up. For the first few days following surgery, it may be useful to have someone to help you with everyday activities.

(I) If you smoke, please avoid smoking for as long as possible, but for at least 2 weeks before the operation. The longer you give up smoking the better. Smoking reduces the amount of oxygen in the blood which is likely to cause problems with wound healing [11].

Postoperative Instructions

(A) You will experience swelling of the face, as well as some bruising which may extend into the neck and chest. This is normal and may take 2–3 weeks to disappear completely. Swelling may make your face feel tight. Over the first 3 days, you may apply ice packs (or bags of frozen vegetables, such as peas, covered with a cloth) to your cheeks for about 20 min every hour. Flannels kept in the fridge are also useful as they can be applied directly to the face [3, 14].

(B) Rarely, drains, which are small plastic tubes to allow fluid to escape from the surgery, may be placed at the time of surgery. These will be removed the day after surgery, before you go home [16].

(C) You will feel drowsy following surgery. It is normal to wake up and doze off during the first day.

(D) Eat a diet consisting of soft food for the first 3 days. You will find it difficult to eat food that requires much chewing. Soups and yoghurts are good examples of soft foods. Drinking fluids through a straw is useful as you do not have to open your mouth too widely.

(E) You may wash your hair 3 days after surgery. It is important that the incisions remain dry for 48 h. Do not have a bath for 1 week after surgery.

(F) You should avoid lying flat, and when sleeping, you should be propped up with several pillows. This helps reduce swelling, by allowing gravity to remove fluid from the face. You may, for example, try two pillows under the head and one under the shoulders.

(G) Limit your activities for 2 weeks after surgery, especially bending, straining, and lifting. During the first 2 weeks, activities such as light house work and gentle walking are fine. Avoid excessive head-turning and any physical exertion. Movements such as these will place strain on the incisions and may cause them to stretch and widen. You may resume activities such as jogging 1 month after surgery [3, 14].

(H) You may return to work when you feel able, though many people allow 2 weeks as most of the bruising and swelling will have disappeared by then.

(I) Please take any medicine that has been prescribed, such as pain killers. If you should have pain that is not relived by the pain killers, please call the surgeon. Do not take aspirin or other medicines that may thin your blood or cause bruising for 1 week after surgery.

(J) The day after surgery, before you are discharged to go home, the surgeon will change your dressings and check the incisions. After you go home, you may remove the dressings in 3 days [17] (Fig. 8.2).

(K) If you should see bleeding coming through the bandages, please call immediately. You will be given the phone numbers of the surgeon, the

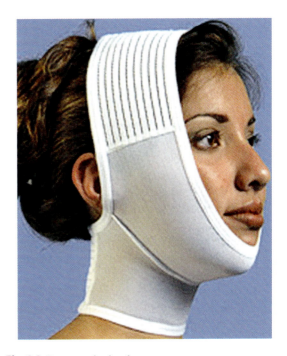

Fig. 8.2 Postoperative bandage

surgeon's assistant, and the hospital, should you have any questions. Please do not hesitate to call at any time. In addition, please call if your pain should continue to get worse or if you should experience a fever [17, 18].

(L) Please do not take alcohol for 1 week after surgery.

(M) Please completely avoid the sun for 3 weeks after surgery as this can increase swelling. After these 3 weeks, please use sun block daily (at least SPF 15) and wear a protective hat. These things are good for your skin in general, as well as to help the healing process after your facelift.

(N) You may have a facial and/or have you hair bleached, tinted, colored, or permed 6 weeks after surgery.

(O) You should expect to return to see the surgeon about 1 week after surgery for a postoperative visit. During this first week, it is usually a good idea to take time off work. At this postoperative visit, as well as inspecting the face and incisions, the surgeon will remove any stitches and skin staples. After this visit, you will also be asked to come see the surgeon after about 6 weeks, to once again check your face and the incisions. If everything is healing well at this point, you may be asked to return for another postoperative visit in several months to 1 year's time for a long-term follow-up.

(P) You may use makeup 1 week after surgery, though there are specialized, medical makeup preparations which may be used immediately once the dressings are removed.

(Q) If you smoke, please try to avoid smoking for as long as possible, but for at least 2 weeks. The longer you can avoid smoking, the better it is for the healing process [11].

(R) For men, because parts of the face may remain numb for the first few weeks, we recommend using an electric razor for shaving. This reduces the chance for cutting the skin and bleeding while wet-shaving.

(S) The final result of the surgery will be evident from about 6–9 months after the operation. By this time, the scars will have softened and faded.

(T) If you also had eye bag surgery to the upper eyelid, you will have that stitch removed at your 1 week postoperative visit. If you had lower eye bag surgery, you may or may not have an incision where stitches will be removed. During this first week, you will be using antibiotic eye drops to lessen the sensation that here is something in your eye and to prevent a very small risk of infection. Your eyes may feel watery. You may wear sunglasses during this time, but you should be careful not to injure the facelift incision near the ear. Normal postoperative swelling and bruising to the upper and lower eyelid areas may take several weeks to resolve completely. During this time, it may also feel tight when closing your eyes. After 2 weeks, you may massage the lower eyelid area with a gentle but firm upward movement. Please do not wear contact lenses for 2 weeks following surgery. Though a dramatic result can be appreciated within the first few weeks, the final result will take about 6–9 months [19–21].

(U) If you had liposuction to the neck, you will notice a very small 2 mm-long incision just under the chin. This will heal without stitches. The dressings used for your facelift incorporate the liposuction area of the neck as well. Normal postoperative swelling and bruising will take several weeks to resolve completely. Over the course of several weeks to months, not only has fat been removed at the time of surgery, but the skin of the neck will progressively tighten and marked improvement will continue to occur. You may perform gentle but firm massage in an upward direction, to both sides of the neck, 2 weeks after your operation [1, 19, 22].

References

1. Stuzin JM. MOC-PSSM CME article: face lifting. Plast Reconstr Surg. 2008;121 Suppl 1:1–19.
2. Chrisman BB. The facelift. J Dermatol Surg Oncol. 1989; 15(8):812–22.
3. Spencer KW. Patient education materials for facelifts and blepharoplasty. Plast Surg Nurs. 1995;15(1):45–7.
4. Henderson JL, Larrabee Jr WF, Krieger BD. Photographic standards for facial plastic surgery. Arch Facial Plast Surg. 2005;7(5):331–3.
5. Marten TJ. High SMAS facelift: combined single flap lifting of the jawline, cheek, and midface. Clin Plast Surg. 2008;35(4):569–603.

6. Terino EO, Edward M. The magic of mid-face three-dimensional contour alterations combining alloplastic and soft tissue suspension technologies. Clin Plast Surg. 2008; 35(3): 419–50; discussion 417.
7. Marten TJ. Facelift. Planning and technique. Clin Plast Surg. 1997;24(2):269–308.
8. Ho T, Brissett AE. Preoperative assessment of the aging patient. Facial Plast Surg. 2006;22(2):85–90.
9. Turpin IM. The modern rhytidectomy. Clin Plast Surg. 1992;19(2):383–400.
10. Tobin HA, Cuzalina A, Tharanon W, Sinn DP. The biplane facelift: an opportunistic approach. J Oral Maxillofac Surg. 2000;58(1):76–85.
11. Ayalp TR. Topical tretinoin and smokers' face lifts. Plast Reconstr Surg. 1998;102(4):1294.
12. Adamson PA, Litner JA. Surgical management of the aging neck. Facial Plast Surg. 2005;21(1):11–20.
13. Kamer FM, Mingrone MD. Deep plane rhytidectomy: a personal evolution. Facial Plast Surg Clin N Am. 2005;13(1): 115–26.
14. Mottura AA. Face lift postoperative recovery. Aesthetic Plast Surg. 2002;26(3):172–80.
15. Destro MW, Speranzini MB, Cavalheiro Filho C, Destro T, Destro C. Bilateral haematoma after rhytidoplasty and blepharoplasty following chronic use of Ginkgo biloba. Br J Plast Surg. 2005;58(1):100–1.
16. Perkins SW, Willaims JD, Macdonald K, Robinson EB. Prevention of seromas and hematomas after face-lift surgery with the use of postoperative vacuum drains. Arch Otolaryngol Head Neck Surg. 1997;123(7):743–5.
17. Teimourian B, Mankani M, Stefan M. A new dressing technique to minimize ecchymoses following face lifts. Plast Reconstr Surg. 1995;96(1):222–3.
18. Basile AR, Basile FV. Transparent dressing for rhytidectomy. Aesthetic Plast Surg. 2001;25(6):454–6.
19. Rohrich RJ, Ghavami A, Lemmon JA, Brown SA. The individualized component face lift: developing a systematic approach to facial rejuvenation. Plast Reconstr Surg. 2009; 123(3):1050–63.
20. Hoefflin SM. Surgical pearls in the management of the aging face from A to Z. Dermatol Clin. 1997;15(4):679–85.
21. Ramirez OM. Classification of facial rejuvenation techniques based on the subperiosteal approach and ancillary procedures. Plast Reconstr Surg. 1996;97(1):45–55.
22. Springer RC. Rhytidectomy: from consultation to recovery. Plast Surg Nurs. 1996;16(1):27–30.

Facial Imaging

John Flynn

9.1 Introduction

There are many variations of the theme of facial imaging and in this chapter the author endeavors to present some of the applications of imaging and some of the pitfalls. One could easily envisage that a chapter with this title will be focussed on photography, especially in the context of a text on facial rejuvenation. In fact this is indeed the case, but there is a wider dimension to straightforward photography. There is a need to consider elements beyond before and after photographs. This would include problems of photo storage and retrieval, issues of privacy and copyright. Consent of the subject to the capture of their image and the subsequent display of that image is an issue often neglected or at least discounted by many practitioners.

The author will try to focus on practical issues and identify problems pertinent to an active clinical esthetic practice. There are many publications which cover in great detail photo-optics, light physics, and tips on taking a great photo. F-stops, aperture, shutter speed do not feature significantly in this chapter.

9.2 The Camera

Digital photography has overwhelmed the print/film version of the art, certainly in the realm of a clinical practice. The choice of camera comes down to digital SLR and the compact digital pocket version.

The digital SLR style owes much to its film version predecessor. This camera allows a great deal of manipulation of variables. The value is of course great flexibility in taking the photo with the right exposure and depth of focus, the challenge however is becoming a master of that very flexibility. There is clearly going to be more onus on the operator. Luckily, most of the newer ones still have a fully automatic function.

Great examples of digital SLR cameras are Nikon and Canon. If, however, you are like me and prefer the "point and shoot" variety then the compact fully automatic digital is worth looking at. There is a plethora of brands and degrees of complexity and sophistication from which to choose (Figs. 9.1 and 9.2).

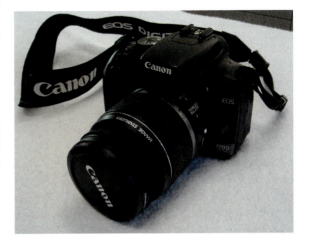

Fig. 9.1 A digital SLR camera with automatic function but also fully selectable for shutter speed, aperture, F stop, and the rest. Most of these cameras also have an interchangeable lens capacity and produce an excellent image

J. Flynn
Cosmetic and Skin Clinic, Suite 1, Level 1, 98 Marine Parade, Southport, Queensland 4215, Australia
e-mail: drflynn@cosmedic.com.au

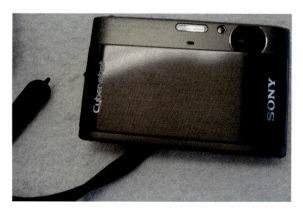

Fig. 9.2 Compact fully automated digital camera. "Point and shoot" camera style

> **Practical Tips**
>
> Digital SLR
>   Be aware of the physical size of the unit. Larger cameras are more trouble to move around. Purchase a good tripod for steady shots. To get best use out of this style of camera it is best to have a dedicated photography space.
>
> Compact Automatic
>   Great if you have to move between clinics, easily transportable. Purchase an extra battery. This is more important than a bigger memory card. Carry a charging unit with you just in case.

9.3 Resolution

Camera resolution is a commonly used selling point with digital cameras. As a general rule the higher the number of pixels the better the resolution and therefore the better the reproduction of the photograph. With more pixels though comes a higher cost of the camera. So how much is enough?

Most often 3 or 4 megapixels is sufficient for most purposes. Used at the highest resolution, each camera has sufficient space on its file storage for up to a hundred or so pictures. If one reduces the resolution on the camera often one can achieve storage of several hundred images. When photos are used only for the clinical record then such an approach is acceptable. However, there are pitfalls if you wish to publish the photos in a journal or if you wish to enlarge them significantly to display a particular feature or simply use a larger screen.

A digital photo of only, say 100 KB, might be very well reproduced on your laptop or office PC. However, if you wish to use that photo projected onto a large screen then the resolution is too poor to display the features properly. In my view, aim for a photo size of 500 KB to 1 MB, this will give the best flexibility. If you take a full face photo and need to display, for example, eyelashes, then you will need a photo size of perhaps 2 MB.

The common concern with many practitioners is the size of the storage files necessary to accommodate very high resolution photos in the numbers pertaining to most busy practices. This is a valid concern but the cost of digital storage is coming down quickly and by considerable margins. However, if your requirement is only your own clinical record, then a lower-resolution photo is acceptable (3–4 megapixel camera). But, if you have an interest in education, presentations, publishing, then invest in a high-resolution camera (anything above 6 is fine).

> **Practical Tips on Resolution**
>
> For clinical records a 3–4 megapixel camera is usually sufficient and will cost almost half the amount of a 8–10 megapixel camera.
>
>   Zoom capacity is very useful. Optical zoom is better than digital zoom. Look for a minimum of ×3 optical zoom. This is common to most cameras. If you can get ×5 optical zoom, then this is about all you should need.
>
>   Macro function is important. Some cameras have an extra close setting called "macro magnifying glass."
>
>   When sending photos via email, your computer program might automatically reduce the resolution for faster transfer. You need to be aware of this because the quality at the other end might not be suitable for the intended purpose.

9.4 Lighting

In the author's view, lighting is the key element to get right to display the subject well and honestly. Paying proper attention to this aspect will improve your photos greatly.

There are a number of lighting options available and the most common is the camera mounted flash. In the compact automatic camera, the flash is front mounted

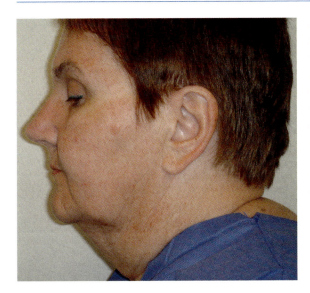

Fig. 9.3 Front mounted flash with compact automatic camera showing shadowing on the background. This also obscures the features and outline of the subject

and therefore strikes the target in a unidirectional mode but also a divergent light stream. Although this produces a well lit surface, there is an increased difficulty with shadowing against the background screen (Fig. 9.3). Poor selection of exposure can easily "wash out" the features of the subject and this type of flash can make a face "flatter" because of the flooding unidirectional light.

The SLR type of camera also comes with an inbuilt camera mounted flash but most also have the capacity for mounting an extra flash. In this circumstance there is an advantage to use a ring flash. As the name suggests, the shape of the flash bulb is a ring which produces a softer and more dispersed light source. Effectively, there are multiple points of light emission and each with a divergent character, and as there is considerable crossover of the light streams, a more diffuse end result is achieved. This gives a more even lighting of the subject and often will decrease the shadowing problems.

In the author's view the best lighting is achieved by high levels of ambient light. In practice, almost always the ambient light comes from above the subject unless one has a dedicated photographic booth. In a booth situation one can place directional flash points from below as well. Most clinicians do not have the available space to dedicate to a properly set up photographic studio with properly placed and coordinated multiple flash points. Additionally, most clinicians will visit different venues and will not have consistent ambient conditions for photography.

The best ambient light is fluorescent with predominance in shorter wavelengths giving a brighter "clean" light. Halogen lights also have a blue predominance and give a good light. Incandescent lamps, commercially available in most buildings, have a predominance of slightly longer wavelengths and give a more yellow light. This is often referred to as a "warm light." Camera flashes are generally a very bright "clean," light with a predominance of shorter wavelengths.

Direct camera flash can "wash out" the finer details on the subject (Fig. 9.4). This is particularly in a facial

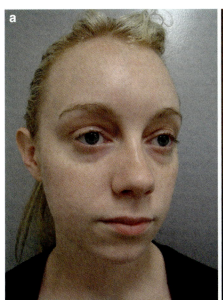
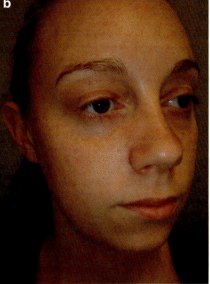

Fig. 9.4 Direct flash can wash out the finer details on a subject. Over exposure will efface the photos hiding natural contours and texture. Note also the differences in color and texture between flash and no flash. (**a**) No flash. (**b**) Same distance with flash

procedure where it is important to show this detail. Especially when the procedure involves improvement of skin texture and complexion these fine details of the skin are important to demonstrate in before and after photographs. Figure 9.5 shows a series of photographs taken at the same sitting, using the same camera and subject. Only the lighting elements have varied. In the first photo taken on a compact automatic, no flash was used. In this photo the color elements are softer because when using only ambient light there is a very diffuse light source. Fine details can be picked up quite easily. Because the light is largely from above, the shadowing in the acne scars is not washed out and provides the contrast necessary to display this feature. From the same position in using the automatic flash the colors are "warmer," that is, more red and yellow on display. This is primarily because the greater amount of light flooding the subject alters the reflection of wavelengths differently and so the camera "sees" more intense color. The problem with this photo is that the flash is reflected quite strongly from the convexity of the malar eminence and almost completely washes out the detail here. The side of the cheek fares better in displaying the acne scars but also the fine shadowing seen in the earlier shot tends to obscure the detail of the acne scarring. Using the same camera and flash, but this time the camera is positioned at one meter and the camera zoom lens is used to create the same framing, the warmer colors are retained and there is more even distribution of light. Still, however, the malar eminence reflects more and does not achieve quite the same detail as the first "no flash" photo.

Why should the camera distance make any significant distance at all? After all light travels in straight lines and is so incredibly fast. All true, but the light from the flash is unidirectional but also divergent and so the intensity of the projected flash diminishes exponentially with distance traveled. So, one can make adjustments for the ambient conditions in varying locations by experimenting with both "flash" or "no flash" and with distance from the subject. There is a limit to this aspect of things though which you will find out in a less clinical setting particularly at night. When used with a flash, the camera also automatically selects a different aperture and shutter speed. If your subject is more than 3 m (10 ft) away then your subject will be almost fully blacked out. Try taking the same shot with the flash off; you might be surprised how well the photo turns out. Remember though the shutter speed is also slower and you need a steady hand.

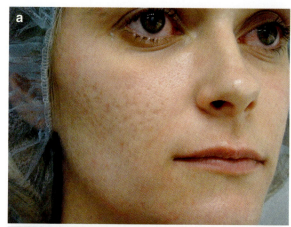

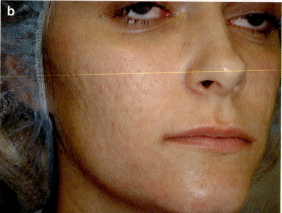

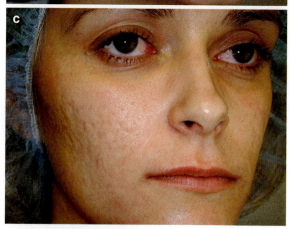

Fig. 9.5 Do not use flash. The "low light" mechanism of the camera will compensate to produce a good quality image with good exposure. (**a**) Compact automatic, no flash, set on macro, camera distance 300 mm. (**b**) Compact automatic, with flash, set on macro, camera distance 300 mm. note some loss of detail and washed out appearance of the malar eminence. (**c**) Compact automatic, with flash, camera distance 1,000 mm and using camera zoom to get a similar framing. Note that the malar eminence is still a little washed out but not as much as the earlier photo. From a purely photographic perspective the subject has more color definition and the end result is a "warmer" image

9 Facial Imaging

> **Practical Tips**
>
> With flash, stand further away and use the zoom capacity of the camera to get the close up view. With good ambient lighting, do not use flash. Most cameras have a "low light compensation," which will still give you a good quality image even when ambient lighting is low.

9.5 Background

The important aspect of clinical photography is to display the subject matter clearly. In very close up shots, the image fills the entire field and so background issues are not as important. With a more distant facial shot the background presents some issues. Too much clutter in the background distracts from the subject (Fig. 9.6).

> **Practical Tips**
>
> Doors and walls provide good blank backgrounds. Avoid a highly reflective background. Avoid window and door frames and watch for door handles. Plain curtains provide good background. Dull plain colors work best: mid-blue, burgundy, grey, and beige.

9.6 Advertising and Ethics

A discussion of advertising and ethics is not out of place in a chapter on facial imaging. The images we generate in our practices, although essential for our own records and our own professional monitoring of results, are often used as marketing tools to attract potential customers. To avoid privacy problems, certain clothes and jewelry that may identify the patient should not be photographed (Fig. 9.7). We have all seen advertising which feature "Before and After" photographs. Such advertising of itself is not out of place and can be a very useful method of conveying accurate information to patients. Used in this manner photographs are a valuable resource. However, the pictorial display needs to be honest and accurate. If not, then it is simply misleading and preys on patient vulnerabilities.

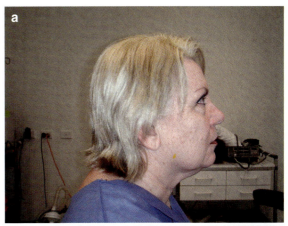
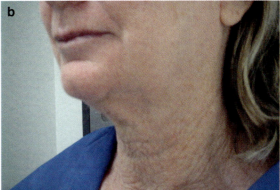
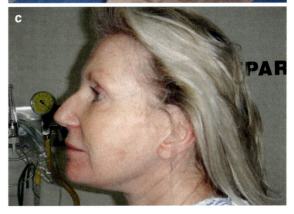

Fig. 9.6 (**a**) A generally cluttered background provides distractions. (**b**) The appearance of straight lines in the background of this photo is a particular concern. (**c**) Sometimes the camera is focused on a particular point in the background and so the subject becomes blurred

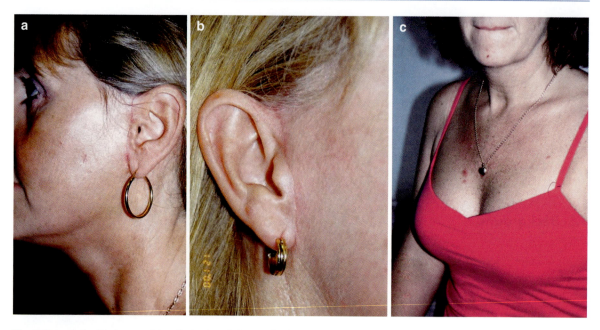

Fig. 9.7 (**a–c**) Avoid photographing distinctive clothes and/or jewellery. Such items could allow identification of the subject

9.7 Before and After Photos

The accuracy and honesty of "Before and Afters" is so important. We want to be able to display our results in an honest and informative fashion. We should not be engaging in cosmetic photography rather than showing off the results of our cosmetic practice. There is nothing wrong with presenting good flattering photographs of patients but we must make a distinction between the great "glamour shot" and the genuine results of our treatments.

The author adheres to a Code of Practice for Advertising which includes Before and After photographs. This is essential for a number of reasons, not the least of which is just simple accuracy and honesty. There are a number of jurisdictions in the world where the Regulatory Authorities are very much against advertising cosmetic procedures because of the inaccuracy often portrayed. This is often considered to influence patients to have a procedure by suggesting better results than what may realistically be obtained.

If the subject of these photos (Fig. 9.8) was to advertise the value of say microdermabrasion (which the patient genuinely has had) then this would be very misleading since the photos also demonstrate the result after microdermabrasion, thread lifting, and fillers to lips. Then consider that the pose, lighting, hair, and makeup differences and it can easily be seen how patients might have the wrong impression of the potential results from microdermabrasion.

Reproduced below is the section of the Code of Practice for the Australasian College of Cosmetic Surgery dealing with Advertising, and I believe it provides an excellent template from which to consider one's approach to advertising and photography.

ACCS Code of Practice Section 2

(Full code available at www.accs.org.au and hit the icon on the Home Page).

2. Advertising and promotion.
2.1 Advertising must not contain false, misleading or deceptive statements, or create misleading impressions about the doctor or clinic or the services offered. It should provide balanced information on the procedures or products advertised and should not suggest these are risk free. Critical omissions can also be misleading.
2.2 Members must not mislead consumers about the need for any procedure.
2.3 Superlatives should not be used in any advertising unless they can be readily proven to be correct and as such are not misleading. For example,

Fig. 9.8 (**a**) Before. (**b**) After. Photographs need a similar pose and lighting and should contain a statement detailing all of the treatments the patient has had to produce this change. If microdermabrasion only is being advertised, this would be false since, in this instance, she had microdermabrasion, thread lifting, and fillers to lips

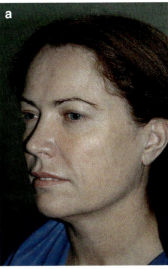
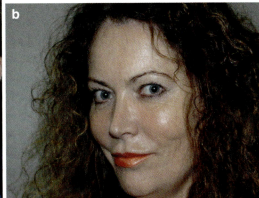

to claim that a particular breast implant has the "least" risk of a specific complication would be acceptable if true and supported by the peer reviewed literature. Such information is of value to consumers. To claim a practitioner is the "best" in any way is not permissible as it is a value judgment, not readily proven, which could mislead consumers.

2.4 Members must be able to substantiate any claims made in their advertising at the time the claims are made.

2.5 Comparative advertising should be used with caution. It can be valuable in conveying information to consumers but it must be correct and readily proven. For example, to claim a type of treatment is safer than another type of treatment is acceptable if true and supported by the peer reviewed literature. Again, such information is of benefit to consumers.

2.6 Photographs may be used to display the results of treatment and or complications. "Before and after" photographs should be presented with similar pose, presentation, lighting, and exposure. Any uncomplicated results shown should be typical and be likely to be reproduced in a similar patient. Photographs must not be altered in any way other than to protect a patient's identity. "Before and after" photographs must be of the advertising doctor or clinic's own patients and contain accurate and informative captions. Where before and after photographs are used the procedure being referred to must be the only change that has occurred to the person being photographed. Further, a clear statement that the procedure being referred to is the only change that has occurred to the person being photographed should be included when photographs are used in advertising.

2.7 Testimonials should not be used in advertisements.

2.8 Medical or surgical procedures should not be offered as inducements or prizes in competitions or contests, or as a way of generating business.

2.9 Offers of gifts or other inducements (e.g., time sensitive discount periods) shall not be used in order to attract potential clients.

2.10 Discounts for early payment should not be used as an inducement to commit to a procedure.

2.11 No member will offer finance facilities as part of the services provided, except a credit card facility. In no circumstances should a member accept any commission from a credit provider.

Cosmetic Photography is the term the author uses to describe "improvements" after treatment, which exaggerate the benefits. Figure 9.9 shows how lower eyelids can be remarkably improved. These photos show what might be a great result from "lower lid" blepharoplasty and repositioning of intraorbital fat. However, in fact, the photos show how manipulating

Fig. 9.9 (**a**) Before. (**b**) After. Good cosmetic photography to show improved lower eyelids. No procedure has been performed simply add flash and a different exposure

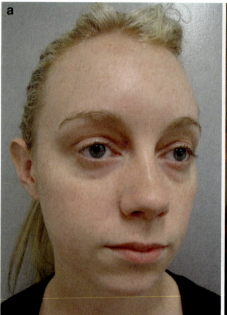
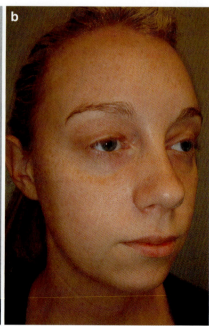

lighting and exposure can give a result. No surgery has been performed on this patient.

Similarly, in Fig. 9.10 we can see a big improvement in periorbital wrinkles and lines which could be purported to be from botulinum toxin or even perhaps fractionated laser resurfacing. In fact, all that has happened here is the patient has relaxed or contracted their orbicularis or simply are smiling. Because the photo is closely cropped, an inexperienced eye will not detect the activation of the muscles involved. When assessing such treatments the photo should have a wider frame so that it can be clear that there is no fudging involved.

In reality, cosmetic treatments, be they surgical or nonsurgical, are very good these days and there is excellent training available in most continents. Photos do not need to be fudged. Results usually speak for themselves and if photos are accompanied by accurate captions and explanations then patients are more likely to harbor realistic expectations and not be misled.

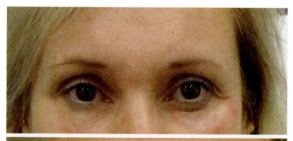
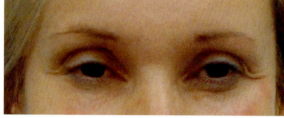

Fig. 9.10 Before and after crows' feet lines. Cosmetic photography, no treatment at all, just relaxation/activation of obicularis muscle. Close cropping of the photo might fool an inexperienced eye

9.8 Consent

In any medical endeavor, it is important to obtain informed consent from the patient. This also includes consent for the use of a photographic image. In my view, it is important to obtain specific consent for the use of photos. We all routinely use before and after photos as part of the patient record. Many consent forms have a general statement to the extent that the patient "consents to the use of photographs for medical record purposes." Such a statement does not extend to the use of photos for advertising or any other purpose. Sometimes the general statement might include "… use of photos for medical records or education purposes." It is imperative to be more specific about the exact nature of the "education purposes." Is it planned to use these photos in a closed "in house" teaching event or for use in a conference? Or is it "education" for potential new patients?

> **Practical Tips for Consent for Photography**
>
> Patients should be asked to consent specifically to the use of their photos for particular purposes:
>
> 1. The doctor's own clinical record
> 2. For use in the doctor's or nurse's office as talking points for other patients
> 3. Display of the photographs in the waiting room
> 4. Use of the photos for medical conference presentations in projected slides
> 5. Publication of photos in magazines, books, newspaper, TV advertisements
> 6. Publication of photos on the practice website or other internet options

All of these scenarios need to be explored specifically with the patient. If this is neglected then the patient will most likely have a strong case against you if they decide to follow legal pathways.

Consent also needs to address the issue of time frame. Is it reasonable to use an image taken and its use consented to several years past? Circumstances may have changed with the patient and a previously given consent may be long forgotten. This may cause difficulties for both the patient and the practitioner. I would urge anyone planning to use an identifiable image of a patient to make sure they have specific, written consent for its use. Secondly, inform the patient that you are about to use their image in the particular format so that they are not caught by surprise by any of their friends who sees the image before they themselves do.

9.9 Special Problems with Consent

Many patients are only too willing to allow their image to be used in a medical teaching format such as a presentation at a medical conference. However, it is becoming more frequent for others in the audience to video or at least take still photos of the presentation. This is a breach of trust; firstly against the doctor presenting the material and secondly against the patient.

The patient gave their permission to their trusted medical practitioner with specific conditions. That consent does not extend to the unknown doctor in the audience who "steals" that image. I personally have had the experience whereby a photo in one of my presentations featured in another doctors advertising.

Another area where one can be caught is with tattoos or particular items of clothing. Although a patient's face may be obscured or another part of the body featured in the photo, distinctive tattoos, a particular piece of jewelry (bracelet, necklace, pendant, etc.) may be identifiable. While it might be argued that even though the patient (or family) might recognize the subject, others would not and thence confidentiality has been honored; the fact that the patient can recognize themselves may translate into a sense of betrayal of trust and lead to serious consequences. We must remember that many of our patients are vulnerable, and with a heightened sense of fear.

9.10 Radiology

No chapter on facial imaging would be complete without some mention of the more purely clinical imaging techniques.

X-ray is the traditional imaging technique which has served very well for many years. It is useful as a quick initial radiologic examination of the facial bones for fractures or in assessing placement of screws/alignment post-surgery (Fig. 9.11). X ray utilizes a high energy electromagnetic beam that penetrates the anatomy in question and impacts onto the x-ray sensitive film plate. Dense structures, such as bone, attenuate the x-ray (block), whereas soft tissue structures let it pass through. The resultant image is one of shades or white/grey. Certainly, soft tissues can be imaged to a degree by lowering the intensity of the beam but this will also sacrifice clarity. Both figures display the clear outline of the bony anatomy but suffer from a confusion of overlying and surrounding anatomical structures making interpretation of anatomy off the main axis of focus much more difficult.

9.10.1 Computed Tomography (CT)

Computed tomography (CT) is an excellent imaging technique for imaging the bones and their alignment in the face (Fig. 9.12). A plain CT shows slices in coronal

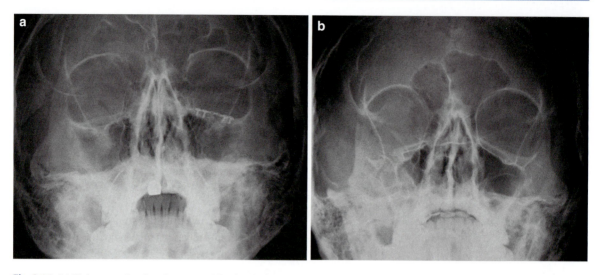

Fig. 9.11 (**a**) Plain x-ray showing placement of fixation device on a lower orbital rim. (**b**) Plain x-ray showing tripod fracture right orbit

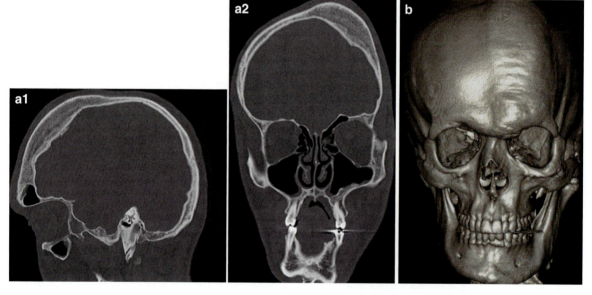

Fig. 9.12 (**a**) Two-dimensional CT of skull showing fibrous dysplasia. (**b**) Three-dimensional view of the same patient above. The three-dimensional view is a compilation of multiple scan slices

or sagittal or even horizontal planes. For composite images, an x-ray source rotates around the face, with x-ray sensors opposite the source collecting the data. The patient continuously moves through the CT tube, whilst the x-ray tube and detectors rotate around the face, enabling three-dimensional data to be acquired. This data in turn can be visualized from multiple orientations. The obvious advantage of CT of the face is the exquisite delineation of bony anatomy with high resolution, with no superimposition of anatomy as per x-ray.

9.10.2 Magnetic Resonance Imaging (MRI)

Magnetic resonance imaging (MRI) is the modality of choice for imaging the soft tissue structures of the face (Fig. 9.13). MRI utilizes a strong magnetic field together with radiofrequency pulses on the resonant frequency of hydrogen to obtain the images. The RF pulses excite the hydrogen atoms of the tissues and in turn these tissues emit a signal which the MRI machine collects to form an image. MRI has excellent definition

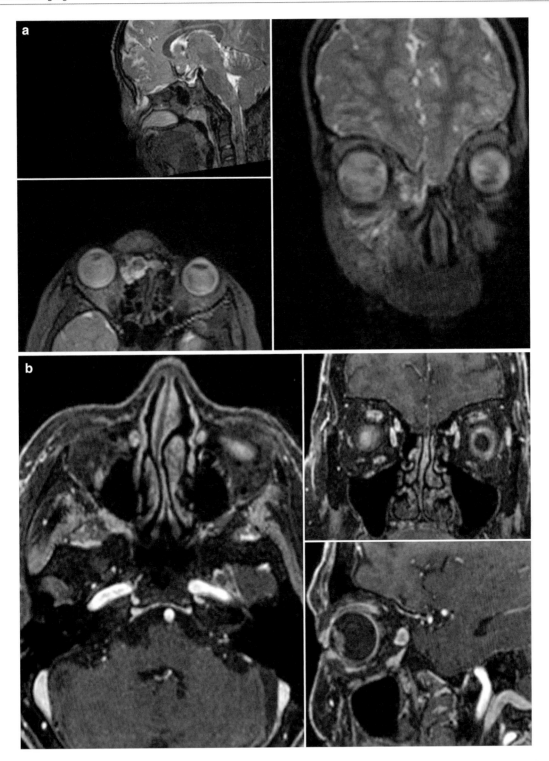

Fig. 9.13 (**a**) MRI showing an encephalocoele. Note the clear delineation of the different soft tissue components of the image. (**b**) MRI showing infraorbital nerve

of soft tissue structures, with better soft tissue characterization than all other imaging modalities. MRI is used primarily to look for soft tissue masses, bony masses, soft tissue anatomy, nerves of the face, and orbits. It is not used for imaging cortical bone, as it has no hydrogen component and appears black (hypodense) on the MRI pictures. CT is best if looking for fractures, bony alignment, etc. MRI is the imaging modality of choice if looking for perineural spread of SCC and can identify extensions into the orbit or oral cavity of this dermatologic tumor. So, as a planning tool, it is very useful in surgery.

Skin Care and Adjuvant Techniques Pre and Post Facial Surgery

10

Anthony Erian and Clara Santos

10.1 Introduction

Modern facial rejuvenation surgery offers patients a wide range of possibilities, including dermatologic treatments which are able to improve skin condition as well as enhancing and maintaining the final surgical result. The skin of most patients who seek facial rejuvenation surgery presents clinical and histological changes secondary to intrinsic aging or extrinsic photo-aging. Many noninvasive and non-ablative dermatologic treatments exist, which are able to improve damaged skin without recovery time and may be administered prior to surgery. Ideally all patients should start receiving local treatment with topical retinoic acid, unless a specific contraindication exists. In my practice, as well as the skin care program, adjuvant techniques such as the light chemical peel, microdermabrasion, or carboxytherapy are commonly used. A combination of these treatments improves skin condition, which will allow patients undergoing facial surgery the best possible results for facial rejuvenation.

A. Erian (✉)
Pear Tree Cottage,
Cambridge Road, Wimpole 43,
SG8 5QD Cambridge, UK
e-mail: plasticsurgeon@anthonyerian.com

C. Santos
Dermatology in Private Practice, Department of Dermatology,
Avenida Brasil, 583 Jardim Europa, CEP 01431-000
São Paulo, Brazil
e-mail: clara_santos@terra.com.br

10.2 Skin Aging

With time, skin ages due to a combination of both intrinsic and extrinsic factors. It is important to recognize the difference between these two different processes. With intrinsic aging, the functional capacity is decreased, the epidermal/dermal junction is flattened, and there is a reduction in dermal thickness. These patients present with skin laxity, wrinkles, and dry skin. Patients with extrinsic aging present initially with an increase in dermal thickness. This is the result of elastotic material accumulating during elatosis. Clinical signs of extrinsic aging are evident as changes such as lines, wrinkles, dryness, flaccidity, hyperpigmentation, seborrheic and actinic keratoses, and solar lentigos. In addition, in almost all cases, neoplastic growths such as basaliomas and epiteliomas develop in these areas of sun exposure and extrinsic aging.

10.3 Techniques

10.3.1 Skin Care Program

Performing facial surgery without preoperative skin treatment is like building a house without a foundation. Omitting postoperative skin treatment is like building a house without the final interior design. In practice, this can be seen in cases where patients, who have significant skin damage, undergo excellent facial surgery, and yet fail to achieve satisfactory facial rejuvenation. Both patient and facial surgeon are disappointed with the suboptimal result, yet this may be avoided if dermatological techniques are employed. Topical treatments are easy and safe to apply as well as afford excellent results when correctly performed. Facial skin is particularly responsive to these treatments and signs of aging may be reversed even in the very elderly patient. All patients who seek a facial cosmetic surgery consultation should have a skin treatment program, whether or not surgery is performed. Figure 10.1 shows a case where eyelid surgery was performed in combination with dermatologic skin care program. Good looking, healthy skin improves self-esteem and confidence, promotes attraction and youthfulness, and offers skin in the best possible condition for surgery.

Local treatment is based on the use of topical agents. There are many products on the market, a lot of which unfortunately promise miracles. It is important to understand that, among these, only very few will be effective. Patients require education, so that they may question the products, which the media promote. Examples include advertisements for light fruit acids that can significantly rejuvenate facial skin, for moisturizers that can eradicate sun damage, or for "special agents" applied to the skin that can "fix" dermal damage.

The local treatment program, which is recommended, employs a minimum of topical agents: an active agent at night, a cleanser morning and night, and a sun protection factor morning and afternoon. In most cases, during the skin preparation before surgery, I avoid moisturizers, tonics, and astringents, as the combination of these with the acid at night leads to skin sensitivity. In addition, moisturizers have no power to restore skin function, they cannot treat nor prevent skin aging, and they cannot stimulate collagen growth as they do not penetrate the dermis. The action of moisturizers is temporary as they fill the space between desquamating skin cells.

10.3.1.1 Tretinoin

Topical tretinoin or retinoic acid has been investigated in randomized studies. Regular daily application has shown the ability to compact the stratum corneum, to increase epidermal thickness, and to decrease melanin content. In the dermis, new collagen formation has been demonstrated [1–3]. According to Kligman [4], tretinoin improves not only the structure of the skin but also influences positively its physiological functions. Tretinoin may be used as a single agent, though in cases of darker skin or in cases of hyperpigmentation, tretinoin may be used with hydroquinone and 1% hydrocortisone (Kligman formula) [5, 6]. As some countries forbid the use of hydroquinone, other available bleaching agents such as kojic acid or azelaic acid may be employed [7–9]. In most cases 0.05% retinoic acid applied at night will benefit the skin preoperatively (Fig. 10.2) as well as maintain the skin postoperatively. When used in this manner, skin youthfulness, shine, and quality can be significantly improved.

Possible reactions during tretinoin treatment should be explained to the patient, so that the commonly witnessed erythema, dryness, and desquamation will not be misunderstood and lead to noncompliance. It is important to explain that this type of irritation is commonly seen in the initial phases of treatment, but that this subsides. I find it particularly important to teach patients how to apply topical agents. In my clinical practice of almost 30 years, I have found that almost no one has applied these agents correctly. The correct way to apply the topical treatment is similar to the "Friendly Peel" technique that will be explained subsequently.

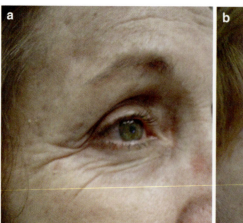 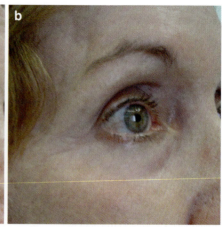

Fig. 10.1 (a) Preoperative. (b) Postoperative eyelid surgery combined with dermatologic skin care program

Fig. 10.2 (*Left*) Preoperative. (*Right*) Postoperative with previous skin care treatment giving optimal skin quality for surgery

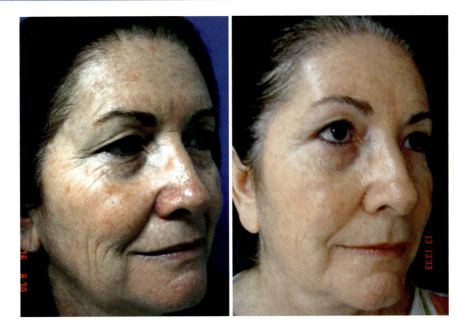

10.3.1.2 Skin Cleansers

Cleansing the skin should be performed gently twice a day, both in the morning and at night. Rather than using multiple agents or scrubbing the skin, an ideal cleansing is performed gently and using a large amount of the product. Many cleansers exist, but it is important to choose one which is pH-neutral and therefore does not change the pH of the skin.

10.3.1.3 Sun Protection

Sun protection may be performed in three different manners: physically, chemically, and in a combined manner. Above all, a sun protector or sunblock should protect the skin against UVB, UVA I, and UVA II radiation [10]. The authors prefer physical sunblocks because they offer better protection, are waterproof, and do not cause skin irritation. Chemical sunblocks can cause a burning sensation when applied to the skin that is undergoing a skin care program or following a resurfacing technique. It is also my belief that this forms a type of chronic irritation to sensitive skin which may worsen or prevent the improvement of melasma.

The authors have also observed in patients with hyperpigmented skin, that the absence of improvement may be related to the suboptimal use of the sun protector. Many patients apply this agent in an amount that is less than ideal or they do not reapply the protector during the day, both of which leave the skin without complete protection. To obtain the best sun protection, the application should be done gently, carefully, and using an adequate amount. Sun protectors should be applied half an hour before going outside and half an hour before applying makeup.

10.3.1.4 Light Chemical Peel or "Friendly Peel"

There are several chemical agents that can be used as a light chemical peel [11–13]. For many years the authors have used a modified retinoic peel named "Friendly Peel" (Table 10.1) for the skin care program. The Friendly Peel can be performed safely in any facial skin, from skin type I to skin type VI. In a combined program, this is the first step, after which, skin care products must be commenced. Unlike other agents, the Friendly Peel does not give rise to the commonly seen burning sensation. Skin sensitivity is also rarely a consideration in this light peel.

The Friendly Peel and the use of the skin care program are best commenced 2 weeks prior to surgery and will recommence after surgery once the sutures have been removed.

Table 10.1 Friendly Peel composition

Substance	Concentration
Retinoic acid	5–10%

If surgery is postponed, the skin care program may continue without interruption. Not only can the Friendly Peel be used for preoperative purposes, but it may be used weekly or biweekly for skin rejuvenation without surgery over the course of 6–12 weeks. Excellent results can be achieved for acne, superficial melasma, fine lines, or when "skin refreshment" is desired. The aforementioned skin care program should be performed between sessions of the Friendly Peel.

During the application of the Friendly Peel, the patient is given a mirror. Not only does this allow the patient to witness the procedure, but it allows the patient to learn the manner in which to apply topical agents at home. After the patient's skin has been washed, it is gently scrubbed with gauze and 70% alcohol. The application begins at the forehead and follows adjacent anatomic units in a sequential manner. An amount equivalent to a kernel of corn is used, distributing it in circular movements. In each unit, 10–20 circular movements are employed, depending on the sensitivity and oiliness of the skin (Fig. 10.3).

This is repeated in order to cover the entire face. The nasolabial folds, chin, and malar-zygomatic zones are demonstrated to the patient as being areas more prone to irritation, therefore less topical agents may be applied. The eyelids, due to their skin's thin and

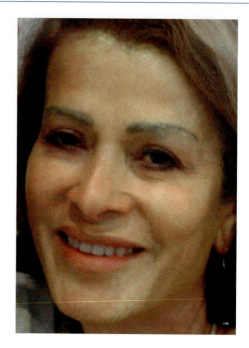

Fig. 10.4 Patient immediately after Friendly Peel. The product must be removed 6–12 h after

sensitive nature, must be treated differently. A smaller amount of peel is used and applied with one or two passes; circular movements are not employed.

The Friendly Peel is left in situ for several hours (Fig. 10.4), until the next morning when it is removed by washing.

A soft redness will be witnessed. After having the Friendly Peel done, the patient begins the skin care program that has been described above. Light skin peeling will be seen on the fourth or fifth day, lasting about 24 h.

It is also important to teach the patient that when signs of sensitivity appear (e.g., with tretinoin), application over this specific area should be stopped until the skin in this area returns to normal. We have found that teaching the patient how to use local treatments has dramatically improved results, so that the common side effect of skin irritation can be minimized or made absent.

The Friendly Peel can also be used as an adjuvant in the treatment of stretch marks or post-inflammatory hyperpigmentation (PIH).

If the skin is more resistant, we often combine the Friendly Peel with Jesenner solution at the same treatment session. This combination of agents enhances the action of each, resulting in a deeper desquamation.

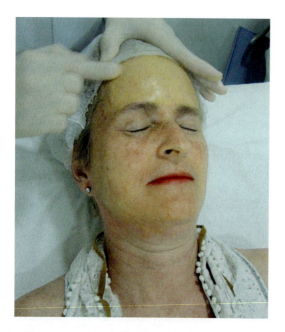

Fig. 10.3 Patient during Friendly Peel session

In grade I acne and for light acne scars, excellent results can be achieved using the combination of the Friendly Peel with microdermabrasion at the same session. Finally, we also combine the Friendly Peel with 10–30% salicylic acid peel, which is especially useful for darker skinned patients with very thick and oily skin. The importance of these treatments is that they offer excellent results with minimal skin irritation and with quick recovery.

Light friendly peel is very good for young as well for elderly patients. It can be especially useful if used in combination with chemical cauterization of certain neoplastic growth such as actinic and seborrheic keratosis (Fig. 10.5).

10.3.1.5 Microdermabrasion

This technique uses aluminum oxide crystals to cause delicate abrasion to the skin surface [14–16]. I first began using this technique in 1993. Similarly to the Friendly Peel, it may be performed as the first procedure before starting the skin program for the surgery and it may be continued after surgery. Microdermabrasion may also be used as a sole dermatologic treatment in weekly or biweekly sessions over the course of 6–12 weeks. Microdermabrasion may also be performed in combination with the Friendly Peel. I prefer this combination, as it enhances the results of skin rejuvenation.

Microdermabrasion uses a device to project aluminum crystals onto the skin surface and negative pressure to re-aspirate them. This removes or peels off the outer surface of the skin. This mechanism allows new skin to form in a safe and pain-free manner and without the need for local anesthesia. Microdermabrasion can be used for a variety of indications, such as in patients with thick skin, melasma, acne scars, superficial wrinkles, and actinic melanosis. As well as the face, it can be used to treat the neck, the décolleté arms and hands, and stretch marks.

After the patient's skin has been washed, it is degreased with gauze and 70% alcohol. This is performed gently in sensitive skin, though with slightly more force in skin which is thicker or oilier. This technique is really safe and presents no real risk to patients. Along many years of practice we have heard only very rare reports of complications like post-inflammatory hyperpigmentation and sensitiveness of the eyes due to the presence of crystals adherent to the cornea. In both cases the complications were related to physician malpractice. When performing microdermabrasion it is necessary to understand that the action must be smooth. Eye protection is recommended to avoid crystals entering the eye (Fig. 10.6).

The technique should be performed step by step to cover all the anatomic units of the face. The skin of the area being treated must be stretched either by the physician's nondominant hand or by the assistant's hands.

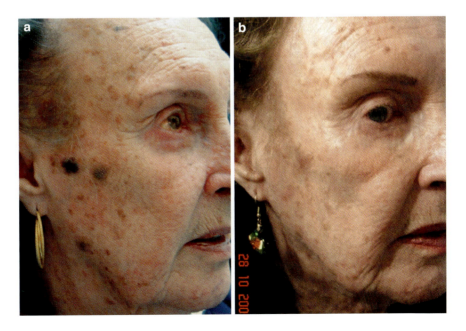

Fig. 10.5 (**a**) Preoperative. (**b**) Postoperative after Friendly Peel and chemical cauterization of actinic and seborrheic keratosis

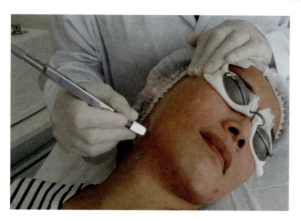

Fig. 10.6 Microdermabrasion session. Patients should wear glasses for protection

There are a variety of pressures that can be administered by the machine, but it is advisable to avoid high pressures and to avoid pushing down excessively hard with the hand piece as these will result in bruising. Movements should be done in at least two directions in each anatomic area. Around the eyes, only one movement is required. Uneven distribution of pressure resulting in uneven abrasion may eventually lead to an irregular pattern to the skin. Once the session is completed, the skin must only be cleansed with water to remove the crystals. This must include the eyes, as crystals may cause eye irritation. Once the skin is clean and dry, the Friendly Peel may be applied. The peel is removed after 6–12 h, generally the following morning. Microdermabrasion is safe, may be employed on any skin surface, and when performed correctly can lead to excellent results in 6 weeks time (Fig. 10.7).

10.3.1.6 Carboxytherapy

Dermatologic injection of carbon dioxide was originally employed at the Thermes de Royat and Marienbad (France), during the 1930s. Its initial purpose was the treatment of peripheral arterial occlusive disease. Laser Doppler flow measurements have shown that topical application of carbon dioxide increases skin blood flow. As well as its initial use, carboxytherapy has been shown to be an excellent noninvasive technique for skin preparation prior to surgery, as well as for skin rejuvenation, scars, and striae. The dermatologic injection of CO_2 results in pseudohypoxemia, leading to mechanisms which increase local tissue. Increased blood flow improves skin elasticity and irregularities, as well as allowing neocollagenesis [17–20].

The area to be treated is cleaned with a local antiseptic. Some patient may experience slight discomfort, but most patients will tolerate this procedure without complaint and without the need of local anesthesia. A small needle (30 gauge) is used to insufflate the carbon dioxide through the

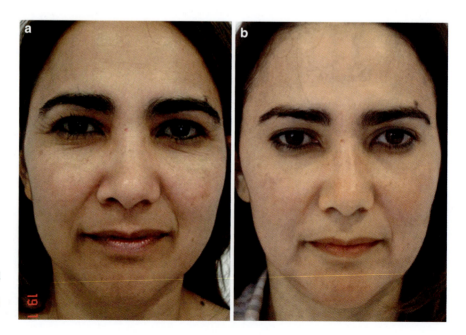

Fig. 10.7 (**a**) Preoperative patient with skin type IV and melasma. (**b**) Two months after microdermabrasion and Friendly Peel

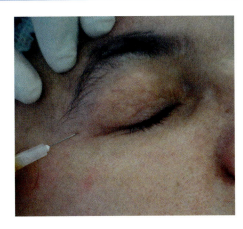

Fig. 10.8 Carboxytherapy session showing localized and temporary bulging eyelid

skin. For the delicate skin of the eyelids, a selected flow of 20 ml/min is adequate, while flows as high as 150 ml/min may be used in other areas. It is important to warn patients that the treated area will bulge slightly due to the insufflation (Fig. 10.8), but that this is temporary.

One session of carboxytherapy may take 10–15 min and there is no need for a recovery period. Carboxytherapy may be performed in combination with other skin rejuvenation techniques. Results are most typically seen after the fifth session. In eyelids, for example, improved skin texture, color, and reduction in prolapsed fat pads may be seen. As well as the face, the neck, chest, and arms can be treated. In combination with techniques such as the CromoPeel or Dermaroller, excellent results may also be achieved in improving striae [21].

10.4 Complications

Due to the noninvasive and non-ablative nature of these techniques, if correctly performed, the risk of complication is minimal. With the local skin treatment, it is important to adequately teach patients how to apply the topical agents and to avoid mixing their prescription with any others agents. Strict avoidance of sun exposure during the treatment is required. If the instructions are not correctly followed, either a suboptimal result or indeed no result will occur. In addition, skin irritation or a burning sensation may be experienced.

With the Friendly Peel, which is an extremely safe agent, very few side effects have been witnessed. This treatment can be safely carried out in all skin types, including very sensitive skins. I have personally never seen a case of PIH. This light chemical peel can be done in combination with microdermabrasion. A few patients may experience mild swelling of the face or a slight subjective yellow tinge to the face, which are temporary.

With microdermabrasion, it is important not to exert excessive pressure on the face and to perform regular movements of the handpiece, in order to avoid irregular patterns, skin damage, and the possibility for PIH development.

Dermatologic Carbon Dioxide Infusion is a highly useful procedure, if properly done. Some patients may develop ecchymosis and temporary bulging, especially on the eyelids.

10.5 Discussion

In order to achieve the best results, some type of local treatment is mandatory. There are numerous agents on the market which promise skin improvement and rejuvenation; however, most of them will not work. Unfortunately, many of these will cause skin sensitivity. I consider tretinoin to be the best agent in terms of skin conditioning and skin rejuvenation. It is also very useful in cases of acne and can be used in all skin types. Its side effects are temporary and can be minimized if the patient understands how to use it and if treatment starts gradually.

The Light Chemical Peel or "Friendly Peel" is used when the skin requires more than a home treatment. It stimulates the skin in a mild manner, hence its name "Friendly." Microdermabrasion can produce epidermal and dermal improvement by outer layer stimulation. In cases where thicker skin, oily skin, or acne skin is present, or in cases where skin needs stronger action, the combination of microdermabrasion and Friendly Peel is excellent. Dermatologic CO_2 infusion is an old technique that has reappeared recently and has an important role when the eye lids, face, and neck require skin improvement.

10.6 Conclusions

Together, Cosmetic/Plastic Surgery and Dermatology play important roles in helping patients achieve their goals of facial rejuvenation. These specialities must work together in order to complement one another. Most surgery will achieve a better result if the skin is properly treated. On the other hand, in many cases, skin treatment alone will not achieve the ultimate goal of face rejuvenation. We see excellent results and patients are highly satisfied when the medical plan and the surgical plan are clearly explained. This avoids misinterpretations and facilitates patient compliance, leading to the best possible results for facial rejuvenation.

References

1. Bhawan J, Serva AG, Nehal K, Labadie R, Lufrano L, Thorne EG, et al. Effects of tretinoin on photodamaged skin a histologic study. Arch Dermatol. 1991;127(5):666–72.
2. Griffiths CE, Finkel LJ, Ditre CM, Hamilton TA, Ellis CN, Voorhees JJ. Topical tretinoin (retinoic acid) improves melasma. A vehicle-controlled, clinical trial. Br J Dermatol. 1993;129(4):415–21.
3. Rendon MI, Gaviria JI. Review of skin-lightening agents. Dermatol Surg. 2005;31(7 Pt 2):886–9.
4. Kligman LH, Crosby MJ. Topical tretinoin enhances corticosteroid-induced inhibition of tumorigenesis in hairless mice previously exposed to solar simulating radiation. Cancer Lett. 1996;107(2):217–22.
5. Gupta AK, Gover MD, Nouri K, Taylor S. The treatment of melasma: a review of clinical trials. J Am Acad Dermatol. 2006;55(6):1048–65.
6. Picardo M, Carrera M. New and experimental treatments of cloasma and other hypermelanoses. Dermatol Clin. 2007;25(3):353–62.
7. Espinal-Perez LE, Moncada B, Castanedo-Cazares JP. A double blind randomized trial of 5% ascorbic acid vs 4% hydroquinone in melasma. Int J Dermatol. 2004;43(8):604–7.
8. Halder RM, Richards GM. Management of dischromias in ethnic skin. Dermatol Ther. 2004;17(2):151–7.
9. Lim JT. Treatment of melasma using kojic acid in a gel containing hydroquinone and glycolic acid. Dermatol Surg. 1999;25(4):282–4.
10. Shaath NA. The chemistry of sunscreens. In: Lowe NJ, Shaath NA, editors. Sunscreens development, evaluation and regulatory aspects. New York: Marcel Dekker; 1990. p. 223–5.
11. Monheit GD. Advances in chemical peeling. Facial Plast Surg Clin North Am. 1994;2:5–9.
12. Monheit GD, Chastain MA. Chemical peels. Facial Plast Surg Clin North Am. 2001;9(2):239–55.
13. Monheit GD. Chemical peels. Skin Ther Lett. 2004;9(2):6–11.
14. Coimbra M et al. A prospective controlled assessment of microdermabrasion for damaged skin and fine rhytides. Plast Reconstr Surg. 2004;113:1438–43.
15. Grimes PE. Microdermabrasion. Dermatol Surg. 2005; 31 (9 Pt 2):1160–5.
16. Lew B, Cho Y, Lee M. Effect of serial microdermabrasion on the ceramide level in the stratum corneum. Dermatol Surg. 2006;32(3):376–9.
17. Ferreira JC, Haddad A, Tavares S. Increase in collagen turnover induced by intradermal injection of carbon dioxide in rats. J Drugs Dermatol. 2008;7(3):201–6.
18. Brockow T, Hausner T, Dillner A, Resch KL. Clinical evidence of subcutaneous CO_2 insufflations: a systematic review. J Altern Complement Med. 2000;6(5):391–403.
19. Ito T, Moor JL, Koss MC. Topical application of CO_2 increases skin blood flow. J Invest Dermatol. 1989;93(2):259–62.
20. Brandi C, D'Aniello C, Grimaldi L, Bosi B, Dei I, Lattarulo P, et al. Carbon dioxide therapy in the treatment of localized adiposities: clinical study and histopathological correlations. Aesthetic Plast Surg. 2001;25(3):170–4.
21. Badran MM, Kuntsche J, Fahr A. Skin penetration enhancement by a microneedle device (Dermaroller) in vitro: dependency on needle size and applied formulation. Eur J Pharm Sci. 2009;36(4–5):511–23.

Part IV
Psychological Aspects

What Is Human Beauty?

Pierre F. Fournier

11.1 Introduction

Paul Valery said, "Health is the silence of the organs" and the World Health Organization said that, "Health is not only the absence of illness but a state of complete mental and social well being." On the other hand, beauty, which Plato placed behind health and before fortune, has not been well defined.

An esthetic surgeon by definition must create or conserve beauty. Surgical techniques abound in the textbooks of Europe north, south and Central America but, in my opinion, artistic teaching on beauty or human beauty is not taught enough.

The esthetic surgeon often finds it difficult to define beauty, he is not alone. Ask different people and the answers vary considerably and, in the main, are not satisfactory. This is why one thought it would be useful to approach the subject from a psychological point of view, and attempt to understand what it is that enters the mind of a person, esthetic surgeon or not, when she perceives, or does not perceive the feeling of beauty. It is important to understand this feeling within us in order to guide us during our operations.

11.2 Beauty

11.2.1 What Is Human Beauty? What Do the Books Say? Dictionaries? Philosophers?

- Right from the start we are told that beauty is about proportion, equilibrium, symmetry. I therefore want to explain beauty objectively and describe the different canons of Egyptian, Greek, and Roman. Apparently the centimeter is not the sole judge, little by little the subjective has entered into the equation.
- Beauty is an ensemble of shapes and proportions, which bring us pleasure and which we admire, but the concept varies according to different cultures.
- Beauty is a balance between shape and volume.
- Beauty stimulates an esthetic feeling within us, pleasing to the eye, a sense of admiration. Some say beauty is a visual pheromone!
- Beauty is a combination of qualities such as form, proportion, and color in a human face (or other object) that delights the sight.
- These last four words are important, beauty does not exist itself, it exists in the eye of the beholder. If something pleases someone, it is beautiful to him. If this same thing does not please another, it is not beautiful to him. It is not that which is beautiful that pleases him, it is that which pleases him that is beautiful.
- David Hume (1711–1776) the Scottish philosopher said, more than 200 years ago, "Beauty is essentially a private and personnel experience. Beauty is in the eye and mind of the beholder." He also said, "Beauty is not a quality of the thing itself but that which exists in the mind of those who contemplate it." Everyone experiences beauty individually.

P.F. Fournier
57 Avenue de Villiers, 75010 Paris, France
e-mail: pierre.fournier27@wanadoo.fr

- Eric Newton: "Beauty is something which gives pleasure, but that which gives pleasure to one person does not necessarily give pleasure to someone else."
- Some philosophers conclude, "that which is beautiful is good, that which is good is beautiful." What the poetess Sappho said a long time ago was "that which is beautiful is good and he who is good will soon become beautiful."
- Our past feelings are partly responsible for how we feel today. Our parents, love, former loves, women, and friends. They remind us of past experiences, and beauty is not represented by the detail but by the whole collection being greater than the sum of its parts. Equally, today's "emotions will be responsible for tomorrow's emotions." The happy and unhappy times of our past life leave permanent impressions guiding our preferences. The faces we have loved during our youth, warm and comforting, continue to live on in our mind.
- Beauty is not only a question of the face, voice, body, or a graceful physique. People are beautiful because of their character, personality, and their ability to bring joy, their capacity to love. We see emerging the notion of charm.
- When we like a face, we like the spirit that animates it and it is not enough to say that someone is physically attractive; a person can be attractive in many ways.
- Beauty and charm are often confused. Cleopatra, George Sand, Louise de la Valliere, and Theodora were famous for their beauty; in fact they were not very beautiful but possessed great charm. Beauty is more an illusion than a reality.
- Beauty is not for the eye but for the mind. "Attraction is in the eye of the beholder," said Hungerford. Steven M. Hoefflin states: "I must correct, attraction in the eye of the beholder, while beauty is shared by all."
- The beauty of the personality eclipses the beauty of the face. We have seen many ways to define beauty and that it is often associated with charm. Charm differs from beauty in that it lasts forever, whereas beauty fades. The English say, "Charm last! Beauty blast!" Finally we see that it is not only the eye that judges whether someone or something is beautiful; it is, above all, the mind and that which we term the heart or inner beauty.
- According to the American sociologist Frumkin, a woman is deemed beautiful according to her "sexual aptitude." Whether she is judged beautiful or not depends not only on the symmetry of her proportions or shape but equally by the potential sexual functions suggested by these attributes, and the sensual emotion is transformed into an esthetic emotion.
- The preceding classic assertions allow us to conclude that the notion of beauty differs according to the culture and the individual, and that it is not exclusively a question of shape, form, and symmetry. A person's personality, charm, and interior beauty powerfully contribute to elicit a pleasing impression in the beholder. The eye is not the sole judge; there is also the spirit and, above all, the heart. The mind is influenced by old memories which reside within us and shape our judgment in the same way that today's experiences will influence the future. This is seen in a phrase of Buddha "Today is the son of yesterday and the father of tomorrow."

Beauty is like an iceberg: only one part of it is visible. We could say that the baits are the face and body; and the hooks are the heart and the mind.

11.2.2 Konrad Lorenz's Theory

Konrad Lorenz, Nobel Prize winner for Medicine and Physiology in 1973, has contributed in a decisive way to the progress of the biology of behavior. It is he who helped us understand human beauty.

In his work "Essays on animal and human behavior" he proposed the drawing, which explains the release of an emotion in both human and animals to care for young. In the left column one sees a child's head and the heads of very young animals, a gerbil, a Pekingese, and a robin red breast. In the column on the right we see an adults head and the heads of the same animals as adults.

If one asks which column is preferred, the left is automatically chosen. Konrad Lorenz concluded from this that beauty is an emotion, an emotion associated with the desire to protect. Only the left column evokes this emotion. This emotion is associated with a desire to protect as much in humans as in animals. It is, he says, the release of an innate behavior. A relatively large head, a disproportionately large forehead, large eyes placed underneath prominent curved cheeks, short thick limbs, a firm elasticity, and awkward movements are the essential defining characteristics of "sweet" and "pretty." These present themselves according to the law of the "summation of excitations" of a small child or "bait," like a dog or a cuddly animal.

On the left are those that give the impression of a "Sweetie" (child, gerbil, Pekingese, red breast), the adults to the right do not elicit this caring reaction (man, hare, hunting dog, blackbird). The conclusion is obvious: beneath the traits of an adult, the face of a child must show through. When a face attract a human it is because the face has childlike characteristics.

Everyone is instinctively attracted by a child's face. The sight of a child's face immediately provokes within us an emotion and this emotion is automatically accompanied by a desire to protect. This is found equally in man and beast. Konrad Lorenz explains that adult animals which are driven to protect their offspring are attracted by "something" which the offspring emanates – a physical trait, a sound, a smell. It is the same with man. There are signals that elicit protection, sympathy, and tenderness.

What are the cues according to Konrad Lorenz? For the small child, the signals are on its head. They are roundness, fullness, curves, the rounded forehead, full cheeks, and the little turned up nose; all these infantile characteristics elicit a desire to protect. An infant's face is associated with purity, sincerity, honesty, and vulnerability.

The adult we see on the right hand column does not elicit these reactions. His face has changed, his head is flattened, the forehead receding, the nose lengthened, and cheeks hollowed. He has lost all his childlike characteristics. He elicits no emotion, no desire to protect. It is the same for adult animals, and the contrast is startling on viewing the two columns: in the man angles have replaced curves with the naso-labial angle, angles of the jaw, external angles of the orbit, and angles of the chin. Designers and painters know this theory well and reveal it in their work aimed at students. Cartoonists know that to touch the hearts of their readers, they must exaggerate certain traits in an adult or child's face, making the head bigger than normal, with a rounded forehead, full cheeks, and shortened limbs.

We see that women maintain their curves, whereas men lose them. We understand therefore that in his interventions a good esthetic surgeon should optimize the traits that, as in a baby or child, evoke reactions of attraction, tenderness, and protection.

Softness, roundness = tenderness.

Again, and this is fundamental to giving the impression of beauty, in the adult face one must find and recognize the traits of a child. However, the traits are not the sole source of the protective reflex; there are also the expressions. These at least have the advantage of being accessible to everyone. Some adults know how useful expressions are in order to please or to move someone. The emotions provoked by the childlike features of Brigitte Bardot were increased by her famous spoiled child "pout." Also well known are the childlike expressions used, and some say abused, by Marilyn Monroe and Audrey Hepburn.

It has been said that Marilyn Monroe made herself up badly to give the impression of a little girl who did not know how to apply her makeup and also that after a long session at the hairdressers she would ruffle up her hair to obtain a certain look of disorder that reminded one of a little girl who had just finished playing.

Also, if women do not have a childlike demeanor and wish to dominate men, men will not feel a protective desire and will be reminded more of their mother than of their wife.

Women, who are more concerned about beauty than are men, may show these childlike expressions consciously or unconsciously. They can appear knowingly or unknowingly shy, fragile, weak, innocent, naïve, ignorant, temperamental, sulky, admiring, curious, etc. Some women highlight apparent weaknesses in order to provoke this protective emotion. Has it not been said that it is the apparent weakness of women that is their strength? Considering that all this has the aim of striking straight to the heart of men, Napoleon I would have said "Women's two weapons are makeup (the significance of this will be discussed later) and tears, as in a helpless little girl." One therefore understands how a child's features on an adult can be moving: freckles, rosy cheeks, a glowing complexion, long eyelashes, blond curls, full cheeks, and full, well-defined full lips.

Today, times have changed, and such "bait" may not be used as often as before since our modern society is becoming more and more egalitarian between men and women.

For men, wearing a side parting of the hair, as sported by many of the great seducers (Clark Gable, Gary Cooper, George Clooney), a "floppy mop" (Leonardo Di Caprio), and shaving every day can only be explained by a desire to resemble a child. It is not necessary to have all these signals; only one is needed to please.

Each individual can always have childlike expressions. As for traits, if one does not have them, they can sometimes be acquired thanks to esthetic surgery. Beauty is not entirely a natural phenomenon. It has long, and especially in our time, been a cultural phenomenon. Humans seek to improve themselves, and women, for whom beauty is more important than for men (men are attracted above all by force and power), improve their beauty and charm with makeup and what we call accessories: glasses; false eyelashes; earrings; hairstyles; highlights; tattoos around the lips, eyelids, and eyebrows (the word "tattoo" should not be used when talking to women, rather semi-permanent implantation of natural pigments!); hats; necklaces; and the invisible accessory, perfume. Some of the more modern accessories have been studied by beauty professionals in order to hide faults: wide arms on modern glasses hide "crow's feet" and a high bridge can accentuate the length of a too short nose. Placed lower down, it reduces the length of a long nose. All these stratagems are explained discreetly and at length in women's magazines. An old proverb summarizes this perfectly: "30% of beauty is made by nature and 70% by nurture, by adornment." The disadvantage of these accessories is that without them one may no longer seem as young or as beautiful.

The desire to make oneself more beautiful is not a trap that women set for men, it is a wish to please, to be better accepted by society and the family. It is agreed that life is harder for a woman than for a man, although great improvements have been made in the last few decades. In addition, makeup gives confidence, a little like the war paint of the North American Indians. Do we not say "change the appearance and you change the person" and "if one prepares, it is for the parade!" Its importance is extreme. Have we not read Sharon Stone state in a women's magazine: "I have never considered myself as a great beauty, only a great magician"? Tyra Banks, a well-known black beauty, said, "I am not ugly but my beauty is a total creation."

We have always had makeup, and to improve a face makeup must be natural, and by increasing it, remind one of the qualities of a young face. Lipstick must make one think of the more intense red of a the lips of a child, who has a faster metabolism; blusher must make one think of a child's rosy cheeks, and powder the pale and velvet skin of youth. This is what Desmond Morris calls over stimulation. Very long false eyelashes are only a reminder of the long lashes of a child. If makeup can improve, badly applied, it can also spoil the beauty of a face. It can be friend or foe. Have we not read in certain ethnology books that it was the witch who was asked to make up ill peoples' faces so that they would not needlessly shock those with whom they lived?

Childlike traits and expressions are therefore important in order to evoke emotion with a desire to protect. There is also the voice, which must be soft and pleasant, like that of a child. A harsh voice, found among many smokers, does not make one think of a child. Clothes must also be pleasing to the eye and to the heart, and have a youthful cut. Does the mini skirt not evoke the long legs of the adolescent? Colors also have to evoke childhood; light colors, such as blue and pink, have always been chosen by old ladies. Of course black is to be avoided. In summary, all the human senses must be solicited, sight, hearing, smell (children have no smell, hence the use of deodorants), and touch; the firmness of the skin is important. Beauty institutes have long understood this and centered their advertising on it. Do we not read in women's magazines: ladies, perhaps you have beautiful breasts, a beautiful stomach, and beautiful legs, but are they firm? Firmness, the elasticity of tissue, is a fundamental quality of children's skin and forms part of its beauty. It can be very expensive to be beautiful: jewels, the beauty accessories, are easily available to those with a sufficient income, but more difficult to obtain for those with a modest budget. This fact explains why medicine and esthetic surgery are popular among those who are not well off and who cannot please with their natural gifts alone, or with the artificial means of the well off. Only being able to please with their bodies, if patients of modest means have acquired or natural defects, they will allow themselves to be operated on more easily as it is their only way of continuing to be pleasing.

The idea of using a child's image is well known. One sometimes wants to sensitize the heart for more mercenary, rather than noble reasons. It is well known that every time one shows a child's face next to a product, distribution is improved and profit increased. Whether it is a medicine or any other product, the number of consumers, if they are sensitive, will increase. Marketers are of course looking for a path to the heart, but also, and above all, to the wallet. The strategy of showing a child's face is used in public awareness campaigns by charity organizations when trying to raise funds for a country in difficulty or in the battle against poverty and misery. It is also well known that a child who begs will receive more handouts than an adult. The Walt Disney films that so enchant their viewers use only small and vulnerable animals; it is always the little mouse, little dog, or little deer that we see, never the adult. This is also the case for toys; it is most often a little animal or a child's head that is used for a doll. As Saint-Exupery said: "It is the heart that is the final judge, not the eye."

It is necessary to know that a physical defect can also evoke a protective desire. Some celebrities or women in politics voluntarily keep a discreet squint, which could easily be corrected by surgery, in order to elicit this famous protective impulse and by this strategy increase their powers of seduction and attraction. They do not want to be operated on. As is also well known, if one of the features on a face is not perfect, other traits should be enhanced in order to lessen the attention paid to the defect and to dazzle the eye with the other traits. If, for example, the eyes are beautiful and the nose ordinary, embellish the eyes even more and the ordinary nose will be noticed less, advise beauticians who, even if they do not know the theory of Konrad Lorenz, do know how to make a face more beautiful. A facial scar can detract from the beauty of a man's face. To avoid the embarrassment that it can provoke in social situations, Passot said: "Give him the Legion of Honor and he will be taken for a hero."

It has also been said: "the defect is standing proud, the featureless eclipes".

Equally, the beautician who does not know the Muller-Lyer illusion of two lines of equal length with arrowheads pointing in different directions at each end knows how to give the illusion of making the eyes look closer together by applying makeup to the internal angle of the eye, or contrarily increasing the apparent distance between the eyes by applying makeup to the external angle. The same applies for making up cheek bones on an either too long or too wide face. The rouge can be placed closer or further apart.

11.3 Conclusion

Why be beautiful? It has been said that this is because of pride, pretentiousness, and a desire to be admired and to be ranked above the others!

The cult of beauty is in fact a culture. Humans are the only animals who do not accept their fate and seek to improve it: to cultivate beauty is to increase your quality of life, to want to make it more beautiful. Progress of civilization in all areas has increased life expectancies, but this does not seem to be enough. People want to be and appear even more beautiful, and this is what has made some say: if medicine has given years to life, it is medicine and esthetic surgery that has given life to years.

Beauty and fashion, it is still said, are external signs of our internal need to express ourselves and to reinvent ourselves, and we have defined fashion as an attempt to apply works of art on the living.

Finally, beyond wanting to be admired, the desire to be beautiful in some stems from a great desire to be loved. This desire to be loved even more is the final message that the followers of the beauty cult want to get across. Konrad Lorenz affirms this: everyone loves children and wants to protect them; this is innate. Can one blame someone for wanting to resemble them to be loved more? His theory is without failings. We must remember that esthetic surgeons must try to reproduce juvenile characteristics in their work when possible and desired in order to elicit emotion and admiration. We have seen the links that exist between beauty and admiration, and the deep reverberations felt by the mind and the soul. This is well summarized by Theodore Gautier: "to admire is to love with the mind, to love is to admire with the heart."

Beauty, as everyone knows, is not eternal, but equally, beauty has no age. One can be good looking at 20, but it is also possible to be irresistible at any age, as Coco Chanel said. Madame de Pompadour stated: "The first requirement of a woman is to please and as time passes this becomes more and more difficult." This reminds me of a very old woman who came to me one day to ask me to do a facelift. In response to the lack of enthusiasm I showed about performing this intervention because of her advanced age, she said very calmly "when one has ceased to please, one must not displease."

In his book *Essays on animal and human behavior*, Konrad Lorenz again offers us two drawings in which he compares the changes that have occurred in animals that have become domesticated, and he evokes a parallel with similar modifications in humans over time and the idea that modern life imposes upon him a sort of "domestication".

11.4 Summary

Konrad Lorenz's theory about human beauty is developed in detail:

- To trigger an emotion, inspiring at the same time a desire to protect, an adult face should have childish features or expressions. The emotion of human beauty is in fact subjective; the personality and the main qualities of the person are also part of the emotion.

We should remember that whenever it is possible and desired, a skilled esthetic surgeon should optimize the features that provoke an attraction reflex of tenderness and protection, like a baby does.

Body Dysmorphic Disorder

Melvin A. Shiffman

12.1 Definition

Body dysmorphic disorder (BDD) is defined as a preoccupation with an imagined or a very slight defect in physical appearance that causes significant distress to the individual. It was first described by Morselli in 1886 [1] who called it "dysmorphophobia." The disorder is manifested in people who dislike some aspect of how they look to such an extent that they cannot stop thinking and worrying about it. To other people these reactions may seem excessive as the supposed problem may not even be noticeable or is related to a very minor blemish such as a mole, or mild acne scarring that anyone else may not even notice. To sufferers of the syndrome the "defects" are very real, very obvious, and very severe.

12.2 Symptoms

1. There is preoccupation with the supposed appearance problem.
2. The patient takes actions to "hide" the defect or avoid situations because they feel ugly and do not want to be seen by others.

Some patients with body dysmorphia realize they look worse to themselves than to others and that their view of their appearance is exaggerated and distorted. Others are convinced that their view of their physical defect is accurate. Some have the feeling that other people are taking special notice of the "defect," that people are staring at it and making fun of it or laughing about it behind their backs when in reality, no one may even notice it. Many sufferers feel ashamed and fear being rejected by others.

Most patients with BDD perform one or more repetitive and often time-consuming behaviors also known as "rituals" that are usually aimed at examining, "improving," or hiding the perceived flaw in appearance. They usually spend a lot of time checking in the mirror to see whether their "defect" is noticeable or has changed in some way. Others will frequently compare themselves with other people or images in magazines or billboards. Some will spend hours "grooming" themselves by applying makeup, changing clothes, or rearranging their hair to "correct" or cover up the "problem." Others attempt to camouflage or hide their defect by wearing a hat, a wig, or sunglasses. In extreme cases, people wear a mask or hood over their head. Some try, by acting or standing in a certain way in public, to make the defect seem less noticeable. Others weigh or measure themselves continually or wear big and baggy clothing to hide what they think are "huge" hips or large breasts. Some may wear many layers of clothing to make themselves appear larger or more muscular, and some men (especially those who suffer from "muscle dysmorphia") lift weights or exercise excessively to try to bulk up. They may eat special diets or use drugs such as anabolic steroids to try to build up their muscles.

Patients with body dysmorphia may approach cosmetic surgeons or dermatologists seeking surgery or medical treatments that place the doctor at risk for a continually dissatisfied patient with whatever is done.

M.A. Shiffman
17501 Chatham Drive,
Tustin, California 92780-2302, USA
e-mail: shiffmanmdjd@yahoo.com

12.3 Consequences of BDD

Some patients with BDD function well despite their distress. Others are severely impaired by their symptoms, often becoming socially isolated by not going to school or work and extreme cases refusing to leave home for fear of being embarrassed about their appearance. It can be especially difficult for sufferers to go to places such as beaches, hairdressers, shopping, or places where the person may feel anxious about how they look. It is not uncommon for patients with BDD to feel depressed about their problem and the negative impact this has on their life. Some become so desperate that they attempt suicide.

Relationship problems are common and many BDD sufferers have few friends, avoiding dates and other social activities or even getting divorced because of their symptoms.

12.4 Associated Disorders

Many patients with BDD also suffer from depression at some point in their life and there is a high rate of depression in families of patients who develop BDD. The patient develops low esteem, feelings of rejection, heightened sensitivity, and of being unworthy.

Other disorders include obsessive compulsive disorder (OCD) such as eating disorders, anxiety disorders, trichotillomania (hair pulling), and abuse of drugs or alcohol.

There is a high rate of suicidal ideation (mean 57.8% of 185 subjects over 4 years) and a mean of 2.6% attempted suicide per year [2, 3].

12.5 Treatment

Serotonin-reuptake inhibitors (SRIs) are a group of medications that appear to be useful and effective in patients with BDS. The SRIs are a type of antidepressant used successfully in the treatment of both depression and obsessive compulsive disorder. These include Prozac, Zoloft, Cipramil, and Aropax.

Cognitive behavioral therapy (CBT) appears to be an effective treatment for BDD [4]. The behavioral component consists of "Exposure and Response Prevention" where the patient exposes their defect in situations which they would usually avoid while response prevention involves helping the patient stop carrying out the compulsive behavior related to the defect. The aim over time is to decrease anxiety involved with that particular avoided situation. The cognitive component addresses the range of intrusive thoughts that accompany the behaviors, or rituals such as mirror checking, in BDS. This focuses on exploring beliefs and values that support and strengthen a person's perceptions about their body. Cognitive restructuring is aimed at developing an understanding of how these strongly held values impact the person's sense of "self" and to progressively build up alternative ways of thinking about the intrusive thought, rather than going through the usual range of behaviors such as mirror checking and reassurance seeking. Restructuring consists of a range of techniques involving making changes to a person's values while not directly questioning the repetitive and intrusive thought the person has about their body.

12.6 Discussion

Understanding BDD and recognizing the patient with this disorder will prevent many misunderstandings between patient and doctor, especially the dermatologist or cosmetic surgeon. The BDD patient presenting for treatment of minimally abnormal skin findings, if recognized, will prevent unnecessary and potentially unsuccessful treatments [5-7]. Many patients with BDD seek cosmetic surgery and the unwary surgeon will invariably have to deal with a dissatisfied patient. Many eventually fall into the cosmetic surgery victim category of "overoperation." Recognition and deferral of surgery for BDD patients is advised because findings have shown the propensity of these patients to litigate, threaten, and even harm or kill their surgeon [8].

12.7 Conclusions

Failure to diagnose BDD in a preoperative cosmetic surgery patient will almost always lead to a dissatisfied patient. The surgeon will have a patient who is continuously dissatisfied with results no matter what is done to correct the perceived deformity. The treatment for the patient with BDD is medications, usually SRIs, or psychiatric care with cognitive behavioral therapy. The surgeon has to identify the BDD patients before surgery and tell them that surgery is not the treatment for their problem and refer them to the psychiatrist for treatment.

References

1. Thomas I, Patterson WM, Szepietowski JC, Chodynicki MP, Janniger CK, Hendel PM, et al. Body dysmorphic disorder: more than meets the eye. Acta Dermatovenerol Croat. 2005; 13(1):50–3.
2. Phillips KA, Menard W. Suicidality in body dysmorphic disorder: a prospective study. Am J Psychiatry. 2006;163(7): 1280–2.
3. Phillips KA, Coles ME, Menard W, Yen S, Fay C, Weisberg RB. Suicidal ideation and suicide attempts in body dysmorphic disorder. J Clin Psychiatry. 2005;66(6): 717–25.
4. Honigman R, Castle DJ. Body dysmorphic disorder – a guide for people with BDD. Victoria: Collaborative Therapy Unit, Mental Health Research Institute; 2003.
5. Buescher LS, Buescher KL. Body dysmorphic disorder. Dermatol Clin. 2006;24(2):251–7.
6. Glaser DA, Kaminer MS. Body dysmorphic disorder and the liposuction patient. Dermatol Surg. 2005;31(5):559–60.
7. Mackley CL. Body dysmorphic disorder. Dermatol Surg. 2005;31(5):553–8.
8. Hodgkinson DJ. Identifying the body-dysmorphic patient in aesthetic surgery. Aesthetic Plast Surg. 2005;29(6):503–9.

Part V

Techniques

Hair Transplantation

Paul C. Cotterill

13.1 Introduction

The most common form of hair loss for both men and women is androgenetic alopecia (AA) and the most common reason for performing hair transplantation is for the surgical correction of male pattern baldness (MPB). However, hair transplantation is available for women with female pattern hair loss (FPHL); eyelash, eyebrow, moustache, beard, and pubic transplantation; and cicatricial alopecia secondary to trauma, burns, rhytidectomy, and inactive inflammatory dermatoses. Current techniques allow for the superior removal, dissection, and placement of hair to yield natural looking results. Available donor hair cannot only come from the back of a permanent fringe of hair bearing scalp, but from other body areas such as the chest, back, and arms, while at the same time leaving, in most cases, undetectable scars.

It is beyond the scope of this chapter to describe in detail the vast amount of knowledge that has developed in this field in such a relatively short period of time since the first punch grafts were performed in the 1950s. This chapter is aimed at the practicing physician who may or may not be performing transplants and desires to learn more about the current state of the art in the field of hair restoration with its many applications both medically and surgically to help people that suffer from hair loss.

13.2 Pathophysiology and Classification

MPB occurs because of a combination of genetics, hormones, and time. MPB is androgen dependent and has a polygenic or multifactorial form of inheritance [1], hence the term, androgenetic alopecia (AA) to describe MPB. Although MPB can be passed on from either side of the family, there is a slightly higher risk through the maternal side. The typical scalp possesses between 90,000 and 140,000 terminal hair follicles, of which 84–90% are in the anagen (growing) phase. Scalp hairs in anagen grow at a rate of 0.35 mm/day, for 3–4 years. Approximately, 10% are in telogen (resting) phase, lasting 3–4 months. There is also a very short catagen (involution) phase lasting 3 weeks in 2% of scalp hairs. In humans, hair growth is asynchronous such that at any one time 50–150 hairs/day are shed as they cycle into telogen. In any area of the scalp a human needs to lose at least 50% of the hair to begin to have the appearance of hair loss. In those affected with AA there is a gradual conversion of terminal hairs (miniaturization) to fine, short, soft, hypopigmented vellus hairs. At the genetically predisposed hair follicle, free testosterone is reduced by the enzyme, 5-alpha reductase, to dihydrotestosterone (DHT). DHT then accumulates in the hair follicle and allows the chemical pathways that produce specific proteins that ultimately lead to hair follicle miniaturization and the eventual total loss of that hair. The role of androgens is less clear with FPHL. Women with FPHL, compared to men with MPB, have less androgen receptor proteins, and 5-alpha reductase enzymes but more estrogen producing aromatase enzymes [2]. This difference can help explain why women have a milder expression of AA compared to men and tend to maintain the frontal hairline.

The specific pattern of hair loss in men with MPB makes diagnosis generally easy. The individual affected

P.C. Cotterill
Private Practice,
21 Bedford Road, Toronto, ON M5R 2J9, Canada
e-mail: paul@drcotterill.com

first notices an increased shedding of scalp hair with an increasing amount of vellus hairs as the process of miniaturization occurs. Norwood's classification [3] of seven types of MPB, while not describing all common patterns of hair loss, is frequently used (Fig. 13.1).

The most common presentation for women with FPHL shows preservation of the frontal hairline with generalized thinning, but not total balding, behind the hairline. The thinning may be limited to the frontal scalp, but in many cases, can also include the rest of the scalp, including the occipital region, which is often spared in men. Ludwig's three grades of thinning [4] have been classically used to describe the pattern of FPHL (Fig. 13.2). More recently, Olsen [5] has described a Christmas tree pattern of thinning to the top of the scalp with frontal accentuation (Fig. 13.3) and is seen as the most common presentation affecting 70% of women with FPHL.

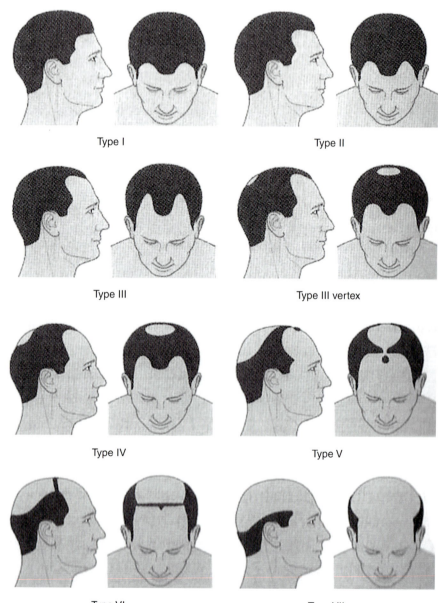

Fig. 13.1 Norwood classification of the common types of male pattern baldness [3]

Fig. 13.2 Ludwig classification of diffuse frontal loss [4]

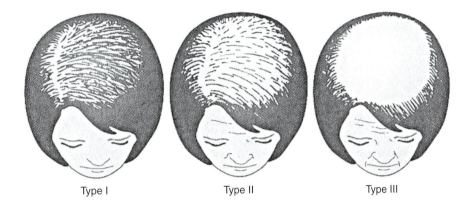

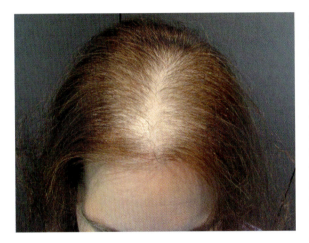

Fig. 13.3 Christmas tree pattern of thinning showing preservation of the hairline and frontal accentuation

13.3 Modern Hair Transplantation and Terminology

Traditional hair transplantation, employing circular punch grafts of 3–4 mm in diameter containing up to 25 hairs or more is largely accredited to Orentreich. In 1995, he published a paper that described the use of small autografts to treat various types of alopecias. The term, "donor dominance" was coined by Orentreich to describe how hair, taken from the permanent rim of scalp in a male with MPB, will continue to grow when transplanted to an alopecic area [6]. In the 1980s, Nordstrom and Marritt [7, 8] introduced one- to two-haired "micrografts," cut down from larger grafts, to refine and soften the frontal hairline to take away from the "plugginess" associated with large circular punch grafts. Later, it was shown that upon close inspection of the scalp, hairs could be seen to be emerging in bundles of one, two, three, and rarely four to five hairs surrounded by a common adventitia (Fig. 13.4). This integral bundle of hair is termed a follicular unit (FU). From this observation came the idea of removing and dissecting out FUs using magnification to allow proper visualization of FUs with the aim of keeping them intact. The advent of follicular unit transplantation (FUT) has led to the superior results now obtainable with modern hair transplantation techniques. A big advantage of FUT over traditional punch grafting, is that a natural result can be achieved even with one session on an otherwise alopecic area. Circular punch grafts were initially, "cut to size," trimming these larger grafts into smaller ones or using parts of two adjacent punch grafts, without paying attention to keeping FUs intact. A number of confusing terms has arisen to describe the various types of grafts. Table 13.1 gives a description of some of the more commonly used terms.

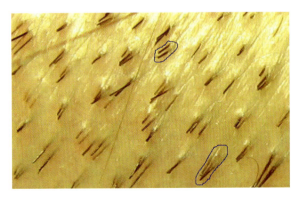

Fig. 13.4 View of scalp hairs emerging in bundles. A two-haired Fu and a three-haired FU are circled

Table 13.1 Graft terminology

Term	Description
Round graft (punch graft)	Traditional circular grafts using punches of various sizes containing 5–30+ hairs
Follicular Unit (FU, FUG)	One- to four-haired, naturally occurring, graft that exists on the scalp as an integral unit surrounded by a common adventitia
Micrograft	A general term to describe a one- to four-haired graft that can be a naturally occurring FU or cut to size using some hairs from adjacent units
Multifollicular unit/graft (MFU, MUG)	Graft with two or more hairs from adjacent FUs
	Commonly three to six hairs. Each utilized FU is intact
Minigraft	Graft that has three to eight hairs, cut to size using parts of two adjacent FUs
Follicular unit pairing	Placing more than one FUG into a single recipient site with three to eight hairs
Follicular unit extraction (FUE)	A one- to three-haired graft extracted from a donor site individually with a 0.7–1.0 mm punch rather than via strip excision. The FUE may be an intact FU or cut from a larger FU

13.4 Nonsurgical Treatment Options

13.4.1 Medications

The only medication that is approved for both MPB and FPHL by the Food and Drug Administration (FDA) is topical minoxidil (Rogaine). While the exact mechanism of action is unknown, minoxidil has been shown to improve the growth of suboptimal hairs in cell culture, is a potassium channel opener, and acts as a vasodilator. Minoxidil is available as a 2% and 5% mixture using isopropyl alcohol as its base. Studies have shown that topical minoxidil can improve hair counts and hair weights [9]. The solution needs to be applied twice a day to a dry scalp. Side effects, occurring in less than 6% of patients, can include flaking and dryness of the scalp. Females should be warned that facial hypertrichosis can occur in 3–5% of women. Additionally, there can be increased shedding of hair for the first 4–6 weeks of use. Once treatment is stopped any benefits are lost within 24 weeks. A 5% minoxidil foam formulation that uses glycerin as its base is now available. The foam formulation has been shown to be better absorbed and has less scalp irritation when compared to minoxidil with isopropyl alcohol.

Finasteride (Propecia) acts as a competitive inhibitor of the type II 5 alpha reductase enzyme. In turn, this acts to decrease the production of DHT at the hair follicles that are genetically predisposed to MPB. Finasteride has FDA approval for MPB in men aged 18–41 [10], but is not appropriate for women of childbearing years due to the possibility of feminization of a male fetus caused by the reduction of DHT. Studies of postmenopausal women have shown a lack of efficacy with 1 mg finasteride [11]. Concentrations of finasteride in the semen of men taking 1 mg daily were shown to be below levels that can cause risk to a male fetus. At a daily 1 mg dose, finasteride, even after 5 years of daily use, can continue to halt or slow hair loss, primarily in the vertex region and in some instances can regrow hair [12]. It is important to stress to male patients that finasteride works best at maintaining hair so that after 1 year of treatment a positive result is considered to be no change in hair counts and physical appearance. As such, compliance can wane after a period of time, so it is important for the physician to offer continued encouragement. The earlier the treatment is initiated in the thinning process, the better.

Finasteride is tolerated very well with sexual function side effects seen in less than 1.8% of men, with a return to normal levels once treatment is stopped. When assessing patients' prostate-specific antigen (PSA) levels, it should be remembered that finasteride will decrease these levels by approximately 50%. Long-term studies in men taking 5 mg finasteride for benign prostatic hypertrophy have shown that there can be a protective value in reducing the risk of prostate cancer [13].

The use of minoxidil and finasteride play an important role in the overall treatment of young men with MBP. At the time of the initial consultation it is important for the physician to map out a plan of action that often includes both surgical treatment and medical treatments. In the young male with ongoing MPB, hair restoration can often be implemented in the frontal scalp, to reestablish a hairline and to frame the face.

However, in men still in their twenties and early thirties, the extent of possible further hair loss can be difficult to predict. Most men have enough donor hair, even into their sixties and beyond, to surgically treat at least the frontal scalp, which is the most important area cosmetically for maintaining the appearance of their actual age. Once the frame of the face is lost, the patient can look 5–10 years older than their apparent age. Since minoxidil and finasteride work best in the younger men with early ongoing hair loss and work best in the vertex regions, which is just the area where the physician should not place grafts, it is a good marriage of surgery and medication. Perform transplants to the frontal scalp and use medications to maintain vertex hair until such time that the front is fully transplanted and /or the thinning pattern is clearly established and it is safe to commit to a portion of the vertex.

The medical treatment of FPHL can also include the use of antiandrogens [14, 15] especially in women with documented elevation of male hormones. Spironolactone, at doses of 100–200 mg/day, has weak antiandrogenic properties that has been used with varying degrees of success to slow down the progression of FPHL. However, there can be the possibility of menstrual irregularities, hyperkalemia, and feminization of a male fetus requiring the necessity of ongoing monitoring and contraceptive measures. Other antiandrogens that have been tried include cyproterone acetate, estrogen and cimetidine. A study by Tosti [16], following premenopausal women with FPHL taking higher dosages of finasteride, 2.5 mg daily in combination with an oral contraceptive, showed that 62% of the group studied had improvement over their hair loss.

Women are also found, much more commonly than men, to have low serum iron and/or serum ferritin levels. It has been shown that improving a low ferritin level with an iron replacement such as ferrous gluconate can improve the benefits of daily minoxidil use and improve hair growth [17]. Additionally, vitamin supplements including biotin and folic acid may help.

13.5 Nonmedical Treatments

Low-level light lasers are being used to stimulate hair growth for MPB and FPHL and have been given approval by the FDA as being a safe device [18]. Currently, more third party studies need to be done in order to show accurate efficacy. However, lasers are beginning to receive more widespread use as an adjunct treatment to surgery and medications for hair loss.

To aid in minimizing the contrast of thinning hair against a pale scalp and to give the appearance of fuller hair, camouflage agents can be used to good affect if there is still hair left in the thinning area. Colored hair sprays (ProTHIK: Aquila International Ltd), colored lotions (COUVRe: Spencer Forrest, Inc), fibers (Toppik: Spencer Forrest, Inc), and powders (DermMatch: DermMatch, Inc) are all available to men and women to achieve the visual impact of more scalp hair.

13.6 Preoperative Consultation

The consultation is the time when the physician determines if the patient is suitable for hair transplantation both physically and mentally. Extra time taken at the consultation is time well spent to determine if the patient's expectations are appropriate. The young male and female patients are especially prone to having inappropriate expectations that the physician must determine and decide if they can be reset or decide if the patient is not appropriate for surgery at all.

The following are important items to be covered at the consultation:

1. History and physical: It is important to know the length of time that hair loss has occurred, patient's age, family history of hair loss, medications that can contribute to hair loss, past and present illnesses, and allergies. The physician needs to make an educated guess as to the future potential thinning and possible worst case scenario. It is important that the patient be educated on not only what may be required now but also what might be required in the future.
2. Once MPB/FPHL is diagnosed, a full explanation of treatment options and adjuncts to hair restoration should be given. Proper medical therapy with minoxidil and finasteride to enhance surgery and maintain hair for a longer period of time should be stressed and incorporated into your treatment plan if possible.
3. For all patients, it is important to know the specific area the patient wants treated and what the physician assesses should be treated. For MPB, draw

a hairline on the scalp with a grease pencil for a focus of discussion. Generally speaking, for a younger male with MPB, concentrate on the frontal scalp only.
4. Photographs with any lines drawn on the scalp to indicate where grafts will be positioned should be taken at the time of consultation or immediately before surgery. Photographs can be invaluable at a later time when assessing the success of a transplant. Patients often forget what they looked like with hair loss and sometimes photos are your chief tool to convince the patient of a successful outcome.
5. Set the expectations of the potential short-term and long-term outcomes: If the patient has early thinning then one session may be appropriate, but as ongoing thinning of the preexisting hair occurs, a second and eventually a third session may be required. If there is complete baldness then stress the need for possibly up to three sessions depending on the density desired. It is essential that at consultation the potential need for further sessions in the future be discussed. Unlike many other cosmetic surgeries, hair restoration patients tend to have a long relationship with their physician often spanning decades. The physician should be cognoscente that what they say one day about the degree of hair loss and the number of sessions and grafts required could come back up for discussion years later.
6. The patient should understand that the end result will never achieve the density the patient had before the onset of thinning. In an otherwise bald area the result achieved can be that of early thinning.
7. Stress that different hair types and hair colors and scalp colors can lead to varying results. Hair characteristics should be assessed and documented. Patients with fine, wavy, salt and pepper hair with a lot of body and a lighter scalp will have a fuller look than patients with straight, black, thin, coarse hair, and a pale scalp.
8. Assess the density and amount of hair available in the donor area compared to the eventual size of the balding area and relay this information to the patient.
9. Emphasize that the limiting factor in hair restoration is the amount of permanent, limited, donor hair available.
10. The donor scar will be camouflaged as long as the hair in the donor region is not shaved off the scalp. There is a limitation as to how short the hair can be.
11. Go over the timing of important stages after a transplant: The crusts/scabs on each graft will have fallen off by 10–12 days. Patients are warned to expect that every hair in each transplanted graft will be shed and start to grow by 3 months. At 6 months there is a cosmetic benefit, but full maturity is not appreciated till after 12 months.
12. There can be significant postoperative effluvium of preexisting hair, primarily in women.
13. Have many representative photographs of your patients available for patients to see and discuss with you.
14. A thorough discussion of the complications and potential side effects must be provided and understood.

13.7 Female Considerations

Females that present with scalp hair loss often present with more complex assessment issues. FPHL, due to the generalized nature of thinning with maintenance of the frontal hairline, can be more of a diagnostic challenge [14]. The history and physical play a much more important role compared to their male counterpart. The chief causes for generalized hair loss that can mimic FPHL include acute telogen effluvium and less commonly chronic telogen effluvium and generalized alopecia areata. Acute telogen can occur from such things as child birth, high fever, general anesthetics, certain medications, rapid weight loss, and thyroid imbalances. It is important to determine the exact time of onset of the hair loss. Low ferritin/or iron levels, in addition to contributing to FPHL, can also contribute to telogen effluvium. Chronic telogen effluvium, usually presenting with no specific trigger, occurs usually in the 40–50 year-old age group. At the consultation, the physician should be looking for signs and symptoms of a testosterone excess syndrome that could be quickening or contributing to FPHL. Blood tests routinely indicated for women include a complete blood count, free thyroxine, serum thyroid stimulating hormone, serum iron, and serum ferritin. If there is a suspicion of testosterone excess, (lowering of the voice, rapid hair loss in the frontotemporal recessions, hirsutism, acne, and menstrual irregularities), then referral to a gynecologist or endocrinologist for appropriate workup are suggested. In addition to a hair pull test, a biopsy is often indicated to help differentiate FPHL from telogen effluvium, alopecia areata, or scarring inflammatory disorders. It is suggested when performing biopsies to do two 4 mm diameter biopsies and request for horizontal sectioning.

Just as important as making the diagnosis of FPHL is determining if the patient is suitable for transplantation and if their expectations are appropriate. Psychological studies have shown that women are much more upset by their hair loss [19]. Men can be satisfied with a thinning look from a frontal scalp transplant and may not desire to transplant the crown at all. Women may not be satisfied with any appearance of thinning at all. Additionally, since typical FPHL is that of generalized thinning and not total loss, once transplanted, there is less of a relative impact or change, when compared to adding hair to a bald male. It is much more important for the physician to take the extra time to assess and set the expectations with women. The physician needs to assess the extent of generalized thinning which can include the occipital potential donor region. Often the thinning area is too large, with too small a potential donor region. If transplantation is to be considered then it is better to settle with making a small area, such as just behind the frontal hairline, discretely thicker. Emphasize that there will still be some degree of see-through to the scalp after treatment, but to a lesser degree. The female patient should be forewarned of the greater risk of postoperative telogen effluvium and the potential benefit of pretreating with minoxidil to help minimize this occurrence.

13.8 Preoperative Instructions

At the time of the initial consultation it is a good idea to advise the patient that they may require up to 1 week off work (Table 13.2). Up to 20% of patients may experience some degree of postoperative forehead swelling and / or facial edema. This can start 2–3 days after surgery and continue for another 2–3 days. Patients are also advised not to play any sports or perform any heavy physical exercise for 1 week postoperatively. The patient should also be warned about the potential visibility of the scabs in the recipient area. The patient is advised to keep the donor hair long enough to easily camouflage the sutures. Blood tests are to be ordered to include hepatitis B, hepatitis C, HIV, a complete blood count, and clotting profile. To minimize the chance of bleeding, patients are told to stop anticoagulants, alcohol, and acetylsalicylic acid products 1 week prior to surgery. Additionally, vitamin E. products and ginkgo biloba should also be stopped. If using minoxidil solution, do not apply an application on the day of surgery to minimize the vasodilatation effect on the local microvasculature. On the day of surgery some physicians advocate an antistaphylococcal antibiotic given 1 h preoperatively. Half an hour prior to surgery a mild tranquilizer or sedative, such as 10 mg p.o. valium or 1–2 mg sl ativan, can be given. At the time of the consultation if there is any indication of a preexisting medical risk, then consent for surgery from either the family doctor or cardiologist should first be obtained. The author suggests that an anesthetist be present for any patient that may have a preexisting medical risk or when intravenous sedation is required.

13.9 Surgical Planning

Hairline design and placement is of critical importance to the successful esthetic outcome of a hair transplant. It is one of the most difficult aspects of the procedure to master, and consequently the area where the most errors are made. The reader is referred to other sources for a thorough treatment of hairline planning [20–23]; however, certain principles should be described.

13.9.1 Men with MPB

It is important to remember when planning a hairline in men that thinning is ongoing throughout life, and that there is a finite amount of hair available from the permanent donor fringe. There may not be enough hair to transplant both the frontal and crown regions. As such, for most men with MPB, it is generally prudent to treat the front one-third to half of the scalp and not treat the crown at all. Another option is to wait until such time as the front is completed before deciding if the patient is concerned with the crown and if there is adequate hair left to treat that area. It is also important to impress upon the patient with early

Table 13.2 Preoperative instructions

BLOOD TESTS
You must have your blood work done at least 2 weeks prior to your surgery date. Our office must receive these results in order to proceed with your scheduled surgery
THE HIV ANTIBODY TEST
As part of your routine preoperative laboratory blood tests, all patients are required to be tested for HIV. The testing and results are kept strictly confidential. We have instituted this additional test because individuals who are infected should not be undergoing elective surgery, which will tax their immune system unnecessarily and perhaps trigger a disease that might otherwise not surface
ANTIBIOTIC PRESCRIPTION
Please have the enclosed prescription for Keflex (a form of penicillin), filled PRIOR to your surgery. If you are allergic to penicillin, please contact our office immediately. Do not take any M.A.O. inhibitor (e.g., Parnate, Marplan, Niamid), Seldane (antiallergy medication), or Nizoral (anti-fungal medication) when taking our prescribed antibiotic
BEFORE YOUR SURGERY CAREFULLY READ and FOLLOW instructions below:
IF YOU LIVE OUT OF TOWN, please make arrangements to stay in town the night before and the night following your surgery. Traffic and/or weather could delay your arrival at our office. If you arrive late, your appointment may have to be postponed
DO NOT BOOK FLIGHTS UNTIL AFTER NOON THE DAY AFTER SURGERY as you will be required to return to the office to have your hair washed. If for some reason you need to be seen very early that day, arrange a time with the booking secretary 1–3 weeks before your appointment
YOU WILL NOT BE ABLE TO DRIVE AFTER YOUR SURGERY as the drugs used during the procedure will impair your driving ability. Arrange for someone to pick you up or take a taxi. It is also a good idea for someone to be with you overnight, following your surgery
HAIR LENGTH, PERMANENTS, AND/OR COLORING. Let your hair grow to 1.5–2 in. in the back and sides for easy coverage of donor areas. Permanents and/or hair coloring may be done up to 1 week prior to surgery, and 2 weeks following surgery.
Two (2) WEEKS PRIOR TO SURGERY:
BE SURE THAT YOUR BLOOD WORK HAS BEEN DONE
ELIMINATE the intake of vitamin E capsules or vitamin pills containing vitamin E
Notify the office if you are using any medications (either prescribed or over-the-counter). It may have to be discontinued or substituted with an alternate drug
ONE (1) WEEK PRIOR TO SURGERY:
DO NOT drink any alcohol (wine, beer, liquors).–not even "just one glass"
DO NOT use marijuana or any non-approved drugs
DO NOT take any aspirin (ASA) or any drugs containing aspirin. You may use tylenol
STOP the use of minoxidil (Rogaine). You may continue to use propecia
DO NOT take any herbal products
THE DAY BEFORE SURGERY:
STOP taking medications such as viagra, levitra, cialis
DO NOT do any strenuous activity, including exercise
THE NIGHT BEFORE SURGERY:
WASH your hair well. If you have long hair, please use a cream rinse. Do not use hair spray or setting lotion
THE DAY OF SURGERY:
TAKE the first dose of antibiotics 2 h prior to your scheduled time of surgery – unless otherwise directed
EAT a good meal before you come for your surgery UNLESS otherwise directed
DO NOT wear any piece of clothing with a tight neckline that has to be pulled over your head. A sweatshirt or jacket with a hood that can be pulled over the head provides an easy way to camouflage the bandage. Female patients may want to bring a scarf

thinning, that even though one session may thicken and treat nicely the frontal scalp for now, a second and possibly third session may ultimately be required as thinning progresses, to yield the density that can be achieved with transplantation.

The scalp can be divided into several important zones (Fig. 13.5), with the three potentially treatable areas being the frontal region, mid-scalp, and vertex (crown).

When recreating a frontal hairline, a line is drawn from the midline anterior most point, or mid-frontal point (MFP). This point usually is placed 7– 11 cm above the midglabellar line, at approximately where the forehead transitions from being vertical to sloping gradually posteriorly (Fig. 13.6). It is best to choose the MFP as superior as is acceptable to both patient and physician. A difficulty that can arise when, typically with the younger male, there is a strong remnant of the immature hairline present as a teenager, which can be as low as 4–6 cm above the midglabellar line. It can be very difficult for the patient to understand why the surgeon is placing a hairline 3 cm to even 6 cm higher than where the patient thinks it should be. This is a chief reason why many physicians wait till a patient is above 25 years of age to start surgery, when the patient is more mature, with better expectations, and the eventual thinning pattern becomes more evident. A curved line is then drawn from the MFP superiorly and laterally to the apex, the highest point of the frontotemporal recessions. As a guide, an imaginary line can be drawn vertically from the lateral epicanthus. The apex is placed at, or medial to, where this line intersects with a line drawn from the MFP. If the apex is placed too low or lateral, and as a consequence the frontotemporal recessions are filled in, this can lead to an unnatural appearance. Continue the line from the apex posteriorly, keeping

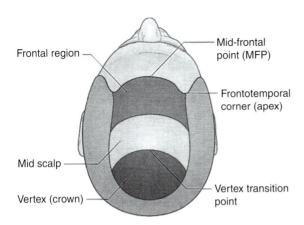

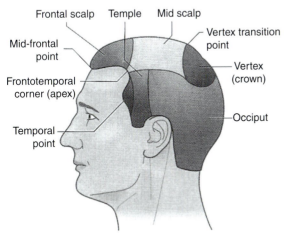

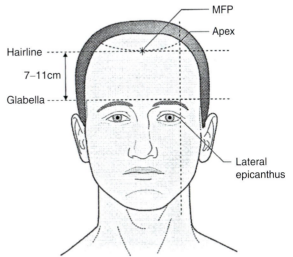

Fig. 13.5 Major zones and landmarks. The three transplantable zones are the frontal region, mid-scalp, and vertex. The mid-frontal point (MFP) is the lowest anterior mid-point of the frontal hairline. The frontal hairline meets the temple at the apex (frontotemporal junction). The vertex transition point is where the horizontal scalp changes to the vertical, and is often the positioning of a posterior hairline when not committing to crown transplantation (Reprinted with permission from Berg and Cotterill [24]. Copyright Elsevier Limited 2009)

Fig. 13.6 The frontal hairline is designed by placing the MFP 7–11 cm above an imaginary line drawn horizontally across the glabella. A *curved line* is drawn from the MFP to meet with a line drawn vertically from the epicanthus, at the highest most point of the frontotemporal recession (*apex*) (Reprinted with permission from Berg and Cotterill [24]. Copyright Elsevier Limited 2009)

the line horizontal with the ground to define the part. A common mistake is to not identify lateral fringe areas of ongoing thinning. It is best to place some, "insurance" hair in the triangles for when the patient goes on to more advanced thinning, keeping in mind that eventual thinning in the parietal region usually ends up in a line often horizontal with the ground (Fig. 13.7).

In some patients, thinning progresses inferiorly into the temporoparietal fringe and recedes. A lateral hump can be created by incorporating the apex with the newly designed lateral hump (Fig. 13.8). The posterior border of the frontal region and mid-scalp region is finished frequently in a curved fashion to re-create a natural appearing posterior hairline when viewed from the back of the patient. When transplanting the frontal and mid-scalp regions the mid-portion of the posterior hairline should not go further than the vertex transition point (VTP). This is the point where the horizontal scalp changes to the vertical (Fig. 13.5). Beyond that point the hair direction begins to change as the hair in the crown begins to form a whorl from where the hair radiates out in a 360° pattern. The appearance of a head of hair, when viewed from the front of the patient is achieved if adequate transplantation is performed to the VTP. After that point any additional hair is not appreciated from the front.

There are a variety of hairline placement patterns depending on the age of the patient, nationality, extent of present and possible further thinning hair loss patterns and expectations. For the very bald or very young patient who may become very bald in the future, an isolated frontal forelock can be planned [25]. This is one of the safest ways to achieve a conservative hairline when there is the concern of present or future extreme limitations in the amount of donor hair relative to a significant balding area. Figure 13.9 demonstrates a frontal forelock in a young male that may go onto extensive hair loss in the future. There is the creation of a natural hairline pattern with an island of central density being created in the middle with less

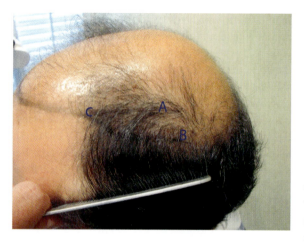

Fig. 13.7 Line CA indicates where transplants are often finished, without anticipating where future hair loss may extend to. Insurance hair should be placed to line CB so that the physician does not need to keep chasing an advancing, thinning triangle of continuing hair loss

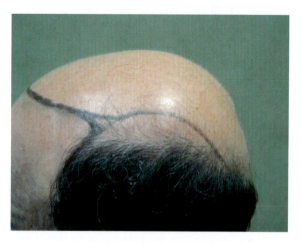

Fig. 13.8 Creating a lateral hump in a lowered temporoparietal fringe allows the frontal hairline to be kept in a natural alignment

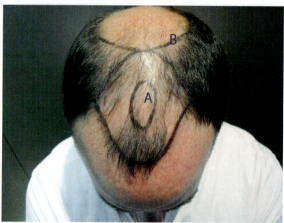

Fig. 13.9 Creation of a frontal forelock in a young male that may go on to extensive balding. The central oval zone is planted most densely with less density toward the fringe. This pattern is meant to stand on its own even if there is significant balding in the future

density laterally without a specific connection to the fringe. This mimics a pattern of hair loss seen naturally in many men with significant balding and does not incur significantly more grafting in the future, if many additional grafts are not available.

13.9.2 The Crown

The front half of the scalp is the most important area cosmetically for most men. Proper transplantation principles dictate that men roughly less than 35–40 years of age should not have their crown treated. Young men should wait until such time as they are older and their thinning pattern is securely established or they have finished treating a previously bald frontal scalp with transplants.

The crown, if transplanted, adds less cosmetic gain compared to the front. Some men are not concerned about the crown as they do not see it and are disinclined to treat that area. Once the frontal scalp has been transplanted, the posterior hairline is designed to mimic the beginning of a naturally occurring bald vertex. When viewed from the rear of the patient then a non-transplanted crown will appear very natural (Fig. 13.10). Other men are concerned with a bald or thinning crown and want that area covered too. However, in the author's experience, many men want some good reasonable density and coverage with the frontal scalp, and for the crown they either are not concerned with that area or will settle with a light coverage to take away from the appearance of a bald dome. By limiting crown transplantation to one or two treatments of light coverage, additional donor hair can be left in reserve for any future hair concerns that may develop over time.

Traditional punch grafting performed from decades ago routinely required three or four sessions of plugs to adequately treat an area and would frequently exhaust the donor area. If further treatments were at all anticipated more posteriorly then the use of scalp reductions, flaps, extenders, or expanders to minimize the crown area by whatever means necessary were often utilized. These procedures are still utilized today by some surgeons in the very bald male to minimize the area of alopecic scalp. There is the concern, however, that with extensive scalp reduction of the bald areas and scalp lifting of the permanent fringe, there can be the occurrence of unnatural hair directions and the presence of an obvious scar that needs to be camouflaged. Due to these concerns of unnatural hair direction, the presence of an obvious scar, in conjunction with the excellent results that can be achieved with just one session of FUT placed on a bald crown,

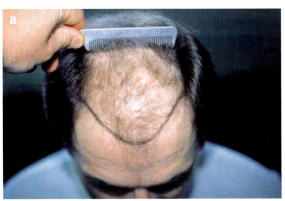
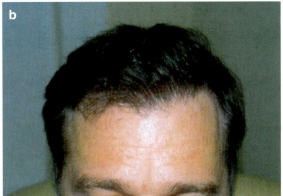
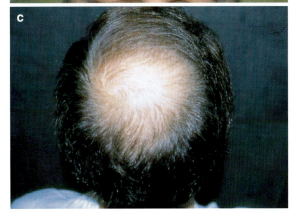

Fig. 13.10 (**a**) A typical frontal hair line has been drawn on with the intent of limiting transplantation to the vertex transition point. (**b**) After transplantation, when viewed from the front, there is the appearance of a full head of hair. (**c**) When viewed from the rear the vertex is still untreated but the posterior hairline looks very natural

reductions, flaps, extenders, and expanders are being used much less frequently today for MPB. However, these procedures are still invaluable in the treatment of extensive scalp hair loss due to trauma, burns, and congenital malformations. The indications and proper uses of these techniques are beyond the scope of this chapter and as such the reader is directed to other reference sources for a full description [26–29].

13.9.3 Females

Females with FPHL present their own unique planning challenges. Typical thinning patterns apparent in women with FPHL differ from men in that there is usually frontal hairline sparing with generalized thinning behind. In many women the thinning can involve most if not all of the potential occipital donor region and as such many women do not have sufficient donor areas of adequate density to warrant transplantation. Often there is evidence of generalized miniaturization of hair follicles throughout the scalp. In those women that maintain adequate density with minimal miniaturization of hair follicles in the occipital region, transplantation can be considered. However, as has been previously described, female expectations as to what can be achieved also come into the equation as to deciding the appropriateness of transplantation. Frequently, the areas to be treated are just behind the hairline to the mid-scalp or filling in the frontotemporal recessions to create a more rounded, feminine appearance (Fig. 13.11). With planning, in women the concern is not so much the possibility of ongoing hair loss that could result in total balding, but of what the patient can expect as a reasonable result with one session. The FUT techniques used today allows for the creation of tiny sites made between preexisting hairs, so as to conserve hair, and to not remove hair, as was the case with the use of traditional 3.25–3.5 mm punch grafts. Women should be warned that they should plan for the possible risk of telogen effluvium postoperatively. Generally, sessions should be smaller than their male counterpart, performing approximately 1,000–1,500 grafts per session. This helps to minimize the risk of telogen and allow for better camouflage using hair in the non-treated area to comb over the temporary crusts in the recipient area.

13.9.4 Selection of Donor Area Site and Size

The decision as to where to choose the donor zone and how much tissue to take can be a difficult concept for the novice surgeon to grasp. It is inherent in any successful hair restoration procedure that any grafts removed will be taken from an area that will be permanent and to not develop male or female pattern hair loss in the future. Otherwise the transplanted hair could eventually fall out and a visible scar could eventually become apparent as the surrounding donor hair disappears. When deciding on where to take the strip and how much to take, one needs to consider the age of the patient as well as the family history to aid in predicting

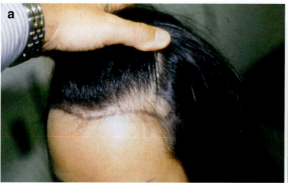
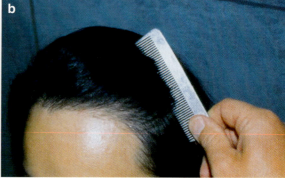

Fig. 13.11 (a) A female with familial high frontotemporal recessions that desires a more rounded feminine hairline. (b) After the hairline has been lowered with transplants into a more feminine position

eventual hair loss. It is helpful to know that most patients have at least the ability to have two to three strips of scalp, 8–10 mm wide, removed from the permanent hair-bearing scalp. In these strips, the average balding male has from 5,000 to 7,000 FUs that can be safely used for transplantation.

In general, the first strip should be removed from the occipital scalp at or above the level of the occipital protuberance. Unger's studies on the size of the safe donor area [30] indicate that an area, for 80% of men under 80, exists that is from 70 mm wide at the midline occipital region extending laterally to 80 mm at its widest point and then narrowing to 50 mm wide in the temporal scalp above the ears.

13.9.5 Estimating Size of Donor Strip

This step takes much experience to be comfortable knowing the size of strip and number of grafts required to transplant the size of area to be treated. Some physicians will choose to transplant all small one- to three-haired FUs, while others will choose a combination of FUs and MFUs. This can alter the size of strip required. The following is an example to illustrate how one might go about determining strip length for a commonly treated area:

1. If one is to transplant the hairline to mid-scalp, the average area to be covered is approximately 60 cm squared. (To more accurately determine the area to be covered a 1 cm^2 transparent grid can be used and the area to be transplanted traced on top of the grid to give the recipient area size.)
2. Assume the density of the average permanent safe donor zone is 100 FU/cm^2. The range is from 60 to 140 FU/cm^2. (To accurately determine the density a trichscope, densitometer, or video microscope can be used to assess donor density.)
3. A decision is made as to what density the surgeon wants to plant the FUs. In an initial session, for the novice surgeon, it is good to know that densities of 25–30 FU/cm^2 will yield a satisfactory appearance and is suggested. In some practices, densities of 50 FU/cm^2 and greater are achieved, but should be reserved for those with adequate staff and expertise.
4. Once the number of follicular units required to transplant the area to be treated is determined then the length of a 1 cm wide donor strip, based on the number of FUs needed, can be estimated.

An example calculation shows that if a frontal hairline and scalp are to be transplanted in a 60 cm^2 area, placing the grafts at a density of 25 FUs/cm^2 then: $(60 \times 25) = 1{,}500$ FUs will be required.

If 1,500 FUs are required from a strip that is 1 cm wide, taken from a donor site with a density of 100 FUs/cm^2: $(1{,}500/100)$ then the strip needs to be 15 cm long.

> **Tip**
>
> For a novice surgeon or surgeon that does transplantation infrequently the average size of a frontal area from hairline to mid-scalp is approximately 60 cm^2. To transplant at densities of 25–30 FU/cm^2, approximately 1,800–2,000 FU grafts (one to four hairs each) are required, taken from an average density donor zone. A 1 cm wide strip should then be removed at approximately 20–22 cm long.

13.10 Anesthesia

For the vast majority of cases, local anesthesia, with or without oral sedation, is the most commonly used form of anesthesia for hair transplantation. Procedures can be performed without any oral sedation or with a mild sedative such as 10 mg of oral valium and/or 2 mg of sublingual lorazepam given 30 min before the start of surgery. Some physicians will use intravenous twilight sedation using midazolam, propofol, or fentanyl. The author has found the need for twilight sedation to be used only in those circumstances when the patient has a strong desire to be totally unaware of what is happening. In those rare circumstances, or when the author feels the patient with a preexisting medical condition could put the patient at risk, an anesthetist will be present for the entire procedure. An automatic blood pressure cuff and pulse oximeter should be used for each surgery and to have available oxygen, a defibrillator, a fully equipped crash cart with emergency medications, and an emergency action plan with staff trained in basic cardiopulmonary life support is essential.

Techniques used to aid in the delivery of local anesthesia to the scalp include topical lidocaine cream, needleless injectors, supraorbital, supratrochlear, occipital nerve blocks, and field blocks. The maximum dose of lidocaine with epinephrine, (7 mg/kg), and bupivacaine (3 mg/kg), must be kept in mind. Epinephrine is commonly used in scalp anesthesia to act as an effective vasoconstrictor and as such can prolong the affect of the local anesthetic. The use of tumescent anesthesia will allow for large volumes of a dilute anesthetic to be administered with minimal chance of toxicity.

Once the donor area has been identified, clipped, and prepared (Fig. 13.12), an initial field block in the occipital donor area is administered using a 10 ml syringe filled with 1% lidocaine with 1:100,000 epinephrine and a 30 gauge, half inch needle. Six to eight small wheels are slowly injected to raise small blebs of solution, about 1 in. apart just at the inferior edge of the clipped hair. To mask the sting of the initial injections, some physicians advocate the use of ice in the area, local vibration, or buffered anesthetics. Once the initial wheels are raised, the operator goes back to each wheel and continues the field block aiming the needle left and right from each already numbed site to fill in the gaps, using a total of 8–10 ml. In this manner, the patient should only feel a mild sting of the initial injections. A tumescent solution is prepared using a 100 ml bag of normal saline adding 5 ml of 2% lidocaine without epinephrine and 0.4 ml of 1:1,000 epinephrine to give a 100 ml tumescent solution of .1% lidocaine with 1:250,000 epinephrine. Using 10 ml syringes with 21 gauge 1.5 in. needles, inject just superior to the block as much tumescent solution as the tissue will take. The intent is to cause maximum tissue turgor in order to lift subcutaneous fat away from underlying arteries and nerves and to keep the tissue firm to minimize transection of follicles during removal of the strip. The high volumes of dilute anesthetics also help to minimize bleeding. The patient is then left for 10–15 min to allow proper anesthesia and vasoconstriction to take place. The patient is then placed in a prone pillow, if a mid-occipital area is to be harvested (Fig. 13.13). Just before the initial strip is removed, an additional 8–10 ml of tumescent solution is injected to allow for further turgor and to test that the area is fully numbed.

The recipient site is anesthetized while the donor strip is being dissected. With the patient in a semi-supine position, a ring block is administered, similar to the initial donor area block, just inferior to the anterior hairline. Up to 10 ml of a 2% lidocaine with 1:100,000 epinephrine mixture is used. One 10 ml syringe is then filled with a mixture made up using 0.6 ml of 1:1,000 epinephrine to 30 ml injectable saline to yield a 1:50,000 epinephrine mixture. The entire recipient area is then plumped up using 10 ml of the 1:50,000 epinephrine

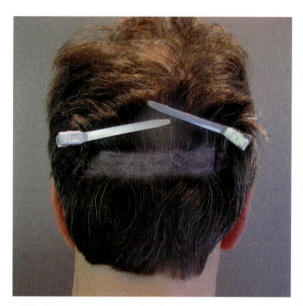

Fig. 13.12 Occipital donor area clipped

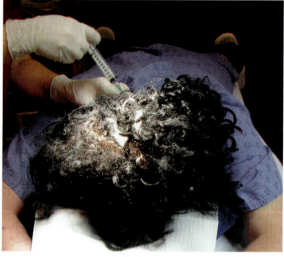

Fig. 13.13 Patient in prone pillow with anesthesia being checked

mixture (and 5–10 ml of further 1% lidocaine where required), to allow for complete anesthesia and hemostasis. If further plumping of tissue is required, injectable normal saline can be used. Some surgeons may also employ additional tumescent anesthesia to minimize damage to the supragaleal vascular plexus during surgery, to improve hemostasis and to expand the recipient sites during surgery allowing for contraction of sites, and minimizing distances between sites, once the tumescent fluid has dissipated. Some physicians will also mix marcaine with lidocaine solutions to give prolonged anesthesia.

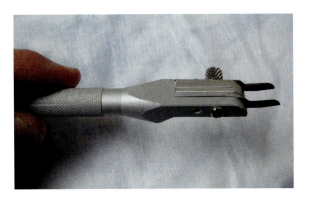

Fig. 13.14 Double-bladed scalpel with four spacers that could accommodate further blades

13.11 Removal of Donor Strip

With the patient seated the donor site is marked and clipped with curved Metzenbaum scissors to 2–4 mm in length. This minimum hair length is required so that hair direction can be continually assessed while removing the donor strip. The shorter hair length also helps to avoid hairs being inadvertently trapped while planting the graft. Once the donor site has been clipped it is then cleaned with alcohol and with a povidone-iodine solution. The area is then anesthetized and allowed to sit for 10–15 min to enable the adrenalin to take effect. (The recipient area anesthetic is administered later in the procedure.) The patient is then placed in a prone pillow. At this stage the donor site is further tumesced. This allows for maximum tissue turgor just before the strip is cut and additionally checks are made for adequate anesthesia. The author prefers to use a single bladed scalpel with a #15 blade to remove a single ellipse that is tapered at the ends. Some surgeons may use double-bladed (Fig. 13.14) or multi-blade scalpels with spacers to allow multiple strips to be excised simultaneously with the aim of reducing the time for dissection. However, studies have shown that there can be more transection of follicles with a multi-blade knife as there is less visualization of the follicles. The strip is cut to 1–2 mm below the level of the hair follicle leaving some subcutaneous tissue to protect the root bulb. Going much deeper will disturb the subcutaneous blood supply and incur more bleeding. The operator must continually assess the angle of the hair follicles and adjust the blade accordingly. The assistant provides counter traction with a tissue clamp to allow easier strip removal.

Once the strip is removed it is immediately placed in chilled saline and handed to the technician for dissection. Figure 13.15 shows the author's technique for strip removal. Any electrocautery, if necessary, is used at this point and any stray hairs or hair spicules are very diligently cleaned from the wound. Undermining is performed when excessive tension on closure is a concern. The author rarely needs to perform undermining as the wound width is generally kept to less than 1.2 cm to allow for easy closure. With minimal tension the scar should heal to being pencil line thin. Some physicians, the author included, will perform trichophytic closure. A 1 × 1 mm wide triangular strip, cut at a 45° angle, is trimmed from the inferior wound edge (Fig. 13.16). This will de-epithelialize one to two hair follicles and when the wound is sutured closed, the superior border will cover the trimmed inferior border allowing the inferior hairs to grow through the scar to allow more enhanced camouflage. The author will perform this in most circumstances where there is minimal tension. If there has been multiple procedures performed in the same area or there is above average tension demonstrated at the time of strip excision, then a standard closure is performed. Physician preference dictates what type of suture is used and if staples are favored. The author uses a running single-layer closure with a 3–0 non-dissolving thread. Sutures are to be removed in 7–10 days.

When subsequent sessions are performed, it is common to re-excise the previous linear scar with the new strip excision to minimize scaring of the donor zone. It should be kept in mind that with subsequent re-excisions, overall tension in the donor zone increases, such that the width of the donor strip should be adjusted

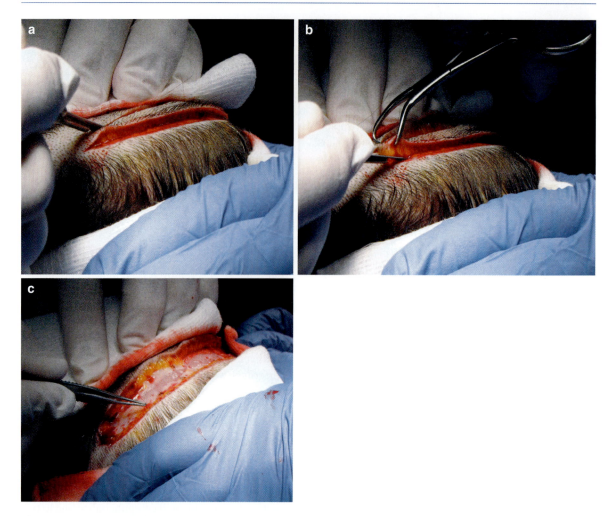

Fig. 13.15 (**a**) Donor strip is incised using a single blade being careful to keep blade parallel to the hair follicles. Notice that the end of the strip is tapered. (**b**) The strip is being dissected out ensuring that the blade is 1–2 mm below level of the follicle bulb leaving some fat surrounding the bulb and avoiding deeper blood vessels and nerves. The assistant applies strong counter traction with the use of the tissue clamp. (**c**) Strip is removed and any stray hairs or hair spicules are removed from the wound

accordingly. When patients return after many years, having had the original punch graft excision technique performed, previous circular punch scars that leave intact hairs between excised rows, and between grafts on the same rows, can be excised. The current strip excision techniques can benefit this type of patient two-fold: (1) By re-excising and minimizing old punch scars and (2) making available more reusable donor hair.

After the wound has been sutured closed, any trapped hairs under the suture are carefully freed. The area is then cleansed with a dilute hydrogen peroxide mixture applied from a spray bottle. At this juncture, if a second strip is to be taken from a temporal site, the patient's head is taken out of the prone pillow and turned to one side for the next excision. Otherwise, if donor excision is complete, then the patient is turned over on to their back to wait while the strip is being dissected until such time as the recipient site is anesthetized.

13.12 Follicular Unit Extraction

Follicular unit extraction (FUE) is a relatively new technique that uses small circular punches to core out donor grafts one at a time. Unlike the original punch

13 Hair Transplantation

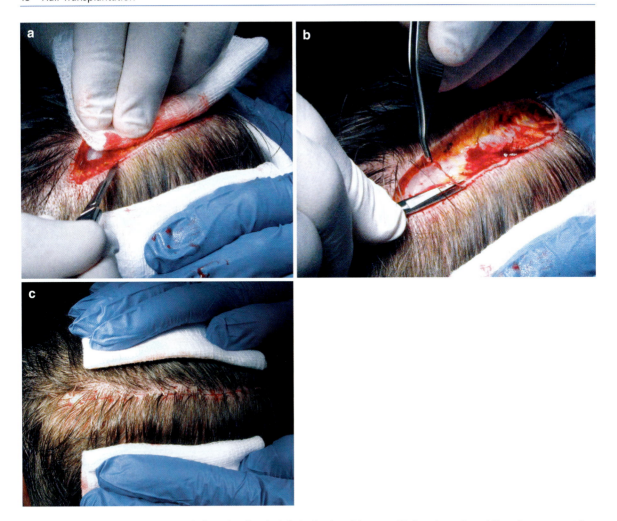

Fig. 13.16 (**a**) Trichophytic closure technique showing the inferior border of the wound being trimmed at a 45° angle to create a triangular strip 1 × 1 mm. (**b**) The strip is being trimmed to de-epithelialize one to two follicular units. (**c**) Following single-layer closure

grafts that were 3.5–4.0 mm in diameter, FUE employs a 0.7–1.0 mm punch. Because the site created is so small, sutures are not required and the wound is allowed to heal by secondary intention.

13.12.1 Indications for FUE

1. Wanting to avoid linear scalp donor site scar
2. Limited recipient area dictating the need for fewer grafts: eyebrow, eyelash, and moustache
3. Due to excessive scarring in donor area, further linear scars are not appropriate
4. Use of non-scalp hair, that is, chest, back, and beard
5. To thicken widened scars in donor area from traditional excisions that cannot be re-excised

13.12.2 Advantages of FUE

1. Tiny 0.7–1.0 mm incision
2. No sutures required
3. No linear scar in donor area
4. No or minimal tension in donor area
5. Possibility of wearing hair in donor area very short

13.12.3 Disadvantages of FUE

1. Higher percentage of follicular transection and ingrown hairs compared to FUT
2. Time consuming and more costly to patient

3. Limited to one- to three-haired follicles that may have been cored out from a larger, previously intact FU
4. Concerns of healing at regional donor sites via secondary intention (i.e., Keloids to chest)

Typically, one to at most three hairs, are removed at a time. An advantage of FUE is that not only can the traditional scalp donor sites be used, but also other body areas such as the chest, back, beard, arm, and leg can be utilized (Fig. 13.17).

The original two-step method for harvesting an FUE graft was to identify a FU and then with a .7–1.0 mm punch, using a rotating motion, score down to the epidermis and upper dermis [31]. The loose graft is then grasped with rat-toothed forceps, and with gentle counter traction on the surrounding tissue, the graft is pulled free. However, since hair direction under the skin can change and hair follicles can splay, transection can frequently occur. Harris has developed a three-step method [32]. Once the initial score 0.3–0.5 mm into the upper dermis is made with a sharp punch, a second blunt punch is inserted into the site and finishes the graft dissection (Fig. 13.18). In this manner, the ability to extract full, intact grafts with less transection is improved. The author currently uses a powered FUE tool which greatly improves the accuracy and speed at which grafts are harvested.

Eyebrow transplants in men are a good example of a use for FUE. Hair taken from the chest has a slower growth rate than donor hair taken from the scalp. As such, chest donor hair transplanted to the eyebrow will have to be clipped less often than hair from the scalp.

With practice, the operator becomes more adept at removing grafts quickly and with less transection. However, it is a time-consuming procedure that is usually performed by the physician and as such can be more costly for the patient. This technique does not yield any better result in the recipient area. Marketing this procedure as scar less can be misleading. Over time, if subsequent sessions to the same area and more grafts are taken, the tiny scars can add up and the ability to shave the hair to a minimal length on the scalp and to not have any visible scar may not be achievable.

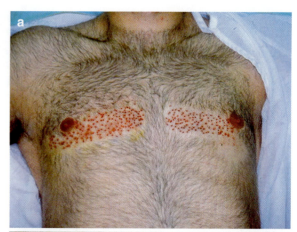
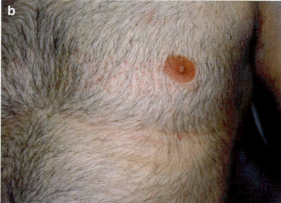
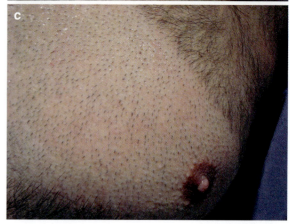

Fig. 13.17 (**a**). Follicular unit extraction using a 1 mm punch. (**b**) One month after surgery the sites are healing well. (**c**) Close-up of healed sites 1 year later

13.13 Graft Preparation

As soon as the first donor strip has been harvested it is immediately placed into chilled saline and given to the technicians for dissection into FUs and MFUs. The importance of keeping the donor tissue moist and cool from the time the tissue is excised until it is replanted into the recipient sites cannot be stressed enough. Graft coolers that have ice in the base, with saline-filled petrie dishes on top, will keep the tissue moist and cool (Fig. 13.19). Graft survival studies have shown that

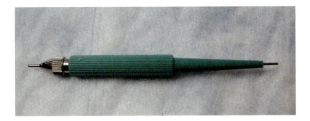

Fig. 13.18 Instrument used for FUE. Sharp disposable 1 mm punch on right and autoclavable blunt punch on left

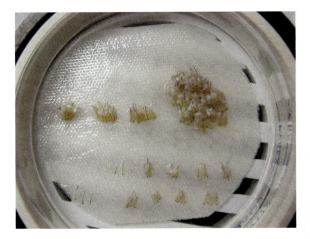

Fig. 13.19 Grafts being kept chilled in a cooler that has ice in its base and chilled saline in petrie dishes above

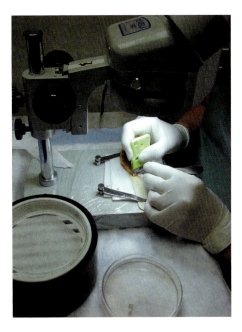

Fig. 13.20 Strip is being slivered into smaller loaves utilizing microscopes

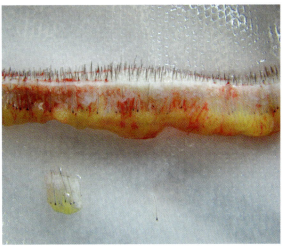

Fig. 13.21 A recently removed strip is shown at the top with a slivered section of the strip on the left, containing several FUs and a fully dissected one hair FU on the right

inadvertent drying of grafts, even after 3 min of air drying on surgical gloves, as could happen in a typical surgery session, can cause serious damage leading to cell necrosis [33]. The ellipse removed from the donor site (Fig. 13.20) is first slivered into smaller strips, one FU wide and several FUs long (Fig. 13.21) under magnification using a stereomicroscope. The smaller slivers are then further subdivided into either FUs or MFUs depending on the needs of the surgery (Fig. 13.22). Technicians will cut the grafts on top of tongue depressors placed on gauze. The tongue depressors act as a firm surface to place the grafts. Other offices may use cutting boards specifically designed for cutting donor tissue. Care must be taken at all times to dissect between FUs and not through FUs so that the integrity of each graft can be maintained. During the dissection process the technicians must be aware of inadvertent graft transection, drying or excessive manipulation of tissue. Technicians can use one-sided razor blades with handles; others use #10 or #11 scalpel blades for dissection. It is important to leave a small amount of adventitial tissue around the bulb of the follicle to maintain viability. Grafts can be described as "chubby" or "skinny" depending on how much surrounding tissue is removed. Physicians that prefer to transplant larger numbers of densely packed grafts prefer the skinny size. However, some studies indicate that as the density of transplanted grafts increase, at a certain point, viability will decrease [34].

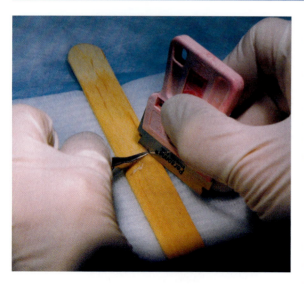

Fig. 13.22 A slivered portion of the strip is now being further dissected into individual FUs using a tongue depressor as a cutting board

mid-occipital and should be taken into account when choosing and sorting grafts.

Graft preparation is definitely a team effort, but it does require the physician in charge to be the team leader. It is apparent that different technicians will have different strengths, whether it be dissecting or planting of the grafts. Proper quality control is important at all times with hair transplantation due to the many steps that can be influenced by the many assistants involved.

13.14 Recipient Site Creation

Incisions can be made with either needles or blades. One to two millimeter circular punches can be used to core out, or thin, traditional unacceptable 3.5–4.0 mm punch grafts from decades ago. Round and slot punches are used rarely now for recipient site creation when one is utilizing modern FUT techniques.

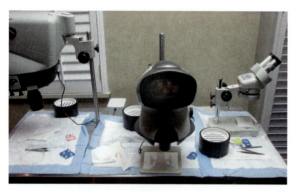

Fig. 13.23 Stereomicroscopes used in graft dissection. Meiji scope is on the right. The left and middle scopes are Mantis scopes. The middle scope is shown with an up lighter

13.15 Graft Orientation: CAG or SAG

Hair in the frontal scalp grows in a forward direction. In order to re-create natural hair direction in the frontal scalp, grafts are oriented to be placed sagittal, or parallel to the direction of the preexisting hair. This is called sagittal angle grafting (SAG). To make these sites, usually 18–21 gauge needles or angled scalpel shaped blades oriented forward, parallel to the natural hair direction are used. In this manner one is able to minimize damage to underlying vasculature and to spare preexisting hair in the area by going between hairs. Coronal angle grafting, (CAG), is a newer technique whereby grafts are placed perpendicular (Fig. 13.24) to the natural forward hair direction when transplanting the frontal scalp [35]. On close inspection of the anterior scalp, (Fig. 13.25), it is observed that although hairs grow in a superior–inferior direction, the hairs in each individual FU are oriented side-by-side, or left to right, perpendicular to the natural hair direction. The benefit of placing FUs in a CAG orientation allows for the appearance of more fullness when viewed from the front and less like hairs lining up behind one another as is seen when a three- to four-haired FU is placed parallel to the angle of preexisting hair direction. This technique usually utilizes small 0.6–1.2 mm flat-edged chisel blades to make the recipient sites and as such is more superficial

Stereomicroscopes (Fig. 13.23) are now used routinely to produce superior grafts with minimal transection rates and should be used by all practicing hair surgeons. Back lighting can also help the technician to visualize the graft and aid in dissection.

The grafts are sorted into number of hairs per graft and kept moist in the chilled saline dishes until time of implantation. To ease in counting, the grafts are kept in bundles of ten. Additionally, the grafts are subdivided by hair texture. Finer one-haired grafts taken in the temples or lower in the occipital area may be used for anterior hairline grafts, with coarser multiple hair FUs used behind the hairline. Hair color in the donor area can also change dramatically from temples to

Fig. 13.24 Traditional orientation of sites for sagittal angle grafting and more recently the coronal angle grafting orientation (Reprinted with permission from Berg and Cotterill [24]. Copyright Elsevier Limited 2009)

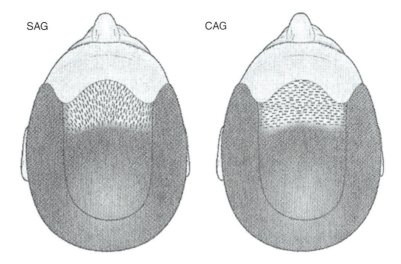

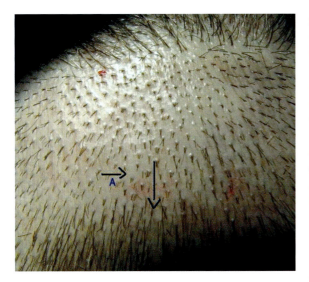

Fig. 13.25 Close-up view of frontal scalp illustrating the superior–inferior hair direction and the perpendicular direction of hairs oriented in each FU. Letter, "A" shows a three-haired FU lined up perpendicular to the overall hair direction (*large arrow*)

required to maximize vasoconstriction, to minimize damage to the underlying neurovasculature, and to increase the surface area of the scalp so that upon dissipation of the fluid one can achieve a greater density of recipient sites. This technique is more inherently difficult and often requires the patient to shave the recipient area to aid in creating the sites.

It is a matter of personal choice whether to use SAG or CAG, dictated by the experience of the physician, the area to be treated, the amount of preexisting hair in the area, and the size, density, and number of grafts to be transplanted. However, for the casual transplant surgeon, it is suggested to use SAG.

13.16 Instruments (Table 13.3)

The decision as to what size of FU the physician will use at what density they will be placed at, and whether to use a needle or blade (Fig. 13.26) is very much physician dependent.

Needles have the benefit of being inexpensive, color coded in sizes ranging from 18 to 22 gauge, and can provide dilatation of a recipient site. The beveled ends can aid in planting grafts and ensuring depth control.

Blades can be either pointed, coming to a tip at the midline (Spearpoint) or laterally (Minde, Sharpoint). The lateral angled blades are intended for SAG where the angle and orientation of the created site is parallel to hair growth with the intent of minimizing disruption of blood vessels deep in the wound.

throughout its length of incision depth compared to the same length of a parallel incision employing a blade that comes to a point, so that there may be less chance of injury to underlying vasculature. But this cannot be said if larger three- to four-haired FUs or MFUs are used. However, when there is significant preexisting hair in the area there is a greater chance of disturbing that hair. As such sites for CAG need to be very small, requiring the use of more skinny FUs as opposed to chubby FUs. Greater tumescence of the recipient site with 1:1,000,000 epinephrine is also

Table 13.3 Suggested equipments needed for a typical hair restoration procedure

1	Two mirrors and black grease pencil for marking hairline on scalp
2	1% and 2% lidocaine with 1:100,000 epinephrine
3	Epinephrine 1:1,000
4	10 cm^3 syringes with 16, 18, 19, 20, 21, 25 g, and 30 gauge needles
5	100 ml bag of normal saline
6	Towel clip
7	Straight iris scissors, 3 in.
8	Needle driver
9	Scalpel handle with #15 blade
10	Straight adson forceps (non-toothed)
11	Aluminum rattail comb – Ellis Instruments
12	Curved Metzenbaum scissors
13	2-O & 3-O Supramed nylon ½ circ, rev cutting, white, non-abs. suture – S Jackson Co., Alexandria, VA
14	Hyfrecator and tips
15	Petrie dishes – Ellis Instruments (with 7.5 × 10 cm telfa pad cut to size inside)
16	Two versi handles for spear tip blades
17	#5 Jeweller's forceps for planting grafts
18	Two Mantis microscopes – Micro-Vid, Huntington Beach, CA
19	Two Meiji microscopes – Micro-Vid, Huntington Beach, CA
20	Tongue depressors to act as cutting boards
21	Personna double edge prep blades and holders
22	Gauze: 4×4 sponge topper Nu-gauze non-woven gauze
23	Hydrogen peroxide 3% with spray bottle
24	Chemical ice packs with covers
25	Petrie dish coolers – Ellis Instruments, Madison, NJ
26	Kerlix dressing
27	Bandana
28	Surgilube – water soluble lubricant
29	Betadine and alcohol for disinfecting scalp
30	Prone pillow – Foam Products Inc., Bronx, NY

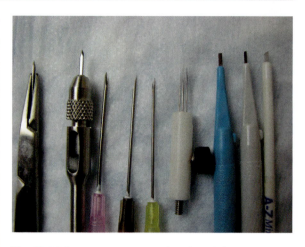

Fig. 13.26 Instruments to create sites: from *left* to *right* – needle driver holding a cutting blade, blade holder with spear tipped blade, three color-coded beveled needles, multi-blade recipient device, flat bladed chisels, and Minde Knife

Chisel blades are flat and rectangular and are used primarily for CAG where the angle of the cutting surface of the blade is perpendicular to the intended direction of hair growth. Chisel blades are not appropriate for SAG as there is a greater ability of the leading edge of the chisel to damage underlying vasculature. Needles and midline blades can be used for both CAG and SAG. Chisel blades are commercially available or can be created and cut to size using single- or double-edged razor blades cut with a blade holder or with a custom cutting tool (CuttingEdge-Surgical.ca).

Depth control is an important aspect in proper recipient site creation. Inadvertent disruption of the blood vessels of the supragaleal plexus can lead to needless interruption of the local blood supply and increased bleeding, which can make planting of the grafts more difficult. With increased bleeding there is also an increased need for additional local anesthetic. Needles have their own built in depth control due to their bevel. Blades can be purchased with handles that aid in depth control or blade-holder handles can be purchased that allows the blade to be positioned for accurate recipient site depth. Needle drivers can also be used as a graft holder and sized to the length of graft to be planted (Fig. 13.26).

Multi-blade recipient devices are used by some physicians to speed up the time required to make thousands of recipient sites and as a way of assisting in creating a template for spacing of the sites. However, there is a risk of damaging any preexisting hair in the area as well as not being able to minutely adjust the angle of each individual blade. The Choi implanter, used in Asia, is an example of an automatic graft placing device that is preloaded with a graft and then, at the time of creating the site, the graft is injected into place.

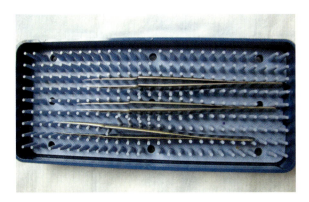

Fig. 13.27 Autoclavable container to store jeweller's forceps that has rubber walls to protect the forceps' tips from being damaged

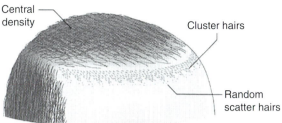

Fig. 13.28 The anterior hairline zone is feathered and made irregular with the use of small groupings of three to five hairs and single, randomly placed hairs (Reprinted with permission from Berg and Cotterill [24]. Copyright Elsevier Limited 2009)

Fine tipped Jeweller's forceps are required for planting to avoid crushing or damaging the grafts. The tips are very fragile and can be easily blunted or nicked in the cleaning process. It is advisable to place a plastic guard over the tip during sterilization. A holding device (Fig. 13.27) can be purchased that holds the forceps safe and secure between rubber cushions during sterilization.

13.17 Re-creating a Natural Hairline

At the beginning of surgery the frontal hairline, which has been agreed upon by both the physician and patient at the time of initial consultation, is drawn on with a black grease pencil employing the proper principles of planning an anterior hairline, (see surgical planning). A photo should be taken at this time if it was not already done at the time of the initial consultation. The aim in creating the recipient sites is to create a zone of naturally increasing density with the irregularities that one sees in a natural hairline. Hairlines that are too abrupt, too sharp, too dense, or too symmetrical can draw the eye to it and appear unnatural. The author will use for the hairline either 19–20 gauge needles, or .8–1.2 mm chisel tipped blades to accommodate single FUs. An initial defined zone of evenly spaced single-haired FUs sites is made just posterior to the drawn hairline. Anterior to this zone, micro-irregularities employing three to four single-haired FUs are utilized in clusters as well as scattering random (Fig. 13.28), single-haired FUs, placed erratically in front and between groupings. In this way the hairline is softened and abrupt straight lines are avoided (Fig. 13.29). What is created is a gradually increasing density in a hairline

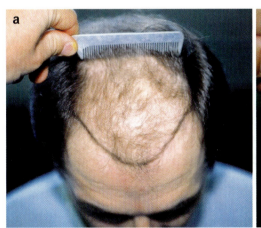
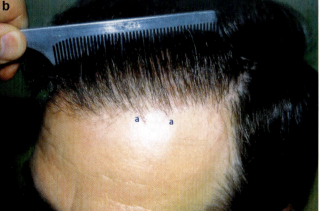

Fig. 13.29 (a) Hairline drawn on before surgery. (b) Completed hairline showing clusters of hairs, "a," with single-haired FUs scattered about randomly with gradually increasing density created behind hairline zone

zone, approximately 5–10 mm in width. With experience, the surgeon will understand that different hair types and colors will dictate a zone that should be wider or narrower. For example, a patient with black, coarse wiry hair and pale skin may require a wider transitional zone to avoided abruptness, while a patient with fine, salt and pepper hair and pale skin will achieve a feathered result with a narrower zone. At a distance one can also appreciate widow's peaks and lateral peaks that can be re-created by using a small number of FUs concentrated in areas at the hairline.

Once the hairline zone has been created then increased density can be achieved posteriorly. For the beginner or surgeon that performs transplants infrequently it can be difficult to know how densely one should attempt to place the grafts. It is suggested that the surgeon practice by drawing a 1 cm^2 box and assess the degree of difficulty of placing grafts at 20, 30, 45, and 75 FU/cm^2. Densities greater than 35 FU/cm^2 are considered dense packing. However, as densities increase the concern of graft viability also increases. With high numbers of densely packed grafts there is also the need for higher numbers of skinnier grafts, with consequently the need for more skilled technicians to assist with the procedure. It should be kept in mind that excellent results can be achieved with densities of 30–35 FU/cm^2 using one- to three-haired FUs and four- to six-haired MFUs. A 1.5–3.0 mm spear tip blade is an example of the type and size of blade required to make a site that will accommodate the larger MFUs. A suggested scenario would be to create a frontal hairline zone with 600 one- to three-haired FUs followed posteriorly by 600 four- to six-haired MFUs. This will yield approximately 4,200 hairs. An oval shaped area at the midline frontal region, just behind the hairline zone, is often densely transplanted to give the illusion of density. This can be achieved with single FUs placed at 30–35 FUs/cm^2 or with MFUs placed slightly farther apart. It should also be remembered that to transplant a bald frontal zone it is wise to instruct the patient they may require two sessions and possibly a third finishing session. While some surgeons will attempt to complete a bald frontal area in one pass using high numbers (3,000–4,500+) of densely planted all one- to three-haired skinny FUs, as well as spacing all the grafts in a CAG orientation, this technique is not recommended for the casual hair transplant surgeon. It would be more prudent, with an equally great result, to split the transplant into two procedures, 1 year apart, of approximately 1,500 FUs each, using a combination of FUs for the hairline zone and a combination of FUs and MFUs for the rest of the anterior frontal scalp.

Pearls: For the novice or casual hair surgeon

1. Limit transplant to front one-third of scalp.
2. If area is bald, split the procedure into two sessions of 1,200–1,500 grafts per session spread 1 year apart.
3. Use a combination of FUs and MFUs.
4. Place grafts using SAG orientation.
5. Use 19 gauge needles or similar sized blades.
6. Place sites at densities of 25–35 FUs/cm^2.
7. Remove donor grafts using strip excision technique.

Pearls: For the novice surgeon for choosing their first patients.

1. Use family or friends.
2. Select a male that is over 50 years of age, with moderate thinning confined to the frontal scalp, such that there is preexisting recipient hair to aid in camouflage.
3. Have excellent hair characteristics: Salt-and-pepper or gray hair color with pale scalp to minimize color contrasts. Fine, wavy or curly hair to yield a feathered hairline with added fullness behind hairline zone.
4. Good to high density in the permanent hair-bearing donor zone.
5. Appropriate expectations as to what to expect from one session.

Just before the recipient sites are made the patient is placed in a semi-supine position. The recipient area is tested for adequate anesthesia and further tumescence is placed by some physicians to aid in graft site creation and to minimize bleeding. The length of the donor graft should be sized so the appropriate length of blade or needle is adjusted accordingly. If one is using SAG then it is essential to follow the direction and be parallel to any preexisting hair in the area in order to minimize the chance of transection of hairs in the immediate area. Any preexisting terminal hairs in the area can be used as a guide for direction. Hair direction at the mid-frontal scalp while growing in a posterior to anterior direction can change markedly as one creates sites from one side of the scalp to the other. As one travels from the midline to the frontotemporal corner, for example, the angle of incisions created should gradually change from a forward direction to laterally and down. The angle that hair exits the scalp at the frontal midline is from 30° to 45° while closer to the temples the exit angel is more acute. The physician must pay close attention to changes in direction and angle of scalp hair as it exits from the scalp. Once all the sites have been made the grafts are planted. Some practices advocate "stick and place," whereby the physician or technician will make a recipient site followed by a second technician immediately placing the graft in the site created (Fig. 13.30). This technique is used in some practices where high numbers of very small sites are made. If all the sites were left to the end to be planted, they may be difficult to find. The author prefers to make all the sites initially and have two to three technicians plant, once the sites are made. However, stick and place can be useful at the end of the session if there are still some final sites to be made between previously planted grafts.

13.18 Planting Recipient Grafts

Planting of the grafts can be done at the same time the recipient incisions are made, (stick and place), or once all the sites are completed. Whatever method the surgeon chooses, hair restoration is definitely a team effort. Compared to any other type of cosmetic surgery, the hair restoration nurse/technician plays an essential part in both the dissection of the donor strip and in the planting of the recipient grafts and as such has a great influence on the successful outcome of the procedure. However, with excellent, well-trained staff there is no need for the physician to plant all the grafts. The time involved would be excessive with no better outcome. However, some essential principles need to be kept in mind. The grafts should be kept moist and cool in chilled saline until such time as they are ready to be planted. Three to five grafts at a time are placed on the glove of the technician's nondominant finger and then planted following the exact angle and predetermined depth of the incision (Fig. 13.31). The graft should not be allowed to subside into the recipient site or pitting could occur upon healing. The graft is left

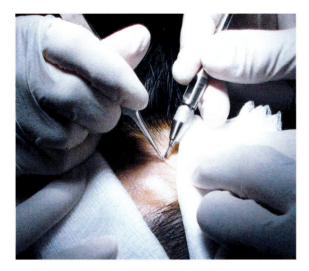

Fig. 13.30 Planting grafts using the "stick and place" method. The physician or assistant makes the site and the graft is then immediately inserted

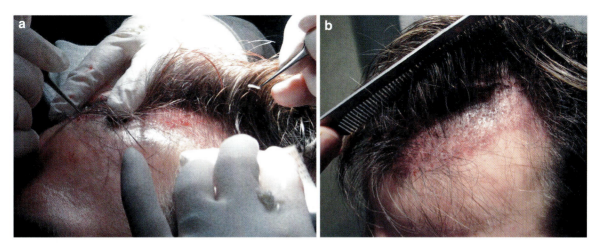

Fig. 13.31 (**a**) Two assistants planting grafts using jeweller's forceps once all the sites have been made by the physician. (**b**) Same recipient site the day after surgery once the hair has been washed to show minimal crusting

slightly elevated above the dermis. If the graft was allowed to sink and another graft was placed on top (piggybacking), an inclusion cyst could form. During the planting process the area is sprayed with a dilute hydrogen peroxide mixture to enhance visibility of the work area and to aid in cleaning off blood clots and any stray hairs or hair spicules that could congregate under planted grafts.

13.19 The Vertex Region

Proper planning principles are crucial when attempting to treat a crown. The very young patient or patient who may become very bald is often best served by not transplanting the crown. However, when treatment is appropriate, the crown presents its own set of design challenges. When transplanting a crown the center of the whorl needs to be identified as that site where the hairs exit the scalp radiating out in a 360° direction. To accurately reconstitute the whorl, the physician needs to find the center of the whorl, or create one if the patient is bald in that region, and make the recipient sites radiating out from that site (Fig. 13.32). In some instances, there are the remains of a whorl to follow; in other circumstances where there is total hair loss the physician must choose an arbitrary whorl.

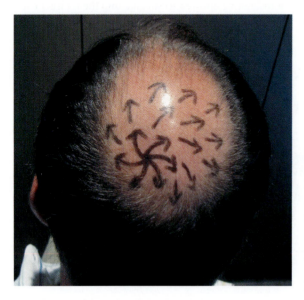

Fig. 13.32 Hair direction when reconstituting the whorl formation in the bald vertex

With the use of two- to three-haired FUs, one session of grafting can give a pleasing light coverage.

13.20 Postoperative Care

It is suggested that following surgery the patient be accompanied home if any intraoperative sedation was used. All patients are called the night following surgery by the physician as well as being seen in the office the morning following surgery to have the hair washed, grafts inspected, and postoperative directions confirmed (Table 13.4).

Postoperative dressings are rarely used anymore do to the small size of grafts and limited postoperative bleeding. Patients are given gauze to be used to apply pressure to any small bleeding areas as well as pads to use against pillowcases to soak up any blood. The patient is advised to take 5–7 days off work or sports, to minimize the chance of knocking out a graft or bleeding. Patients are given baseball caps when they leave the day of surgery to help keep the scalp clean and to avoid accidental injury. There may be some degree of forehead swelling, which is common when the anterior scalp is transplanted. It is suggested that the patient sleep at a 45° angle for the first three nights and to use the supplied chemical ice pack, with sleeve to prevent burning the skin, for the first 2–3 days on the forehead region. Many physicians advocate the use of postoperative oral steroids, or intralesional steroids to minimize the chance of facial edema. Antibiotics are also employed, usually just for the day of surgery, since infections are rare.

There should be no discomfort during the procedure if adequate anesthesia is used. Postoperatively, there can be some discomfort usually in the donor area due to do the pulling of the sutures. There is remarkably little discomfort in the recipient region. Patients are typically given prescriptions for acetaminophen with codeine and acetaminophen with oxycodone, as well as diphenhydramine as an antinauseant. There should be no prescription medication required after the night of surgery. At most, a patient may require acetaminophen or ibuprofen for 2–3 days after surgery.

The day following surgery, the patient's scalp and hair is washed at the office so that the patient can be instructed in general hair care and to help remove any superficial blood clots that may have appeared

Table 13.4 Postoperative instructions

Immediately following surgery:

1. DO NOT DRIVE, the medication you receive can impair your reflexes and driving could be dangerous

2. Have something substantial to eat

3. Take the antibiotic as directed

4. You will be given the following medications:

    Pain pills: take as directed on the package and when needed. If you are having pain 1 h after you have taken the pain medication from package #1, take two tablets from package #2

    Gravol: take with the stronger pain pills or if you feel nauseated

5. Do not take aspirin or any drugs containing aspirin

6. Do not drink alcohol on the day of surgery or while taking any medication

7. Do not lift anything over 10 lbs and do not exercise

8. Do not bend your head below your waist or bend your head down to read

9. Rest for the remainder of the day and when sleeping keep your head at a 45° Do not lie flat. This will help to reduce any swelling that may occur

10. If you have a bandage, do not lift or try to look under the bandage. If the bandage slips off, DO NOT BE CONCERNED. DO NOT try to put it back on. Leave it as is, and allow the Doctor or Nurse to deal with it the following day

11. If any bleeding should appear apply firm steady pressure over the bleeding area for 10 min with the gauze given to you. You can keep pressure on a suture area by tying the sticky bandana given to you around your forehead to hold the gauze in place. If there is any bleeding that does not stop easily with pressure call Dr. Cotterill

12. The Doctor will call you during the evening but, if an emergency should occur, he may be reached at the emergency number on the top right hand side of this page

13. You will have been given some green absorbent pads to put on your pillow case to absorb any small amount of blood that may come from the suture line

For the first 2 weeks after surgery:

1. Your hair will be washed on the day after surgery and all surgical areas will be checked. If you had a bandage it will be removed. Your appointment time is written at the top of page 1. Occasionally, there is a small amount of bleeding from the surgical areas. If this should happen, apply gentle pressure to the bleeding area with the gauze we give you, for 5–10 min

2. To help prevent swelling:

    - Apply an ice pack (we will give you a reusable ice pack), to your forehead and temples, for 10–15 min, every hour, for the first 2 days (if possible). Use the protective sleeve for the ice pack provided for you. Direct contact of the chemical ice pack with skin could cause freezer burn. If swelling develops, keep applying the ice pack, as frequently as possible, until the swelling subsides. DO NOT PLACE THE ICE PACK DIRECTLY ON THE GRAFTS OR STITCHES

    - Sleep at a 45° for 3 days or until any there is no swelling in the area

    - Note: If swelling occurs, there is no further treatment or medication available – nature must take its course. It will gradually subside over a 3–7 day period

3. Beginning on the second day after surgery and until your stitches are removed, you should wash your hair twice a day, in the following way:

    - Fill the bathtub with warm water and lay back until the water covers the stitched areas. Epson salts can be added to the bath water

    - Soak and gently massage the areas for 10 min

    - Then apply shampoo (nothing medicated) TO BOTH THE FRONT AND THE BACK OF YOUR HEAD and gently massage. Rinse well with clean water

    - After the stitches are removed wash your hair daily until all the crusts have fallen off

    - Note: You may have a shower but do not let the water beat directly on the grafts for 7 days

(continued)

Table 13.4 (continued)

4.	To encourage the crusts to fall off, we will give you some packages of "surgi-lube" (a water soluble lubricant) to apply sparingly to both the larger crusts in the recipient area (where the grafts are) and the donor area (where the stitches are) using a clean finger. Apply the "surgi-lube" three times a day; once in the morning, after you wash your hair and after you apply the Rogaine, if you are using it (see instruction #5), once in the afternoon and once before you go to bed
5.	Sometimes the use of Rogaine (Minoxidil, Apogain) postoperatively will result in fewer hairs temporarily falling out and/or will stimulate hairs in the grafts to grow a little faster. It will not grow more hairs. It is not necessary to use it but if you wish to use Rogaine postoperatively, a prescription will be given to you. Spray the transplanted area twice a day, after you wash your hair and before you apply the "surgi-lube", for 5–6 weeks. Do not apply Rogaine the morning of surgery
6.	Your sutures (stitches) will be removed in 7 days. Your appointment time is written on the top of page 1. If you are unable to return to our office to have your sutures removed, you may make alternate arrangements with someone qualified to remove sutures. We will provide a diagram of where your sutures are and a description on how they should be removed
7.	No exercise, sports activities, or strenuous work for 1 week
8.	No heavy lifting or weightlifting for 2 weeks
9.	To prevent infection, avoid exposure to dirt in the air at work or play for 2 weeks following surgery. If you do begin exercising after 7 days, or engage in activities that cause you to perspire, please wash your hair as soon as possible after the activity. Bacteria can grow quickly in any moist warm area and may cause infection in an area not completely healed. If you experience any redness, or "pus pimples" please call Dr. Cotterill

Additional information

Healing and crusts

Immediately after surgery the transplanted grafts can look white, red, or blue. This is very normal and you should not be concerned. Leave the transplanted area open to the air as much as possible; avoid the use of hats and hairpieces unless absolutely necessary

Crusts will soon begin to form over the grafts. These crusts are part of the normal healing process. They may look and feel like hard dry tissue or they may look like a scab that forms over a cut. DO NOT PICK AT OR OTHERWISE TRY TO REMOVE THEM. They will fall off on their own 1–3 weeks after surgery. There may be some hair attached to these grafts – do not be alarmed, the hair root is firmly embedded in the skin. If all the crusts have fallen off after 3 weeks, please call Dr. Cotterill

You may gradually expose the transplanted area to the sun, but AVOID SUNBURN

Transplanted hair regrowth

DO NOT expect any hair growth for 3 months. Some patients may have hair growth as soon as 6 weeks, but this is unusual. Hair grows at approximately 0.5 in./month. It will take 6–9 months before the full cosmetic benefit is reached

You may experience some temporary shedding of the non-transplanted, preexisting hair in the recipient area. If you do, be assured that it is temporary, and any shed hair will all start to regrow by 2–3 months after surgery

Numbness

Decreased sensitivity is nearly always temporary and will resolve on its own in 6–9 months

Swimming

You may swim in a clean lake, clean private pool, or ocean after 3 days. Wait 2 weeks before swimming in a public pool or lake of uncertain cleanliness

Vitamins

There may be some benefit to taking vitamin supplements postoperatively

Immediately following surgery: vitamin C, 2,000 mg (2 g) per day for at least 14 days

24 h following surgery; vitamin E 800 I.U., per day for at least 14 days and multi-vitamin/mineral supplements

Hair products

Shampoo – NOTHING MEDICATED. We suggest Modern Organic Products (MOP) shampoo and conditioner, or alternatively, Ionil (no tar), Redkin, Nexxus, or Neutrogena (available in drugstores)

Conditioner – may be used with every second washing

Table 13.4 (continued)

Light hair spray (non-alcohol based, if possible), gels and mousses – may be used when you begin shampooing your hair but as little as possible for the first week and must be washed off daily
Hair coloring and perms – should be avoided until all the crusts have fallen off; generally 2 weeks
Haircuts – after the crusts have fallen off
Camouflage
Camouflage must only be used to cover up the recipient area for a few hours, when absolutely necessary, that is, important meeting or function you must attend
We suggest:
1. Any water-based makeup
2. Lancôme "Maquicontrole" (available at large department stores)

overnight. A water soluble lubricant is applied to the donor area/suture line for the first week, every time the patient has washed and dried their hair. This is to aid in dissolving crusting. Vitamin E oil can also be applied to the suture line to aid in healing; however, oil is not water soluble and can be greasy. Patients are instructed to gently wash their hair by soaking in the tub twice a day for 6 days. Epson salts can be added to the bath water to aid in healing. The crusts on the grafts will start to flake off at 4–5 days, and should be all removed by 10–12 days postoperatively. Patients are instructed to lightly massage the recipient grafts with their finger pads. The grafts should only come out inadvertently if the area is picked excessively with the fingers or hit. Even pressure with gauze would stop any bleeding.

Patience may resume daily applications of 5% minoxidil on the scalp starting the day after surgery. Minoxidil used for 6 weeks postoperatively may help to minimize telogen of any preexisting hair after surgery and encourage the grafts to grow in 2–4 weeks sooner than average. Patients can cut, perm, or color their hair 1 week prior to surgery and starting 2 weeks post surgery. Patients return to the office 7–10 days after surgery to have their sutures removed. Patients are then called 1 month after surgery to inquire about their progress and then are called again at 10–12 months after surgery for a follow-up appointment.

13.21 Complications

A positive outcome in hair restoration surgery is a combination of proper surgical technique on the part of the physician and surgical assistants, in addition to proper expectations on the part of the patient. It is paramount to a successful outcome that the physician assesses the patient's expectations and sets the expectations at the time of the initial interview. Complications are divided into surgical complications/side effects and cosmetic/esthetic complications.

13.21.1 Surgical Complications/Side Effects

1. Bleeding can occur intraoperatively. However, with appropriate operative infiltration of local anesthetic with epinephrine and the use of electrocautery, ligation, or direct pressure, bleeding is minimal. Postoperative bleeding in the donor or recipient area, while rare, is easily controlled with pressure.
2. Infections are rare and occur in less than 0.1% of patients in either the donor or recipient area. If suspected, a culture should be taken and a topical/oral antibiotic given, as well as instructing the patient to apply hot saline compresses. Sterile folliculitis typically occurs in the recipient area up to 3 months post transplant. This can be as a result of trapped hairs or fragments of grafts.
3. Inclusion cysts occur when grafts are placed or buried too deeply in the recipient site or when a second graft is placed on top (piggybacked), on an unseen previously transplanted graft at the time of implantation. The area should be incised and the contents expressed.
4. Postoperative facial/forehead edema occurs within the first few days postoperatively and can last up to a week, and in some cases can be severe. Many

physicians use corticosteroids as well as instruct the patient on elevation and judicious use of cold compresses.

5. Telogen/anagen effluvium can occur in the recipient and donor area. The majority of transplanted hairs in most patients are shed within the first 2–3 weeks after surgery and will begin to grow in 3 months. Temporary shedding of preexisting hair can also occur, beginning soon after surgery and can last for 2–4 months. In the author's experience, women are affected more commonly, in up to 40% of surgeries. It is important to warn the patient of the risk of temporary thinning. Some physicians will treat patients with a minoxidil solution for 6–10 weeks after surgery to help speed up hair growth and to minimize temporary loss. However, since there can be an increased shedding stage lasting 4–6 weeks when first initiating minoxidil treatment, it is wise to start minoxidil several months before a surgery, especially in women.

6. Abnormal scars in the donor area are rare if proper care is taken to minimize tension on closure of the wound as well as instructions to the patient on proper post-surgery wound care. Hypertrophic or keloidal scars can be treated with intralesional corticosteroids or revised at a later time. If there is a family history of keloids then it is prudent to perform a test graft in advance of surgery. Scarring of the recipient area can occur if the grafts are placed too high, "cobble-stoning" or too low, "pitting". Both of these complications can be avoided with proper planting techniques.

7. Postoperative pain is typical within the first 24 h postoperatively and is usually associated with tension upon closure of the donor wound. Acetaminophen tablets with 30 mg codeine (Tylenol #3), and oxycodone are typically given following surgery, with most patients commonly requiring Tylenol #3.

8. Hypoesthesia occurs due to cutting of the superficial sensory nerves during surgery, but is less frequent now with the use of tumescent anesthesia that lifts the tissue away from many sensory nerves. Hypoesthesia lasts 6–12 months and in some cases small spots of permanent decreased sensitivity can persist. Neuralgias during the healing process can occur but are usually self-limiting. Rarely a neuroma can occur, generally in the occipital donor region, due to nerve injury. Triamcinolone acetonide injected into the area can often relieve the problem.

9. Arteriovenous (AV) fistulas occur in approximately 1:5,000 surgeries and can occur in both the donor and recipient areas. The majority of AV fistulae will resolve spontaneously in 3–6 months, or if there is a concern of rupture, the vessels can be ligated.

10. Dehiscence, pruritus, hypopigmentation, and hyperpigmentation are all very rare occurrences. Necrosis of the recipient area has been reported, when large numbers of densely packed grafts has been attempted. However, with proper surgical technique this complication is still very rare.

13.21.2 Cosmetic/Esthetic Complications

1. Improper hairline placement is the number one reason why patients present from elsewhere with a complaint. The positioning of a hairline that is too low or too curved at the frontal temporal recessions is a common mistake. Often young patients will present with a strong idea of the hairline they want, usually the hairline they had as a teenager, which is often too low for a mature, adult male.

2. Improper planning regarding the extent of the recipient area to be treated, especially in the young male, is another common complication for the inexperienced surgeon. Attempting to place grafts in the frontal scalp as well as the vertex region in a young male could result in a very poor transplant that can take years to develop or show itself as the surrounding hair slowly recedes. The amount of permanent donor hair must always be kept in mind when planning a transplant, especially in the younger male.

3. Improper graft selection, positioning and angling are all important concepts and techniques that if not followed will yield a poor esthetic result.

4. Inappropriate expectations can lead to the complaint of a poor result on the part of the patient, no matter how well the surgery turned out.

5. Inappropriate hair color match in a transplanted frontal area can occur if a patient, for example, with black hair has all the donor hair taken from the mid-occipital region and then the patient's hair turns prematurely gray/white in the temporal areas. Newly transplanted hair, especially in patients with fine hair, can initially grow kinkier than the preexisting hair. However, over time this tends to resolve.

13.22 Examples of Applications for Hair Transplants

13.22.1 Male Pattern Baldness

Hair transplants can be used in young patients to thicken deepening recessions or in the older male with extensive baldness. As has been discussed, principles in planning need to be applied carefully so as to select the appropriate patient based on age, family history, hair type, and expectations. Figure 13.33 illustrates the growth of one session of 2,200 follicular unit grafts in a male in his 20s. Care must be taken to limit the grafting to the frontal area and to stress that further sessions will likely be required as he ages.

Figure 13.34 shows a male that started transplantation in his 70s. He had worn a hair piece for most of his life and finally decided he "just wanted hair." In this type of patient, one can be more aggressive with the size of area to be treated since the thinning pattern is very well established and the patient has excellent hair characteristics.

13.22.2 Female Pattern Hair Loss

Women that have typical FPHL with maintenance of the frontal hairline usually have less of a dramatic change after transplants (Fig. 13.35), therefore it is very important that the patients understand what to expect with a treatment. However, because of the presence of a hairline and more preexisting hair, relative to their male counterpart, women can have an easier time of camouflaging the sessions.

13.22.3 Transplants After Rhytidectomy

Scarring and hair loss can occur after rhytidectomy at the temples with loss of side burn hair, anterior-superior to the ear, behind the anterior hairline, as well as behind the ear in the lower/lateral occipital region. Figure 13.36 shows a female that had a face lift in her late 20s that resulted in an extensive unnatural lift to her anterior hairline and scarring behind.

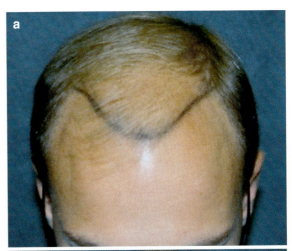
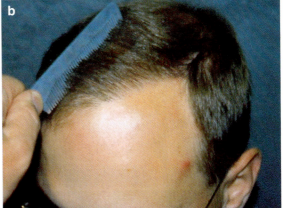
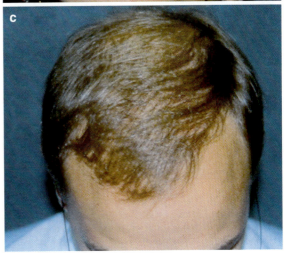

Fig. 13.33 (**a**) A male in his 20s has a hairline drawn on to show conservative placement. Transplanting will be limited to frontal scalp only. (**b**) After one session of 2,200 FUs. A second and potentially a third session are planned. (**c**) Hair combed forward to show light coverage. This patient has minimal contrast of hair to scalp. If the patient had black, course hair, the scalp would show through even more, necessitating even more the need for another session

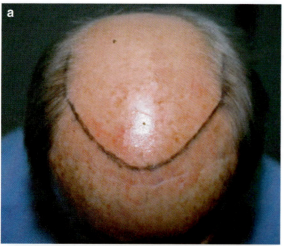
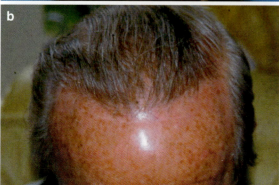
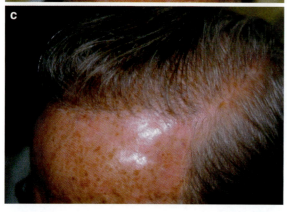

Fig. 13.34 (a) Seventy-eight-year old male before first session showing extensive baldness. (b) After three sessions to the frontal scalp and one session to the crown of approximately 6,000 FUs and MFUs. (c) This patient has ideal hair characteristics: fine, salt and pepper hair with some wave to give added body, and a pale scalp with a well-established thinning pattern

13.22.4 Transplants After Burns

Extensive burn patients can benefit from transplantation after scalp extenders or expanders have been tried (Figs. 13.37 and 13.38). Typically, fewer grafts per session are performed with the grafts spaced farther apart, to encourage proper revascularization and take of the grafts.

13.22.5 Repairing and Updating Previous Transplants

Procedures performed before the advent of FUT when large plugs were used still present today and can be very nicely updated with current techniques. Inappropriate hairlines and graft selection still occurs and can be softened with use of single-haired follicular units (Fig. 13.39). Isolated, inappropriately large, or improperly placed traditional circular plugs can be cut out by performing an FUE technique to thin out or to completely remove the graft. Or the unwanted large grafts can be cored out completely and sutured, or lasered.

13.23 Non-scalp Areas

The use of single-haired FUs has allowed almost any part of the body to benefit from transplants. Eyebrows are transplanted commonly to increase thickness due to genetic loss, over plucking, or scarring (Figs. 13.40 and 13.41). Traditional donor areas include the lower occipital region and temples with the aim of matching the texture of the transplanted hair. It is important to stress that the transplanted scalp hair will have to be trimmed every 5–7 days. Due to the greater tendency for scalp hair to have more curl and wave compared to eyebrow hair, it can be a challenge to find hairs that are straight. Errant eyebrow hairs can often be "trained" to lie flatter to the skin. Techniques to train eyebrows include applying clear mascara to the eyebrow to make them stick in one place or by using an eyebrow brush that has a small amount of hair spray put on the brush and then brushing the eyebrows in the direction you want them to fall. The physician, at the time of making the sites, should be very careful to keep the angle of placement very oblique with the skin. When appropriate, other body areas, such as the chest in men, can be used. The chest hair has the added benefit of not growing as long as scalp hair and as such trimming of the transplanted hair is less frequent.

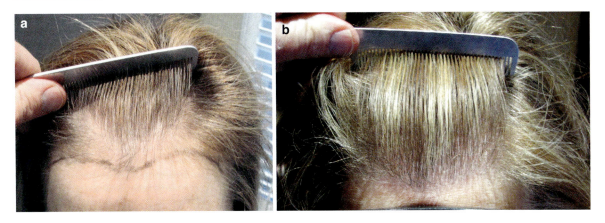

Fig. 13.35 (**a**) Typical FPHL showing hairline marked to indicate that grafts will be placed at the hairline and behind. (**b**) After one session of approximately 1,200 FUs and MFUs. The hair is colored lighter to give the appearance of added fullness

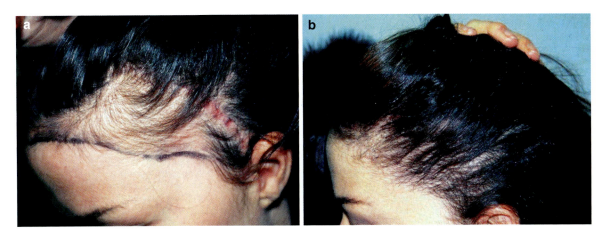

Fig. 13.36 (**a**) Preoperative, showing scarring and hair loss from a previous face lift. The temporal hairline was lifted extensively. Hairline is drawn on to show where the new hairline will be created. (**b**) After two sessions of approximately 2,500 FU and MFUs. The scar is hidden by hair growing in front of and into scar

Eyelash transplants are typically performed for congenital loss, trauma, or burns [36]. There are more potentially serious complications with eyelash transplants compared to other types of hair transplants. This includes scarring, cysts, infections, entropion, and ectropion. As such, the author suggests caution when considering eyelash transplants for routine cosmetic enhancement. The FDA recently gave approval for an ophthalmic solution, bimatoprost 0.03%, previously used for glaucoma, as a new treatment for hypotrichosis of the eyelashes. The solution is to be applied daily to the lash line of the lids and has been reported to lengthen, thicken, and darken the eyelashes. Side effects, reported in 4% or less of patients, include itching and redness to the eye. Less common side effects include skin darkening, eye irritation and dryness, and redness of the eyelids.

Other non-scalp areas that can benefit from transplants include the pubic region (Fig. 13.42), moustache (Fig. 13.43), beard, and chest.

13.24 Transgendered Patients

Hair restoration surgery for the transgendered (TG) patient is almost always for male to female patients. The TG patient seeks hairline feminization which involves creating a rounded frontotemporal recession

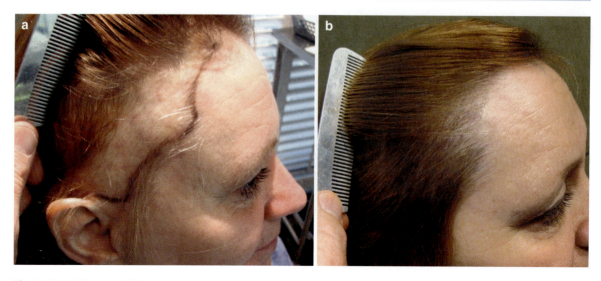

Fig. 13.37 (**a**) Scarring hair loss as a result of a grease burn at age 2. (**b**) After two sessions of a total of 1,200 FUs and MFUs. Fewer grafts, placed farther apart than average were performed to take into account the lessened blood supply

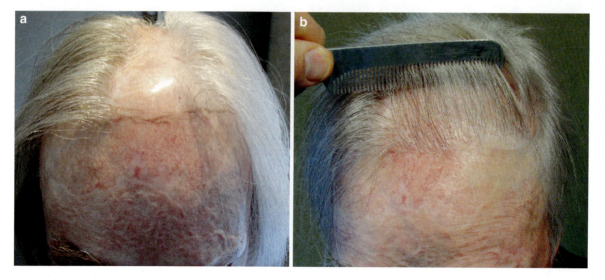

Fig. 13.38 (**a**) Before first session. This patient was involved in a plane crash and suffered extensive burns to his face, scalp, and body. Subsequent scalp reductions or expanders to minimize the scalp scarring were inadvisable due to the tightness of the skin. (**b**) After two sessions of a total of 1,350 FUs and MFUs. Grafts can grow very well when the placement of the grafts and the timing of sessions are appropriate

and a lowered mid-frontal point for the anterior hairline (Fig. 13.44). The TG patient is often undergoing other facial cosmetic surgeries that should be timed with any hair transplantation (Fig. 13.45). Often the MPHL is too severe and the patient may not be happy settling for a frontal frame to the face or less than total coverage, which may be satisfactory in a typical male. Expectations are often higher in the TG patient and as such a full hair piece or wig may be more appropriate.

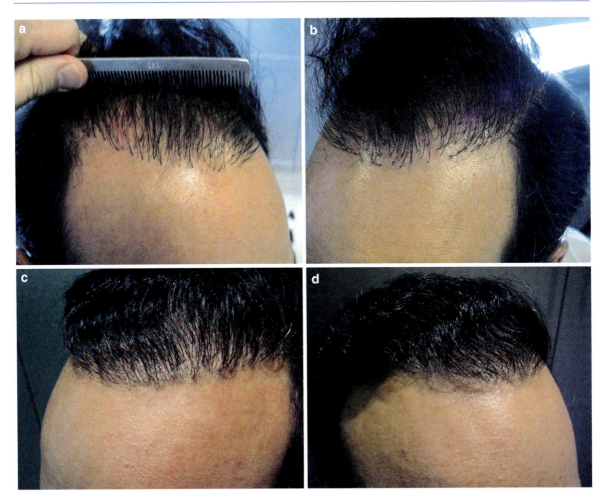

Fig. 13.39 (**a**, **b**) Patient had one session of poorly selected large grafts placed too far apart to create a very unnatural hairline. Adding to the improper placement is the patient's coarse, black hair, which makes creating a feathered, soft hairline a challenge. (**c**, **d**) After a session of approximately 1,900 FUs and MFUs. The hairline is softened considerably with the use of one-haired FUs placed at the hairline zone, but a further refining session is suggested

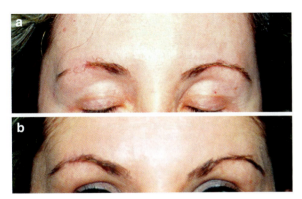

Fig. 13.40 (**a**) This patient had a tumor removed from the right eyebrow causing scarring hair loss. (**b**) After one session of single-haired FUs

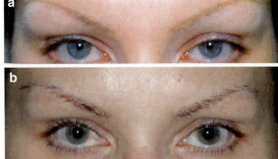

Fig. 13.41 (**a**) A young woman that was always unhappy with her low eyebrows, such that she shaves and plucks preexisting hairs and draws on desired eyebrows with pencil. (**b**) After one session of 180 FUs to define new eyebrows. The hairs must be kept short to maintain appropriate length and to minimize any curl

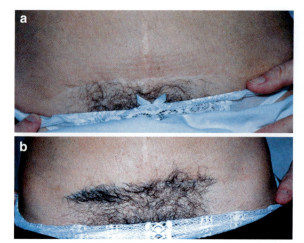

Fig. 13.42 (a) There is a scar from previous abdominal surgery. (b) After one session of grafting (Reprinted with permission from Berg and Cotterill [24]. Copyright Elsevier Limited 2009)

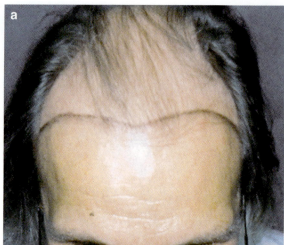

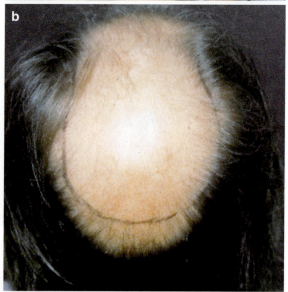

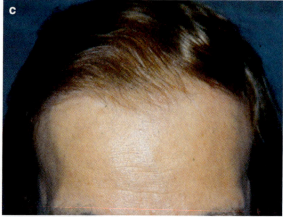

Fig. 13.44 (a) TG patient before first session showing feminine hairline desired. (b) TG patient before surgery showing extent of MPB involvement. (c) After two sessions with hairline showing. (d) After two sessions with hair brushed forward to illustrate amount of coverage achieved

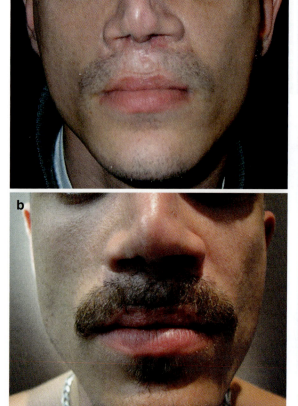

Fig. 13.43 (a) Patient with scarring from previous cleft lip repair. (b) After one session and the hair has grown in

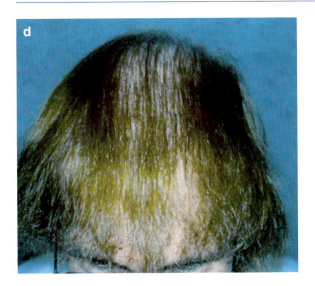

Fig. 13.44 (continued)

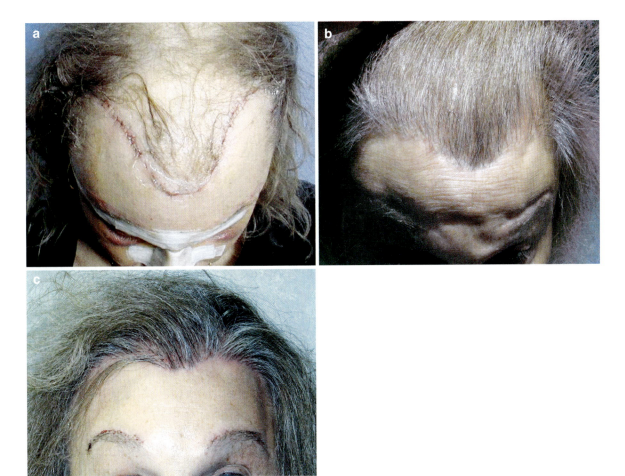

Fig. 13.45 (**a**) TG patient before transplant as well as showing recent scalp advancement and nasal/brow work. (**b**) After two sessions of grafting, hair is pulled back to show new feminine hairline and camouflage of scalp advancement scar. (**c**) Recent grafting to thicken eyebrows and cover incision scars. (Reprinted with permission from Berg and Cotterill [24]. Copyright Elsevier Limited 2009)

13.25 Conclusions

The physician utilizing the modern principles and techniques of hair transplantation practiced today is able to deliver, consistently, very cosmetically acceptable and natural results. This chapter has presented the currently practiced principles of planning and design, how to create a transplant, as well as discussed the importance of patient education and incorporating nonsurgical therapies into a hair restoration practice. In the future, exciting new advances in hair multiplication and gene therapy may be available to assist, even further, those affected with hair loss and allow many more people to benefit from hair transplantation.

References

1. Kuster W, Happle R. The inheritance of common baldness: two B or not two B? J Am Acad Dermatol. 1984;11(5 Pt 1):921–6.
2. Sawaya ME, Price VH. Different levels of 5alpha-reductase type I and II, aromatase, and androgen receptor in hair follicles of women and men with androgenetic alopecia. J Invest Dermatol. 1997;109(3):296–300.
3. Norwood OT. Male pattern baldness: classification and incidence. South Med J. 1975;68(11):1359–65.
4. Ludwig E. Classification of the types of androgenetic alopecia (common baldness) occurring in the female sex. Br J Dermatol. 1977;97(3):247–54.
5. Olsen EA. The middle part: an important physical clue to the diagnosis of androgenetic alopecia in women. J Am Acad Dermatol. 1999;40(1):106–9.
6. Orentreich N. Autografts in alopecias and other selected dermatological conditions. Ann NY Acad Sci. 1959;83:463–79.
7. Nordstrom RE. Micrografts for improvement of the frontal hairline after transplantation. Aesthetic Plast Surg. 1981;5:97–101.
8. Marritt E. Transplantation of single hairs from the scalp as eyelashes. Review of the literature and a case report. J Dermatol Surg Oncol. 1980;6(4):271–3.
9. Olsen EA, Dunlap FE, Funicella T, Koperski JA, Swinehart JM, Tschen EH, et al. A randomized clinical trial of 5% topical minoxidil versus 2% topical minoxidil and placebo in the treatment of androgenetic alopecia in men. J Am Acad Dermatol. 2002;47(3):377–85.
10. Kaufman KD, Olsen EA, Whiting D, Savin R, DeVillez R, Bergfeld R, et al. Finasteride in the treatment of men with androgenetic alopecia. Finasteride Male Patient Pattern Hair Loss Study Group. J Am Acad Dermatol. 1998;39(4 Pt 1):578–89.
11. Price VH, Roberts JL, Hordinsky M, Olsen EA, Savin R, Bergfeld W, et al. Lack of efficacy of finasteride in postmenopausal women with androgenetic alopecia. J Am Acad Dermatol. 2000;43(5 Pt 1):768–76.
12. Finasteride Male Pattern Hair Loss Study Group. Long-term (5 year) multinational experience with finasteride 1 mg in the treatment of men with androgenetic alopecia. Eur J Dermatol. 2002;12(1):38–49.
13. Thompson IM, Goodman PJ, Tangen CM, Lucia MS, Miller GJ, Ford LG, et al. The influence of finasteride on the development of prostate cancer. N Engl J Med. 2003;349(3):215–24.
14. Olsen EA. Female pattern hair loss. J Am Acad Dermatol. 2001;45(3 Suppl):S70–80.
15. Price VH. Treatment of hair loss. N Engl J Med. 1999;341(13):964–73.
16. Iorizzo M, Vincenzi C, Voudouris S, Piraccini BM, Tosti A. Finasteride treatment female pattern hair loss. Arch Dermatol. 2006;142(3):298–302.
17. Rushton DH, Ramsay ID. The importance of adequate serum ferritin levels during oral cyproterone acetate and ethinyl oestradiol treatment of diffuse androgen-dependent alopecia in women. Clin Endocrinol. 1992;36(4):421–7.
18. Avram MR, Leonard RT, Epstein ES, Williams JL, Bauman AJ. The current role of laser/light sources in the treatment of male and female pattern hair loss. J Cosmet Laser Ther. 2007;9(1):27–8.
19. Cash TF, Price VH, Savin RC. Psychological effects of androgenetic alopecia: comparisons with balding men and with female control subjects. J Am Acad Dermatol. 1993;29(4):568–75.
20. Norwood OT, Taylor BJ. Hairline design and placement. J Dermatol Surg Oncol. 1991;17(6):510–8.
21. Norwood OT. Patient selection, hair transplant design and hair style. J Dermatol Surg Oncol. 1992;18(5):386–94.
22. Unger WP, Beehner ML, Knudsen R, Parsley WM. Basic principles and organization. In: Unger WP, Shapiro R, editors. Hair transplantation. New York: Marcel Dekker; 2004. p. 81–164.
23. Parsley WM, Rose P. Science of hairline design. In: Haber RS, Stough DB, editors. Hair transplantation. Philadelphia: Elsevier; 2006. p. 55–71.
24. Berg D, Cotterill PC. Hair transplantation. In: Alam M, Gladstone HB, Tung RC, editors. Requisites in dermatology, cosmetic dermatology. Philadelphia: Elsevier; 2009. p. 187–232.
25. Beehner ML. A frontal forelock/central density framework for hair transplantation. Dermatol Surg. 1997;23(9):807–15.
26. Seery GE, Unger MG, Marzola M, Cattani RV. Alopecia reduction procedures. In: Unger WP, Shapiro R, editors. Hair transplantation. New York: Marcel Dekker; 2004. p. 709–63.
27. Frechet P. Scalp extension. In: Unger WP, Shapiro R, editors. Hair transplantation. New York: Marcel Dekker; 2004. p. 765–94.
28. Seery GE, Juri J, Anderson RD, Epstein MD, Rabineau P. Flap procedures. In: Unger WP, Shapiro R, editors. Hair transplantation. New York: Marcel Dekker; 2004. p. 795–830.
29. Brandy DA. An evaluation system to enhance patient selection for alopecia-reducing surgery. Dermatol Surg. 2002;28(9):808–16.
30. Unger WP, Cole J. Donor harvesting. In: Unger WP, Shapiro R, editors. Hair transplantation. New York: Marcel Dekker; 2004. p. 301–5.
31. Rassman WR, Bernstein RM, McClellan R, Jones R, Worton E, Uyttendaele H. Follicular unit extraction: minimally invasive surgery for hair transplantation. Dermatol Surg. 2002;28(8):720–8.

32. Harris J. Follicular unit extraction: the SAFE system. Hair Transpl Forum Int 2004;14(5):157,163–164.
33. Gandelman M, Abrahamsohn PA. Light and electron microscopy of follicular unit grafting: studying iatrogenic injury of follicles. In: Unger WP, Shapiro R, editors. Hair transplantation. New York: Marcel Dekker; 2004. p. 279–81.
34. Unger WP, Beehner ML. Studies of hair survival in grafts of different sizes with additional hair survival studies and conclusions. In: Unger WP, Shapiro R, editors. Hair transplantation. New York: Marcel Dekker; 2004. p. 261–79.
35. Hasson V. Perpendicular angle grafting. In: Haber RS, Stough DB, editors. Hair transplantation. Philadelphia: Elsevier; 2006. p. 117–25.
36. Gandelman M, Epstein JS. Hair transplantation to the eyebrow, eyelashes, and other parts of the body. Facial Plast Surg Clin North Am. 2004;12(2):253–61.

Ablative Laser Facial Resurfacing

P. Daniel Ward and Jessica H. Maxwell

14.1 Introduction

The laser has now become one of the most commonly used means of achieving facial rejuvenation [1]. Although other methods of resurfacing, such as dermabrasion and chemical peels, are still frequently used, the laser's ability to offer controlled delivery of energy with more predictable results has led to its adoption by many plastic surgeons as the standard method of performing facial rejuvenation. This chapter will provide a brief overview of basic laser physics as it relates to the skin, a description of the lasers commonly used, a description of the technique used in laser resurfacing, and a discussion of the complications associated with laser resurfacing.

The first laser used for facial resurfacing was the carbon dioxide (CO_2) laser [2]. Its continued use today stands as a testament to its durability as a technique that provides good results for the majority of patients. The wavelength of the CO_2 laser is 10,600 nm and primarily targets water. The other laser used for facial resurfacing, the erbium:yttrium-aluminum-garnet (Er:YAG) laser, also has water as its primary chromophore. The wavelength of the Er:YAG laser is 2,940 nm, which corresponds to the peak absorption of energy by water, resulting in absorption that is around ten times greater than the CO_2 laser.

Since the epidermis is approximately 90% water, delivery of light at wavelengths that target water results in heating of the water, which is vaporized with subsequent heat transfer to the surrounding extracellular matrix and the collagen therein. Delivery of heat to collagen in the skin leads to denaturation of the proteins and, as healing progresses, the formation of new collagen and other extracellular matrix proteins helps tighten skin and reduce rhytids. Delivery of too much energy, however, can lead to damage to the reticular dermis and an overabundant expression of collagen and subsequent scarring. Thus, choosing a proper amount of energy to be delivered to a particular region is a critical component of laser facial resurfacing, because delivery of too little energy results in inadequate treatment, and delivery of too much energy leads to scarring [1–7].

The amount of energy delivered by the laser is typically measured in joules and the amount of energy delivered by the laser per surface area of tissue is measured in joules per square centimeter. This latter term is defined as the fluence of the laser. In addition to the fluence of the laser, the other variable that is important is the pulse duration, which is defined as the amount of time that the tissue is exposed to the electromagnetic radiation from the laser. Complete cooling must occur between passes with the laser to minimize the chance that unwanted heat will be conducted to adjacent tissues and result in undesirable effects. The thermal relaxation time is the amount of time required for complete tissue cooling to occur. For the CO_2 and Er:YAG lasers, a very high energy level is utilized allowing for a very short pulse duration, which is on the order of 1,000 μs or 1 ms. The power density of

---

P.D. Ward (✉)
Division of Facial Plastic and Reconstructive Surgery,
Division of Otolaryngology – Head and Neck Surgery,
University of Michigan, 50 North Medical Drive, 3C120
School of Medicine, Salt Lake City, UT 84132, USA
e-mail: pdanielward@hsc.utah.edu

J.H. Maxwell
Department of Otolaryngology – Head and Neck Surgery,
University of Michigan Medical School,
1500 E. Medical Center Drive, Taubman 1904 D,
Ann Arbor, MI 48109-0312, USA
e-mail: jmhooton@med.umich.edu

Reprinted with Permission of Springer, Berlin

the laser, measured in watts, takes all three of the above variables into account and is commonly used to describe the energy delivered by the laser.

In addition to the physics of the laser, individual patient characteristics must also be considered including skin type, possible wound healing or scarring history, the patient's age, the thickness of the patient's skin, and the region to be treated. The most commonly used skin type classification system is the Fitzpatrick classification, which is described as follows:

Class 1: Very fair skin, never tans, always burns
Class 2: Fair skin, mildly tans, nearly always burns
Class 3: Medium skin tone, tans, sometimes burns
Class 4: Medium-dark skin, tans, still may occasionally burn
Class 5: Dark skin, tans intensely, rarely burns
Class 6: Darkest skin, tans intensely, never burns

Patients with skin class 4–6, are at high risk for dyschromia post-resurfacing and are thus rarely candidates for laser facial resurfacing. Any possible wound healing concerns should be assessed as should the thickness of the patient's skin. Finally, the regions of skin that are to be treated must also be considered. For example, the thin skin of the eyelids will require less energy than the thicker and appendage-rich skin of the cheek regions. This last consideration will influence the laser settings used as well as the number of passes of the laser. The energy of the first pass of the laser is nearly completely absorbed by epidermal water; however, once this layer has been removed, passes of the laser into dermal layers, which have less water content, results in greater heating of surrounding tissues leading to more injury with each pass.

14.2 Technique

14.2.1 Preoperative Preparation

Resurfacing of patients with darker skin types leads to a much more unpredictable result and is not routinely performed. All patients who desire laser resurfacing of the face should be informed that the procedure is one that is capable of producing unpredictable results, especially in terms of final results, recovery time, and complications [8]. Pretreatment of the skin is commonly recommended and may include sun avoidance, hydroquinone, isotretinoin, and glycolic acids. Sun avoidance is particularly important due to the theoretical risk of sun-induced melanocyte activation, which may result in unpredictable post-procedure pigmentary changes [8].

Prophylactic antivirals should be initiated in all patients and is routinely started 2 days prior to the procedure and continues for 14 days or until reepithelialization is complete. The risk of viral eruption following resurfacing is approximately 5% [7, 9–11]. Prophylactic antibiotic use is much more controversial and variable [12]. Many surgeons use pre- and post-procedure antibiotics routinely, whereas others use them only on a case-by-case basis. Many surgeons will also provide patients with prophylactic antifungal medications.

Preoperative photographs can be a helpful tool to help patients remember their preoperative appearance and can be used to document the patient's progress (Figs. 14.1 and 14.2). Cosmetic units may be marked in the preoperative holding area when the patient is in the upright position. This helps ensure that no error in marking will occur, as may happen when the patient is in the supine position due to skin movement. In addition, marking prior to the procedure helps avoid the temptation of marking intraoperatively, which may result in permanent tattooing if ablated skin is exposed to ink.

14.2.2 Carbon Dioxide Laser

Although initially invented in the 1960s, use of the carbon dioxide laser was limited due to long pulse durations, which led to unwanted thermal diffusion and subsequent scarring [1]. The development of lasers, capable of much shorter pulse durations (less than 1 ms), led to much more controlled and reproducible results. Now, the carbon dioxide laser is typically used for rhytids in the shallow- to medium-depth range and is particularly useful for treating solar and actinic damage. Tissue ablation depth is approximately 50–100 μm and the thermal diffusion injury range is 35–50 μm. Settings used for the carbon dioxide laser vary; however, standard settings are density of 4–5 with an energy delivery of 80–90 mJ that corresponds to a power of 45–60 W [8].

The laser is passed over the areas of the face to be treated with care taken to the different skin depths in different regions of the face. The level of ablation that is

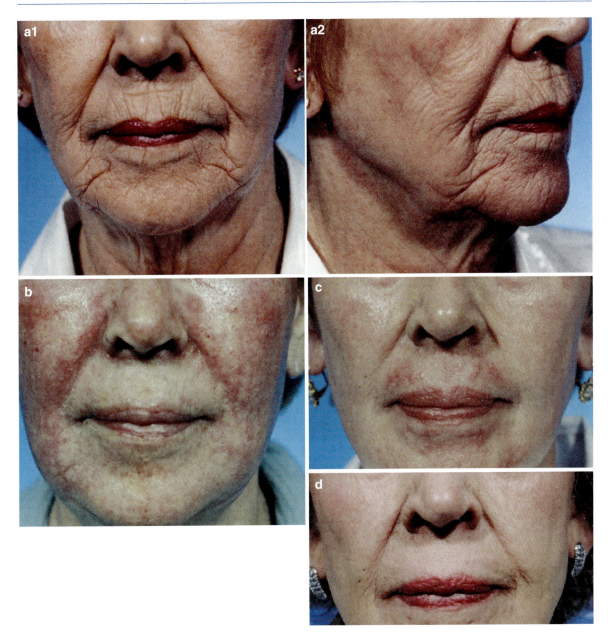

Fig. 14.1 (**a1**) Preoperative frontal view. (**a2**) Preoperative 3/4 view. (**b**) Six days after CO_2 laser resurfacing. (**c**) Six months postoperative. (**d**) Nine years postoperative (Photos courtesy of Shan R. Baker, MD)

required is dependent on the skin thickness, degree of rhytidosis, and the patient's age. This latter point is important to remember, because aging is associated with thinning of the skin. The depth of ablation can be determined by the color of the underlying ablated tissue. A pink color indicates the upper papillary dermis, whereas a gray color indicates the upper reticular dermis, and a chamois appearance with pinpoint bleeding indicates the mid-reticular dermis. Secondary passes over regions are usually performed with a lower energy, for example, 60–70 mJ, with a density of 4. Second passes are used for deeper wrinkles that require more than one pass to reach the base of the rhytid. A moist saline-soaked gauze sponge can be used to remove ablated tissue between each pass of the laser. Blending of the treated skin with non-treated regions is important,

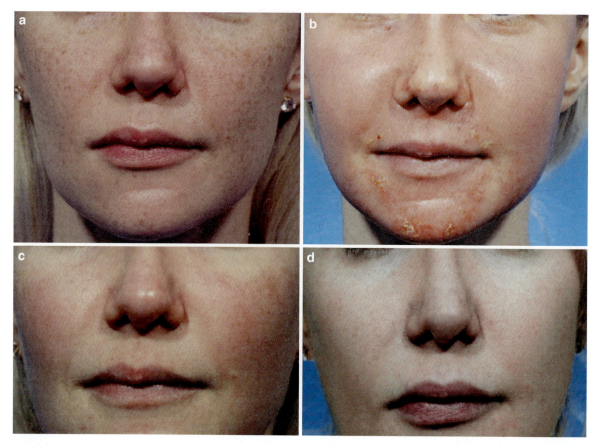

Fig. 14.2 Patient who underwent CO_2 laser resurfacing due to concerns about freckles. (**a**) Preoperative. (**b**) Seven days postoperative. (**c**) Five and a half months postoperative. (**d**) Two years postoperative (Photos courtesy of Shan R. Baker, MD)

because nearly all patients will develop some degree of hypopigmentation postoperatively [8].

14.2.3 Erbium Laser

The erbium laser has a wavelength of 2,940 nm, which corresponds to a point on the water absorption curve that is approximately ten times greater than that seen with the wavelength of the carbon dioxide laser [1]. The clinical relevance of this difference is a laser with a much greater safety margin secondary to less tissue injury to the surrounding tissues. This leads to a decreased improvement in rhytids compared to the carbon dioxide laser; however, it is also associated with less postoperative erythema, shorter recovery time, less scarring, and decreased risk of pigmentary changes. Greater thermal injury can be achieved by increasing the duration of the pulse.

The procedure of resurfacing with the erbium laser is similar to that described with the carbon dioxide laser. Again, the depth of ablation must be carefully monitored to avoid too deep ablative treatment and scarring. The classic color changes described above for the carbon dioxide laser are not seen. Instead, pinpoint bleeding should be used as an indicator that the depth of ablation is in the papillary dermis. Ablative debris must be removed after each pass. However, the erbium laser is not associated with thermal stacking allowing for overlapping of passes.

Due to the decreased thermal diffusion, the erbium laser has less tissue penetration than the carbon dioxide laser. Utley demonstrated that the erbium laser penetrated 20 μm with the first pass, whereas the carbon dioxide laser had a penetration depth of 62.5 μm [13]. These differences allow anesthesia for resurfacing with the erbium laser to be performed with local or even topical anesthesia if the level to be resurfaced is superficial. Otherwise, for deeper peels, local anesthesia with sedation or general anesthesia may be necessary.

14.2.4 Postoperative Care

Reepithelialization post-laser resurfacing is enhanced with the use of occlusive dressings, which are thought to maintain humidity and subsequently enhance fibroblast function and migration. These dressings must be changed daily for the first 3–7 days. Ointments may be used, but care must be taken to avoid contact dermatitis that can occur as a result of continued exposure to these agents. After reepithelialization is complete, the patient may begin to use mild, hypoallergenic makeup to help conceal the underlying erythema. Moisturizers that are fragrance-free should be utilized to improve hydration. The most important aspect in postoperative care is complete sun avoidance. This should be followed for at least 2–3 months or until all postoperative erythema has resolved. Exposure to sunlight during this healing period may be associated with melanocyte activation and increased pigmentary abnormalities.

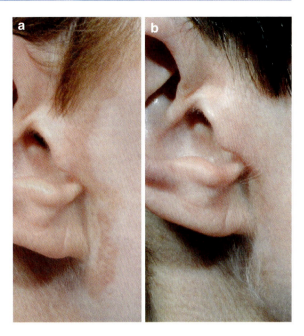

Fig. 14.3 (**a**) Patient with postoperative hypopigmentation demonstrated at line of demarcation between treated and untreated skin. (**b**) Patient is able to disguise line of demarcation with makeup (Photos courtesy of Shan R. Baker, MD)

14.3 Complications

Infection is always a concern with any surgical procedure, especially one with a wound as large as the entire face. Much has been written about viral infections, but both bacterial and fungal etiologies should be considered. Viral infections are typically marked by pain that occurs at the latter portion of the reepithelialization process. These outbreaks can occur despite the use of antiviral medication and should be treated with antiviral doses typically used to treat zoster infections. Bacterial infections are also associated with pain and are also concerning, because they may result in profound scarring. Fungal infections are more likely when dressing changes are not performed frequently enough or when exudate is not completely removed with the dressing change.

All patients experience some degree of transient hyperpigmentation that lasts for 1–2 months. Hyperpigmentation that persists beyond this time may be treated with hydroquinone, retinoic acid, mild topical steroids, and, most importantly, continued avoidance of sunlight [8]. Nearly all patients will also experience some degree of hypopigmentation post-procedure. This occurs in 10–30% of patients. The implications of this effect can be minimized with feathering of the treated and non-treated skin (Fig. 14.3). Unfortunately, this effect is permanent and unpredictable, although there is an association between the degree of rhytid improvement and hypopigmentation. Patients may camouflage the line of demarcation with makeup.

The most troublesome and feared complication of laser resurfacing is scarring. This can be minimized by adopting a conservative approach to help decrease the likelihood of deep dermal penetration [14]. Treatment typically consists of steroids and vascular lasers [1, 9].

14.4 Discussion

The carbon dioxide and erbium lasers provide improved precision and more consistent results compared to chemical peels and have less risk of aerosolized particles compared to dermabrasion. Further technological advances are likely to continue to improve these treatments leading to safer and more effective treatment of rhytids and solar damage of the face.

One key technology not discussed in this chapter is non-ablative rejuvenation, which promises shorter recovery times by treating the dermis and avoiding injury to the overlying epidermis [1, 15, 16]. This results in neocollagen production and secondary dermal remodeling. Many new treatments are available that target different chromophores within the dermis [1].

An additional technology that bears mention as a promising new method is the fractionated technique of thermolysis. This technique works by emitting light of 1,500 nm in tiny zones, which when applied to skin targets water and creates microscopic thermal injury "cylinders" surrounded by healthy, non-injured tissue. The treated cylinders are rapidly reepithelialized by the surrounding non-injured tissue resulting in a recovery time of approximately 24 h. Multiple treatments are required, but patients enjoy the benefits of shorter recovery time with improvement in rhytids and solar injury [17–20].

14.5 Conclusions

The laser is a valuable tool in the facial plastic surgeon's armamentarium. The ideal laser treatment for facial resurfacing will be one that allows improvement in facial rhytids and solar aging with short recovery time and less pain. The rapid improvements in technology that occurred over the past 10–15 years are expected to continue into the next decade and beyond. This time will be an exciting one for those involved in the care of patients who desire improvement in the appearance of their facial skin as new technologies are discovered that maximize results while minimizing side effects and recovery time.

References

1. Alexiades-Armenakas MR, Dover JS, Arndt KA. The spectrum of laser skin resurfacing: nonablative, fractional, and ablative laser resurfacing. J Am Acad Dermatol. 2008; 58(5):719–37.
2. Arndt KA, Noe JM. Lasers in dermatology. Arch Dermatol. 1982;118(5):293–5.
3. Bernstein LJ, Kauvar AN, Grossman MC, Geronemus RG. The short- and long-term side effects of carbon dioxide laser resurfacing. Dermatol Surg. 1997;23(7):519–25.
4. Alster TS. Cosmetic laser surgery. Adv Dermatol. 1996; 11:51–80; discussion 81.
5. Alster TS, Garg S. Treatment of facial rhytides with a high-energy pulsed carbon dioxide laser. Plast Reconstr Surg. 1996;98(5):791–4.
6. Alster TS, Lewis AB. Dermatologic laser surgery. A review. Dermatol Surg. 1996;22(9):797–805.
7. Alster TS, Nanni CA. Famciclovir prophylaxis of herpes simplex virus reactivation after laser skin resurfacing. Dermatol Surg. 1999;25(3):242–6.
8. Ward PD, Baker SR. Long-term results of carbon dioxide laser resurfacing of the face. Arch Facial Plast Surg. 2008;10(4):238–43; discussion 244–245.
9. Ratner D, Tse Y, Marchell N, Goldman MP, Fitzpatrick RE, Fader DJ. Cutaneous laser resurfacing. J Am Acad Dermatol. 1999;41(3 Pt 1):365–89.
10. Nanni CA, Alster TS. Complications of carbon dioxide laser resurfacing. an evaluation of 500 patients. Dermatol Surg. 1998;24(3):315–20.
11. Nanni CA, Alster TS. Complications of cutaneous laser surgery. A review. Dermatol Surg. 1998;24(2):209–19.
12. Walia S, Alster TS. Cutaneous CO_2 laser resurfacing infection rate with and without prophylactic antibiotics. Dermatol Surg. 1999;25(11):857–61.
13. Utley DS, Koch RJ, Egbert BM. Histologic analysis of the thermal effect on epidermal and dermal structures following treatment with the superpulsed CO_2 laser and the erbium:YAG laser: an in vivo study. Lasers Surg Med. 1999; 24(2):93–102.
14. Fitzpatrick RE, Smith SR, Sriprachya-anunt S. Depth of vaporization and the effect of pulse stacking with a high-energy, pulsed carbon dioxide laser. J Am Acad Dermatol. 1999;40(4):615–22.
15. Bjerring P, Clement M, Heickendorff L, Egevist H, Kiernan M. Selective non-ablative wrinkle reduction by laser. J Cutan Laser Ther. 2000;2(1):9–15.
16. Rostan E, Bowes LE, Iyer S, Fitzpatrick RE. A double-blind, side-by-side comparison study of low fluence long pulse dye laser to coolant treatment for wrinkling of the cheeks. J Cosmet Laser Ther. 2001;3(3):129–36.
17. Rinaldi F. Laser: a review. Clin Dermatol. 2008; 26(6): 590–601.
18. Hasegawa T, Matsukura T, Mizuno Y, Suga Y, Ogawa H, Ikeda S. Clinical trial of a laser device called fractional photothermolysis system for acne scars. J Dermatol. 2006; 33(9):623–7.
19. Manstein D, Herron GS, Sink RK, Tanner H, Anderson RR. Fractional photothermolysis: a new concept for cutaneous remodeling using microscopic patterns of thermal injury. Lasers Surg Med. 2004;34(5):426–38.
20. Rokhsar CK, Fitzpatrick RE. The treatment of melasma with fractional photothermolysis: a pilot study. Dermatol Surg. 2005;31(12):1645–50.

Photorejuvenation

15

Kenneth Beer and Rhoda S. Narins

15.1 Introduction

The concept for rejuvenation of the face by using light sources has been present since the advent of laser technologies. Lasers used to accomplish this goal include the ablative (CO_2 and erbium) and non-ablative lasers. However, the sequelae associated with ablative lasers and lack of compelling efficacy associated with non-ablative lasers created a realization that non-laser light source might be the best means of accomplishing facial photorejuvenation. These pulsed light sources began to become popular in the cosmetic surgery community in 2004 and have since undergone various refinements.

Benefits of photorejuvenation are numerous and include: improvements of the tone and texture of the skin, diminished pigment irregularity, reduction of vascular lesions, improvement in the appearance of fine lines and wrinkles.

Intense pulsed light (IPL) differs from laser light in a number of theoretical and clinical aspects. Whereas laser emissions are coherent beams of the same wavelength and frequency, intense pulsed light contains light with a variety of wavelengths. Intense pulsed light used for photorejuvenation is light containing 500–1,200 nm [1]. As such, it targets numerous chromophores within the epidermis and dermis including melanin, vascular structures, collagen, and other structures. The use of filters to limit the spectra of light emitted enables one to focus on one particular aspect of the skin when using this device. Since the process of photoaging (and thus of photorejuvenation) affects each of these, it is worthwhile to consider the interaction of intense pulsed light as it interacts with each.

The actual IPL device consists of a flashlamp light source that produces polychromatic light [2]. Depending on the desired wavelength, filters may be introduced to remove light of a specific wavelength. It is this capability that enables IPL to provide diverse types of treatments with one device and is partially responsible for the popularity of IPL with physician and nonphysician practitioners alike.

One hallmark of aging skin is the pigmentary irregularity frequently seen after photodamage has occurred. The degree of pigment present is a function of the skin type of the individual in question, the amount of ultraviolet exposure they have sustained, mitigating treatments such as the use of topical retinoids, bleaching creams, chemical peels, or cosmeceuticals and the capacity for intrinsic rejuvenation that a given individual possesses.

Hypopigmentation associated with photodamage is, at present, not treated with intense pulsed light with any degree of success. To date, attempts to stimulate melanocytes to produce pigment once they have undergone apoptosis have not resulted in restoration of a normal complement of pigment producing cells within the basal layer of the epidermis.

Hyperpigmentation associated with a variety of conditions including photodamage, pregnancy, and post-inflammation has been more effectively treated with

---

K. Beer (✉)
The Palm Beach Esthetic Center, 1500 North Dixie Highway, Suite 303, West Palm Beach, FL 33401, USA
e-mail: kenbeer@aol.com

R.S. Narins
Dermatology Surgery and Laser Center, Clinical Professor of Dermatology, New York University Medical Center,
New York, NY, USA

Reprinted with permission of Springer, Berlin

A. Erian and M.A. Shiffman (eds.), *Advanced Surgical Facial Rejuvenation*,
DOI: 10.1007/978-3-642-17838-2_15, © Springer-Verlag Berlin Heidelberg 2012

photorejuvenation. The absorption spectrum for melanin is continuous and thus IPL is well suited for this indication. Actinic lentigines, melasma, and post-inflammatory hyperpigmentation may be treated with IPL. When treating hyperpigmentation, it is critical to insure that patients have not had any significant ultraviolet exposure for the preceding several weeks (2–4), have used either broad spectrum sunscreen or physical barrier sunblocks, and that they have no planned sun exposure for a few weeks after the procedure. Prior sun exposure will prime the melanocytes to respond to the IPL by making more pigment as does sun exposure, following the treatment.

Skin types I, II, and III tend to develop telangiectasias with increased sun exposure and aging. In addition, these types of skin are prone to rosacea as the skin ages. IPL can address many of the vascular proliferations seen with both of these problems. Since hemoglobin has a series of absorption peaks including 585, the light from IPL is readily absorbed. One study evaluating the use of IPL for rosacea-associated telangiectasias found significant improvement after five treatments, each 3 weeks apart [3].

The addition of porphyrins to the skin may increase efficacy of this treatment [4]. This treatment is known as Photodynamic Therapy or PDT. The addition of this photosensitizer has increased the energy absorption for IPL, rendering it more effective at treating the various stigmata of photoaging. Various protocols may be utilized, each involving cleansing of the skin prior to application of the Amino levulinic acid (ALA) for an amount of time that may vary between 15 and 60 min. Energy levels and filters for IPL depend on the skin type, degree of damage present, degree of erythema present, tolerance for downtime by the patient, and goals of the treatment. The marriage of IPL with ALA may provide for highly effective photorejuvenation.

Under the microscope, photoaging is associated with disorganization and atrophy of the epidermis, degeneration of the papillary and reticular dermis as the collagen and elastic fibers diminish, and a host of other subtle and overt changes [5]. At a subcellular level, IPL treatments stimulate production of type I collagen transcripts [6]. Devices that optimize this collagen production stimulate elastin production, and remodeling will enhance the ability of IPL machines to perform photorejuvenation. The addition of medications such as low-dose antibiotics including doxycycline may inhibit collagenase and addition of this medication may improve patient outcomes.

IPL has been useful in reversing several of these signs of aging and it is in this category of photorejuvenation that the potential may be the greatest. After observations that non-ablative lasers in the 585 nm spectrum were able to cause collagen remodeling, other methods of accomplishing the same goals were investigated. Goldberg et al. demonstrated the efficacy of IPL for the treatment of rhytids, and since that time various devices and protocols have been utilized for this goal [7]. It is anticipated that this indication will most likely remain extremely popular.

15.2 Technique

The techniques for using IPL for photorejuvenation are as varied and diverse as the number of machines and operators using them and the goals of a treatment regimen for a given patient. Perhaps the most important part of the technique for photorejuvenation is the one that is sometimes overlooked – the consultation and consent process. During the consultation, it is important to listen to what the potential patient is saying about his or her expectations and tolerance for risk and downtime. One signal that the non-ablative photorejuvenation might be the wrong procedure for a particular patient are statements indicating that they want to "get rid" of wrinkles or that they want a nonsurgical facelift. Many of the patients that have these types of expectations are fed by the reports of various procedures in the popular media. Since these types of reports tend to present only the best cases, patients that demand these results are most likely going to be disappointed and thus, are not good candidates unless one can educate them about the realities of the procedure. Other signs that a patient might not be a good candidate for photorejuvenation are similar to warning signs to heed for any cosmetic patient: patients that speak poorly of other physicians, patients that are financially stretched for the procedure and cannot financially afford adjunct treatments such as Botulinum toxins or fillers that might be needed for optimal outcomes, and interactions with ancillary staff that simply gives reliable staff a sense of dread toward the individual.

Consent for photorejuvenation should include discussions of the risks, need for multiple treatments, the fact that each session has a cost, confirmation that the patient is required to avoid the sun, inform the physician if she is pregnant or has certain types of photosensitive diseases, and other relevant considerations for the type of procedure being performed. Many physicians recommend photographic documentation of the patient's baseline, and this should be seriously considered for each patient.

For a particular device, the initial technical considerations are the parameters for the treatment. The first parameter to consider is the reason the patient is undergoing the treatment. Since many devices are capable of emitting light from 400 to 1,200 nm, filters that limit the wavelengths emitted are used to emit light most appropriate for each indication. For instance, when treating vascular or red lesions, filters are used to limit the light emitted to wavelengths that will be efficacious. Other filters may be used when melanin is the target.

Once the proper handpiece is selected, energy settings must be considered. When beginning a treatment with a type I or II skin type that has not been exposed to recent ultraviolet light, settings can be at the upper end of recommended parameters. Darker skin types will need to be treated at the lower end of these settings.

The fluence, pulse duration, and size of the spot are technical considerations whose parameters change with each device. The presence and type of skin cooling available also help to determine the settings for each treatment. Depending on the manufacturer, fluences from 15 to 90 J/cm^2 may be used. Spot size must be selected to best suit the area being treated and these may be as large as several centimeters or small as a few millimeters. Prior to using any IPL device, it is imperative to familiarize oneself with the particular recommendations and literature that are specific for it.

At each treatment, makeup and sunscreen should be removed before the treatment begins. A topical anesthetic cream may be applied for half an hour and removed before treatment begins. Once the treatment is completed, chemical free sunscreen should be applied if the patient will have any outdoor exposure. The patient should be positioned comfortably and the operator should be able to readily access the area undergoing treatment. Eye protection must be worn during the procedure.

Using a double-stacked IPL pulse instead of a single pulse may result in improvements in erythema, skin roughness, and in hyperpigmentation [8]. This protocol, using the Lux G handpiece from Palomar, suggests that operator variables may strongly influence outcomes when treating the visible signs of aging and suggests that using two-stacked pulses is better than a single pulse when treating photoaging. Future devices or techniques will likely expand on this finding. Other devices, including the Quantum Intense Pulsed light (Lumenis, Santa Clara, CA), the Ellipse system (Candela, Wayland, MA), and several other systems offer a variety of light filters that are suitable for treating multiple skin issues including photorejuvenation, hyperpigmentation, telangiectasias, rosacea, and a host of other skin conditions. It is anticipated that advances in skin cooling, power delivery, and light filters will continue to make these products more effective and more versatile.

Prior to treatment, a chilled gel is applied to the skin. Following a few pulses of the treated area, inspection of the skin must be performed to insure that there are no blisters or incipient burns that are occurring. At the completion of the treatment, ice or cool gel packs may be applied to reduce the swelling. Posttreatment care instructions are provided, and documentation that this has been completed should occur in the patient's record.

Treatments for photorejuvenation are usually separated by 2–4 weeks. Most devices recommend that a series of between four and six sessions are scheduled for maximum benefit.

Combining photorejuvenation with other types of cosmetic procedures may enhance the outcomes from each procedure and this is one technical consideration that only recently has begun to be explored. Carruthers and Carruthers [9] reported improvement of pore size, dyspigmentation, telangiectasias, and skin texture when Botulinum toxin A was used concomitantly with IPL.

15.3 Complications

Complications that may occur with IPL for photorejuvenation include common ones such as swelling, bruising, and transient erythema and less common ones including hyperpigmentation, infection, burns, and scarring. The incidence of transient crusting is reported as 2%, and Goldman et al. note that this superficial crusting is self-limited, lasting approximately 1 week [2]. The same authors report a 4% rate of purpura and a rate of swelling of 25% and these are consistent with the experience of the authors [2]. Both purpura and swelling occur at a much higher rate in areas such as the eyelids, and care should be taken when treating the upper cheek/lower eyelid area.

The incidence of scarring is rare and it usually is the result of using excessive energy or from using the IPL device on someone that has been exposed to sun. Infections from herpes simplex may occur after treatment of an area prone to outbreaks and prophylaxis with antiviral medication is recommended for patients with a history of herpes. Bacterial infections are extremely rare with non-ablative photorejuvenation and they may be the result of patients that excoriate the skin following treatment. Any infection in a treated patient should be treated with appropriate antibiotic or antiviral medication. A single case of a vesiculobullous eruption, following IPL, performed by a nonphysician has been reported [10]. In this instance, the patient sustained significant vesicles and bulla that were thought to be a function of poor technique although other etiologies were also entertained.

In order to minimize the risks of complications, patient education and screening are important. Patients with increased ultraviolet exposure should not be treated as they are at significant risk for transient hyperpigmentation as well as for scarring due to the increased epidermal melanin with increased absorption of energy.

15.4 Discussion

The popularity of non-ablative photorejuvenation with physicians, nonphysician providers, and with patients attests to the excellent results, thereby increasing the demand for these types of treatments. Each of these devices, in conjunction with industry, is searching for better outcomes with less downtime. Recent IPL devices are now approaching the goal of improving photoaging with minimal risk and downtime.

Since IPL is a broad spectrum of light that can be administered with varied levels of fluence, its potential for treating telangiectasias, fine lines, hyperpigmentation, skin surface roughness, and other signs of aging continue to be realized (Fig. 15.1).

Results for the treatment of small blood vessels as well as the erythema associated with rosacea have approached those obtained with pulsed dye laser with significantly less posttreatment purpura. The IPL is also useful for maintenance after using other lasers such as the Vbeam or NdYag. While not as dramatic as the outcomes that follow ablative skin resurfacing, the marked reduction of risk when compared to the latter procedure has made IPL extremely popular for the treatment of fine lines and skin surface roughness. The improvements of collagen fibers have been documented and modifications of both devices and protocols (including the adjunctive use of medications to foster collagen production) will continue to enhance outcomes. One likely scenario that will enhance non-ablative photorejuvenation will be the combination of various types of light for synergistic outcomes. Fractional ablation, infrared light, and radiofrequency are among the possible candidates for this. Results from one study have suggested that combing IPL with Botox will yield dramatically better results than the sum of their parts would suggest likely. Undoubtedly, other combinations including the use of other types of type A toxin, the use of fillers to stimulate collagen remodeling and to fill deep rhytids will also be explored.

Photoaging may stigmatize the skin with production of pigment on the face, neck, and dorsal hands. Poikilodermatous changes on the neck as well as the chest, arms, legs, and other parts of the body are amenable to treatment with IPL, and handpieces that can treat this are presently in use. The lentigines on the dorsal hands and face that serve notice of a life spent in the sun are also effectively treated with IPL, and the use of this device, in combination with prescription bleaching creams (including those with combinations of hydrocortisone, tretinoin, and hydroquinone) and sun blocks, have dramatically improved the appearance of both. Skin surface irregularity and roughness are similarly restored to a more youthful appearance following treatment with IPL and it remains to be considered whether pretreatment with topical vitamin C, tretinoin, green tea, or oral medications may enhance the outcomes obtained and if so, what the optimal parameters are.

One problem with the use of IPL for the treatment of photoaging involves not the actual devices but the regulations governing them. In many states, the use of these devices is not regulated to any large extent. This, in conjunction with what can graciously be termed "overly enthusiastic" marketing to the masses of nonspecialists that comprise the larger market for

Fig. 15.1 (**a**) Pretreatment. (**b**) Posttreatment following photorejuvenation

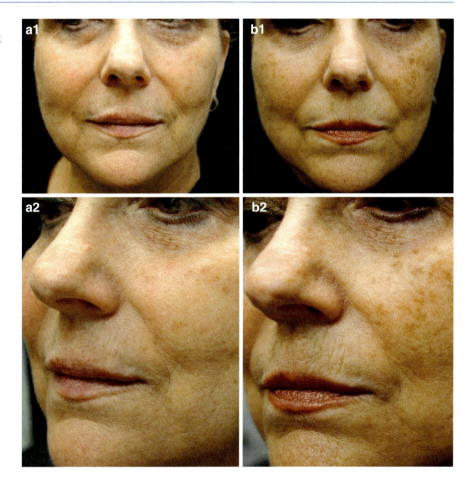

several of the manufacturers has led to a proliferation of devices placed in the hands of those least educated about the potential for harm that may ensue from their use. Scarring, hyperpigmentation, hypopigmentation, and a host of other complications that may occur under the best of circumstances have become more frequent as the treatment of photoaging has been moved (to a large degree) from the dermatologist's office to the mall. Regulations to govern the use of these devices including the need for supervision will, at some point, catch up with the technology and marketing, and this will hopefully bring the situation back into a balance that favors patient safety. Likewise, seminars that train nonspecialists may eventually become liable for the damages that these practitioners cause. This may have a chilling effect on the seminars that exchange official looking certificates designed to confer credibility for the price of the course.

15.5 Conclusions

Non-ablative photorejuvenation is here to stay because it is safe and effective. Enhancements to the technology will continue to improve the ability of the devices to treat the signs of aging. Improvements in technique, including the use of double-stacked pulses and the adjunctive uses of other procedures and medications, will increase the efficacy of the devices used. Regulations and public awareness campaigns will serve to decrease the complications associated with usage by nonphysicians and nonspecialists.

The use of these devices has transformed cosmetic dermatology by providing a safe and effective means to renovate the surface of the skin. Outcomes associated with these devices will continue to improve with refinements in training, techniques, and technology.

References

1. Marmur E, Goldberg D. Nonablative skin resurfacing. In: Dover J, Alam M, Goldberg D, editors. Procedures in cosmetic dermatology: lasers and lights, vol. 2. Philadelphia: Elsevier; 2005. p. 29–30.
2. Goldman M, Weiss R, Weiss M. Intense pulsed light as a nonablative approach to photoaging. Dermatol Surg. 2005; 31(9 Pt 2):1179–87.
3. Mark K, Sparacia R, Voight A, Marenus K, Sarnoff D. Objective and quantitative improvement of rosacea associated erythema after intense pulsed light treatment. Dermatol Surg. 2003;29(6):600–4.
4. Gold MH. The evolving role of aminolevulinic acid hydrochloride with photodynamic therapy in photoaging. Cutis. 2002;69(6 Suppl):8–13.
5. Hernandez-Perez E, Ibiett EV. Gross and microscopic findings in patients submitted to nonablative full face resurfacing using intense pulsed light. Dermatol Surg. 2002; 28(8):651–5.
6. Zelickson B, Kist D. Pulsed dye laser and photoderm treatment stimulate production of type I collagen and collagenase transcripts in papillary dermis fibroblasts, (abstract). Lasers Surg Med Suppl. 2001;13:33.
7. Goldberg DJ, Cutler KB. Nonablative treatment of rhytids with intense pulsed light. Lasers Surg Med. 2000;26(2): 196–200.
8. Kligman D, Zhen Y. Intense pulsed light treatment of photoaged skin. Dermatol Surg. 2004;30(8):1085–90.
9. Carruthers J, Carruthers A. The effect of full face broadband light treatments alone and in combination with bilateral crow's feet botulinum toxin type A chemodenervation. J Dermatol Surg. 2004;30(3):355–66.
10. Sperber B, Walling H, Arpey C, Whitaker D. Vesiculobullous eruption from intense pulsed light treatment. Dermatol Surg. 2005;31(3):345–8.

Superficial and Medium-Depth Chemical Peels

Benjamin A. Bassichis

16.1 Introduction

Chemical peeling of facial skin has become an integral part of the armamentarium for resurfacing aging, sun-damaged, and diseased skin. The desire to reverse the aging process has generated tremendous interest throughout history. Ancient texts describe the application of substances to the skin in an attempt to rejuvenate the appearance. More recently, many factors have contributed to the explosion of popularity of skin resurfacing procedures including the excess ultraviolet exposure both naturally and via tanning booths, the aging baby boomer cohort, youth-centric culture, smoking, ozone layer depletion, and the prevalence of both hot and cold weather outdoor recreations, which have all had a significant effect on people's skin health and premature wrinkling.

The modern body of knowledge regarding chemical agents began with the description of a variety of agents still in use today by Unna [1], including salicylic acid, resorcinol, phenol, and trichloroacetic acid (TCA). Over the ensuing century, peeling became popularized by nonmedical practitioners and cosmeticians who attracted increasing attention because of the rejuvenating results they achieved. Subsequent scientific studies of chemical peels by the medical community have further delineated the indications and limitations of these procedures and improved safety and efficacy. We are currently in an era of rapid development of new techniques for skin enhancement and rehabilitation, some of which offer the possibilities of dramatic results, with minimized discomfort and diminished downtime [2].

There are many products currently available for chemical resurfacing of the skin, from over-the-counter superficial peeling agents to deep peeling chemicals that should only be applied by a physician in a controlled setting [3]. Many of these products and procedures have proven very successful in improving the quality and appearance of facial skin. The goal of chemical peeling is to remove a controlled uniform thickness of damaged skin to improve and smooth the texture of the facial skin by removing the superficial layers and stimulate a wound healing response. In response to the chemical injury, fibroblasts in the papillary dermis increase production of collagen and growth factors. The collagen increase in turns thickens the dermis, which enhances the tensile strength of the skin and yields the clinical appearance of rejuvenation.

16.2 Skin Anatomy

The approach to chemical resurfacing of the skin necessitates a thorough knowledge of skin anatomy and normal wound healing. The skin is composed of two mutually dependent layers, the epidermis and dermis, which reside on a layer of subcutaneous adipose tissue. The epidermis is the most superficial layer of the skin and provides a critical barrier of protection. The epidermis is composed of keratinocytes in four layers: the stratum corneum, stratum granulosum, stratum spinosum, and stratum basale.

B.A. Bassichis
Department of Otolaryngology – Head and Neck Surgery,
University of Texas – Southwestern Medical Center,
5323 Harry Hines Boulevard, Dallas, TX 75235, USA and
Advanced Facial Plastic Surgery Center, 14755 Preston Road,
Suite 110, Dallas, TX 75254, USA
e-mail: drbassichis@advancedfacialplastic.com

Reprinted with Permission of Springer, Berlin

The stratum corneum is the outermost layer of the epidermis and is shed about every 2 weeks. Providing significant protection to the skin, it is formed from flattened, anucleate keratinocytes filled with mature keratin. Depending on the area of the body, the stratum corneum varies in thickness, with the eyelid being the thinnest and the palms and soles the thickest. The cells of the stratum granulosum contain dense basophilic keratohyalin granules, hence the granular layer. These granules are comprised of lipids, which along with the desmosomal connections help form a waterproof barrier that functions to prevent fluid loss from the body. The stratum spinosum keratinocytes contain numerous desmosomes on their outer surface that provides the characteristic spiney or prickled appearance of the cells in this layer. The stratum basale or basal layer, the deepest layer of the epidermis, contains basal cells whose replicative effort replaces the cells of the superficial layers every 2 weeks. The basal layer also contains melanocytes, which provide pigmentation in the skin.

The epidermis is avascular and thus dependent on the underlying dermis for nutrient delivery and waste disposal by diffusion through the dermoepidermal junction. In addition to thermoregulation, the dermis functions to sustain and support the overlying epidermis. The dermis is divided into two zones, the upper papillary dermis and the deeper reticular dermis. The dermis contains numerous fibroblasts that are responsible for secreting collagen, elastin, and ground matrix that provide the support and elasticity of the skin. Also, present in the dermis are a variety immune cells that are involved in defense against foreign invaders passing through the epidermis.

As we mature, the skin undergoes changes over time. The epidermal layer tends to thin and atrophy. The stratum corneum becomes disorganized and less effective as a protective barrier to the external environment. The dermoepidermal junction flattens and exhibits fewer papillae. However, the most significant changes occur in the dermis as it thins with age. The amount of ground substance and collagen fibers decreases, and elastic fibers degenerate and become irregular, making the skin less resistant to deformational forces. As the relatively inelastic epidermis loses dermal volume and support beneath it, fine wrinkles form.

After a chemical peel removes the superficial skin, the epidermis regenerates from the epidermal appendages located in the remaining dermis. This process begins within 24 h of wounding and is usually complete in 7–10 days. The new epidermis shows greater organization and vertical polarity, with the disappearance of actinic keratoses and lentigines. Dermal regeneration is a slower process but is usually complete within several months. Chemical peeling has been shown to improve the quality of the dermis with the formation of a dense, homogenous 2–3 mm band of parallel collagen fibers [4].

Histological sections of skin after a chemical peel procedure reveal a layer of new, denser connective tissue above the older, degenerated elastotic tissue. Clinically, this results in the effective ablation of the fine wrinkles and a diminution of pigmentation. Dermal ground substance is decreased, and telangiectasias are absent. Increased angiogenesis occurs in the dermis, which is thought to aid the appearance of the skin by adding a warm glow. The overall result is soft supple skin that appears more youthful with fewer rhytids and dyschromias. These clinical and histological changes are long lasting (15–20 years) and may be permanent in some patients.

16.3 Technique

16.3.1 Patient Selection

Indications for more superficial chemical peels include dyschromias, comedonal acne, and for skin refreshing. Indications for medium and deep peels are treatment of actinic changes, fine rhytids, pigmentary dyschromias, selected superficial scars, and acne vulgaris and rosacea.

Thorough evaluation and photo documentation prior to chemical peeling is vital for a successful outcome. This includes consideration of the severity of actinic damage, depth and number of rhytids, and need for additional or alternative procedures. Patients with deep rhytids and excess or lax facial skin are likely best served by traditional rhytidectomy. However, patients with severe sun damage and fine to medium rhytids are optimal candidates for chemical peeling. Some patients may benefit from both procedures as rhytidectomy addresses skin quantity, whereas peeling treats skin quality. The procedures are not recommended for simultaneous application. A minimum of 3 months between chemical peel and other surgical procedures is advised to permit complete wound healing.

Skin type, quality, color, ethnic background, and age are important factors that should be considered prior to chemical peel. Patients should be evaluated using Fitzpatrick's scale of sun-reactive skin types (Table 16.1), which denotes a patient's sensitivity to ultraviolet radiation and existing degree of pigmentation. Fitzpatrick's type I patients always burn and never tan. Type II describes patients who only tan with difficulty and usually burn. Type III patients usually tan, but sometimes burn. Type IV patients tan with ease but rarely burn. Fitzpatrick type V patients tan very easily and very rarely burn, and type VI patients tan very easily and never burn [5]. Patients with lighter skin types often tolerate chemical peeling with minimal pigmentary alterations, whereas individuals with darker skin are at a higher risk for either hyper- or hypopigmentation problems after chemo exfoliation.

Another useful grading system for pretreatment classification is the Glogau system describing four types of photoaging (Table 16.2). According to the individual patient's classifications, skin type, and problems, the type and depth of the peels can be customized to suit the patient's needs [6].

Patients must have realistic expectations and the physician must understand what can be accomplished with chemical peeling. A successful peel procedure is a result of good communication between patient and surgeon. Superficial skin resurfacing cannot achieve flawless skin. Rather the goal of chemical peeling is to improve the appearance of the skin as much as possible.

In addition to the physical examination, a thorough medical history and review of systems should be obtained in patients considering chemical peel. Preexisting cardiac, hepatic, and renal disease may influence treatment decisions and choice of peeling agents. A history of melasma, recent pregnancy, exogenous estrogens, oral contraceptives, other photosensitizing medications, or an unwillingness to avoid the sun may portend post-peel hyperpigmentation problems. The patient's medication use, skin sensitivities, and allergy history must also be documented.

In patients with a history of herpes simplex virus (HVS) infections, prophylactic antiviral therapy should be initiated at least 1 day before the peel procedure and continued until reepithelialization is complete. With the ubiquity of HSV, some authors advocate prophylaxis for all patients undergoing chemical peels beyond the superficial dermis. Any existing lesions should be allowed to heal completely prior to proceeding with a chemical peel [7].

A history of prior recent resurfacing by any modality or other facial surgical procedures is another important possible contraindication. Caution is warranted when resurfacing an area with vascular compromise secondary to a recent procedure.

Patients with collagen vascular disease, history of hypertrophic scarring or keloid development, advanced HIV disease, and general poor mental and physical well-being may be poor candidates for chemical peeling.

Compliance with the post-peel regimen is necessary to ensure normal wound healing and to avoid complications. Patients likely to be noncompliant or unable to avoid sun exposure because of occupation

Table 16.1 Fitzpatrick skin types

Skin type	Skin color	Tanning response
I	Very white or freckled	Always burns, never tans
II	White	Usually burns, tans with difficulty
III	White to olive	Mild burn, average tan
IV	Brown	Rarely burns, tans easily
V	Dark brown	Very rarely burns, tans very easily
VI	Black	Does not burn, tans very easily

Table 16.2 Glogau classification of photoaging

Group I – Mild	Group II – Moderate	Group III – Advanced	Group IV – Severe
Age 28–35	Age 35–50	Age 50–60	Age 65–70
No keratoses	Early actinic keratoses	Obvious actinic keratoses	Actinic keratoses/skin cancer
Little wrinkling	Early wrinkling-smile lines	Wrinkling at rest	Wrinkling/laxity
No scarring	Mild scarring	Moderate acne scarring	Severe acne scarring
Little makeup	Small amt makeup	Always wear makeup	Makeup cakes on

are unsuitable candidates. Men are less optimal candidates for chemical peels as their thicker, oilier skin promotes uneven penetration of the chemical agents. Patients with decreased numbers of epithelial appendages from radiation therapy or isotretinoin (Accutane) use are also poor candidates because of slower healing and an increased likelihood of scarring. Recent use of Accutane is considered a contraindication to medium or deep peels. It is recommended to wait at least 1 year after stopping Accutane prior to embarking on chemical peel procedures. This allows for regrowth of epithelial appendages, which are essential for post-peel reepithelialization. While the technique of chemical peeling is relatively simple, the real challenge lies in appropriate patient and peeling agent selection.

16.3.2 Pretreatment

Once a patient is appropriately selected to undergo a chemical peel, informed consent, including a detailed discussion of possible complications, is obtained. The patient should have the procedure and the recovery process explained in detail before the peel is performed. Especially for medium and deeper peels, patients should receive postoperative instructions in advance so they may prepare for the recovery period. Some physicians also routinely prescribe oral antibiotics in advance for the postoperative period [8].

Some authors recommend preconditioning the skin in order to maximize results from a chemical peel. The exfoliative agent transretinoic acid (tretinoin, Retin-A, Renova) may be helpful to facilitate uniform penetration of the peeling agent and promote more rapid reepithelialization. Retin-A promotes thinning of the stratum corneum with shedding of keratinocytes, disperses melanin throughout epidermis, and induces activation of dermal fibroblasts.

Pretreatment with hydroquinone 4–8% blocks can be useful when treating dyschromias or Fitzpatrick types Type III–VI. Hydroquinone functions by blocking tyrosinase from forming precursors for melanin.

Many patients tolerate the chemical peels without any sedation or analgesia. If needed, patients can be offered oral diazepam or celecoxib (Celebrex) 1 h before the peel. Both EMLA and ELA-Max have been shown to decrease the discomfort felt during medium-depth combination chemical peeling without influencing either the clinical or the histopathologic result [9]. Reassurance and a cooling fan are always helpful for patient comfort throughout the procedure.

Patients are instructed to avoid makeup for 24 h before the peel. Prior to the peel, the patient should thoroughly clean their face with non-residue soap the evening before and morning of the procedure. The patient is instructed not to apply makeup or moisturizers. The skin is cleansed in the physician's office immediately prior to the procedure with acetone, ether, Freon, or isopropyl alcohol to remove any residual cosmetics, oil, or debris. Although a vigorous degreasing is important, care must be taken not to abrade the skin as this may cause increased uptake of the chemical, and thus an uneven peel. Some authors have also suggested the use of povidone-iodine or Septisol prior to the alcohol or acetone wash. This cleansing step is important to ensure uniform penetration of the peeling agent.

16.3.3 Technique

A variety of chemical agents can be used to accomplish chemo exfoliation for facial rejuvenation. The effect of the peel is secondary to the depth of epidermal-dermal injury incurred. Thus, in selecting a peel one must factor in the depth of injury needed for the desired result, the pigmentary changes associated with each agent, the toxicities, and the individual physician's experience and comfort with the various agents.

Chemical peeling is generally classified by the depth of penetration into superficial, medium, and deep peels. Superficial peels typically have a depth of penetration of 0.06 mm removing the most superficial stratum corneum and stratum granulosum. Medium depth peels penetrate to a clinical depth into the papillary and upper reticular dermis, approximately 0.45 mm. Deep peels target the mid-reticular dermis with a depth of penetration of 0.6 mm [10]. The process of healing after a chemical peel primarily involves coagulation and inflammation, followed by reepithelialization, granulation tissue formation, angiogenesis, and a prolonged period of collagen remodeling. It is this prolonged process of remodeling that accounts for the continuing clinical improvement in the months after the procedure.

Application of most peeling agents is similar. Before application, the skin to be treated is first cleansed with acetone or alcohol. Because most chemical peels are lipophobic, this facilitates greater depth and promotes even distribution of the peel. The peel is carefully applied to the subunits of the face with gauze or a cotton-tipped applicator. To ensure a consistent effect, it is important to apply the chemical evenly and avoid pooling of the agent on the face. The peel should be delicately blended with the neighboring untreated skin by feathering the edges to prevent a discrete line of demarcation.

16.3.4 Superficial Peels

Superficial chemical peeling is an exfoliation of the stratum corneum or entire epidermis to promote epidermal regrowth with a more rejuvenated appearance. Superficial chemical peeling is a treatment with many benefits and few risks or side effects. It can be performed on individuals of all ages, as early as ages 25–30, when the first effects of photoaging become evident. Superficial chemical peels can minimize fine lines resulting from sun damage, acne, and rosacea. Repeat superficial peels may be required to achieve optimal effects. Patients must be counseled that multiple superficial peels do not equal a medium or deep chemical peel. Superficial peeling agents include alpha hydroxy acids such as glycolic acid 20–50%, salicylic acid, Jessner's solution, and 10–30% TCA.

16.4 Alpha Hydroxy Acids

Alpha hydroxy acids (AHAs) have been used for thousands of years to improve the appearance of the face. Cleopatra herself is rumored to have used the debris of the bottom of wine barrels for facial rejuvenation. AHAs function by promoting keratinocyte discohesion in the granular cell layer; causing increased cell turnover. Commonly used AHAs are derived from fruit and dairy products, such as glycolic acid from sugar cane, lactic acid from fermented milk, citric acid from fruits, tartaric acid from grapes, and malic acid from apples. Glycolic acid is currently the most commonly used AHA.

The efficacy and penetrating depths of AHAs are dependent on their concentration, the vehicle, and the pH. Over-the-counter AHA products containing 3–10% glycolic acid or other naturally occurring organic acids cause exfoliation over several weeks and may be used as a pre-peel primer to potentiate the effects of higher concentration peel procedures or other resurfacing modalities.

Professional grade AHA peels are usually 50% or higher. Unlike other peeling agents, penetration of alpha hydroxy acids is time dependent. The time to peel is dependent on both the concentration and the pH of the acid. Higher concentrations and lower pH's require shorter peeling periods. The alpha hydroxy acid peel is applied with a sponge or gauze, systematically proceeding from one facial region to another. After placement of an AHA preparation, the skin becomes erythematous. The mild stinging and redness typically disappears 1 h after treatment. Development of a white frost is not a desirable outcome of an alpha hydroxy acid peel as it denotes penetration depth into the dermis. Removal of the agent is achieved by rinsing with water or neutralization with an alkaline solution such as sodium bicarbonate. Deeper than intended peeling may occur if neutralization is not performed within the correct time. The subsequent exfoliation takes place over a few days and reepithelialization is usually complete within 7–10 days. Multiple treatments may be required to achieve the desired results and should be spaced several weeks apart to allow epidermal recuperation. Alpha hydroxy acid peels produce the least profound results of the chemical peeling agents; however, they are associated with the lowest frequency of complications.

AHAs, such as glycolic acid, can also be mixed with facial cleaners or creams in lesser concentrations as part of a daily skin-care regimen to improve the skin's texture or maintain results following a resurfacing procedure.

16.5 Salicylic Acid

Beta hydroxy acids, also known as salicylic acids, provide a safe, mild rejuvenation to skin. Salicylic acid functions via keratolysis, is lipid soluble, and has a predilection for sebum-containing cells making it an excellent peel for comedonal acne. In addition to acne, salicylic acid is helpful in treatment of oily skin, textural changes, melasma, and post-inflammatory pigmentation with minimal side effects. Another benefit of salicylic acid is that it does not need to be neutralized. After applying salicylic acid to the skin, salt formation on the skin is seen.

16.6 Jessner's Peel

Jessner's solution is a combination of salicylic acid, lactic acid, and resorcinol in alcohol (Table 16.3) [11]. Considered a mild-medium peeling agent, this formulation was designed to minimize the toxicities inherent to each individual agent. This solution must be stored in a dark bottle as light will discolor the solution and cause staining. Repetitive layers of Jessner's solution may be applied to affect a slightly deeper peel. Jessner's solution peeling action is through intense keratolysis. Its ability to disrupt the barrier function of the epidermis makes it an ideal primer for TCA peels, allowing the TCA to penetrate effectively and evenly [11]. Independently, Jessner's solution is an easy to use peeling agent without timing restriction. Skin sloughing occurs within 2–4 days after application with subsequent epidermal regrowth.

16.6.1 Medium Depth Peels

Medium-depth chemical peeling is defined as controlled damage to the papillary dermis, which can be performed in a single procedure [12]. Indications for medium-depth peel include destruction of epidermal lesions and actinic keratoses, resurfacing moderately photoaged skin, correction of dyschromias, and repair of mild acne scars. Although agents such as pyruvic acid or full-strength phenol can be used to achieve a medium depth peel, the classic agent is TCA.

Table 16.3 Jessner's solution formula

Resorcinol	14 g
Salicylic acid	14 g
85% Lactic acid	14 ml
95% Ethanol (qs)	100 ml

16.7 Trichloroacetic Acid

TCA is a versatile chemo exfoliative agent, in that it can be used as a superficial intermediate-to-deep peeling agent in varying concentrations. The depth of penetration of a TCA peel corresponds to increasing concentrations of TCA. At lower concentrations of 10–35% TCA, only a superficial peel is rendered. The results of superficial depth TCA peels include mild reversal of fine wrinkles and improvement in dyspigmentation with less recovery period and risk than deeper TCA peels or peel combinations.

At higher concentrations, such as 50% and above, TCA behaves comparably to a phenol peel. However, the depth of the wound to the reticular dermis with 50+% TCA increases concurrently with the rate of scarring and dyschromias. Many authors feel that 35% is the highest concentration of TCA which can be reliably used. Therefore, to safely improve epidermal penetration to the desired medium-depth peel, 35% TCA is usually preceded by a superficial keratolytic agent such as solid CO_2, Jessner's solution, or 70% glycolic acid. Two proprietary TCA-based agents, the TCA Masque (ICN Pharmaceuticals, Costa Mesa, California) and the TCA Blue Peel (Obagi), are also commonly used.

TCAs peeling mechanism of action at lower concentrations is via protein precipitation. TCA is a keratocoagulant that produces a frosting or whitening of the skin, which is dependent on the concentration used. Level I frosting, which is defined as erythema with streaky whitening of the face, is the endpoint for superficial resurfacing. Level II frosting is described as even white-coated frosting with patches of erythema showing through. Level III frosting, clinically signifying penetration through the papillary dermis, is a solid white enamel frost with minimal visible erythema. Level III frosting should be reserved for regions exhibiting severe actinic damage.

The dosage of TCA applied is dependent on the amount of agent used, the concentration, and the physician's technique. For example, vigorous rubbing of the agent, as compared with blotting, yields a deeper penetration. The systematic application of TCA with a sponge or brush involves treating the face in a sequence of subunits. During the procedure, if frosting is not uniform, reapplication may be performed until the desired level is reached. To achieve effective treatment of the whole face, certain areas and lesions require specialized care. Thicker keratotic areas may necessitate additional or more vigorous application of the TCA for deeper penetration. Eyelid skin is treated with the patient's head elevated and the eyes closed. The TCA is carefully applied with a semidry applicator extending to within 2–3 mm of the lid margin. With many variables involved, which can be specifically adjusted according to the patient's skin type and the areas being treated, the medium-depth TCA peel can be individualized for each patient.

Appropriate analgesia is necessary as TCA application is associated with an intense burning sensation that resolves within half an hour. Patient comfort may also be improved by cooling the face with a fan and by applying iced saline soaked sponges prior to moving from one facial region to another. Once the procedure is completed, skin sloughing proceeds for several days, and reepithelialization occurs within 7–10 days. Patient discomfort can be controlled with oral pain medications. An advantage of the TCA peels is that the solution is neutralized by the body's serum, and there is no other associated toxicity.

16.8 Adjunctive Measures

In patients susceptible to hyperpigmentation, pretreatment with a bleaching agent may be preventive. Hydroquinone, an isomer of resorcinol and phenol, is commonly used. Other bleaching agents include kojic acid and azelaic acid.

Individuals with more significant laxity of deeper skin structures may benefit from other facial rejuvenative procedures including rhytidectomy, browlift, and/or blepharoplasty in appropriately selected patients. Simultaneous facelift and chemical peel are generally approached with caution as there is a higher likelihood of full-thickness flap loss when peeling over elevated flaps.

Other adjunctive cosmetic procedures include treatment of dynamic wrinkles with Botox and filling very deep furrows or scars with facial fillers.

16.9 Postoperative Care

Postoperative care is designed to provide an ideal environment for moist wound healing. Initially, a generous amount of bland ointment, such as Aquaphor, petroleum jelly, or A&D ointment, is applied to the entire treatment area. This serves as an occlusive ointment, which protects and hydrates the skin. The use of more heavily formulated products can irritate the delicate, healing skin and interfere with the peeling process. Crisco vegetable shortening historically had been used quite successfully, but has since been reformulated and now may actually be irritating. Patients are instructed to reapply the ointment throughout the day or night, any time the face feels tight or dry. The initial inflammatory response is an erythematous and edematous reaction lasting from 12 to 36 h. During this period, patients may experience marked edema of the periocular region as well as the entire face. As the outer layers begin to shed, the patient is allowed to shower and gently wash the face with a mild cleanser. After showering, the face should be patted dry and a new coating of ointment applied.

Patients are instructed not to pick at the face during the recovery period. For best results, the patient should allow the skin to peel independently and resist the temptation to assist the peeling process. The use of loofahs, natural facial sponges, skin brushes, or any skin exfoliants is forbidden as manipulation of the skin prior to complete reepithelialization can result in prolonged erythema, bacterial infection, and scarring. Cool clean compresses and elevation of the head of bed can provide symptomatic relief of discomfort. The skin is generally reepithelialized by 7–10 days postpeel, at which point makeup can be applied. A formal consultation with an esthetician is valuable in educating patients on how to camouflage resolving erythema. Skin care services such as superficial peels and micro dermabrasion are not to be resumed until 3 months after a medium-deep peel. Medium-depth chemical peels need not be repeated for at least 1 year. Sunscreen is crucial to prevent further actinic damage and to prevent hyperpigmentation. The patients should be meticulous in avoiding sun exposure during this period, as any sun damage during this delicate recovery time could prolong post-procedure erythema and the wound healing process.

Following chemical peeling, some practitioners prescribe topical agents containing platelet products or growth factors. Although these products have been reported to improve wound healing, no randomized controlled clinical trials presently support their use in this specific setting. Further research is necessary to determine the clinical utility of these agents in the chemical peel process.

16.10 Complications

Chemical peeling may result in a profound rejuvenation of facial skin; however, this treatment is not without potential complications. Results and complications are generally related to the depth of wounding, with deeper penetration peels providing more marked results and a concomitant higher incidence of complications.

When the resurfacing agent removes the epidermis and a portion of the dermis, an important immunologic barrier between the patient and the environment no longer exists. An occlusive dressing, a topical ointment, or the body's own exudate provides some protection; however, the healing wound is more susceptible to both bacterial and fungal infections than the undisturbed skin. Delayed healing can be seen secondary to viral, bacterial, and fungal infections. Although bacterial infections are relatively rare, these infections can be avoided with the use of perioperative antiviral and antibiotic medications and good wound care. Infectious complications demand vigilance and aggressive therapy with oral and topical antibiotics. Staphylococcus and Streptococcus are the most common culprits when bacterial infections occur. Pseudomonas infections occasionally occur and may be recognized by Wood's lamp examination. Treatment of pseudomonas infections includes cleansing with 0.25% acetic acid and appropriate antibiotics. The trauma of the resurfacing procedure may reactivate a viral infection (e.g., herpes simplex). Persistent pain after the peel may be an indication of secondary herpetic infection. Preoperative prophylaxis for HSV is prudent as herpes infections have been documented in patients with no prior history of outbreaks. Herpes exacerbations are treated with oral and topical antivirals until resolution. The physician must be vigilant for signs of infection to prevent scarring.

Cicatricial complications may be cosmetic failures alone or they may complicate a case by imposing a functional deficit on a patient, particularly in the periorbital area. Scarring is one of the most significant complications following chemical peel. Care must be taken to properly screen patients. The use of Accutane in the last year or two, history of keloid formation, radiation therapy, and collagen vascular disease all may predispose to scarring and may make the patient a poor candidate for chemical peel. Scarring is unusual when the chemical agent is properly mixed and when the skin is effectively cleansed of all surface debris. Nevertheless, scarring may occur if multiple passes of the peeling agent are applied to a single area during the same session. An initial pass weakens the barrier and can permit a subsequent pass of the chemical to penetrate to a deeper level in the skin. Patiently waiting for frosting to occur can prevent this technical error. Delay in wound healing may lead to scarring, a severe complication requiring close follow-up and aggressive early treatment. Topical or intralesional steroids, silicone sheeting, pressure dressing, and scar massage may improve outcome. Scar excision or dermabrasion may be necessary in cases of persistent unsatisfactory results.

Pigment changes after resurfacing are the most frustrating to the surgeon and the patient because they can occur despite proper patient selection and excellent technique. They are also among the most common complications. Pigment complications after chemical peels may involve either hyper- or hypopigmentary changes. Erythema generally subsides within 90 days, but may persist as hyperpigmentation. Patients at increased risk are those taking oral contraceptive pills, exogenous estrogens, or other photosensitizing medications or patients with a history of posttraumatic hyperpigmentation. Hyperpigmentation after a chemical peel is best avoided by careful patient selection. Test spots may be performed on darker-skinned patients before the peel. The application of topical hydrocortisone or a short course of systemic steroids may lead to earlier resolution. Other treatments including transretinoic acid, glycolic acid, or hydroquinone can be useful in reducing pigmentary changes after the peel. Accompanying pruritus may be treated with oral antihistamines. Following chemical peeling, the skin is typically hypersensitive to the sun, which may be a source of additional hyperpigmentation. Sun avoidance and daily sunscreen application following the peel should be strongly endorsed to minimize pigmentary alterations. Pre- and posttreatment with a bleaching agent, such as hydroquinone, may minimize this problem in the susceptible patient.

Hypopigmentation is a late sequela of resurfacing and is extremely difficult to treat. Hypopigmentation is the result of melanocyte destruction or inhibition. Melanocytes are not capable of regeneration or division. It is encountered most frequently following phenol peeling, which has caused many clinicians to abandon phenol in favor of other peeling agents. Most noticeable in darker skinned patients, hypopigmentation may be difficult to assess until post-procedure erythema has subsided, at which point the condition may have unfortunately become permanent. Care must be taken upon initial application of the peel agent to feather the margins to avoid a sharp border between the treated and untreated areas. This may be accomplished either by using a less concentrated formulation or by applying less of the peeling agent in these regions. Camouflage makeup may conceal this and other pigmentary disturbances. When a line of demarcation is apparent between peeled and unpeeled areas of the face, the untreated skin may be resurfaced. Feathering a chemical peel into the neck can help blur the demarcation between the jaw and the neck.

Milia commonly develop after a chemical peel. Their appearance 2–3 weeks after a peel may be secondary to the use of occlusive ointments used during the healing period. They may spontaneously resolve or require removal by mild exfoliation or lancing.

Although uncommon, marked conjunctivitis and corneal abrasions have been reported after seepage of 35% TCA into the eye of a patient undergoing peel application. Chemical peel solutions must be applied extremely carefully in the periorbital regions to avoid ocular complications, which can be quite grave if not addressed in a timely manner [13].

Systemic complications from chemical peels resurfacing are quite uncommon, yet potentially disastrous. Toxic shock syndrome (secondary to Staphylococcus aureus infection), has been rarely reported, and can occur in association with any infected wound. Most often, toxic shock syndrome begins on the second or third day after treatment often presenting with fever, a desquamating rash, and hypotension. Treatment includes hospital admission, supportive care, aggressive cleansing of the wound, and antibiotics.

16.11 Discussion

The art of facial chemical peels encompasses a wide variety of chemical agents and application techniques. When a standardized technique is used, it is possible to quantify the therapeutic effects and to predict the outcome reliably. Variations of chemical peels will be used as clinicians try to achieve better results. If possible, variations from standard techniques should be scientifically studied and quantified to establish their safety and efficacy. Using careful clinical assessment and technique, one can safely and reliably undertake facial chemical peeling to combat photoaging.

16.12 Conclusions

Expertly performed chemical peels with healthy wound healing can achieve a significant reduction in facial rhytids, dyschromias, solar changes, acne, and superficial scarring. The best results for a chemical peel rests both with the cosmetic surgeon as well as the patient. The need for explicit pretreatment education and stringent posttreatment care cannot be overemphasized. Ultimately it is a combination of the surgeon's technique and the patient's compliance with the wound care instructions that determines the overall result. Setting realistic expectations for patients is imperative to the success of the chemical peeling process and will serve to maximize patient satisfaction (Figs. 16.1–16.3).

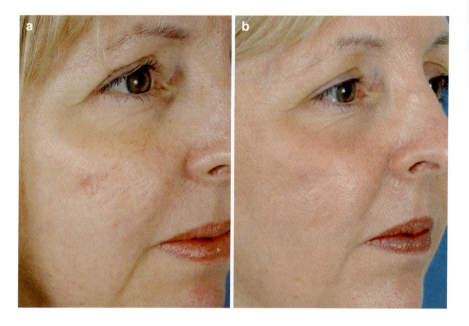

Fig. 16.1 Forty-eight-year-old female. (**a**) Prior to treatment. (**b**) Three months after 35% TCA medium-depth chemical peel

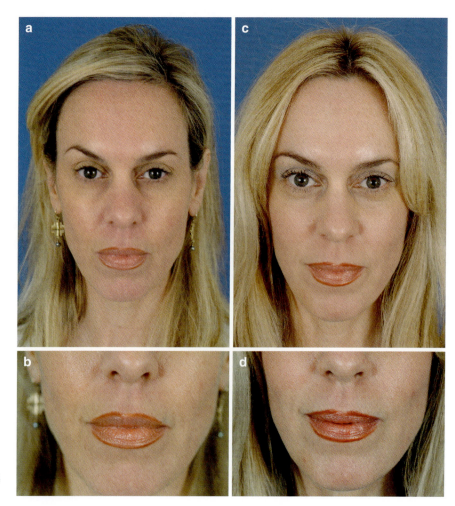

Fig. 16.2 Forty-nine-year-old female. (**a**, **b**) Prior to treatment. (**c**, **d**) After 35% medium-depth peel

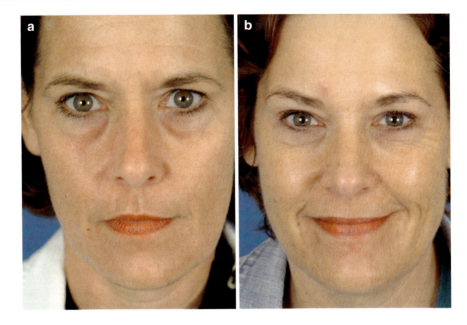

Fig. 16.3 Forty-seven-year-old female. (**a**) Prior to treatment. (**b**) After superficial chemical peel

References

1. Unna PG. Die histopathologie der hautkrankheiten. Berlin: Hirschfeld; 1894. p. 816–20.
2. Hirsch RJ, Dayan SH, Shah AR. Superficial skin resurfacing. Facial Plast Surg Clin North Am. 2004;12(3):311–21.
3. Fulton JE, Porumb S. Chemical peels: their place within the range of resurfacing techniques. Am J Clin Dermatol. 2004; 5(3):179–87.
4. Rubin M. Manual of chemical peels. Philadelphia: J.B. Lippincott; 1995.
5. Fitzpatrick TB. The validity and practicality of sun-reactive skin types I through VI. Arch Dermatol. 1988;124(6): 869–71.
6. Glogau RG. Aesthetic and anatomic analysis of the aging skin. Semin Cutan Med Surg. 1996;15(3):134–8.
7. Sabini P. Classifying, diagnosing, and treating the complications of resurfacing the facial skin. Facial Plast Surg Clin North Am. 2004;12(3):357–61.
8. Manuskiatti W, Fitzpatrick RE, Goldman MP, Krejci-Papa N. Prophylactic antibiotics in patients undergoing laser resurfacing of the skin. J Am Acad Dermatol. 1999; 40(1): 77–84.
9. Koppel RA, Coleman KM, Coleman WP. The efficacy of EMLA versus ELA-Max for pain relief in medium-depth chemical peeling: a clinical and histopathologic evaluation. Dermatol Surg. 2000;26(1):61–4.
10. Matarasso SL, Glogau RG. Chemical face peels. Dermatol Clin. 1991;9(1):131–50.
11. Monheit GD. The Jessner's-trichloroacetic acid peel. An enhanced medium-depth chemical peel. Dermatol Clin. 1995;13(2):277–83.
12. Halaas YP. Medium depth peels. Facial Plast Surg Clin North Am. 2004;12(3):297–303.
13. Fung JF, Sengelmann RD, Kenneally CZ. Chemical injury to the eye from trichloroacetic acid. Dermatol Surg. 2002; 28(7):609–10.

Deep Phenol Chemical Peels

17

Michel Siegel and Benjamin A. Bassichis

17.1 Introduction

In the early 1960s, Baker and Gordon [1, 2] reported their experience with phenol chemical face peeling. Their initial technique involved "taping" or occluding the skin after phenol application, to prevent evaporation and increase the penetration of phenol. In 1985, Beeson and McCollough [3] reported their technique without taping. Almost half a decade later the debate continues. Regardless of the technique used, phenol chemical peeling continues to offer a method of achieving spectacular results for skin rejuvenation. When performed properly and with appropriate patient selection, the complication rate remains low. As with any method of skin resurfacing, the goal involves the production of a controlled and predictable, partial thickness chemical injury. In the case of phenol, penetration is to the superficial dermis, without ablation of the pilo-sebaceous unit.

M. Siegel
Facial Center for Plastic Surgery, 902 Frostwood,
Suite 168, Houston, TX 77024, USA and
7700 San Felipe #420, Houston, TX 77063, USA
e-mail: drsiegel@houstonfaces.com

B.A. Bassichis (✉)
Department of Otolaryngology – Head and Neck Surgery,
University of Texas – Southwestern Medical Center,
5323 Harry Hines Boulevard, Dallas, TX 75235, USA and
Advanced Facial Plastic Surgery Center, 14755 Preston Road,
Suite 110, Dallas, TX 75254, USA
e-mail: drbassichis@advancedfacialplastic.com

17.2 Patient Selection

The most important factor in achieving a good result with phenol chemical peeling is the selection of the proper patient. Because of the depth of penetration with phenol, some degree of injury to the pigment producing cells will occur, resulting in hypopigmentation or depigmentation of the skin. In order to camouflage this appearance, patients with lighter skin will have a better result. It is not who is a good candidate but who should not undergo phenol chemical peeling. Patients with Fitzpatrick skin type V and VI are very poor candidates, as any hypopigmentation will be obvious. Also red haired freckled Fitzpatrick type I patients are poor candidates. Due to the freckling, hypopigmentation in this category of patients will be more obvious as a freckled and "non-freckled" zone is created. Asian patients, notorious for pigmentary problems are poor candidates for phenol resurfacing. Male patients with their thicker and oilier skin are less than ideal candidates. Patients with a long history of sun exposure will make poor candidates, as a line of demarcation may be obvious after peeling due to their mottled skin appearance of the non-peeled areas. Having excluded these categories of patients, the more ideal patients are non-freckled Fitzpatrick types I and II. Type III and IV can be cautiously done as long as the patient understand the possible risks of depigmentation.

17.3 Technique

Phenol chemical peeling can be either done as a regional peel, periorbital and/or perioral, or as a full-face peel. Regional peels are done in the office after

---

Reprinted with permission of Springer.

the patient's medical history has been reviewed and they are deemed good candidates for phenol peeling. Either topical anesthetic cream placed 30 min prior to the procedure to the region to be peeled, or a local block with 1% xylocaine with 1:100,000 of epinephrine are satisfactory for performing the procedure in the office.

Full-face peeling must be performed in an accredited facility where intravenous (IV) access is available, the patient can be sedated, the cardiac status of the patient can be continuously monitored, and immediate intervention is accessible if needed.

Skin preparation is the most important step regardless of the area to be treated. The skin must be thoroughly washed with soap to remove any traces of makeup and dirt. This is followed by skin degreasing with 100% medical grade acetone soaked gauze. It is extremely important to remove all skin oils to ensure even penetration during the peel. Once the skin has been degreased, the peeling is performed with a freshly made mixture of the phenol. The traditional Baker–Gordon mixture (Table 17.1) yields an 88% phenol solution. The solution is made by the physician in the office prior to each procedure to prevent changes in concentration from evaporation and mixed multiple times during the procedure to prevent settling.

The mixture is applied with dampened cotton tip applicators using a rolling motion into the skin, ensuring to paint the area evenly and to use each applicator only once. One pass per area is performed, allowing the skin to become frosty white, a sign of mid-dermal penetration. After waiting approximately 30 s, any areas with signs of poor penetration will be self-evident, and a limited second pass to these areas is undertaken.

The limits of perioral peeling are as follows: laterally to the nasolabial folds, inferiorly feathering 2 cm below the border of the mentum, and feathering at the vermillion border of the lips.

For periorbital peeling, the orbital subunits are marked and the patient is placed at a 45% angle position. Cotton tip applicators placed at the medial and lateral canthus to prevent tears from running down and possibly mixing with the phenol producing a stronger concentration. Along the upper lid no phenol is placed along the tarsus. When peeling the lower lids the patient is instructed to fix their eyes on a superior point at the ceiling to increase the taughtness of the skin. The lid border is marked to 3 mm. Any time a periorbital peel is performed the sedation is kept to a minimum so the patient is cooperative and awake enough to complain of pain in case phenol contacts the cornea. Cool saline is kept on hand in case ocular irrigation becomes necessary. Because of the anesthetic properties of phenol, discomfort during the initial application is self-limited and no further medication is given to the patient.

To avoid the possibility of cardiac arrhythmias from full-face peeling the patient's cardiac status is continuously monitored and the procedure is lengthened approximately 2 h by peeling the face as subunits. Each subunit is peeled separately with a 20 min interval between subunits to prevent rapid absorption of the phenol solution. Because of the renal clearance of phenol, normal renal function is essential thus blood urea nitrogen (BUN) and creatinine are obtained prior to the procedure. The patient also receives about 2 l of IV fluids to enhance renal excretion of phenol during the peel procedure. Full-face peeling is recommended in the following order: forehead, periorbital, cheeks, perioral area, and nose. Because the action of this peel is of coagulation, no neutralization of the acid is required. At the conclusion of the procedure, Vaseline is placed along the peeled areas, providing a "semi-occlusive" dressing. However, nonocclusive phenol peeling can be achieved by avoiding any petroleum-based ointments after the procedure.

Patients undergoing full-face phenol peeling are started on anti-herpetic medication 3 days prior to the peel and are given antibiotics after the procedure. Patients undergoing regional peeling will be given antiviral drugs only with a history of cold sores.

Some patients will experience a severe burning sensation after the procedure, lasting 6–7 h. For regional peeled patients, pain and antianxiety medications will give some relief. For full-face peeled patients, IV pain management is preferred. The pain and burning associated with this procedure usually subsides after 8 h.

During the first 7–10 days after the peel the patient is instructed to wash their face three to four times a day

Table 17.1 Baker–Gordon phenol mixture

3 ml USP liquid phenol
2 ml tap water
8 drops of Septisol liquid soap
3 drops of croton oil

with vinegar, followed by application of a petroleum-based ointment. The vinegar mixture decreases the risk of fungal infection. After reepithelialization, usually after the seventh to tenth day, the patient is permitted to wash their face with a noncomedogenic, non-perfumed soap followed by application of a skin moisturizer and sunscreen. It is imperative that patients are counseled on avoiding sun exposure to prevent developing dyschromias. Any itching may be controlled with antihistamines.

Patients are followed very closely for erythema persisting after 12 weeks. Any signs of prolonged erythema are treated with a 3-week course of 2.5% hydrocortisone applied to the face twice per day.

17.4 Complications

With proper patient selection and diligent technique the complication rate with phenol chemical peeling should be low. It is important to differentiate between true complications and transient post-peel reactions. Because of the depth of penetration of phenol there will invariably be injury to the pigment producing cells. Because recovery of these cells is unpredictable, proper patient selection is imperative.

Poor feathering of the peel will result in a suboptimal cosmetic result due to an obvious demarcation line. Feathering too low in the neck will not only cause this, but also an increased risk of scarring because of the paucity of adnexal structures below the jaw line.

It is important to counsel patients before a phenol peel about the length of erythema associated with this procedure. It is not uncommon for patients to experience erythema from 4 to 12 weeks post peel. Make up may be applied after 2 weeks to conceal redness, but patients should be followed closely to treat persistent erythema with topical steroids.

The use of sunscreen for a minimum of 6 months after a peel is vital to prevent hyperpigmentation from sun exposure. Patients need to be educated that their post-peel skin is highly sun sensitive, thus suntanning and excess sun exposure after a phenol peel is not advised.

The most common problem after a phenol peel is transient hyperpigmentation. The darker the patient, the more likely this may occur. Hyperpigmentation is usually seen around the third to fourth week post peel. The most important step in preventing this is avoiding sun exposure. The first signs will be marked by erythema followed by the appearance of blotchy skin spots. A treatment regimen of Retin-A and hydroquinone is started and patients are seen at intervals of 2 weeks. Patients not responding to this regimen are offered a TCA peel.

The most feared complication of a phenol peel is post-peel hypertrophic scarring (HS). HS results from violation of tissues deep to the reticular dermis. It may be the result of a treated herpes simplex virus (HSV) infection, peeling of tissues with poor adnexal structures, like the neck, or performing multiple passes on the face with phenol solution. Fortunately, HSV leading to hypertrophic scarring is rare as this infection responds well to antiviral therapy. The best treatment though is prevention. Patients with a history of cold sores, or patients undergoing full-face phenol chemical peeling should be treated prophylactic ally with antiviral therapy. Hypertrophic scarring, once diagnosed should be aggressively treated with intralesional and topical steroids.

Patients should be monitored for signs of infection in the post-peel period. Bacterial infections are usually a result of poor facial hygiene. Anti-staphylococcal oral antibiotics will usually resolve this problem. Fungal infections are rare as the patient keeps the pH of the skin in the acidic range using daily vinegar treatments.

Patients with a history of cold sores or undergoing full-face peeling should be started on prophylactic therapy to prevent HSV breakouts. If the patient develops an HSV outbreak post peel, the oral dose of antiviral medication is doubled.

Milia formation is a sequelae rather than a complication. They represent small superficial inclusion cysts, usually lasting days to weeks. Most will spontaneously resolve, but the larger ones can be "unroofed" with an 18-gauge needle.

One should be careful to perform this type of peel on patients with previous history of blepharoplasty, or patients with lower lid laxity as these patients may develop an ectropion. Most will resolve, but corrective surgery may be needed in some instances.

17.5 Conclusions

Phenol chemical peeling has been safely performed for almost half a century. Phenol chemical peeling is a means of providing a controlled and predictable

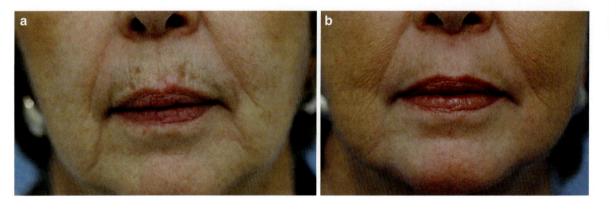

Fig. 17.1 (a) Before. (b) After deep phenol chemical peel

chemical injury to the skin (Fig. 17.1). Microscopically, phenol induces new collagen and elastins formation as well as the reorganization of melanocytes within the basement membrane. Clinically, the results of phenol chemical peeling are significant and long lasting.

Proper patient selection and counseling regarding the length of recovery is the key to excellent results and happy patients. Because of the properties of phenol, it is imperative that the patient be in good health prior to the procedure. Phenol is absorbed through the skin, detoxified in the liver, and excreted by the kidneys. Poor renal or hepatic function will result in toxic levels of phenol producing cardiac arrhythmias. Thus, patients with poor renal function, liver problems, or heart conditions may not be the best candidates for this resurfacing modality. The safety of the patient remains the number one priority. Healthy patients undergoing full-face chemical peeling should have their cardiac function continuously monitored, and application of phenol should be performed in increments of facial subunits with rest in between applications to prevent cardiac problems.

There are certain conditions because of which phenol chemical peeling produces poor to minimal results, and patients with these conditions are not offered phenol peeling as an option. These include: capillary hemangiomas, facial telangiectasia, port wine stains, thermal burns, deep-pitted acne scars, and hypertrophic scars. Phenol peeling is not performed on Fitzpatrick types V and VI, or type I with freckles, due to the abnormal hypopigmentation with severe demarcation changes. Phenol should not be applied to areas with minimal to none adnexal structures, like the neck, chest, and hands due to the high risk of hypertrophic scarring.

With the proper technique, patient selection, and counseling about the recovery time, phenol chemical peeling remains a safe and effective means of skin resurfacing.

References

1. Baker TJ, Gordon HL. The ablation of rhytides by chemical means. A preliminary report. J Florida Med Assoc. 1961; 48:451–4.
2. Baker TJ, Gordon HL, Seckinger DL. A second look at chemical face peeling. Plast Reconstr Surg. 1966;37(6): 487–93.
3. Beeson WH, McCollough EG. Chemical face peeling without taping. J Dermatol Surg Oncol. 1985;11(10):985–90.

Chemical Blepharoplasty

Clara Santos

18.1 Introduction

Surgical blepharoplasty can solve skin flaccidity and fat bags around the eyes, but crow's feet and dark circles are not solved by surgery alone. Chemical peeling is a technique used to renew the skin at the skin surface in order to destroy selected layers of the epidermis and/or dermis [1, 2]. Chemical blepharoplasty can be the sole procedure in certain cases of eyelid rejuvenation or it may be performed approximately 3 months after surgical blepharoplasty, in order to offer a maximum result. This technique may be also indicated as the sole procedure in patients who have constitutional borderline scleral show, in whom surgical blepharoplasty may lead to complications.

To perform chemical blepharoplasty a specific buffered phenol solution named Exoderm [3] (composed of 12 components, including phenol, resorcin, citric acid, and a variety of natural oils) is used in the periorbital and eyelid skin. This solution will effectively melt the epidermis. Due to the presence of oils in the solution, percutaneous absorption is gradual and controlled [4–7]. Melanocytes are only partially destroyed and a self-limiting arrest of the solution in the mid-dermis will guarantee an excellent peeling effect without dermatologic or systemic toxicity. As a result of this exfoliation, tighter skin with less or no wrinkles will be seen in the periorbital and eyelid area. The dark circles around the eyes will also disappear, leading to a fresh and healthy "pink" skin color [8, 9].

18.2 Skin Preparation

As with any other peeling technique, skin preparation or conditioning is of particular importance. The skin should be prepared in advance, as it leads to homogeneous penetration of the peeling agent. This improves healing and there is also less risk of post-inflammatory hyperpigmentation. It is important to prepare the eyelid and periorbital area as well as the face. In addition to the chemical blepharoplasty, the facial skin can benefit from a medium peel done concomitantly.

For facial skin, preparation is commonly performed with the following, where a gel/cream is the vehicle for medication delivery:

Tretinoin	0.05%
Hydroquinone	3%
Hydrocortisone	1%

For periorbital and eyelid skin, a similar but weaker formulation is recommended:

Tretinoin	0.025%
Hydroquinone	2%
Hydrocortisone	0.05%

Skin preparation or conditioning should ideally be performed a month before the procedure. In cases where a month of conditioning is not possible, a shorter period of 2 weeks may be acceptable in patients with lighter skin. In the case of patients with darker skin, it

C. Santos
Dermatology in Private Practice, Department of Dermatology,
Avenida Brasil, 583 Jardim Europa, CEP 041431-000
São Paulo, Brazil
e-mail: clara_santos@terra.com.br

is wise not to perform peeling unless a full month of preparation has been completed. If there is a delay to the peeling procedure, it is advantageous to continue the conditioning regimen for longer than 1 month.

As tretinoin and hydroquinone (or other bleaching agents such as kojic acid or azelaic acid) have the potential to cause skin irritation, the patient should be instructed to start applying these formulations gradually. Beginning every other night for 7–10 days is recommended, after which the skin will have developed a better tolerance and the skin preparation should be applied daily. This local treatment should be discontinued 2 days prior to the procedure in patients with sensitive skin.

18.3 Skin Evaluation and Chemical Agent Selection

It is important to remember that there are differences within the skin within the eyelid and periorbital area. The upper lid shows local and textural differences, which can be divided into three regions. The upper third displays thicker skin that is lighter in color; the medium third displays thin skin and is the region with the darkest pigmentation; and the lower third or tarsal skin displays the thinnest skin which can also be darkly pigmented (Fig. 18.1). Though these differences exist, it would be impossible to apply three different agents of different concentrations to each separate area. The agent of choice is the characteristic of a self-limiting arrest or self-blockage mechanism within the mid-dermis. Using this solution, eyelids can be evenly peeled without the need of using different solutions or concentrations within such a small area. One of the most important aspects of skin beauty is evenness in color and texture, so that performing a facial medium-depth chemical peel, in addition to the chemical blepharoplasty, will achieve excellent results in this regard.

18.4 Anesthesia and Sedation

Chemical blepharoplasty is an ambulatory procedure and is safe due to the buffers present in the Exoderm solution; however, it is recommended that the procedure be performed in an operating room setting, as the patient will receive intravenous sedation and analgesia in order to control pain and burning.

18.5 Details of the Procedure

It is recommended that a medium-depth facial peel be performed in combination with the chemical blepharoplasty in order to achieve the best possible facial rejuvenation results. Before the peel has begun, the patient's skin is deeply cleansed using water and a neutral skin cleanser. One drop of Lacrilube® ointment is placed in each eye, the excess of which is removed, should it encroach on the periorbital or eyelid skin. The skin to be treated is degreased with gauze and 70% alcohol. This is performed in a gentle manner, and when the gauze is almost dry, the periorbital and eyelid areas are degreased, which avoids excessive trauma to those areas. Facial nerve blocks may be carried out using 2% lidocaine without epinephrine. If pre-procedure skin preparation has not been carried out in the weeks prior to the peeling, or if the patient's skin is thick, Jessner's solution may be applied in one or two coats to the face and one coat to the eyelid areas. Ideally, a medium-depth peel is then performed on the face, with the eyelid areas remaining for the chemical blepharoplasty.

After the facial peel has been completed, Exoderm solution is applied to the eyelid and periorbital areas,

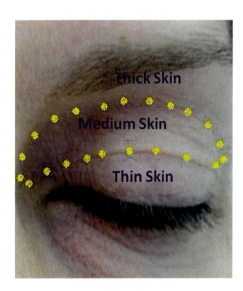

Fig. 18.1 On upper lid, the medium and lower thirds shows differences in thickness and coloration

including the crow's feet. It should be remembered that performing a chemical peel is an art form, part of which relies on working carefully and gently. During this, it is important to squeeze the cotton tip applicator against the Exoderm solution bottle in order to remove excess liquid. When applying the solution to the skin, the cotton tip applicator should not be pressed down with excessive pressure. It is useful to have a cotton ball in the nondominant hand in order to wipe off excess fluid from the skin after each area has been treated. Application should begin on inner cantus of the upper third of the upper eyelid and should extend until the crows' feet. After the upper third has been treated, the medium and lower thirds will follow (Fig. 18.2). During this stage, it is imperative that the patient's eyes remain closed.

Once the upper eyelid has been completed, the lower eyelid is treated. Unlike with the upper eyelid, the patient is asked to open the eye, and to look up and back. This maneuver improves lower lid exposure and moves the ocular globe away from the surgical field (Fig. 18.3).

Though tears may occur, unlike with trichloracetic acid (TCA) and other some agents, they will not leave marks on the skin. Once completed, a thin coat of bismuth is applied. On the lower eyelid, in order to enhance the action of the solution, and in particular in the area of the crow's feet, Micropore® is placed for 24 h (Fig. 18.4). After 24 h, the Micropore® tape is removed, and a thin coat of bismuth is applied for 1 week.

18.6 The Postoperative Period

The only medication that need be given to the patient is analgesia. Routine use of antibiotics is not required. Antiviral medication is also not routinely prescribed, unless the patient has a prior personal history of herpes simplex infection. Soon after the peel has been performed, the eyelids will become swollen. Over the course of the following 48 h, the swelling will often become more pronounced, and will eventually begin to decrease after 72 h. Tearing of the eyes is common at this stage. Cylodex® should be used every 6 h to avoid eye irritation. The Exoderm solution liquefies the epidermis within the initial 24 h, after which regeneration occurs between the second and eighth day. Four days

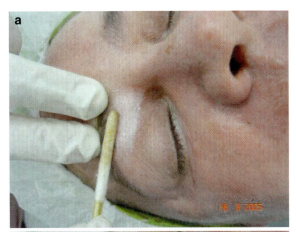
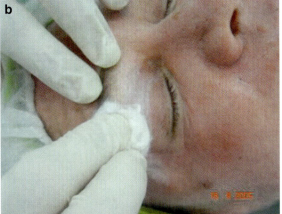
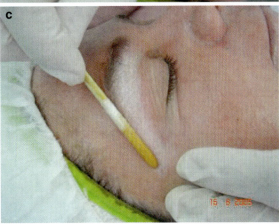

Fig. 18.2 Upper lid chemical blepharoplasty. (**a**) stat in internal upper third, then (**b**) medial upper third and finally (**c**) external upper third. The eyes are kept closed

following the procedure, facial skin where the medium-depth peel has been performed will begin to peel off (Fig. 18.5). During this time, the patient is requested to apply Vaseline® ointment on an hourly basis, in order to massage the old, peeling skin until this is complete.

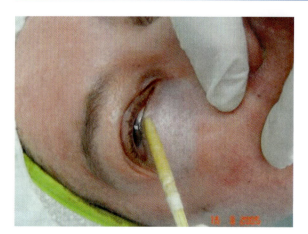

Fig. 18.3 Lower lid chemical blepharoplasty, starts internal canthus and goes to external. The eyes are kept opened

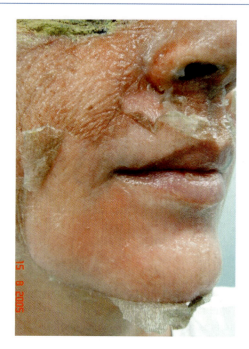

Fig. 18.5 Skin peeling on the fourth day following a medium-depth chemical peel

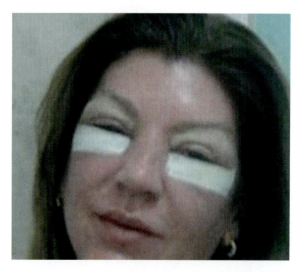

Fig. 18.4 Completion of chemical peel. There are uniform erythema to the face, fine bismuth coat on the upper eyelid, and Micropore® tape on the lower eyelid

The patient is advised not to apply Vaseline® to the eyelids, as these areas require 8 days to peel.

Once the facial skin peeling has finished, 1% hydrocortisone cream should be applied two or three times a day for 1 week. Thereafter, the pre-peeling conditioning regime, that was described earlier, should recommence. Eight days after the procedure, the patient should begin applying Vaseline® ointment to remove the bismuth layer. One percent hydrocortisone cream should be applied twice a day to the eyelids and the periorbital area for the first week, after which the same pre-peeling skin protocol is begun. After the peeling skin has been removed on the fourth day, the skin will display a new, fresh, and healthy pink color. After removing the periorbital and eyelid bismuth layer on the eighth day, this skin will also display a new and fresh, though slightly red color. This difference in skin color will gradually disappear over the course of 2–3 months. It is very important to reassure the patient that this difference in color is a normal reaction to the fact that both deep and medium peels were performed. Patients may use makeup after sun protection has been applied to the skin (Fig. 18.6).

18.7 Complications

Chemical blepharoplasty is associated with excellent results and a high level of patient satisfaction. The reason for this is that, with the Exoderm solution, systemic complications and permanent dermatologic complications are not seen as they are with other phenol peels [10, 11]. Chemical blepharoplasty is a safe and an easily performed procedure. It is important that patients be educated to expect significant swelling of the face and eyelids, and that this is normal and temporary.

18 Chemical Blepharoplasty

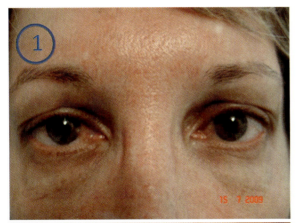
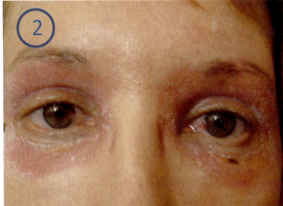
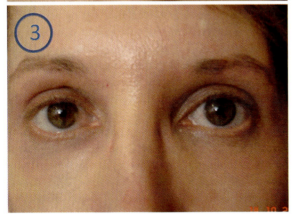

Fig. 18.6 Blepharoplasty properly performed. (**1**) Pre-procedure. (**2**) Eight days following chemical peel. (**3**) Forty-five days post-procedure. After couple of months skin color tends to get evenness

18.7.1 Ectropion

Patients may experience temporary ectropion lasting 2–3 months. This is unlike the ectropion seen after surgical blepharoplasty, which may be permanent. Significant ectropium may however occur in patients who have undergone previous lower eyelid surgical blepharoplasty or in patients with a preexisting borderline or frank ectropion.

18.7.2 Post-inflammatory Hyperpigmentation

Post-inflammatory Hyperpigmentation (PIH) may occur after a chemical peel, particularly in patients with darker skin (Fig. 18.7). This complication is rare due to the aggressive use of pre-chemical peel skin conditioning, as well as the prompt resumption of this conditioning post-procedure, as described above.

18.7.3 Pseudo-Adhesion/Pseudo-Web Formation

During the initial postoperative period, at around the fourth day, the patient may describe some difficulty in completely opening the eyes. In this instance, the bismuth has become thicker in nature and acts like a pseudo-adhesion/pseudo-web, preventing complete upper eyelid movement. This is easily ameliorated by teaching the patient to apply a thin coat of Vaseline® ointment over the bismuth once or at most twice a day for 1 or 2 days. It is important to instruct the patient to only use a thin coat; otherwise the bismuth layer will be removed too soon.

18.7.4 Web Formation

In the author's experience, there were three cases where patients had scratched their upper eyelids post-operatively. Two cases had scratched the lid and one, in particular, the upper inner eyelid. In the first two cases, healing occurred normally without scar formation, though this healing process was slow. In the third case, where the upper inner eyelid was scratched, a web formed and this was successfully treated with early corticosteroid intralesional injections. In patients

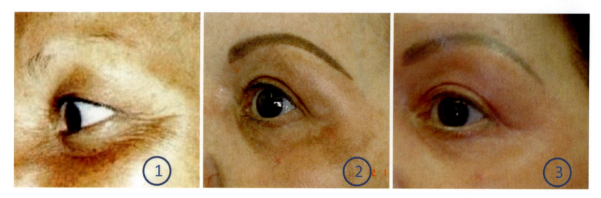

Fig. 18.7 (**1**) Pretreatment (2004). (**2**) Post-inflammatory hyperpigmentation (*PIH*) (2006). (**3**) After treatment for PIH (2006)

who present with pruritus during the healing phase, an antihistaminic drug should be prescribed to avoid scratching.

18.7.5 Eyelid Skin Infection

The author's experience has seen one case of a localized infection to the eyelid skin. This case was treated with Ciprofloxacin for 1 week. The healing process was delayed beyond the normal 8 days, though without permanent complications. At the time that the bismuth layer was removed, an eyelash was found below the infected lid, and described as the inciting event.

18.8 Discussion

Today, more than ever, the public cares about appearing healthy and attractive. Eyes play an important role in the overall expression of the face. Eyes display feelings and emotions, and may be considered the window to the sole. Aging of the region surrounding the eyes may make a patient appear either sad or tired. In the distant past, eyelid surgery was performed in order to remove lesions, though the last 60 years saw aesthetic surgical blepharoplasty blossom. Eyelid rejuvenation surgery has many indications and when properly done brings excellent results. There are, however, some features of the eyelids and periorbital area that surgery cannot solve, such as dark circles and crow's feet. In terms of surgical blepharoplasty, the upper eyelids often show a better result than the lower ones. Chemical blepharoplasty is a new and unique tool that may be complementary to surgical facial or eyelid rejuvenation, as well as the sole option in selected cases. It is important to state that when chemical blepharoplasty is going to be complimentary to facial or eyelid surgery, there must be a delay of 3 months between procedures.

18.9 Conclusion

Periorbital and eyelid rejuvenation can be performed as a single intervention using the unique dermatologic approach described above, or in combination with surgery. The advantage of this combination technique, in selected cases, is to promote a complete and deep rejuvenation of aging, both clinically and histologically [12]. Plastic or cosmetic surgery, in combination with dermatological techniques, can enhance the results of each other, increase patients' satisfaction, and avoid certain complications. For example, a patient may be dissatisfied when facial or eyelid surgery was technically well done, but the skin still does not display beauty and a healthy shine. In this case, a dermatologic approach is also required in order to remove the remaining signs of aging such as fine wrinkles or blemishes.

References

1. Baker TJ. Chemical face peeling and rhytidectomy. A combined approach for facial rejuvenation. Plast Reconstr Surg. 1962;29:199–207.

2. Baker TJ, Gordon HL. The ablation of rhytids by chemical means: a preliminary report. J Fla Med Assoc. 1961;48:451–4.
3. Fintsi Y. Exoderm – a novel phenol-based peeling method resulting in improved safety. Am J Cosmet Surg. 1997;14:49–54.
4. Hetter GP. An examination of the phenol-croton oil peel. Part I: Dissecting the formula. Plast Reconstr Surg. 2000;105(1):227–39.
5. Hetter GP. An examination of the phenol-croton oil peel: Part II. The lay peelers and their croton oil formulas. Plast Reconstr Surg. 2000;105(1):240–8.
6. Hetter GP. An examination of the phenol-croton oil peel: Part III: The plastic surgeons' role. Plast Reconstr Surg. 2000;105(2):752–63.
7. Hetter GP. An examination of the phenol-croton oil peel: Part IV: Face peel results with different concentrations of phenol and croton oil. Plast Reconstr Surg. 2000;105(3):1061–3.
8. Gatti JE. Eyelid phenol peel: an important adjunct to blepharoplasty. Ann Plast Surg. 2008;60(1):14–8.
9. Epstein JS. Management of infraorbital dark circles. A significant cosmetic concern. Arch Facial Plast Surg. 1999;1(4):303–7.
10. Truppman ES, Ellenberry JD. Major electrocardiographic changes during chemical face peeling. Plast Reconstr Surg. 1979;63(1):44–8.
11. Rullan PP. The 2-day light phenol chemabrasion for deep wrinkles and acne scars: a presentation of face and neck peels. Am J Cosmet Surg. 2004;21:199–209.
12. Kligman AM, Baker TJ, Gordon HL. Long-term histologic follow-up of phenol face peels. Plast Reconstr Surg. 1985;75(5):652–9.

Facial Implants

Benjamin A. Bassichis

19.1 Introduction

Over the past few decades, there has been a paradigm shift in the approach to the treatment of facial aging. This philosophical shift has consisted of a departure from older "subtractive" facial surgery techniques to newer "restorative" techniques and procedures to evoke more beautiful natural-looking results.

Older methods of facial rejuvenation consisted primarily of removing (subtracting) skin and fat and pulling tissues tight. In many instances, this led to a skeletonized and more aged, and operated-upon appearance. We now recognize that it is not only the skin that needs to be addressed to correct the signs of facial aging, but facial soft tissues, including subcutaneous tissue, fat, and facial bones that lose volume and projection over time.

The major architectural promontories of the facial skeleton, including the malar-midface region, nose, and chin, provide the structural foundation for aesthetic facial beauty. The overall harmony of the face is largely determined by the balance, size, shape, and position of these structural fundamentals. A cosmetic surgeon may be able to add facial implants to the facial skeleton to accentuate the areas of the cheekbone or chin. These skeletal augmentations re-drape and tighten the skin of the face as well as reorchestrate the elements of facial balance and proportion for an improved cosmetic result. Depending on an individual's specific aesthetic requirements, implant procedures can be performed solo or in combination with other facial plastic procedures to provide a more healthy and youthful appearance. Implant placement surgeries are performed with hidden or invisible incisions so there are no visible scars and the results are immediately evident [1].

Proper selection of implants requires a working knowledge of general size, thickness, and material composition of available implant types. Alloplastic facial implants offer the surgeon many advantages over autogenous tissue, including easy availability of material and simplicity of the operative procedure. Care must be taken to select the proper implant characteristics for the desired aesthetic result, as each synthetic material has unique properties. With all implant types and materials, careful surgical technique is essential to minimize the risks of complications [1].

In the past, a variety of substances have been used for soft tissue and bony augmentation, including autogenous elements such as iliac and rib bone grafts and nasal cartilage. Varied alloplastic materials including ivory, acrylic, and precious metals remain solely of historical interest. Advancements in biomaterial science have promoted the use of novel, alloplastic implant materials for facial skeletal augmentation [2]. There are several general features that contribute to the biocompatibility of an implant. An ideal implant is comprised of materials that do not elicit a chronic inflammatory response or foreign body reaction, are non-immunogenic, inert in body fluids, and noncarcinogenic. Implant materials must also be nondegradable, yet malleable, such that the shape and position are sustained over time.

B.A. Bassichis
Department of Otolaryngology – Head and Neck Surgery,
University of Texas – Southwestern Medical Center,
5323 Harry Hines Boulevard, Dallas, TX 75235, USA and
Advanced Facial Plastic Surgery Center,
14755 Preston Road, Suite 110, Dallas, TX 75254, USA
e-mail: drbassichis@advancedfacialplastic.com

Reprinted with Permission of Springer, Berlin

There are many materials used for alloplastic implants including silicone elastomers, expanded polytetrafluoroethylene (e-PTFE), high-density porous polyethylenes, methylmethacrylate, nylon mesh material, bioglass and alumina ceramics, and hydroxyapatite-calcium phosphate material [2]. Currently, the most commonly used materials are solid silicone and expanded polytetrafluoroethylene. Both materials have performed well in terms of the incidence of infection and lack of bony resorption tendencies (when positioned in the correct plane of dissection).

Improved understanding of tissue-implant interface biology has encouraged the development of bioactive implants which allow for biologic bonding of tissue to implant, which permits natural tissue regeneration as opposed to chronic foreign body or inflammatory reaction. Evolving material technologies have permitted the creation of better implants; however, the ideal alloplastic material has yet to be formulated [3]. The most significant burden still remains in accurate facial analysis, assessment, and planning to achieve a good surgical outcome.

19.2 Technique

Surgical technique affects both the short-term and long lasting outcomes in facial skeletal augmentation. General surgical principles relating to implantation technique such as avoidance of contaminated fields, use of perioperative antibiotics, and meticulous intraoperative handling of the implant materials are vital to the success and safety of the operation. Careful preoperative assessment of the recipient site should determine whether adequate vascularity and soft tissue coverage are present.

19.2.1 Midface Implants

Prominent malar eminences are a canon of beauty in many cultures, conveying the youthful appearance of facial fullness. A hypoplastic flat malar area can make the face appear tired and contributes to a prematurely aged countenance. This tired, sunken look can be secondary to midface hypoplasia and/or atrophy and ptosis of the soft tissues. It can also be accentuated by an over-resected facelift procedure. The goal of midface augmentation is to restore the appearance of youth and beauty by enhancing structure and facial contour.

The majority of patients are unaware of the contribution the midface provides in terms of overall facial harmony; instead, many patients focus on the nose, eyes, or lax facial skin. The facial plastic surgeon can educate patients by illustrating how malar augmentation can restore a youthful and balanced facial contour. In patients lacking bony substructure, rhytidectomy alone does not provide sufficient rejuvenation. Volume restoration by means of midface augmentation in conjunction with facelift can provide the scaffolding for a more optimal redraping of facial tissues to achieve a more successful rejuvenation. Malar implantation enhances rhytidectomy or rhinoplasty results by further improving facial balance and harmony.

The majority of malar augmentations are performed on an elective basis. General indications for malar augmentation include posttraumatic and posttumor resection deformities, congenital deformities, aged face with atrophy and ptosis of soft tissues, unbalanced aesthetic facial triangle, a very round full face or a very long narrow face, and midface hypoplasia. Patients may present with changes associated with aging, such as hollowing of the cheeks and ptosis of the midfacial soft tissue. Malar implants can augment cheek hollows and grooves associated with inferior displacement of the malar fat pad and soft tissues secondary to volume depletion of aging. Patients with midface hypoplasia gain aesthetic benefit from enhanced facial volume. Patients with mild hemifacial microsomia may also show improvement. Other patients may request facial augmentation to produce a dramatic high and sharp cheek contour. Flat, thin, and round faces all benefit from malar augmentation, as it balances the face to create a more aesthetically appealing appearance.

Facial analysis, incorporating photographic documentation, is a critical component of patient selection for malar augmentation. Several techniques of facial measurement analysis of the malar region exist; however, the exact location for augmenting the malar eminence is not universally agreed upon, as the type of malar deficiency varies from patient to patient.

After the determination of appropriate implant size to be used, the patient can undergo the procedure.

The most common technique used is via an intraoral route. No external incisions are made on the face. The initial step is to adequately mark the patient, determining the planned placement of the implants. The precise anesthetic solution used is not as important, as long as it contains epinephrine. After infiltration on both sides, a 1.5 cm sublabial incision is made in the vertical direction through all layers down to the bone. Horizontal incisions for the approach are discouraged. Once this incision has been made, a periosteal elevator is used to dissect the periosteum off the bone. Many authors favor the use of fixation to help secure the implant. The author prefers to use precise subperiosteal pockets for implant placement. Therefore, wide undermining is not required, but careful, deliberate creation of pockets allows for precise localization. The infraorbital nerve is not compromised during the dissection. Depending on the implant, the lateral dissection may be extended to the zygomatic arch. Submalar implants or combined implants will necessitate a more inferior dissection from the arch over the masseter muscle. The correct plane of dissection is over the glistening white fibers of the muscle.

Prior to implant placement, an antibiotic solution is used to irrigate the cavity. A 4–0 chromic suture is passed through the lateral edge of the implant. Using an Aulfricht retractor, the lateral extent of the pocket is identified and the same suture is passed through to the skin surface. With a gentle amount of tension, the implant is inserted into the pocket. The assistant gently pulls on the suture, while the surgeon is guiding from medial to lateral direction. The suture is then gently tied over a bolster, which will be removed after 5 days.

The pocket will "shrink-wrap" around the implant over the next 24–48 h. The incisions are closed in two layers. Attention to detail during the closure cannot be overemphasized as any saliva that penetrates into the wound can lead to infection.

Besides the intraoral route, there are other approaches that may be preferred by other surgeons. The subciliary approach, through a lower blepharoplasty incision, may be used to place smaller implants, especially implants used to augment the nasojugal fold. During facelift surgery, penetration can be made through the subcutaneous musculoaponeurotic system (SMAS) and then carried down to the bone. A subperiosteal pocket can be formed from lateral to medial. This technique limits the access for implant positioning.

19.2.2 Mandibular Implants

The chin has a prominent role in anchoring facial symmetry and aesthetics. Along with the nose, it is a primary determinant of facial balance, especially in consideration of the facial profile. The features of the chin can determine characteristics of the face and even perceptions of personality where a long chin implies strength and power, and a short, small chin portrays weakness.

Abnormalities of the chin are commonly present in patients pursuing cosmetic facial surgery. Chin deformities are the most common abnormality of the facial bones, with microgenia being the most common abnormality but with the lack of an associated functional deficit, microgenia often remains untreated. Most commonly, patients present requesting rhinoplasty and are unaware of their associated chin deficit.

When a patient is considered for chin augmentation with an alloplastic implant, it is important to carefully select the proper implant size and shape. Some alloplastic chin implants, particularly silicone, will heal with the formation of a fibrous capsule resulting in thickening of the overlying skin and soft tissues. This should be taken into account when calculating the size of the augmentation. Women are most judiciously treated with under correction, to avoid the necessity of removal of an implant that is perceived as too large. This is rarely the case in male patients, where a strong chin is viewed as a positive facial feature [4].

Severe microgenia is a contraindication to augmentation mentoplasty. Other contraindications include labial incompetence, lip protrusion, shortened mandibular height, severe malocclusion, and periodontal disease.

As with all procedures in facial plastic surgery, thoughtful preoperative analysis is crucial to a successful outcome. This analysis involves careful three-dimensional evaluation of the face as a whole, with specific attention directed toward the chin, lips, and nose [5]. The patient is examined from all angles, accompanied by precise photo documentation in the standard views. Face shape and length and the relationship of the chin and nose to the face are examined. The chin is analyzed for its soft tissue components and its bony structure. Chin projection and width are noted as is the position and depth of the labiomental fold. Labial competence and lip position are evaluated. The lower lip should be located posterior as related to the upper lip. The lower lip should also be in alignment with the anterior-most projection of the chin.

The technique of implant placement for anterior mandible augmentation can be performed through an intraoral or an external route. Similar to the midface augmentation, a precise subperiosteal pocket will allow for minimal migration of the implant. The external approach is preferred by the author, through either a previous scar in the submental region, or through a 1.5 cm incision in the submental crease. The implant is placed along the inferior edge of the mandible. Preoperative marking delineate the midline, inferior edge of the mandible, and lateral extent of the dissection. The lateral dissection is usually carried out 5 cm on each side, but is dependent on the specific implant used. Once the area is infiltrated with local anesthetic, the submental crease incision is performed. The dissection is carried down through skin and subcutaneous tissue to the periosteum. The midline, inferior edge of the mandible is found and the dissection proceeds superiorly in a supra-periosteal plane for approximately 1.5 cm. During this portion of the dissection, the attachment of the mentalis muscle is carefully dissected. At this point, a 15 blade is used to vertically incise the periosteum. Using a Freer elevator, the dissection is extended 5 cm laterally on both sides. The mental nerve is not routinely identified, but caution is warranted if dissection is superior to the inferior edge of the mandible. The central cuff of periosteum will be used for fixation of the implant to provide a small amount of protection against anterior bone remodeling. After the pocket is created, an antibiotic solution is used to irrigate the cavity. The implant is carefully placed into the pocket on its side and then the opposite side is folded over onto itself to allow for placement.

Once the implant has been positioned, a 5–0 polydiaxanone (PDS) suture is used to fixate the implant to the periosteum in two places. The next layer of wound closure involves reattaching the cut edges of the mentalis muscle back to the periosteum, also performed using 5–0 PDS suture. The following two layers of closure involve the subcutaneous tissue and skin. With meticulous wound closure technique, the incision is very well tolerated by the patient.

19.3 Complications

The complications of using implants for facial augmentation include infection, extrusion, malposition, bleeding, persistent edema, abnormal prominence, seroma, displacement, and nerve damage. Most of the complications are due to technical error, not due to the implant material used. Extrusion of the implants should not occur if the implants were not forced into the pockets. There should be no folding or spring in the implant after placement. Impaired nerve function, usually temporary, is caused by trauma to the tissues overlying the dissection. Bone erosion beneath the implant can occur, and is more commonly seen in mandibular implants. As long as the implant is in correct position, there have been no reports of clinical significance.

Disfigurement is a risk following a failed implant. This can occur with the formation of a capsule, contracture and scarring, or an abnormally draped mentalis muscle. In the event of a failed implant, treatment is removal. This requires removal of the capsule or debridement of the wound in case of infection. Implant replacement is not recommended. Rather, the patient can be reevaluated and recommended for osteoplastic genioplasty.

19.4 Discussion

The role of skeletal changes in facial aging has brought to light the importance of volume restoration in facial rejuvenation. Many patients seek surgery to improve the appearance and balance of facial features to restore a youthful visage. Complete and detailed facial analysis with appropriate patient expectations is vital in all patients undergoing cosmetic surgery. Alloplastic facial implants offer the facial plastic and reconstructive surgeon many advantages over autogenous tissue, including availability of allograft materials and simplification of the surgical procedure. With all implant types and materials, careful surgical technique is crucial in minimizing the risks of extrusion and infection. Both cheek and chin implants can serve to replace lost volume with relative simplicity and low morbidity (Figs. 19.1 and 19.2).

19 Facial Implants

Fig. 19.1 (**a**) Postoperative and (**b**) preoperative chin implant

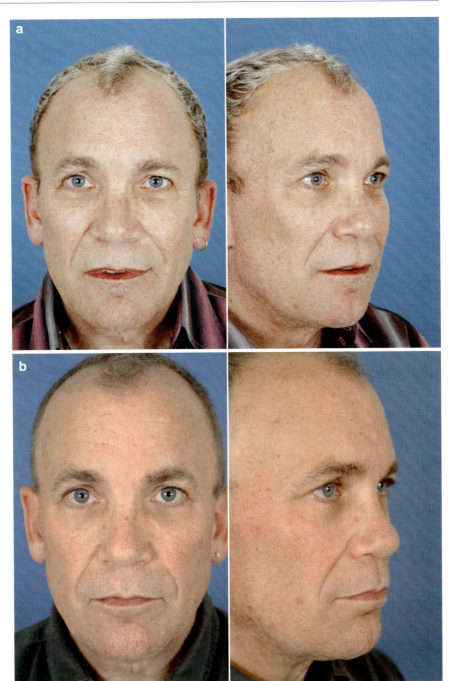

Fig. 19.2 Twenty-six-year-old male. (**a**) Preoperative and (**b**) postoperative chin implant and rhinoplasty

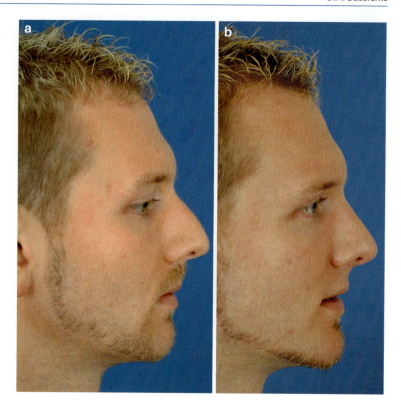

19.5 Conclusions

In the properly selected patients, alloplastic facial implantation can yield highly satisfying results and may complement other facial plastic surgical procedures.

References

1. Eppley BL. Alloplastic implantation. Plast Reconstr Surg. 1999;104(6):1761–83.
2. Friedman CD, Costantino PD. Alloplastic materials for facial skeletal augmentation. Facial Plast Surg Clin North Am. 2002;10(3):325–33.
3. Friedman CD. Future directions in alloplastic materials for facial skeletal augmentation. Facial Plast Surg Clin North Am. 2002;10(2):175–80.
4. Frodel JL. Evaluation and treatment of deformities of the chin. Facial Plast Surg Clin North Am. 2005;13(1):73–84.
5. Terino EO. Facial contouring with alloplastic implants: aesthetic surgery that creates three dimensions. Facial Plast Surg Clin North Am. 1999;7:55–83.

Injectable Facial Fillers

Donald W. Buck II, Murad Alam, and John Y.S. Kim

20.1 Introduction

Now, more than ever, patients are enlisting the help of plastic surgeons to reduce the visible signs of aging. According to the American Society of Plastic Surgeons (ASPS), the number of cosmetic procedures performed in the USA has increased 393% from 1992 to 2002. This increase includes both surgical and nonsurgical procedures, and reflects worldwide trends.

The process of aging is quite complex and involves the following three important factors: global facial volume loss, dynamic and static wrinkles and folds caused by the repetitive movement of facial muscles, and laxity induced by the force of gravity. Generally, the process becomes apparent in the mid- to late 30s, when the eyelids droop, and wrinkles and fine lines appear around the eyes and mouth. As we age into our sixth decade of life, the wrinkling continues, the jaw line begins to sag, and the neck and nasal tip drop.

Traditionally, facial rejuvenation has focused on tightening skin through surgical resection and resurfacing. In recent years, however, a major shift in facial rejuvenation has occurred, with increasing emphasis on minimally invasive cosmetic improvement. Today, plastic surgeons can combat the effects of aging with a variety of non-incisional methods, primarily through the use of facial fillers. A multitude of soft-tissue fillers exist today, each with their own recipe of chemical components, indications, and effectiveness. A thorough knowledge of the properties of these facial fillers is imperative for plastic surgeons treating patients with cosmetic complaints.

20.2 Historical Background

The search for the ideal facial filler began over a century ago, when Neuber [1] was first to describe autologous fat transfer for facial defects in 1893. Just a few years later, reports surfaced regarding the use of paraffin injections for cosmetic enhancement. This technique enjoyed considerable popularity until patients began to develop severe foreign body and granulomatous reactions. The use of liquid silicone for cosmetic purposes was popularized in Germany, Switzerland, and Japan in the 1940s. Beginning in the 1960s, it was also being used successfully in the USA. Despite its success as a soft-tissue filler, reports of significant complications and adverse events have precluded its approval for cosmetic purposes in the USA and Europe.

In the 1980s, the development and use of bovine collagen for cosmetic purposes welcomed a new era of soft-tissue augmentation. Over the past 5 years alone, the number of approved facial fillers in the USA and abroad has expanded rapidly. The most widely used dermal filler products fall into four broad categories: autologous fats, collagens, hyaluronic acids (HA), and biosynthetic polymers.

In addition to the categories based on their chemical makeup, facial fillers can be grouped according to their longevity or degree of permanence after injection. Non-permanent fillers are temporary, producing short-lived results and eventually undergoing resorption.

D.W. Buck II (✉) and J.Y.S. Kim
Division of Plastic and Reconstructive Surgery, Northwestern University, Feinberg School of Medicine, 675 N. St. Clair Street, Galter 19-250, Chicago, IL 60611, USA
e-mail: dwbuck2@yahoo.com

M. Alam
Department of Dermatology, Northwestern University, Feinberg School of Medicine, Chicago, IL, USA

Fillers of this type will require repeated injections for long-term results. Semipermanent fillers typically last longer than most non-permanent fillers, but can be expected to experience some resorption as well. Only permanent fillers can be expected to produce long-term results with a single injection. As the name implies, these products will persist within the tissue indefinitely; a characteristic that might raise concerns regarding safety and the potential for long-term side effects.

Although injectable facial fillers can offer an efficacious alternative to the surgery for the aging face, they also have their limitations. It is important for the plastic surgeon to recognize specific circumstances which may be best managed with an alternative to fillers, including superficial contour defects too shallow for fillers, areas with significant skin laxity in which filler injection may result in lumpiness, and deep defects or folds in areas of dynamic movement which may result in filler dislodgement or visible implants.

20.3 Available Facial Fillers

There are currently many soft-tissue fillers on the market today (Table 20.1). As stated above, these fillers fall within one of four major categories: autologous implants, collagens, hyaluronic acids, and biosynthetic polymers.

20.3.1 Autologous Fat

Despite Neuber's successful use of autologous fat for soft-tissue augmentation in 1893, its use declined until the late 1970s. This decline was most likely due to the limited reproducibility of results; however, with the advent of suction lipectomy and improved harvesting techniques, autologous fat grafts have regained significant popularity. Overall correction and duration are similar to that of bovine collagen, although a high rate of resorption can occur.

20.3.2 Collagen

Collagen is a major component of human connective tissues such as bone, cartilage, skin, and vasculature. The injectable forms consist of varying concentrations of purified bovine or human collagens. Bovine collagen, harvested from cattle skin, was the first Food and Drug Administration (FDA) approved product for soft-tissue augmentation in the USA. Prior to the development of hyaluronic acid fillers, collagen was the "gold standard" injectable filler. As the name implies, newer human collagens are derived from cadavers or laboratory cultures of human fibroblast cells. These collagens have gained popularity due to the reduced risk of hypersensitivity and immunologic reactions when compared to their bovine counterparts.

20.3.3 Hyaluronic Acids (HAs)

Like collagen, hyaluronic acid (HA) is also a major component of connective tissues. HAs are especially prevalent within the human dermis, where it provides a scaffold for collagen development. The main functions of HA include hydration, lubrication, and stabilization of connective tissues. During the aging process, the amount of HA within the connective tissues decreases, leading to a reduction in cell hydration, elasticity, and movement. In its natural form, injectable HA lasts only 1–2 days as a result of local degradation. Fortunately, Biotechnical companies have been successful in creating stabile HA molecules with longer-lasting effects. Most plastic surgeons would agree that the HA filler, Restylane, is currently the most commonly used facial filler worldwide.

20.3.4 Synthetic Polymers

Synthetic compounds are gaining favor as soft-tissue augmentation agents for several reasons: overall cost-effectiveness, consistency of formulation with the possibility for reproducible mass production, limited immunogenicity, and the potential for long-term effects. As discussed previously, one of the first synthetics on the market was silicone. Despite a track record of excellent cosmetic results, reported problems with migration and foreign body reactions have precluded its approval for injectable cosmetic purposes within the USA and Europe. Synthetic facial fillers are typically composed of a biosynthetic polymer

Table 20.1 Available facial fillers (With permission from Buck et al. [8])

Filler type	Name (Manufacturer)	Indication	Durability	Advantages	Disadvantages	Market status
Autologous products	Viable fat	Deep defects	Variable – months to years	Abundant supply, safe, inexpensive	Donor site morbidity, variable reproducibility, requires processing	No FDA/EEA approval required
	Autologous collagen/autolagen (Collagenesis, Beverly, MA; Isolagen, Exton, PA)	Moderate to deep defects	Months to years	Processed from excised skin, can be stored up to 6 months, safe	Donor morbidity, painful, costly	FDA approved/CE mark
Bovine collagens	Zyderm 1 (3.5% dermal collagen) (INAMED, Santa Barbara, CA)	Superficial defects, fine lines, acne scars	2–4 months	Safe, reliable, contains lidocaine, ease of administration	Allergic reaction in 1–3%, short-term results, requires skin testing prior to use, reactivation of herpes is possible with lip injections	FDA approved/CE mark
	Zyderm 2 (6.5% collagen) (INAMED, Santa Barbara, CA)	Moderate defects, deeper acne scars, lip augmentation	2–6 months	Same as Zyderm 1	Same as Zyderm 1	FDA approved/CE mark
	Zyplast (3.5% crosslinked collagen) (INAMED, Santa Barbara, CA)	Deep defects, lip augmentation	2–6 months	Same as Zyderm 1, more viscous and resistant to degradation	Can cause skin necrosis if used in glabella, allergies in 3%, requires skin testing	FDA approved/CE mark
Cadaveric collagens	AlloDerm (acellular human dermis, comes in sheets of varying sizes) (LifeCell, Branchburg, NJ)	Deep wrinkles or scars, lip augmentation	6–12 months	Safe, no allergy testing required	Expensive, surgically implanted, often causes temporary swelling, occasionally palpable, shrinkage with time	FDA approved/CE mark
	Cymetra (micronized, injectable form of AlloDerm) (LifeCell, Branchburg, NJ)	Deep wrinkles or scars, lip augmentation	3–6 months	Safe, no allergy testing required, contains lidocaine	Can cause skin necrosis if used in glabella, costly, often clumps within needle	FDA approved/CE mark

(continued)

Table 20.1 (continued)

Filler type	Name (Manufacturer)	Indication	Durability	Advantages	Disadvantages	Market status
Cell-cultured collagen	Cosmoderm (35 mg/ml collagen) (INAMED, Santa Barbara, CA)	Superficial defects, shallow wrinkles and acne scars	3–4 months	Safe, no allergy testing required, contains lidocaine	Short-term results, the more common side effects include cold symptoms (4%), flu symptoms (2%)	FDA approved/CE mark
	Cosmoplast (35 mg/ml crosslinked collagen) (INAMED, Santa Barbara, CA)	Deeper defects and wrinkles, lip augmentation	3–4 months	Same as Cosmoderm	Same as Cosmoderm	FDA approved/CE mark
Avian-derived hyaluronic acids	Hylaform gel (INAMED, Santa Barbara, CA)	Moderate defects, lip augmentation	3–4 months	Safe, reliable, no allergy testing is required	Short-term results, immunologic reactions in patient allergic to avian products (eggs)	FDA approved/CE mark
	Hylaform plus (INAMED, Santa Barbara, CA)	Moderate to deeper defects, facial wrinkles, and folds	3–4 months	Same as Hylaform gel	Same as Hylaform gel, superficial injection may lead to skin discoloration	FDA approved/CE mark
Bacterial cultured hyaluronic acids	Restylane/Restylane Fine (Medicis, Scottsdale, AZ)	Superficial (Restylane Fine) to moderate defects, deeper wrinkle reduction, nasolabial folds, glabellar creases, lip augmentation	6–12 months	Safe, reliable, predictable results, no allergy testing required, longer lasting than bovine collagens	Rare immunologic reactions, higher incidence of bruising, pain, and post-procedure swelling vs. bovine collagens, higher cost	FDA approved/CE mark
	Perlane (Medicis, Montreal, Canada)	Deeper defects, shaping facial contours, lip augmentation	6–12 months	Same as Restylane	Same as Restylane	FDA approved/CE mark
	Captique (INAMED, Santa Barbara, CA)	Superficial defects, fine lines and wrinkles	3–6 months	Safe, no allergy testing required, similar to Restylane	Relatively new product, short-term results	FDA approved/CE mark
	Juvederm 18, 24, 30 (L.E.A. Derm, Paris, France)	Superficial (18), moderate (24), and deep (30) defects	3–6 months	Safe, predictable results, no allergy testing needed	Short-term results, rare immunologic reactions, relatively new product	FDA approved

20 Injectable Facial Fillers

Synthetics	Sculptra (poly-L-lactic acid microparticles) (*Dermik Laboratories, Berwyn, PA*)	Deep defects	1–2 years	Long-term results, safe	Rare foreign body reaction, limited US results studies	Approved for lipoatrophy; off label for cosmetic purposes/CE mark
	Radiesse (calcium hydroxyapatite microspheres) (*Bioform Medical, Franksville, WI*)	Deep defects, nasolabial folds, vertical lip lines, acne scars, marionette lines, volume restoration around cheeks	1–2 years	Long-term results, no allergy testing required, no concern for antigenic or inflammatory reactions	Can rarely develop nodules if injected superficially	FDA approved/CE mark
	Artecoll/ArteFill (polymethyl-methacrylate microspheres in 3.5% bovine collagen and 0.3% lidocaine) (*Artes Medical, San Diego, CA*)	Deep defects, glabella, nasolabial folds	Permanent after nearly 50% resorption	Unrivaled longevity, probably safe, but reports of persistent erythema at injection site	Palpable if placed superficially or excessively – thus avoid injecting into the lips and areas with thin overlying skin, requires allergy testing	Preliminary FDA approval for cosmetic purposes/CE mark
	Reviderm intra (Dextran beads in a hylan gel) (*Rofil Medical International, Breda, The Netherlands*)	Deep defects, lip augmentation	Months to years	Long-term results, safe	Post-procedural swelling, relatively new product to USA	Not FDA approved/CE mark
	Silicone/Silikon-1000 (liquid silicone) (*Alcon Laboratories, Fort Worth, TX*)	Deep defects, lip augmentation	Permanent	Permanent, safe, long clinical experience	Migration, foreign body reactions, poor reputation	Off label for cosmetic purposes
	Endoplast 50 (Elastin and Collagen) (*Laboratories Filorgra, Paris, France*)	Deep defects, lip augmentation	12 months	Long-term results	Allergy tests required, limited experience	Not FDA approved/CE mark
	Bio-Alcamid (96% water, 4% poly-alkyl imide) (*Pur Medical Corp, Toronto, Canada*)	Deep defects	Permanent	Long-term results, removable, no allergy testing required, bio-compatible	Limited experience, inflammatory reactions, infectious complications, migration	FDA Approved/CE mark for HIV lipoatrophy
	Aquamid (polyacrylamide hydrogel) (*Contura International*)	Deep defects, lip augmentation	Permanent	Long-term results, compound plasticity	High rate of granuloma formation, infectious complications	Not FDA approved/CE mark

Source: Adapted from Johl [2], Murray [3], Broder [4], Eppley [5], Sengelmann [6]

(e.g., poly-L-lactic acid, calcium hydroxyapatite, polymethylmethacralate) combined with an injectable carrier, such as hydrogels, micro-beads, and liquids.

While synthetic polymers may lead to longer-lasting results, it is this very persistence that may also raise concerns over long-term side effects or adverse events.

20.4 Technical Considerations

Most injectable fillers are supplied with a syringe and needle. The needle size, which is generally determined by filler viscosity, can be exchanged with an alternate choice based on surgeon experience. In general, the smallest needle that can deliver the filler appropriately is ideal to limit pain upon injection.

When injecting, the appropriate needle depth is dependent on the defect or wrinkle depth. For example, superficial defects require shallow injection, with the needle tip barely entering the skin, whereas moderate and deeper defects require injections at the level of the mid or deep dermis or at the dermal-subcutaneous junctions, respectively. Blanching typically occurs with superficial and sometimes moderate depth augmentation. Gentle massage of the product after insertion can ensure even correction; however, it is important to avoid aggressive or prolonged massage which can lead to product displacement. As a general rule, as the defect depth increases, products with higher viscosity should be used; whereas less viscous materials are more appropriate for shallower defects.

20.5 Injection Techniques

There are four commonly reported techniques for filler injection: serial puncture, threading, fanning, and crosshatching (Fig. 20.1). There is no algorithm for choosing one injection technique over another. This decision is typically surgeon dependent and related to experience, defect size and location, as well as the particular filler being used.

For serial puncture, the skin is held taut and the needle is inserted to the appropriate depth. The product is then delivered in a small bolus to fill the defect, and the needle is subsequently removed. If delivering filler within a particular rhytid, the needle can be reinserted along the defect and a new bolus injected. This technique is commonly used for lip augmentation, or superficial placement of fillers along a particular wrinkle.

In the threading technique, the needle is inserted into the defect and tunneled along it at the appropriate depth. As the needle is withdrawn, the product is delivered in a slow, continuous fashion until the needle is completely removed from the skin. This technique is

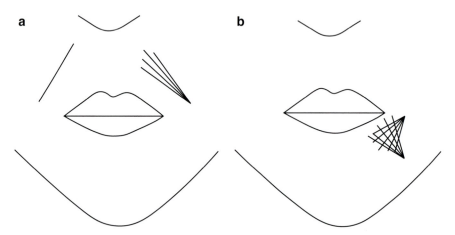

Fig. 20.1 Diagram of common filler injection techniques. (**a**) Threading and fanning – In the threading technique, the needle is tunneled through a defect at the appropriate depth and the filler is injected as the needle is withdrawn. In the fanning technique, multiple threads are injected using a single insertion point without removing the needle from the skin. (**b**) Crosshatching – The fanning technique is used with a secondary injection point occurring perpendicular to the primary injection threads. This technique is useful for injection of larger defect areas (With permission from Buck et al. [8])

commonly used for lip augmentation, as well as nasolabial fold injection.

The fanning technique is similar to the threading technique, but the direction of the needle is continually changed in a radial fashion and new lines are injected without ever withdrawing the needle tip.

Crosshatching involves a series of threads injected in a perpendicular fashion to each other to cover the surface area of a defect. The fanning and crosshatching techniques are generally used to fill larger defect areas.

20.6 Post-procedural Considerations

Following injection, the following immediate posttreatment guidelines are recommended. Cold compresses can be applied, and if desired reapplied, for 24–48 h to reduce swelling. Strenuous physical activity should be avoided after injection. Patients should also be told to minimize aggressive facial movement or massaging/manipulation for several hours after implant placement. They should avoid excessive sun exposure until superficial erythema and swelling disappears.

In patients with a history of cold sores or susceptibility to infections, prophylactic antibiotic or antiviral courses should be considered. Aspirin, nonsteroidal anti-inflammatory drugs (NSAIDs), and/or other blood thinning medications, including herbal medications, should be avoided for 24–48 h before and after injection to limit the potential for localized hematoma formation, unless necessary for patient well-being.

20.7 Facial Filler Complications

Soft-tissue augmentation via facial filler injection is not without risks. There have been many reports within the literature detailing complications associated with facial filler use. Interpreting the literature for a particular filler is often frustrating at it is increasingly common to find reports of contradictory efficacy and side effect profiles. Although most side effects to facial fillers are transient and minor in nature, it is important to discuss these complications with patients prior to injection.

Bleeding is commonly associated with patient anticoagulation due to concurrent and/or recent use of aspirin, nonsteroidal anti-inflammatory drugs, or blood thinning medications. In addition, the use of large bore needles and injection of highly vascular areas, like the lip, can also increase the risk of bleeding.

Infectious complications are rare; however, patients with susceptibility to infection or a history of herpes simplex infections may be candidates for prophylactic antiviral and/or antibacterial therapy.

Acute allergic reactions are a serious concern for fillers containing bovine and other xenogenic components. To minimize this risk, product recommendations for allergies and allergy testing should be followed. Patients who have had a prior hypersensitivity reaction to a specific filler should not, again, be treated with that filler. Given the availability of injectable human collagen, allergy testing prior to bovine collagen injection is now mostly of historical interest.

Post-injection pain is common, and can be reduced using the smallest needle possible for injection. For less viscous fillers, this may be a 30-gauge or 32-gauge needle; more viscous fillers may require a 27-gauge needle (e.g., calcium hydroxylapatite), or even a 25-gauge needle (poly-L-lactate) to avoid clumping or clogging. Topical or regional anesthesia, including nerve blocks, can be used as needed. Some injectables may contain small amounts of lidocaine as part of their injection carrier. Caution should be employed when using local injectable anesthesia as this may alter and obscure contour defects.

In general, all fillers create some form of histologic reaction that generally evolves over time. This inflammatory reaction is of particular concern for the semi-permanent and permanent fillers as their persistence may lead to a more chronic inflammatory process. More severe granulomatous reactions can also occur, and have been reported even with more biologic products, such as the hyaluronic acids [7]. Granulomas can often be treated with simple excision.

Improper injection technique can also lead to complications. If filler is inappropriately injected at the incorrect skin depth, location, or volume, a myriad of unwanted skin changes can occur including palpable bumps, contour deformities, and superficial beading. These unwanted changes may resolve slowly.

Of the common injectable fillers, only Cosmoderm or Zyderm is appropriately injected so superficially as to cause a florid white blanch. Significantly, initial reports have shown that laser or energy device treatment over soft-tissue augmentation materials appears not to damage, deform, or destroy the implants, or cause adverse tissue reactions.

Serious complications are rare, but can include anaphylactic reactions, skin necrosis, blindness, and death.

20.8 Conclusions

Injectable facial fillers offer an excellent alternative to surgery in the management of facial aging, wrinkling, and contour defects in select cases. Fillers are ideal for patients seeking a safe, minimally invasive, and affordable means of maintaining a youthful appearance. It is imperative for the plastic surgeon to have a thorough knowledge of all available products and their properties. This knowledge will enable optimal filler-defect pairing, thereby maximizing efficacy and overall patient satisfaction.

References

1. Neuber F. Fetttransplantation. Chir Kongr Verhandl Dtsc Gesellch Chir. 1893;22:66.
2. Johl SS, Burgett RA. Dermal filler agents: a practical review. Curr Opin Ophthalmol. 2006;17(5):471–9.
3. Murray CA, Zloty D, Warshawski L. The evolution of soft tissue fillers in clinical practice. Dermatol Clin. 2005;23(2):343–63.
4. Broder KW, Cohen SR. An overview of permanent fillers and semipermanent fillers. Plast Reconstr Surg. 2006;118(3S):7S–14S.
5. Eppley BL, Dadvand B. Injectable soft-tissue fillers: clinical overview. Plast Reconstr Surg. 2006;118(4):98e–106e.
6. Sengelmann RD, Tull S. Dermal fillers. Available at http://www.emedicine.com/derm/topic515.htm. Accessed 29 Mar 2007.
7. Honig JF, Brink U, Korabiowski M. Severe granulomatous allergic tissue reaction after hyaluronic acid injection in the treatment of facial lines and its surgical correction. J Craniofac Surg. 2003;14(2):197–200.
8. Buck DW, Alam M, Kim JY. Injectable facial fillers for facial rejuvenation: a review. J Plast Reconstr Surg. 2009;62(1):11–8.

Recommended Reading

Alam M, Yoo SS. Technique for calcium hydroxylapatite injection for correction of nasolabial fold depressions. J Am Acad Dermatol. 2007;56(2):285–9.

Alam M, Levy R, Pavjani U, Ramierez JA, Guitart J, Veen H, et al. Safety of radiofrequency treatment over human skin previously injected with medium-term injectable soft-tissue augmentation materials: a controlled pilot trial. Lasers Surg Med. 2006;38(3):205–10.

American Society of Plastic Surgeons. 2002 Cosmetic surgery trends. Available at http://www.plasticsurgery.org/public_education/loader.cfm?url=/Commonspot/security/getfile.cfm&PageID=6069. Accessed 29 Mar 2007.

Andre P, Lowe NJ, Parc A, Clerici TH, Zimmermann U. Adverse reactions to dermal fillers: a review of the European experiences. J Cosmet Laser Ther. 2005;7(3–4):171–6.

Baumann L, Kaufman J, Saghari S. Collagen fillers. Dermatol Ther. 2006;19(3):134–40.

Glicenstein J. The first "fillers", vaseline and paraffin. From miracle to disaster. Ann Chir Plast Esthét. 2007;52(2):157–61.

Kanchwala SK, Holloway L, Bucky LP. Reliable soft tissue augmentation. A clinical comparison of injectable soft-tissue fillers for facial-volume augmentation. Ann Plast Surg. 2005;55(1):30–5.

Kaufman MR, Miller TA, Huang C, Roostalen J, Wasson KL, Ashley RK, et al. Autologous fat transfer for facial recontouring: is there science behind the art? Plast Reconstr Surg. 2007;119(7):2287–96.

Lam SM, Azizzadeh B, Graivier M. Injectable poly-L-lactic acid (Sculptra): technical considerations in soft-tissue contouring. Plast Reconstr Surg. 2006;118(3 Suppl):55S–63S.

Lowe NJ, Maxwell CA, Patnaik R. Adverse reactions to dermal fillers: review. Dermatol Surg. 2005;31(11 Pt 2):1616–25.

Matarasso SL, Carruthers JD, Jewell ML. Restylane Consensus Group: consensus recommendations for soft-tissue augmentation with nonanimal stabilized hyaluronic acid (Restylane). Plast Reconstr Surg. 2006;117(3 Suppl):3S–33S.

Monheit GD, Coleman KM. Hyaluronic acid fillers. Dermatol Ther. 2006;19(3):141–50.

Narins RS, Beer K. Liquid injectable silicone: a review of its history, immunology, technical considerations, complications, and potential. Plast Reconstr Surg. 2006;118 (3 Suppl):77S–84S.

Rapaport MJ, Vinnik C, Zarem H. Injectable silicone: cause of facial nodules, cellulites, ulceration and migration. Aesthet Plast Surg. 1996;20(3):267–76.

Rohrich RJ, Rios JL, Fagien S. Role of new fillers in facial rejuvenation: a cautious outlook. Plast Reconstr Surg. 2003;12(7):1899–902.

Zimmerman U, Clerici TJ. The histologic aspects of fillers complications. Semin Cutan Med Surg. 2004;23:241–50.

Botulinum Toxin for Facial Rejuvenation

21

George J. Bitar, Daisi J. Choi, and Florencia Segura

21.1 Introduction

Botulinum toxin has evolved over the last few years becoming both the patient and the plastic surgeon's best friend! Botox® Cosmetic is a household name, often referenced in movies, reality television shows, and the news, and lauded by many as a miracle antiaging drug. It is no wonder then, that Botox® Cosmetic is now interwoven into the fabric of our society. It works quickly with minimal downtime and is relatively painless in reducing facial wrinkles. The use of botulinum neurotoxin is the most common noninvasive cosmetic procedure in the USA with five million treatments performed in 2008. This figure represents a 537% increase in these procedures as compared to the year 2000 [1]. In addition, a new commercially available botulinum toxin, Dysport®, has been approved by the FDA for facial wrinkle treatment as an alternative to Botox® Cosmetic. Therefore, it is very important to have an understanding of the botulinum toxin's chemical properties, mechanism of action, commercial preparations, and clinical data regarding its administrations in order to avoid complications and to deliver maximal aesthetic results to one's patients.

G.J. Bitar (✉)
Assistant Clinical Professor, George Washington University,
Medical Director, Bitar Cosmetic Surgery Institute,
3023 Hamaker Ct, #109 Fairfax, VA 22031, USA
e-mail: georgebitar@drbitar.com

D.J. Choi and F. Segura
Bitar Cosmetic Surgery Institute, Northern Virginia,
8501 Arlington Blvd. Suite 500, Fairfax, VA 22031, USA

21.2 History

Classic botulism was first observed by Julius Kerner, a medical officer, who reported symptoms of skeletal and gut muscle paralysis, myadriasis, and maintenance of consciousness after the ingestion of improperly preserved foods in 1820 [2]. More than a century later, in 1973, Scott et al. described the first clinical application of botulinum toxin while investigating nonsurgical treatments of strabismus in a primate model [3, 4]. Subsequently, botulinum toxin type A was discovered to have widespread applications as a neuromuscular blocker in neurology, orthopedics, gastroenterology, and ophthalmology, eventually earning Food and Drug Administration (FDA) approval for disorders involving the facial nerve, adult strabismus, and blepharospasm in 1989 [2]. Cosmetic use of botulinum toxin type A is largely credited to Carruthers and Alistair in 1987, when they observed the aesthetic improvements and lessening of glabellar lines after injecting the neurotoxin into patients with blepharospasm [5]. This led to subsequent clinical trials and FDA approval of the use of Botox® Cosmetic to improve the appearance of glabellar lines in April 2002. Over the next few years, Botox® Cosmetic gained worldwide popularity as a safe and effective drug to treat facial wrinkles. Off-label usage for other facial muscles became widespread, and satisfaction was reportedly high and consistent. In April 2009, the FDA announced the approval of a new botulinum toxin type A formulation, Dysport®, for two separate indications: the treatment of cervical dystonia and the temporary improvement in the appearance of moderate to severe glabellar lines. The latter is currently being marketed by Medicis in the USA for its aesthetic indications. Dysport® has been used for cosmetic purposes in the UK since 1991 and has been approved in 27 other countries for aesthetic use with over two million single treatment cycles [6].

21.3 Chemical Overview

Botulinum neurotoxins are produced by the gram-positive anaerobic bacterium Clostridium botulinum (Fig. 21.1). Various strains of this bacterium exist, resulting in eight immunologically distinct serotypes: A, B, C1, C2, D, E, F, and G, seven of which are associated with paralysis [7, 8]. Botulinum neurotoxin types A and B have been extensively studied and are the only two to be used routinely for clinical purposes [9]. Currently, type A is the only serotype approved by the FDA for cosmetic purposes.

Botulinum toxin serotypes are synthesized as macromolecular complexes containing 150 kDa neurotoxin molecules as well as one or more nontoxin proteins [10]. The exact structure and molecular weight is determined by the clostridium strain that produced the neurotoxin and its particular serotype [10]. Furthermore, the percentage of active neurotoxin differs between the various serotypes [10]. Botulinum toxin type A forms a 500 kDa protein complex and 95% of its neurotoxin molecules are in the active form [10]. The 150 kDa neurotoxins can be converted into their active form by endogenous or exogenous proteases that nick the toxin into two polypeptide fragments, a 100 kDa heavy chain and 50 kDa light chain, that remain linked by a disulfide bond [10, 11]. The 100 kDa heavy chain portion of the active neurotoxin is responsible for binding of botulinum neurotoxin to membrane receptors at peripheral cholinergic nerve terminals [10, 12]. Once bound, the entire 150 kDa neurotoxin undergoes endocytosis and subsequent conformational change whereby the 50 kDa light chain moves out of the vesicular compartment and into the cytosol [10, 13]. Once in the cytosol, the light chain portion of the active neurotoxin acts as a zinc-dependent endopeptidase that inactivates one or more proteins of the SNARE complex, thereby inhibiting vesicular exocytosis [10, 14].

In comparing various preparations of botulinum toxin for medical use, it is important to consider the percentage of nicked versus unnicked neurotoxin, as the unnicked toxins may allosterically inhibit binding of nicked toxin to its intended receptor sites, thereby decreasing its potency [9]. Botulinum toxin type A is the most commonly used serotype for cosmetic practice because of its potency which is generated by endogenous proteases [10, 15]. Other serotypes, such as type B, may only be partially nicked and, therefore, not as potent when recovered from bacterial cultures [10, 16]. Clinical preparation of type B and other partially nicked or unnicked serotypes often require an additional "nicking step" where the unnicked toxin is exposed to exogenous proteases to increase the percentage of active neurotoxin [10] The active neurotoxin can be inactivated by heat, 85°C (185°F) or greater, for 5 min [17].

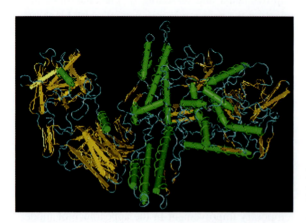

Fig. 21.1 Crystal structure of botulinum neurotoxin serotype A [6] (US National Library of Medicine Molecular Modeling Database http://www.ncbi.nlm.nih.gov/Structure/mmdb/mmdbsrv.cgi?uid=11100)

21.4 Specific Mechanism of Action

Botulinum neurotoxin causes temporary muscle paralysis by inhibiting acetylcholine release at peripheral cholinergic nerve terminals [17]. The various serotypes act via different intracellular molecules at presynaptic nerve endings. Botulinum toxin type A specifically cleaves SNAP-25 of the SNARE complex, preventing vesicles from anchoring and fusing with presynaptic membranes, thereby blocking acetylcholine release at the neuromuscular junction [4, 17]. The various neurotoxin serotypes cleave different intracellular SNARE proteins or the same protein at different sites [10]. Proper intramuscular injections of botulinum toxin type A at therapeutic doses cause partial chemical denervation of muscle fibers resulting in localized reduction of muscle activity [17]. This is not a permanent effect, as new nerve endings form and recovery of acetylcholine transmission gradually occurs. As such, the effects of botulinum neurotoxin are temporary, and muscle activity should start returning within 4–6 months.

21.5 Onset and Duration of Paralysis

Although each botulinum neurotoxin has its unique onset of paralysis, period of clinical efficacy, and time of recovery, many generalities can be made in regards to the most commonly used serotype, type A [4]. Once facial muscles are injected with botulinum neurotoxin type A, clinical effects start becoming noticeable within 48–72 h, and paralytic effects peak during the following 7–14 days followed by approximately 90 days of steady results [4]. By the end of this period, new neuromuscular junctions and axonal sprouts will have replaced the nonfunctional junctions, so reinjection is generally recommended in 3–4 months [18]. The amount of time between injections will vary depending on which facial area is being treated. Stronger facial muscles, such as the corrugator supercilii and procerus muscles, may require more frequent treatments than the weaker orbicularis occuli, as an example. Furthermore, anatomical differences, genetics, age, gender, and skin quality may affect botulinum injection results. Questions still remain regarding the very long-term effects of botulinum toxin on muscle potency as more research needs to be conducted in this area.

21.6 Preparation of Botox® Cosmetic

Standard units of measurement for botulinum toxin are important to assess the potency of various serotypes. Units of biological activity (U) for botulinum toxin serotypes are determined according to a mouse lethality assay, where 1.0 U represents the amount of neurotoxin complex protein that is lethal in 50% of female mice following an intraperitoneal injection [7].

The most frequently used formulation of botulinum neurotoxin type A includes the 900 kDa formulation (Botox® Cosmetic; Allergan; Irvine, California). Botox® Cosmetic is packaged in a vial containing 100 U of vacuum-dried neurotoxin complex (approximately 4.9 ng of protein), 0.5 mg of human albumin, and 0.9 mg of sodium chloride for a composite pH of 7.0 [17]. Botox® Cosmetic requires reconstitution with non-preserved sterile 0.9% sodium chloride before clinical use [17]. Reconstituted Botox® Cosmetic should be "clear, colorless and free of particulate matter" [17]. Members of the Botox® Cosmetic consensus panel noted that most clinicians use a dilution of 2.5–3.0 ml of 0.9% non-preserved saline per vial to obtain a reconstituted solution at a concentration of 4.0 Units/0.1 ml [18]. They also noted that a number of dilutions are acceptable and depends on practitioner preference as well as the total number of units to be injected [18]. The authors dilute 100 U of Botox® Cosmetic in 4.0 ml of non-preserved sterile 0.9% saline to simplify the process of loading syringes and injecting with consistency. In this case, 1.0 ml will contain 25 U of Botox® Cosmetic which will simplify calculations of how much Botox® Cosmetic is injected in each area. The dosage can be adjusted based on each individual patient's anatomy and, ultimately, their results.

Unopened 100 U vials of Botox® Cosmetic are stable for up to 24 months when refrigerated at 2–8°C [17]. Since botulinum toxin type A solution does not contain a preservative, it should be administered within 4 h after reconstitution [17]. The manufacturer recommends use of the entire reconstituted product within 4 h when stored at 2–8°C for maximum efficacy [17]. Clinically, we have noted that Botox® Cosmetic stays effective even when administered after the recommended 4 h have elapsed. One study demonstrated that reconstituted botulinum toxin type A maintains its efficacy and potency in treatment of glabellar frown lines for up to 6 weeks with proper storage at 4°C [19].

21.7 Preparation of Dysport®

Dysport®, a 500–900 kDa formulation (Dysport®; Medicis; Scottsdale, Arizona) [4] of botulinum toxin type A, was originally launched in 1991 and was approved by the US FDA in April 2009. Similar to Botox® Cosmetic, Dysport® has shown a good safety profile and low incidence of treatment failures. Although both Dysport® and Botox® Cosmetic contain botulinum toxin type A, they differ in their process of manufacture and potency determination, method of purification, and formulation. Consequently, Dysport® and Botox® Cosmetic should be regarded as individual botulinum toxin type A products with their own individual unit dosing requirements rather than generic equivalents [20].

Dysport® is formulated by fermentation of the bacterium Clostridium botulinum. The neurotoxin is recovered through a series of steps including chromatography, precipitation, dialysis, and filtration [20]. The recovered complex is then dissolved in an aqueous solution of lactose and human serum albumin which is then filtered and freeze-dried [20]. Unlike Botox® Cosmetic, the lactose in Dysport® acts as a bulking agent [20]. Therefore, the product seen in the vial resembles a small cake of white powder facilitating its reconstitution with saline prior to clinical use [19]. Dysport® is packaged as a freeze-dried powder in a single-use vial in which 5.0 U contains 12.5 ng of protein, 2.5 mg of lactose, and 125 µg of albumin [21]. Each 300 U vial of Dysport® is to be reconstituted with 2.5 ml of 0.9% sterile, preservative-free saline before injection [21]. Reconstituted Dysport® should be a clear and colorless solution [21]. Dysport® is stable for 1 year when refrigerated at 2–8°C [21]. Once reconstituted, Dysport® should be stored in the original container at 2–8°C and used within 4 h of reconstitution [21].

21.8 Comparing Botox® Cosmetic and Dysport®

Botox® Cosmetic and Dysport® differ in terms of their preparation and formulation, including the method of extraction, diluents and stabilizers used, and recommended volume of injection [22]. One of the main differences in their formulations is the protein concentration. Dysport® contains 12.5 mg of protein per 500 U whereas Botox® Cosmetic contains approximately 5.0 mg more protein per 100 U [17, 21]. This is significant since botulinum toxin proteins can cause an immune response at high doses. An immune response can lead to the development of neutralizing antibodies that prevent the effects of the neurotoxin [23]. Therefore, protein load and potential for antibody formation are two factors that physicians must bear in mind when choosing a formulation for botulinum toxin therapy. Additional research is needed to determine the clinical significance of lower protein load of Dysport® as compared to Botox® Cosmetic.

Due to manufacturing differences, a single unit of Botox® Cosmetic differs in potency from a single unit of Dysport®. This results in a marked difference in dosing between these two products. Since Botox® Cosmetic has been the most widely used botulinum toxin type A preparation, the clinical efficacy of Dysport® is described in reference to it. Clinical studies have described doses of Dysport® that can be 2.5–6 times higher compared to doses of Botox® Cosmetic when treating the same condition [24, 25].

The difference between the potency units of Botox® Cosmetic and Dysport® remains a controversial issue despite 15 years of clinical studies. The manufacturer of Botox® Cosmetic supports higher conversion ratios, 4–5:1 (Dysport®: Botox® Cosmetic), which is the current consensus among medical faculty. On the other hand, the manufacturers of Dysport® argue that a lower conversion factor of 3–2.5:1 (Dysport®: Botox® Cosmetic) is just as efficacious [26].

It has also been suggested from clinical studies that Dysport® is likely to diffuse further from the injection site than Botox® Cosmetic and that the Botox® Cosmetic formulation provides a longer dose ratio of 2.5:1 (Dysport®: Botox® Cosmetic) [10, 27]. However, these data are heavily contested and more research is needed regarding this topic. Since its use in 1991, Dysport® has been shown to be effective and safe in treating the upper face, but long-term safety data regarding diffusion and other effects in aesthetic indications are much more limited than for Botox® Cosmetic.

21.9 Botulinum Toxin Type A Injection and Follow-Up Care

In order to minimize common local reactions to botulinum toxin therapy (i.e., bruising), it is recommended that patients refrain from taking medications that inhibit clotting such as vitamin E, aspirin, and nonsteroidal anti-inflammatory drugs 10–14 days before treatment. Pain is commonly reported by patients as a result of botulinum toxin type A injections and can be markedly reduced by pretreating the area with ice for 5 min prior to injection or applying a local anesthetic cream such as betacaine, or both. Pre- and posttreatment application of ice is a safe, cost-free, and effective skin analgesic that has been shown to significantly decrease pain perception, swelling, and bruising as well as the duration required to complete a series of injections [28]. Patients should be instructed not to massage the injection sites to avoid unintentional diffusion of the botulinum toxin [4]. Mode of injection may vary between physicians. The authors recommend injecting with a 1.0 ml syringe and a 30 gauge needle for ease of injection, consistency, and minimal pain to the patient.

More research is needed regarding the effects of exercise on botulinum toxin injections. According to the American Society of Plastic Surgeons (ASPS), 28% of its members from one particular study permit their patients to exercise immediately after treatment [9]. An additional 50% allow exercise later the same day of treatment, and the remaining 22% recommend waiting until the following day [9].

21.10 Locations of Treatment

In the upper face, botulinum toxin type A is indicated for treatment of wrinkles caused by the hyperdynamic muscular action of the corrugator supercilii and procerus muscles (glabellar wrinkles), the orbicularis oculi muscles (lateral canthal fold wrinkles or crow's feet), and the frontalis muscle (forehead wrinkles). In the lower face, botulinum toxin type A is used to treat the wrinkles formed by the orbicularis oris, the mentalis, and the platysma with its corresponding transverse neck lines. When treating each area, it is important to track injection location, number of injection points, and total units of botulinum toxin used. This section discusses recommended doses of Botox® Cosmetic for different locations of treatment based on the results of consensus recommendations from a study conducted by the ASPS [9].

21.10.1 Upper Face

The three principal areas of Botox® Cosmetic treatment in the upper face are the frontalis muscle, which contributes to formation of transverse forehead lines, the corrugator supercilii and procerus muscles, which contribute to formation of glabellar lines (Figs. 21.2 and 21.3), and the orbicularis oculi muscles, which contribute to formation of crow's feet (Fig. 21.4). Consensus recommendations on number of Botox® Cosmetic units for treating the upper face has decreased overall; however, the range of injection points remains unchanged. For transverse forehead lines, the recommended range of Botox® Cosmetic units is 6–15 U for women and 6–15 U or greater for men [9]. This is a marked decrease from older recommendations which suggested using 10–20 U for women and 20–30 U for men. The recommended range in number of injection points for transverse forehead lines remains 4–8.

To treat the corrugator and procerus muscles of the glabellar complex, 10–30 U of Botox® Cosmetic is recommended for women versus 20–40 U for men [9]. The recommended range of injection points for the glabellar lines remains 5–7, although men may require more sites. It is important to inject the whole length of the corrugator muscle extending to the area above the pupil, otherwise the wrinkle correction may be incomplete. When there are furrows in the glabellar region, supplementing botulinum toxin injections with filler, such as a hyaluronic acid, may improve the results by addressing the dermal component of the wrinkle, whereas the botulinum toxin addresses the muscle component. The two injectables may be done simultaneously or on separate visits.

The current recommended dosage for treating crow's feet is 10–30 U of Botox® Cosmetic for women and 20–30 U of Botox® Cosmetic for men [9]. The crow's feet are the only facial muscles where recommended doses are relatively unchanged for women and increased for men. The recommended range of injection points for crow's feet remains 2–5 per side. The pattern of wrinkles varies tremendously in this area. One must be able to differentiate wrinkles caused by sun damage versus wrinkles caused by hyperdynamic muscle activity. Botulinum toxin is very effective for treating the latter; however, skin wrinkles may need to be addressed by fillers, surgery, laser treatments, or other modalities.

At our institute, the amount of Botox® Cosmetic injected is usually based on each individual's anatomy and prior clinical experience with Botox® Cosmetic, when applicable; however, we have tended to see better results when injecting the forehead in the 20–25 U range for both men and women. This observation holds true for all three areas of the upper face.

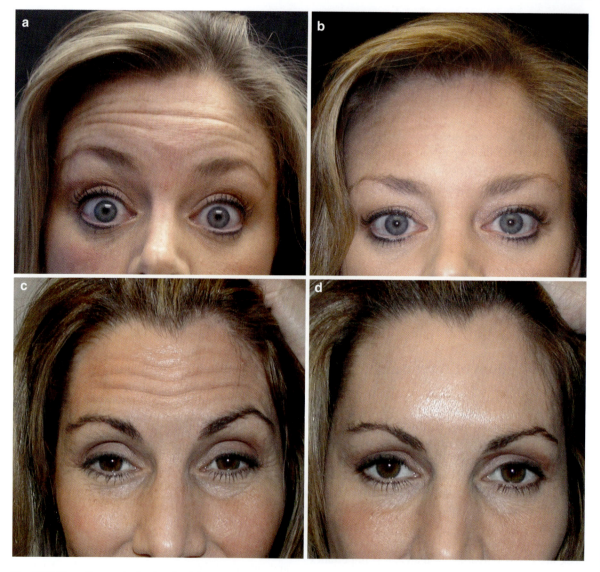

Fig. 21.2 Frontalis muscle (forehead wrinkles) treatment with Botox® Cosmetic. (**a**, **c**) Pretreatment. (**b**, **d**) Posttreatment

21.10.2 Midface

The current consensus for treating the midface is that volume restoration via fillers produces a more aesthetically pleasing result over rhytid reduction using botulinum toxin. In treating areas of the midface, such as malar smile lines and nasolabial folds, the majority of medical faculty from the ASPS study advised against the use of botulinum toxin alone to avoid causing a frozen look or an inability to smile [9]. The exception is malar wrinkles as an extension of crow's feet, where the injection of botulinum toxin can be done more medially when injecting the crow's feet.

21.10.3 Lower Face

Treating the lower face with botulinum toxin is not as readily accepted by plastic surgeons as treating the upper face because of alternative methods of treatment, lack of consistently great results, or a combination of these reasons. Botox® Cosmetic is currently recommended

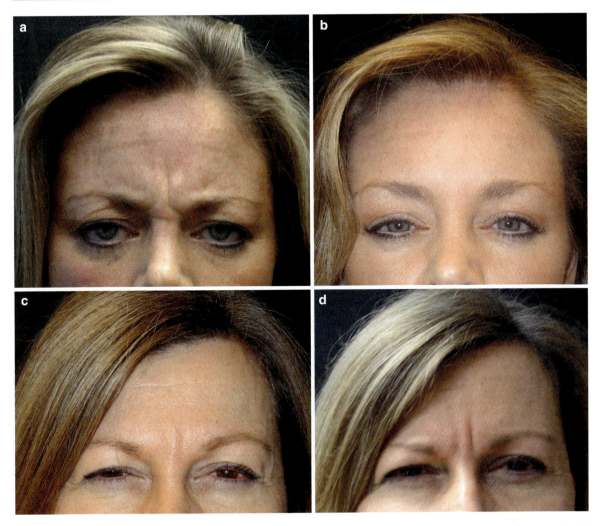

Fig. 21.3 Corrugator and procerus muscles (glabellar wrinkles) treatment with Botox® Cosmetic. (**a, c**) Pretreatment. (**b, d**) Posttreatment

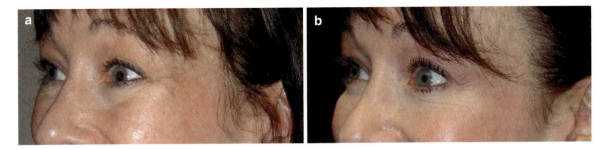

Fig. 21.4 Orbicularis oculi (crow's feet wrinkles) treatment with Botox® Cosmetic. (**a**) Pretreatment. (**b**) Posttreatment

for treating three targeted muscles of the lower face. These include the orbicularis oris, which contributes to the development of perioral wrinkles with aging, the mentalis, which leads to formation of an irregular chin contour due to muscle hyperactivity (Fig. 21.5), and the platysma bands, which become more prominent with aging. For perioral wrinkles, the consensus recommendation is 4–5 U of Botox® Cosmetic for both men and women, and two to six injection points total for both lips [9]. In treating the mentalis area, 4–10 U of Botox® Cosmetic is recommended for both men and women, and one to two injection points [9]. To treat the platysma bands and corresponding horizontal neck lines, the recommended dosage is 40–60 U of Botox® Cosmetic total per neck (about 10 U per band on average) [9]. The recommended number of injection points for this area is 2–12 per band for women and 3–12 per band for men. At our institute, we tend to favor fillers and surgical correction for the lower face over the use of botulinum toxin.

21.11 New Frontiers for Botulinum Toxin in Facial Rejuvenation

Now that botulinum toxin has become a staple of the plastic surgery world, it is not all that surprising that it is being used in cosmetic treatments outside of its conventional use in reducing facial wrinkles. One example is the use of botulinum toxin in treating excessive gingival display or "gummy smile" (Fig. 21.6) as an alternative to surgery. The elevator muscles of the upper lip include the levator labii superioris, levator labii superioris alaeque nasi, levator anguli oris, zygomaticus major and minor, and depressor septi nasi [9]. At our institute, we inject about 25 U total of Botox® Cosmetic to the levator labii superioris and orbicularis oris muscles to resolve a "gummy smile."

Another emerging trend is the use of botulinum toxin for masseter reduction in treating facial widening [9]. According to the ASPS, clinicians who treat this area use anywhere from 10–50 U of Botox® Cosmetic per side; however, 25–30 U per side is generally recommended [8]. In treating facial widening with botulinum toxin, the underlying cause should be the masseter muscles and not mandibular bony prominence [9].

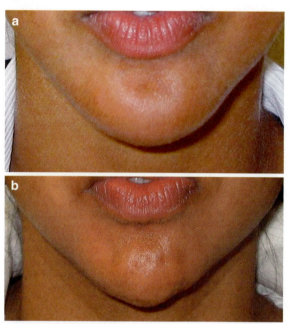

Fig. 21.5 Mentalis (dimpled chin) treatment with Botox® Cosmetic. (**a**) Pretreatment. (**b**) Posttreatment

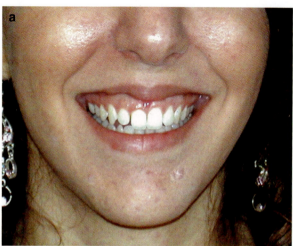 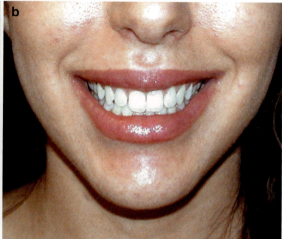

Fig. 21.6 Excessive gingival display (gummy smile) treatment with Botox® Cosmetic. (**a**) Pretreatment. (**b**) Posttreatment

21.12 Contraindications

Botulinum toxin is contraindicated for patients with known hypersensitivity to any ingredient in the formulation, including albumin [17]. It should not be used in treating special patient populations with known neuromuscular disorders and peripheral motor neuropathies such as multiple sclerosis, Eaton–Lambert syndrome, and myasthenia gravis since further muscle paralysis may exacerbate muscle weakness [4, 17].

Since Botox® Cosmetic is considered a category C drug, it should be avoided in women who are pregnant or breastfeeding. Also, the physician should be cautious when using Botox® Cosmetic in patients who have had surgery in the target area since muscles may have been repositioned or weakened, and also in patients who have any inflammatory skin conditions at the injection site [29]. Furthermore, people who have had an allergic reaction to tetanus immunization should refrain from having Botox® Cosmetic injections in case of an allergic reaction.

Dysport® is contraindicated for patients with any of the above stated hypersensitivities to botulinum toxin preparations. Dysport® is also contraindicated in patients known to have allergies to cow's milk protein since Dysport® may contain trace amounts of these proteins [21].

21.13 Avoidance of Potential Pitfalls

General complications associated with botulinum toxin treatment include mild erythema at the site of injection that may last a few hours due to needle sticks. Ecchymosis may last a few days and most commonly occurs when injecting crow's feet, where the skin is thin and the veins are more superficial. Ecchymosis can be reduced by advising patients to avoid taking any aspirin or other anticoagulants prior to treatment as well as applying local anesthetic cream and/or ice packs to the injection site before and after treatment. Asymmetry may occur and may have a prolonged effect, but will self-correct when the botulinum toxin wears off.

In the upper face, a significant concern when injecting botulinum toxin is the migration and diffusion of the toxin from the target muscle to unintended muscle groups. One of the most common complications in the upper face is brow ptosis, which can be caused by the following reasons. The first possible reason is excessive diffusion of the toxin in the frontalis muscle. This complication may be avoided if injection is given no closer than 1 cm above the bony orbital rim in the mid-pupillary line and avoiding overtreatment of the frontalis by using low doses of botulinum toxin [9]. Brow ptosis may also occur if the patient has upper eyelids with weak muscles and redundant skin which cause dependence on forehead muscles to elevate the upper eyelids. In this situation, complication can be avoided by abstaining from botulinum toxin treatment altogether or performing an upper blepharoplasty prior to treatment with botulinum toxin.

Another reported complication is eyelid ptosis and diplopia, resulting when botulinum toxin diffuses to the levator palpebrae superioris [30]. In more severe cases, dry eye and eye pain can result when the toxin affects the innervation of the lacrimal gland via the petrosus major nerve [29]. Such complications have been shown to occur more commonly during therapeutic uses of botulinum toxin type A, such as in the treatment of blepharospasm, where higher doses of the botulinum toxin are injected as compared to cosmetic treatments [31]. Therefore, using lower doses and more dilute concentrations of a botulinum toxin A formulation may reduce complications [32]. If a patient develops ptotic or droopy eyelid, one treatment used by plastic surgeons is Iopidine® (apraclonidine 0.5%) eye drops. Iopidine® is an α2-adrenergic agonist that is indicated for glaucoma patients needing intraocular pressure reduction. It is also effective as a short-term treatment for eyelid ptosis by contracting Müller's muscle, which helps elevate the upper eyelid. At our institute, we recommend applying one or two drops to the affected eye three times daily until ptosis resolves.

In the lower face, one particular complication is partial lip ptosis, after administration of botulinum toxin to the periocular region for treatment of crow's feet, caused by weakening of the zygomaticus major muscle [30]. Complications of botulinum toxin treatment in the lower face may result in an asymmetric smile, mouth incompetence, drooling, flaccid cheek, reduced proprioception, and difficulties in speech if the perioral muscles are overly paralyzed [33]. It is recommended that patients who depend on full function of the perioral muscles (i.e., musicians) not be treated with botulinum toxin in the lower face [33]. Potential complications of platysma band injection are dysphagia and neck weakness [34]; however, these complications require further investigation. Due to the variety of potential complications that exist, botulinum toxin injections demand a full understanding of each individual patient's face by the physician administering the treatment.

21.14 Long-Term Safety of Botulinum Toxin Type A

Botox® Cosmetic is one of the most widely studied drugs in history and has proven to have an excellent safety profile. Patients should be informed about the potential complications of botulinum toxin type A. However, they should also be made aware of the low probability of these effects and reminded that most adverse effects are slight and temporary. One study demonstrated long-term safety of botulinum toxin type A based on a retrospective analysis of 50 patients who had Botox® Cosmetic treatments for facial wrinkles for up to 9 years [35]. Less than 1% of the total 853 sessions in this 9 year period resulted in a treatment-related unfavorable outcome [34]. Of these events, five were determined to be treatment-related [35]. Therefore, a substantial amount of research and clinical experience supports the safety and effectiveness of Botox® Cosmetic as a noninvasive cosmetic procedure. Dysport® has also demonstrated to be an efficacious and safe treatment for the upper face, but there is less data on Dysport® as it has just recently been approved by the FDA.

21.15 Conclusions

Botox® Cosmetic has been hailed a miracle drug due to its good safety profile, low incidence of treatment failures, and remarkable age-defying results. As the most common, minimally invasive cosmetic procedure in the year 2008, the Botox® Cosmetic treatments have been very popular. With a new competitor on the scene, Dysport®, the demand for these two products will continue to rise. Thus, it will be critical for the plastic surgeon to have a good understanding of facial anatomy and the wrinkles caused by various facial muscles in order to provide reasonable surgical and nonsurgical treatment options. Furthermore, it will become increasingly necessary for the plastic surgeon to be equipped with a thorough knowledge of botulinum toxin's basic science, new formulations, and the most recent literature concerning its administration in order to be at the frontline of competing botulinum toxin treatments as well as avoid complications and deliver maximal aesthetic results to patients.

References

1. American Society of Plastic Surgeons. ASPS 2008 statistics on cosmetic minimally-invasive procedures. Available at http://www.plasticsurgery.org/Media/stats/2008-US-cosmetic-reconstructive-plastic-surgery-minimally-invasive-statistics.pdf. Accessed on 13 Jul 2009.
2. Scott AB. Development of botulinum toxin therapy. Dermatol Clin. 2004;22(2):131–3.
3. Scott AB, Rosenbaum A, Collins C. Pharmacologic weakening of extraocular muscles. Invest Ophthalmol. 1973;12(12):924–7.
4. Adelson RT. Botulinum neurotoxins: fundamentals for the facial plastic surgeon. Am J Otolaryngol. 2007;28(4):260–6.
5. Carruthers A, Carruthers J. History of the cosmetic use of botulinum A exotoxin. Dermatol Surg. 1998;24(11):1168–70.
6. FDA approves Dysport® for therapeutic and aesthetic uses [press release]. Available at http://www.dysport.com/inthenews.html. Accessed 29 Jun 2009.
7. Thakker MM, Rubin PA. Pharmacology and clinical applications of botulinum toxins A and B. Int Ophthalmol Clin. 2004;44(3):147–63.
8. Hauser RA, Wahba M. Botox® Injections. Available at http://emedicine.medscape.com/article/1271380-overview. Accessed 26 Jun 2009.
9. Rohrich RJ. Advances in facial rejuvenation: botulinum toxin type A, hyaluronic acid dermal fillers, and combination therapies–consensus recommendations. Plast Reconstr Surg. 2008;121 Suppl 5:5S–30S.
10. Aoki KR, Guyer B. Botulinum toxin type A and other botulinum toxin serotypes: a comparative review of biochemical and pharmacological actions. Eur J Neurol. 2001;8 Suppl 5:21–9.
11. Das Gupta BR, Sugiyama H. Role of protease in natural activation of Clostridium botulinum neurotoxin. Infect Immun. 1972;6(4):587–90.
12. Dolly JO, Black J, Williams RS, Melling J. Acceptors for botulinum neurotoxin reside on motor nerve terminals and mediate its internalization. Nature. 1984;307:457–60.
13. Pellizzari R, Rossetto O, Schiavo G, Montecucco C. Tetanus and botulinum neurotoxins: mechanism of action and therapeutic uses. Philos Trans R Soc Lond B Biol Sci. 1999;354:259–68.
14. Stecher B, Weller U, Habermann E, Gratzl M, Ahnert-Hilger G. The light chain but not the heavy chain of botulinum type A toxin inhibits exocytosis from permeabilised adrenal chromaffin cells. FEBS Lett. 1989;255:318–25.

15. Matarasso A, Deva AK. Botulinum toxin. Plast Reconstr Surg. 2002;109:1191–7.
16. Das Gupta BR, Sugiyama H. Molecular forms of neurotoxins in proteolytic Clostridium botulinum type B cultures. Infect Immun. 1976;14(3):680–6.
17. Allergan, Inc. Botox® Cosmetic [botulinum toxin type A) purified neurotoxin complex (Package Insert). Irvine: Allergan; 2008.
18. Carruthers J, Faigen S, Matarrasso SL. Consensus recommendations of the use of botulinum toxin type A in facial aesthetics. Plast Reconstr Surg. 2004;114(Suppl):1S–22S.
19. Hexsel DM, de Almeida AT, Rutowitsch M, et al. Multicenter, double-blind study of the efficacy of injections with botulinum toxin type A reconstituted up to six consecutive weeks before application. Dermatol Surg. 2003;29(5):523–9.
20. Markey AC. Dysport®. Dermatol Clin. 2004;22(2):213–9.
21. Dysport® [package insert]. Scottsdale: Medicis Aesthetics; 2009.
22. Mclellan K, Das RE, Ekong TA, Sesardic D. Therapeutic botulinum type A toxin: factors affecting potency. Toxicon. 1996;34(9):975–85.
23. Critchfield J. Considering the immune response to botulinum toxin. Clin J Pain. 2002;18(Suppl):S133–41.
24. Nussgens Z, Roggenkamper P. Comparison of two botulinum-toxin preparations in the treatment of essential blepharospasm. Graefes Arch Clin Exp Ophthalmol. 1997;235:197–9.
25. Odergren T, Hjaltason H, Kaakkola S, et al. A double blind, randomised, parallel group study to investigate the dose equivalence of Dysport® and Botox® in the treatment of cervical dystonia. J Neurol Neurosurg Psychiatry. 1998;64(1):6–12.
26. Sampaio C, Costa J, Ferreira JJ. Clinical comparability of marketed formulations of botulinum toxin. Mov Disord. 2004;19 Suppl 8:S129–36.
27. Lowe P et al. Comparison of two formulations of botulinum toxin type A for the treatment of glabellar lines: a double-blind, randomized study. J Am Acad Dermatol. 2006;55(6):975–80.
28. Sarifakioglu N, Sarifakioglu E. Evaluating the effects of ice application on the pain felt during botulinum toxin type-A injections; a prospective, randomized, single-blind controlled trial. Ann Plast Surg. 2004;53(6):543–6.
29. Frankel AS, Markairian A. Cosmetic treatments and strategies for the upper face. Facial Plast Surg Clin North Am. 2007;15(1):31–9.
30. Ferreira MC, Salles AG, Gimenez R, et al. Complications with the use of botulinum toxin type A in facial rejuvenation; report of 8 cases. Aesthet Plast Surg. 2004;28(6): 441–4.
31. Cote TR, Mohan AK, Polder JA, et al. Botulinum toxin type A injections: adverse events reported to the US Food and Drug Administration in therapeutic and cosmetic cases. J Am Acad Dermatol. 2005;53(3):407–15.
32. Bennett JD, Miller TA, Richards RS. The use of Botox® in interventional radiology. Tech Vasc Interv Radiol. 2006;9(1): 36–9.
33. Carruthers J, Carruthers A. Complications of botulinum toxin type A. Facial Plast Surg Clin North Am. 2007;15(1):51–4.
34. Niamtu J. Complications in fillers and Botox®. Oral Maxillofac Surg Clin North Am. 2009;21(1):13–21.
35. Klein AW, Carruther A, Fagien S, Lowe NJ. Comparisons among botulinum toxins: an evidence-based review. Plast Reconstr Surg. 2008;121(6):413–22.

History of Fat Transfer

Melvin A. Shiffman

22.1 Introduction

The history of autologous fat augmentation gives insight into the development of fat transfer for both cosmetic and non-cosmetic problems. Transplantation of pieces of fat and occasionally diced pieces of fat advanced to removal of small segments of fat by liposuction after the development of technique by Fischer and Fischer reported in 1975.

22.2 History

Neuber [1] reported the use of small pieces of fat from the upper arm to reconstruct a depressed area of the face resulting from tuberculosis osteitis. He concluded that small pieces of fat, bean or almond size, appeared to have a good chance of survival. Czerny [2] used a large lipoma to fill a defect in the breast following resection of a benign mass. The transplanted breast, however, appeared darker in color and smaller in volume than the opposite breast. Verderame [3] observed that fat transplants solved the problem of shrinkage at the transplant site. Lexer [4] reported personal experience with fat transplants and found that larger pieces of fat gave better results. Bruning [5] used fat grafts to fill a post-rhinoplasty deformity by placing fat in a syringe and injecting the tissue through a needle.

Tuffier [6] inserted fat into the extrapleural space to treat pulmonary conditions. Biopsy of the fat 4 months post transplant showed most of the fat was resorbed and replaced by fibrous tissue.

Straatsma and Peer [7] used free fat grafts to repair postauricular fistulas and depressions or fistulas resulting from frontal sinus operations. Cotton [8] used a technique of broad undercutting and insertion of finely cut fat which was molded to fill defects.

Peer [9] noted that grafts the size of a walnut appear to lose less bulk after transplanting than do smaller multiple grafts. He also found that free fat grafts lose about 45% of their weight and volume 1 year or more following transplantation due to the failure of some fat cells to survive the trauma of grafting as well as the new environment. Fat grafts are affected by trauma, exposure, infection, and excessive pressure from dressings [10]. Peer [10] stated that microscopically, grafts appear like normal adipose tissue 8 months after transplantation.

Liposuction was conceived by Fischer and Fischer in 1974 [11] and put into practice in 1975 [12].

Fischer and Fischer [13] first reported removal of fat by means of 5 mm incisions using a "rotating, alternating instrument electrically and air powered." This allowed aspiration of fat through a cannula. Through a separate incision, saline solution was injected to dilute the fat. In 1977 [14] they reviewed 245 cases of liposuction with the "planotome" for treatment of cellulite in the lateral trochanteric areas. There was a 4.9% incidence of seromas despite wound suction catheters and compression dressings. Pseudocyst formation, which required removal of the capsule through a wider incision and the use of the planotome, occurred in 2% of cases.

The advent of liposuction spurred a move toward using the liposuctioned fat for reinjecting areas of the

M.A. Shiffman
17501 Chatham Drive,
Tustin, California 92780-2302, USA
e-mail: shiffmanmdjd@yahoo.com

body for filling defects or augmentation. Bircoll [15] first reported the use of autologous fat from liposuction for contouring and filling defects. Illouz [16] claimed he began to inject aspirated fat in 1983. Johnson [17] stated that he began in 1983 to use autologous fat injection for contouring defects of the buttocks, anterior tibial area, lateral thighs, coccyx area, breasts, and face. Bircoll [18] presented the method of injecting fat that had been removed by liposuction. Krulig [19] asserted that he began to use fat grafts by means of a needle and syringe. He called the procedure "lipoinjection." He began to use a disposable fat trap to facilitate the collection process and to ensure the fat's sterility. Newman [20] stated that he began reinjecting fat in 1985. The idea of utilizing the aspirated fat, which was otherwise wasted, was an attractive idea and other surgeons began to make use of the aspirate to augment defects and other abnormalities.

The American Society of Plastic and Reconstructive Surgery (ASPRS) Ad-Hoc Committee on New Procdures produced a report on September 30, 1987, regarding autologous fat transplantation [21]. The conclusions were:

1. Autologous fat injection has a historical and scientific basis.
2. It is still an experimental procedure.
3. Fat injection has achieved varied results and long-term, controlled clinical studies are needed before firm conclusions can be made regarding its validity.
4. Fat transplant for breast augmentation can inhibit early detection of breast carcinoma and is hazardous to public health.

Coleman and Saboeiro [22] reported success in fat transfer to the breast and concluded that it should be considered as an alternative to breast augmentation and reconstruction procedures. Two of 17 patients had breast cancer diagnosed by mammography, one 12 months and one 92 months after fat transfer to the breast.

Now fat transfer to the breast area is being used outside the breast itself, into the pectoralis major muscle and behind and in front of the muscle. The fat is also being used to augment tissues around the breast following treatment for breast cancer.

Although most of the fat transfer procedures are for augmentation of tissues, there has been a surge of the use of fat for non-cosmetic procedures.

References

1. Neuber F. Fettransplantation. Chir Kongr Verhandl Deutsche Gesellsch Chir. 1893;22:66.
2. Czerny V. Plastischer ersatz der brustdruse durch ein lipoma. Chi Kong Verhandl. 1895;2:126.
3. Verderame P. Ueber fettransplantation bei adharenten knochennarben am orbitalrand. Klin Monatsbl Augenh. 1909; 47:433–42.
4. Lexer E. Freie Fettransplantation. Deutsch Med Wochenschr. 1910;36:640.
5. Bruning P. Cited by Broeckaert TJ, Steinhaus J. Contribution e l'etude des greffes adipueses. Bull Acad Roy Med Belgique. 1914;28:440.
6. Tuffier T. Abces gangreneux du pouman ouvert dans les bronches: hemoptysies repetee operation par decollement pleuro-parietal; guerison. Bull Mem Soc Chir Paris. 1911; 37:134.
7. Straatsma CR, Peer LA. Repair of postauricular fistula by means of a free fat graft. Arch Otolaryngol. 1932;15:620–1.
8. Cotton FJ. Contribution to technique of fat grafts. N Engl J Med. 1934;211:1051–3.
9. Peer LA. The neglected free fat graft. Plast Reconstr Surg. 1956;18(4):233–50.
10. Peer LA. Loss of weight and volume in human fat grafts. Plast Reconstr Surg. 1950;5:217–30.
11. Fischer G. The evolution of liposculpture. Am J Cosmet Surg. 1997;14(3):231–9.
12. Fischer G. Surgical treatment of cellulitis. Third Congress International Academy of Cosmetic Surgery, Rome, 31 May 1975.
13. Fischer G. First surgical treatment for modeling body's cellulite with 35 mm incisions. Bull Int Acad Cosmet Surg. 1976;2:35–7.
14. Fischer A, Fischer G. Revised technique for cellulitis fat reduction in riding breeches deformity. Bull Int Acad Cosmet Surg. 1977;2(4):40–3.
15. Bircoll M. Autologous fat transplantation. The Asian Congress of Plastic Surgery, February 1982.
16. Illouz YG. The fat cell "graft": a new technique to fill depressions. Plast Reconstr Surg. 1986;78(1):122–3.
17. Johnson GW. Body contouring by macroinjection of autologous fat. Am J Cosmet Surg. 1987;4(2):103–9.
18. Bircoll MJ. New frontiers in suction lipectomy. Second Asian Congress of Plastic Surgery, Pattiyua, Thailand, February 1984.
19. Krulig E. Lipo-injection. Am J Cosmet Surg. 1987;4(2): 123–9.
20. Newman J, Levin J. Facial lipo-transplant surgery. Am J Cosmet Surg. 1987;4(2):131–40.
21. American Society of Plastic and Reconstructive Surgery Committee on New Procedures. Report in Autologous Fat Transplantation, 30 Sep 1987. Plast Surg Nurs. 1987; Winter:140–1.
22. Coleman SR, Saboeiro AP. Fat grafting to the breast revisited: safety and efficacy. Plast Reconstr Surg. 2007;119(3): 775–85.

Role of Fat Transfer in Facial Rejuvenation

Anthony Erian

23.1 Introduction

Fat transfer (autologous fat grafting) has increased in popularity for soft tissue augmentation despite perceived drawbacks of unpredictable results. In facelifting and facial rejuvenation, it has improved the author's aesthetic results tenfold as it addresses the soft tissue loss and atrophy that accompanies aging that a standard facelift does not address (Fig. 23.1). This has many advantages over the list of injectables both permanent and nonpermanent on the market.

Fat grafting is a concept that existed since 1893. It gained popularity over last two decades with the development in liposuction techniques. It also gained recognition for being the natural approach to restore a youthful look to face. It can be performed as an isolated procedure or in conjunction with different types of facial rejuvenation surgical and nonsurgical procedures. Despite the clinical optimism associated with fat transfer, there remains an uncertainty among practitioners regarding the viability of transferred fat.

Fat transfer is known by variety of names, commonly used are fat transfer, fat injections, fat grafting, micro-lipoinjection, and autologous fat grafting. It is considered safe due to the autologous property and fat graft survival duration. Though it is more invasive and expensive than available semipermanent and permanent synthetic fillers, it has least reported complications and longer survivability.

The credit of introducing the concept of fat transfer goes to Neuber [1] who used a small piece of upper arm fat to augment the depression on a patient's cheek caused tuberculosis. In 1895, Czerny [2] reported breast augmentation by using a fatty tumor from the patient's lumbar region, or lower back, to a breast defect. The use of autogenous abdominal fat to correct deficits in the malar area and chin was reported in 1909 by Verderame [3]. In 1919, Marchand [4] reported that large central portion of grafted fat is nonviable by the tenth week, with proliferation from the peripheral fat.

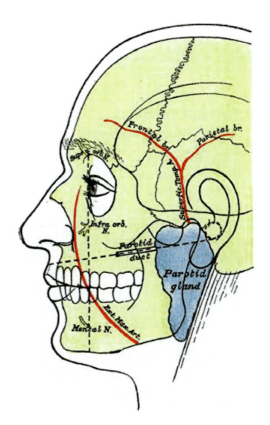

Fig. 23.1 Surface anatomy of trigeminal nerve branches and parotid duct

A. Erian
Pear Tree Cottage, Cambridge Road,
Wimpole 43, SG8 5QD Cambridge, United Kingdom
e-mail: plasticsurgeon@anthonyerian.com

His study was based on histological examination of the grafted tissue in humans. The idea of fat injection came into practice from 1920. Neuhof in 1923 [5] claimed that transplanted fat adopts the similar course as transplanted bone, that is, replacement of grafted fat with fibrous tissue or newly formed cells. In 1950, a publication by Peer [6] contradicted the findings of earlier publications regarding survival of grafted fat and believed that durable fat cell are more concentrated in the center. He also noted larger percentage of weight and mass loss in that grafts sectioned into multiple small segments than single autologous fat grafts of equal size.

With the innovation in techniques of liposuction in 1980s, the idea of fat transfer for facial rejuvenation readily flourished. Illouz [7] published the idea of the transfer of liposuction aspirate fat in 1984. Later Ellenbogen [8] introduced the technique of fat transfer popularized by the name of free pearl fat autografts in a variety of atrophic and posttraumatic facial deficits. Despite all the controversial reports regarding the survivability fat graft, the basic facts remain the same, that is, patient selection, comorbid factors, blood supply of recipient site, and safe and reliable technique. Despite the lack of hard evidence regarding the survivability and longevity of fat grafting it is still widely practiced procedure in the field of cosmetic surgery.

23.2 Relevant Anatomy and Pathophysiology

With refinements in technique, fat grafting has become the procedure of choice for an array of problems, including facial scarring, lip augmentation, and nasolabial fold and glabellar furrows). Although fat grafting and other types of grafting are still not perfect, they have come a long way.

The knowledge of anatomy is the key to any surgical procedure. A surgeon with sound anatomical knowledge can avoid certain iatrogenic complications related to the procedure. A detailed description of facial anatomy is beyond the scope of this chapter. However, one of the complications of fat transplant is injury to the nerves or other vital structure, namely, parotid duct.

Most anatomists agree that face has six layers, namely, skin, subcutaneous fat, SMAS (superficial musculoaponeurotic system), muscular layer, parotideomasseteric fascia, and retaining ligaments (zygomatic osteofasciocutaneous ligaments, mandibular osseocutaneous ligament and masseteric fasciocutaneous ligaments). The face is supplied mainly from branches of external carotid (facial and superficial temporal artery) and internal carotid arteries (ophthalmic artery). The venous drainage runs along arteries. The facial vein can communicate with cavernous sinus through ophthalmic vein or pterygoid plexus. The lymphatic drainage is mainly through superficial and deep cervical nodes.

The terminal branches of trigeminal nerve division's, that is, the supraorbital branch of the ophthalmic nerve, the infraorbital branch of the maxillary nerve, and the mental branch of the mandibular nerve emerge from corresponding foramina on the face (Fig. 23.1). A vertical line drawn from supraorbital foramen through the interval between the two lower premolar teeth will pass through infraorbital and mental foramina. The supraorbital foramina lies approximately 3 cm from midline. The infraorbital foramina lies 1 cm below infraorbital margin and the mental foramina lies midway between the upper and lower borders of the mandible in adults. In children, it lies near the lower border and near the upper border in older people.

The surface marking of the parotid duct is the horizontal line from the lower end of tragus to midway between the ala of nose and red margin of the lip (Fig. 23.1). The duct is 5 cm long and ends opposite the upper second molar tooth.

The facial nerve divides into five terminal branches, namely, temporal or frontal zygomatic, buccal, marginal mandibular, and cervical (Fig. 23.2). Among these, frontal and marginal mandibular are more at risk of

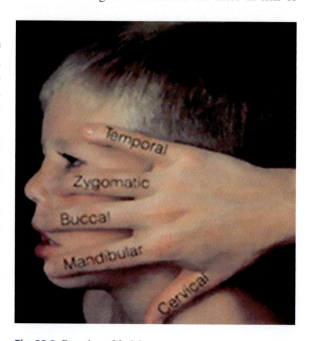

Fig. 23.2 Branches of facial nerve

injury. The frontal branch lies along the line drawn from infra-tragal notch to 1.5 cm above the lateral eyebrow. The zygomatic branch runs along zygomatic arch. The buccal branch runs along parotid duct. The mandibular (or marginal) division lies along the body of the mandible (80%) or within 1–2 cm below (20%). The marginal branch lies deep to the platysma along most of its course. Approximately, 2 cm lateral to oral commissure it becomes more superficial and ends on the under surface of the muscles. Injury to the marginal branch results in paralysis of the muscles that depress the corner of the mouth. The cervical branch supplies platysma and runs behind the posterior border of mandibular ramus. These nerves are likely to get injured when the fat graft is placed below the muscle or above periosteum.

23.3 Clinical Applications

There are six areas that are the best areas for fat transfer in the face (Table 23.1; Fig. 23.3).

Table 23.1 Areas that need fat

1. Trough area
2. Nasolabial
3. Marionette lines
4. Cheeks
5. Brows
6. Chin area

23.3.1 Harvesting the Fat

Under twilight anesthesia the area is marked from which fat would be taken. The commonest areas are:

1. Submental area during facelift.
2. Abdomen, upper and lower. The author prefers the upper abdominal area.
3. Outer or inner thighs.
4. Inner knee.
5. Sacral area.

The area is marked in black, the entry site in red, and the highest point of the fat in red.

Local infiltration is done using lignocaine with 1:200,000 adrenaline at the point of entry. Inject the area with tumescent infiltration about 20–30 ml depending on the amount of fat required to be removed. You will only need to aspirate 20–30 ml of fat (Fig. 23.4). With a sharp 15 blade make a puncture wound using a 10 ml syringe and a small aspiration cannula 2–3 mm (Fig. 23.5). Insert 1 ml of saline in the syringe and cannula to act as a buffer and remove

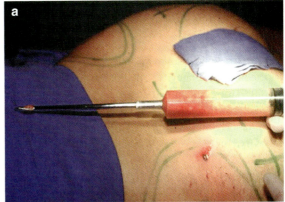
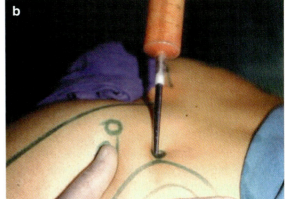

Fig. 23.4 Aspirate 20–30 ml of fat

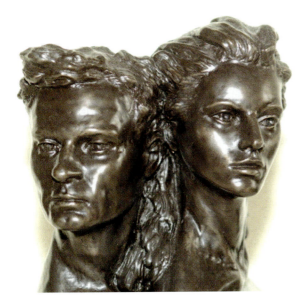

Fig. 23.3 Areas that need fat

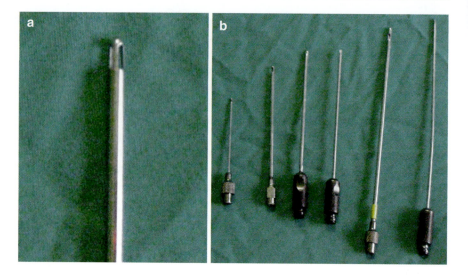

Fig. 23.5 (**a**) Mercedes cannula (**b**) collections of cannulae i use in different parts of neck

the dead space to minimize injury to the fat cell. Pull the plunger about 1 cm and you will get pure fat.

23.3.2 Preparation

The syringes are kept upside down in the rack for 10 min to remove all the excess blood and plasma oil, and then you are ready to inject (Fig. 23.6). The fat is not centrifuged or washed as there is no evidence that it prolongs its longevity. The author does not expose the fat to the open air and does not use additives to the fat like growth factors insulin or insulin growth factor igf-1 or any nutrients such as polyethylene glycol, or hyperbaric oxygen that has been used in some practices.

23.4 Applications and Injection Techniques

23.4.1 Injection Methods

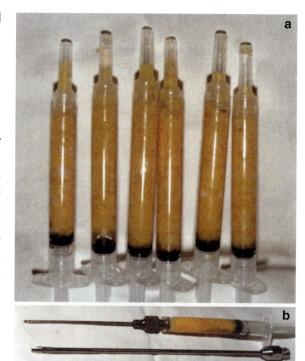
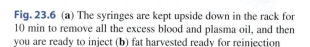

Fig. 23.6 (**a**) The syringes are kept upside down in the rack for 10 min to remove all the excess blood and plasma oil, and then you are ready to inject (**b**) fat harvested ready for reinjection

The techniques for fat injection have evolved but are currently based on the principle that fat survival is based on the proximity to a blood supply. It is believed that fat within 2 mm of an arterial supply will survive but fat placed beyond that distance will necrose and leave only scar tissue. Therefore, in an attempt to maximize the surface area of the graft that is in contact with vascularized tissue, many authors describe a "fanning-out" technique to lay down small particles of fat in multiple tunnels. Another important detail in the injection technique involves creating a tunnel on insertion and injecting only during withdrawal of the cannula (Fig. 23.7). There is variability with regard to cannula size and other alternative techniques believed to improve graft success. Many authors have described using a 14-gauge blunt tip or curved microcannula for injection, whereas others have used a 2–3 mm cannula for reinjection.

The common principle in the injection technique is to maximize the fat tissue surface area that is in contact with well-vascularized tissue. The author uses the "Pearl" technique by using droplets of fat in a multilayer fashion starting from the periosteum upward to avoid irregularity (Figs. 23.8–23.11).

23.5 Complications

Complications include swelling, lumpiness, infection, pain, discomfort, and unsatisfactory long-term results.

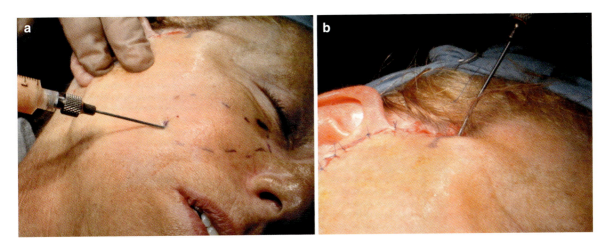

Fig. 23.7 Injection technique

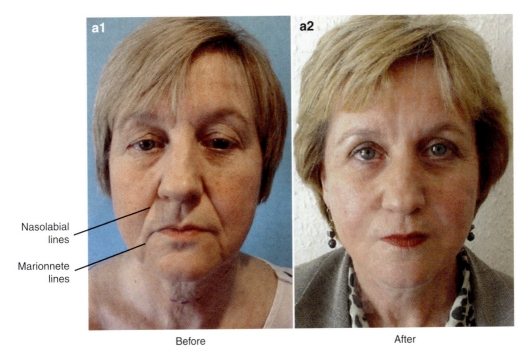

Fig. 23.8 Marionette lines. (**a**) Preoperative. (**b**) After fat transfer to nasolabial and marionnete lines

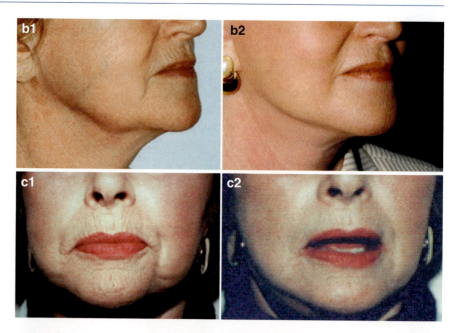

Fig. 23.8 (continued)

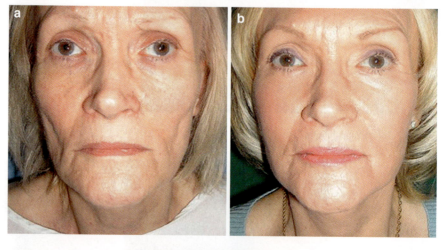

Fig. 23.9 Cheeks.
(**a**) Preoperative.
(**b**) After fat transfer

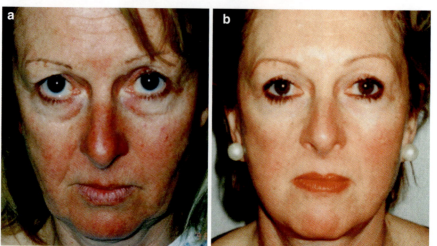

Fig. 23.10 Trough area.
(**a**) Preoperative.
(**b**) After fat transfer

Fig. 23.11 Brows and cheeks. (**a**) Preoperative. (**b**) After fat transfer

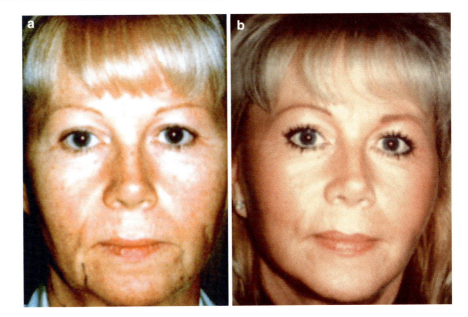

References

1. Neuber F. Fettransplantation. Chir Kongr Verhandl Dtsch Ges Chir. 1893;22:66.
2. Czerny V. Plastischer Ersatz der Brustdruse durch ein Lipom. Zentralbl Chir. 1895;27:72.
3. Verderame P. Ueber Fetttransplantation bei adharenten Knochennarben am Orbitalrand. Klin Monatsbl Augenheilkd. 1909;47:433.
4. Marchand F. Ueber die Veranderungen des Fettgewebes nach der Transplantation. Beitr Pathol Anat Allg Pathol. 1919;66:32.
5. Neuhof H. The transplantation of tissues. New York: D. Appleton & Co; 1923.
6. Peer LA. Loss of weight and volume in human fat grafts: with postulation of a "cell survival theory. Plast Reconstr Surg. 1950;5:217–30.
7. Illouz YG. L'avenir de la reutilization de la graisse apres liposuccion. Rev Chir Esthet Lang Franc. 1984;9:36.
8. Ellenbogen R. Free autogenous pearl fat grafts in the face – a preliminary report of a rediscovered technique. Ann Plast Surg. 1986;16(3):179–94.

Cosmetic Surgical Rejuvenation of the Neck

L. Angelo Cuzalina and Colin E. Bailey

24.1 Introduction

The history of neck rejuvenation began with simple skin excision and then progressed to modification of the platysma and the extraction of subcutaneous fat. Bourguet [1] described the first surgical platysmaplasty through a submental incision in 1928. In 1964, Aufricht [2] described a lateral plication of the platysma to the mastoid fascia. Other important concepts came from Connell's [3] work that demonstrated the need to modify subplatysmal structures such as bulging fat, ptotic submandibular glands, and prominent digastric muscles. In 1988 Feldman [4] described his corset platysmaplasty. This technique is now commonly used to flatten the submental plane and prevent a concave hollow after subplatysmal lipectomy. Of course, Klein's [5] development of tumescent anesthesia and influence on microcannular liposuction technique gave surgeons another tool to recontour the neck. This set the stage for Courtiss [6] to demonstrate that removal of submental fat with liposuction can, in the correct patient, redrape and recontour the skin of the neck without redundancy.

Over the last decade there has been an exponential increase in the number of new nonsurgical procedures that are designed to rejuvenate the aging neck. Most of them are marketed as being minimally invasive with no down time, yet at the same time providing maximal safety and effectiveness. A popular example includes the use of radiofrequency energy for skin tightening [7]. Applying thermal energy to the dermis is thought to stimulate new collagen formation, which will ultimately result in skin contraction. Laser lipolysis represents another recent innovation that is believed to help with skin tightening through the application of thermal energy, while at the same time enhance the sculpting effect of liposuction. There are also claims that laser-assisted liposuction may provide for more rapid healing and patient recovery [8]. Even Botulinum Toxin Type A has been used to diminish the appearance of unsightly platysmal bands [9]. Another procedure that has received much attention in the realm of neck rejuvenation is mesotherapy. This involves the injection of strategically placed small doses of phosphatidylcholine and deoxycholate (with or without additional homeopathic ingredients) to dissolve fat [10]. While all of these procedures may have some role in neck rejuvenation it is clear that the literature supporting their efficacy and durability is not mature [11, 12]. Just as important is the fact that these procedures do not address the problems of bulging subplatysmal fat, or provide effective long-term solutions for age-related changes of the platysma and submandibular glands. Our goal in writing this chapter is to describe our approach to treating age-related changes of the neck. Even though these patients present with a wide variation of abnormalities, we will provide a simplified approach to stratify the patients to undergo either microcannular liposuction, or some form of submentoplasty, with or without rhytidectomy (Fig. 24.1). The authors have found that an excellent aesthetic outcome that is durable can consistently be provided.

L.A. Cuzalina (✉)
Tulsa Surgical Arts, 7316 East 91st Street,
Tulsa, OK 74133, USA
e-mail: angelo@tulsasurgicalarts.com

C.E. Bailey
Bailey Cosmetic Surgery and Vein Centre,
1075 Nichols Road, Street 5,
Osage Beach, MO 65065, UK
e-mail: cebailey@baileyveinandskincare.com

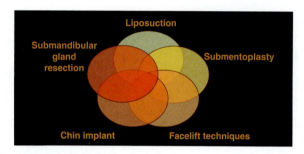

Fig. 24.1 A cosmetic surgeon must have a thorough knowledge of all options in neck surgery to determine what is the best treatment plan for maximum aesthetic results

24.2 Patient Assessment

Prior to any surgical procedure, taking an accurate and focused history along with the performance of an appropriate physical exam is essential. During this time one must develop a clear understanding of the patient's concerns while simultaneously establishing whether the patient has realistic expectations. As with all cosmetic procedures, reviewing pictures from when the patient felt like they looked their best can be helpful. During the physical exam on cosmetic surgery patients it is very easy to focus on the aesthetic concerns and forget that occasionally a coexistent pathologic abnormality may be present. The physician who evaluates a patient for contour irregularities of the neck or submental fullness must remember that pathologic processes either benign or malignant within the thyroid, salivary glands and or lymph nodes are possible. Suspicious lesions should be dealt with appropriately. Once the physician is certain that there are no pathologic changes he or she should feel comfortable proceeding with the aesthetic evaluation.

The first thing to evaluate is the patient's skin and its tone. A study by Gryskiewicz [13], stated that the most accurate predictor of poor skin retraction with cervicofacial liposuction is the presence of a crepe paper skin texture, which is characterized by a crisscross pattern of fine creases. This is thought to represent a loss of dermal skin elasticity (Fig. 24.2). The most dramatic skin retraction after closed cervicofacial liposuction is seen in patients younger than 40 (Fig. 24.3). Patients in the age group of 60 and above can however see very pleasing results with this technique if they have adequate skin tone. Another limiting factor in achieving an excellent result with cervicofacial liposuction is the amount of

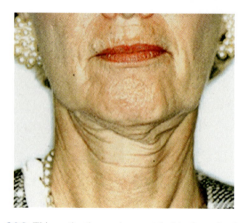

Fig. 24.2 This patient's cervicomental skin has clearly lost dermal elasticity and will not respond well to liposuction even if excess adipose tissue was present. She is an ideal candidate for a basic facelift

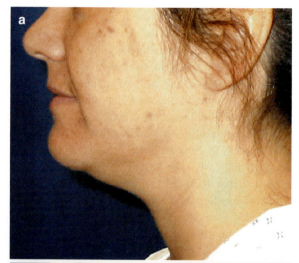

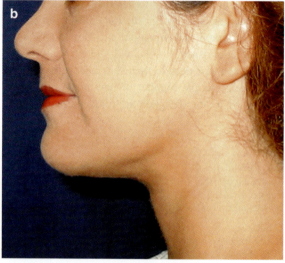

Fig. 24.3 (**a**) Preoperative 27-year-old female. (**b**) One year postoperative following basic microcannular liposuction superficial to the platysma. This is a good example of a Type I neck that is ideal for liposuction only

Fig. 24.4 (*Left*) Preoperative 37-year-old. (*Right*) Two months postoperative following aggressive submentoplasty. Significant subplatysmal fat was directly excised under fiber optic illumination. No liposuction was performed until the entire flap was elevated to maintain adequate fat on the skin for redraping

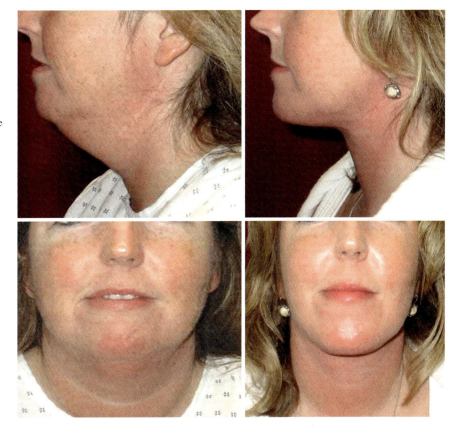

subplatysmal fat that is present. Determining precisely how much subplatysmal fat is present can be difficult. One technique is for the surgeon to pinch the skin gently with his or her fingers, and the observed residual fullness in the neck represents subplatysmal fat. Little has noted that if the submental tissue moves up and down with swallowing then the bulk of the tissue is subplatysmal [14]. Patients with very obtuse cervical-mental angles almost always have significant subplatysmal fat. Also, patients with extremely heavy necks typically have the majority of fat stored in the subplatysmal space (Fig. 24.4). Subplatysmal fat tends to be more firm and fibrous than preplatysmal fat and is more resistant to liposuction. In addition, access to the subplatysmal space with closed liposuction is potentially dangerous making and open approach preferable. Therefore, submentoplasty is necessary to rejuvenate the neck with significant subplatysmal fat (Fig. 24.5). Next, we assess chin projection while viewing the patient laterally. In females the chin should just touch or be no more than 2 mm behind an imaginary line that is perpendicular to Frankfurt's line. This perpendicular line runs vertically through

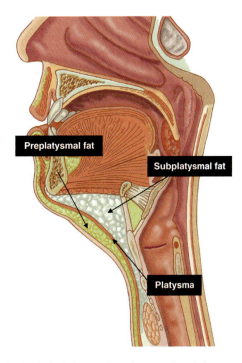

Fig. 24.5 Limited degree of cervicomental angle improvement that would be possible if only preplatysmal fat underwent liposuction and the subplatysmal fat was not addressed in a patient with an obtuse chin–neck angle

Fig. 24.6 The horizontal line demonstrates "Frankfurt Horizontal" (FH), which should be maintained parallel with the floor. Two perpendicular lines from FH can be used to estimate the need and size of chin implant required. The ideal position for most females is just behind the lower lip vermillion border

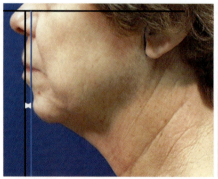
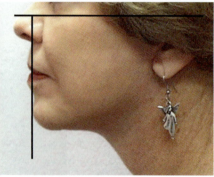

Size of chin implant needed estimated   6 months past chin implant & facelift

the vermillion border of the lip (Fig. 24.6). For men, the chin should touch the vertical line or project up to 2 mm beyond. At this point one should also try to determine the level of the hyoid/thyroid complex. Usually, it resides at the C4 level. A normal, aesthetically pleasing cervicomental angle is 105°–120° [15]. When the hyoid/thyroid complex is low, an obtuse cervicomental angle is created which limits the final aesthetic outcome that can be achieved. Sometimes, one can improve the appearance of an obtuse neck with the placement of a chin implant. The most important reason to recognize a low hyoid/thyroid complex is to counsel the patient regarding this finding, thus ensuring that the patient has realistic expectations regarding the outcome of the procedure.

Another common finding in the aging neck is platysmal banding. With age, the thickness of this muscle diminishes as does its tone. The resultant laxity along with midline atrophy appears as platysmal banding. When seen in the midline, the bands represent the dehiscence of the medial edges of the platysma. Although the bands may have developed some laxity they are still capable of contracting and have some static tone. This is demonstrated by the fact that they become less noticeable when injected with strategically placed botulinum toxin Type A. When evaluating the platysma, it is important to remember that platysmal bands are often not seen with the patient in repose. Asking the patient to animate and contract their platysma with a grimace may give one a better view of platysmal banding. If one does not see platysmal banding at rest and only with animation, removal of subcutaneous fat will leave them exposed. Therefore, these patients are not ideally suited for liposuction alone. Other contour irregularities that patients find displeasing include jowling, ptotic submandibular glands, and prominent digastric muscles. The ideal treatment for significant jowling is cervicofacial rhytidectomy and patients need to be appraised of this fact. Mild improvement can be achieved via submentoplasty and microcannular liposuction although one needs to stay superficial with suctioning to decrease the chance of marginal mandibular nerve injury. If submandibular gland ptosis is noted within the submental triangle one must decide whether resection is warranted. Prominent digastric muscles also need to be recognized during the initial patient evaluation. While subtotal resection is an option to deal with prominent digastric muscles the authors have been less satisfied with the results and have abandoned the technique because of unacceptable scarring, fibrosis, and contour irregularities. One should focus on not removing too much fat in this area. In addition, it is important to have an appropriate preoperative discussion with the patient regarding realistic expectations when prominent digastrics are present. Finally, one should also evaluate the patient for asymmetry and include these findings in the discussion.

There are several classification schemes that one can use to categorize a patient's neck for surgical rejuvenation. Dedo's [16] Type I–VI classification is often quoted and is useful, but we find that most patients can easily fit into several different classes using this approach. The authors' simplified classification matches physical exam findings with the appropriate operative procedure(s). It also takes into account the need for chin implant, orthognathic surgery, and submandibular gland treatment.

24.3 Cuzalina and Bailey Cosmetic Neck Classification

Type I – Liposuction only (patient has good skin tone, minimal subplatysmal fat, no platysmal banding, normal submandibular glands, and minimal to no jowling)

Type II – Submentoplasty with or without liposuction (Patient has fair skin tone, subplatysmal fat bulging, and/or platysmal banding with minimal to no jowling.)

Type III – Rhytidectomy only (Patient has jowling and neck laxity with or without significant preplatysmal fat and the platysma has minimal laxity.)

Type IV – Rhytidectomy with submentoplasty with or without liposuction (Patient has significant jowling, facial cutis laxis, and either major platysmal banding or heavy subplatysmal fat for submentoplasty.)

Types I–IV may be followed by the letters A, B, or C. (A) The patient has microgenia or retrognathia and requires a chin implant or orthognathic surgery, (B) The patient has submandibular gland excessive fullness and may require submandibular gland resection, (C) The patient has a low hyoid position or obtuse chin neck angle and may have limited improvement capability that requires counseling (Fig. 24.7).

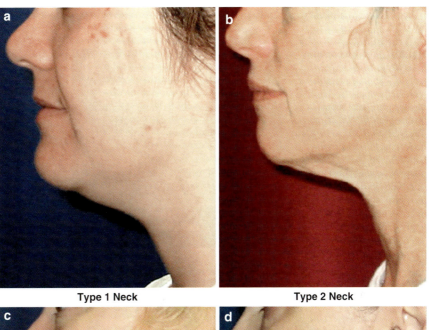

Fig. 24.7 Cuzalina and Bailey cosmetic neck classification. The four common neck classifications based on procedures required. (**a**) Type I requires liposuction only. (**b**) Type II is best treated with submentoplasty alone. (**c**) Type III can be treated with a facelift alone. (**d**) Type IV requires a facelift and submentoplasty combined. Subclassification A, B, and /or C can be added, where A represents chin weakness, B represents submandibular gland fullness, and C represents a low hyoid position

Therefore a patient listed as Type IV AB would be a patient who requires a facelift with submentoplasty, chin implant along with submandibular gland resection (Fig. 24.8).

The goals in rejuvenation of the aging neck are:

1. To restore a more youthful cervicomental angle
2. To redrape and tighten the skin within the cervical/submental region
3. To eliminate or decrease platysmal banding
4. To correct any deficiency in chin projection
5. To correct or improve skin laxity
6. To enhance the length and sharpness of the mandibular border
7. To soften or eliminate any contour irregularities associated with aging and fatty changes

24.4 Anatomy

When performing submentoplasty or submental liposuction one must have an understanding of some key anatomic features of the neck in order to avoid complications and ensure an aesthetic outcome. The platysma (Greek for flat object or plate) is a vestigial muscle that originates in the fascia of the pectoralis major and inserts above the inferior border of the mandible. It is innervated by the lateral cervical nerves. Cadaver dissections by Cardoso de Castro [17] have demonstrated that there is a decussation in the midline in 75% of people (Fig. 24.9).

With age, fat can accumulate above the platysma and below. The fat above the platysma is easily removed

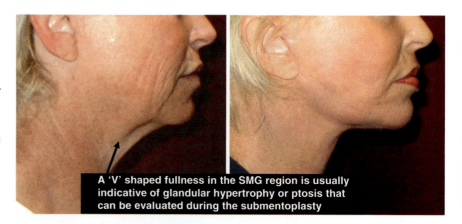

Fig. 24.8 (*Left*) Preoperative 57-year-old. (*Right*) Three months following a facelift with submentoplasty, chin implant and partial submandibular gland (SMG) resection. The patient has a Type IV AB neck. Type IV necks require both a facelift and submentoplasty because of both extreme skin laxity, jowling and platysmal laxity. Subtype A indicates a weak chin and B implies SMG excess

A 'V' shaped fullness in the SMG region is usually indicative of glandular hypertrophy or ptosis that can be evaluated during the submentoplasty

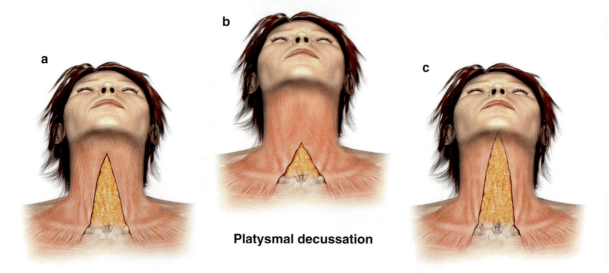

Fig. 24.9 (**a**) Type I: 75% of patients have limited decussation of the platysma extending 2–3 cm below the mandibular border. (**b**) Type II: 15% of patients demonstrate decussation of the platysma from the mandibular border to the thyroid cartilage. (**c**) Type III: 10% of patients demonstrate no decussation of the platysma

with liposuction. Subplatysmal fat is more fibrous and is slightly whiter in color. In the cheek area the superficial musculoaponeurotic system (SMAS) is its equivalent. This fat is more efficiently removed via sharp or electrocautery dissection. Below the subplatysmal fat the anterior digastric and mylohyoid muscles are visible. Within the subplatysmal space one will also encounter the anterior jugular veins. When dissecting under the platysma one must be vigilant to avoid these veins as they may cause troublesome bleeding. The posterior border of the platysma often runs parallel and just in front of the external jugular vein. At this location the external jugular vein crosses the sternocleidomastoid muscle as the vein moves toward the central portion of the clavicle. The midline of the hyoid bone is the landmark used prior to making a back-cut to mobilize the platysma. The hyoid also marks the inferior limit of platysmal resection in most cases. Submandibular glands are located underneath a layer of cervical fascia in the subplatysmal space lateral to the lateral border of the anterior digastric muscle. A more detailed description of this anatomy will be provided in the section on submandibular gland resection.

An important nerve that is most at risk for injury during submentoplasty or liposuction of the neck is the marginal mandibular nerve branch of the facial nerve. Injury to this nerve results in weakness of the ipsilateral lower lip depressor muscles (depressor labii inferioris, mentalis, and depressor anguli oris). The nerve leaves the anteroinferior edge of the parotid gland and runs deep to the platysma as either one main nerve trunk (40%) or as two branches (50%) or as three to four branches (10%) and then travels either above or below the mandible. Occasionally, the nerve runs 1–2 cm below the mandibular border shortly after exiting the parotid but proceeds back above the border of the mandible at the antegonial notch as it crosses over the facial artery. Baker and Conley wrote that in their clinical experience the nerve is usually 1–2 cm below the lower mandibular border but can be as much as 3–4 cm below it [18]. Dingman and Grabb noted in their cadaver series that posterior to the facial artery the nerve passed above the inferior mandibular border in 81% of dissections. Anterior to the facial artery all of the marginal mandibular nerve branches innervating the mouth depressors passed above the lower border of the mandible [19]. Approximately 2 cm from the lateral corner of the mouth the nerve becomes more superficial and enters the undersurface of the depressors [20, 21, 22].

24.5 Liposuction

Upon completion of the patient's aesthetic analysis a decision can be made to proceed with liposuction alone or in combination with submentoplasty or with submentoplasty and rhytidectomy. The most suitable patient for isolated submental and cervical liposuction has no platysmal banding, (at rest or with animation) minimal subplatysmal fat, no jowling and excellent skin tone. In addition, the ideal patient will have a good hyoid/thyroid position and a lack of submandibular gland ptosis.

In the past, surgeons used large spatulated cannulas and sought to remove as much fat as possible. This often lead to pleasing early results but in some cases significant scarring, contour irregularities, and even a skeletonized look resulted with the passage of time. The authors approach is to use microcannulas of approximately 2–3 mm in size. These smaller cannulas facilitate the sculpting process and decrease the likelihood of contour irregularities. Our goal is to leave a uniform 4–5 mm of fat behind.

Recently laser lipolysis using YAG (yttrium–aluminum–garnet) technology has become popular. The technology continues to evolve with different manufacturers claiming the benefits of different wavelengths. The touted benefits include better skin retraction, less bleeding and bruising, and a shorter recovery time.

The goal of this technique is to use laser energy to emulsify the fat prior to suctioning while heating the dermis which also may aid in skin contraction. The authors have used both 1,320 and 1,064 nm wavelengths and feel that there may be some benefit in small areas such as the neck. Much more needs to be learned about laser lipolysis. Specifically, what is the optimal wave length and ideal amount of energy delivery needed for collagen tightening while at the same time avoiding injury? The technology is further limited by its substantial cost. Presently, we look forward to the publication of definitive studies. Essentially the most important thing required to achieve an excellent neck contouring result in the Type I patient is superb skills with microcannular liposuction and the ability to choose the correct patient.

24.6 Tumescent Anesthesia

Tumescent anesthesia was developed by Cosmetic Dermatologist Jeffrey Klein in 1985. Essentially Klein demonstrated that when dilute lidocaine solution is combined with Epinephrine; liposuction can be safely performed under local anesthesia. Since that time Tumescent anesthesia has been incorporated into virtually every aspect of cosmetic surgery. The power of the technique is that it is safe, while at the same time providing profound long lasting anesthesia with a marked reduction in blood loss. This fact makes tumescent anesthesia useful with general anesthesia as well as with sedation or as a stand-alone technique. A review of the Physicians' Desk Reference will show that the maximum safe dose of lidocaine is 7 mg/kg when used with epinephrine. This is actually an extrapolated dose limit that was established by a letter to the Food and Drug Administration in 1948 from Astra Pharmaceuticals. The letter stated that the safe dose for lidocaine "was probably the same as that for procainamide" [22].

Exhaustive and well-executed studies by Klein have demonstrated that the maximum safe dose for using dilute lidocaine with liposuction is 35 mg/kg [23]. Peak lidocaine levels occur 12–24 h after administration for body liposuction but may occur as early as 3–4 h after facial tumescent anesthesia because of the increased blood flow in the face. In a study of 20 patients receiving approximately 50 mg/kg, peak levels were less than 3.5 μg/ml. (The toxic threshold for lidocaine is 5 μg/ml) With the tumescent technique, studies have also shown that up to 4,000 ml of fat can be removed safely in one session [24]. When larger volumes of fat are removed the physiologic insult increases exponentially. Large volume liposuction is associated with potentially massive intravascular volume shifts and an increase in cardiac complications, deep venous thrombosis, and pulmonary embolism. Neck and facial liposuction is considered small volume liposuction and usually less than 100 ml of fat is removed.

Lidocaine's main effects are due to decreased conductance through the sodium channels which results in neural blockade and an antiarrhythmic effect. Lidocaine is hepatically metabolized and renally excreted, 10% of which is unchanged. Therefore, one should beware of the patient with undiagnosed liver disease such as a case of occult cirrhosis.

There are many drugs that may affect lidocaine metabolism. Any drug that is metabolized by the cytochrome P450 3A4 (CYP3A4) system can increase the likelihood of lidocaine toxicity. The most common drugs that will affect lidocaine degradation include the proton pump inhibitors, benzodiazepines (lorazepam is an exception), serotonin reuptake inhibitors (Zoloft, Prozac, Lexapro, Celexa, Paxil, etc.), macrolide antibiotics and calcium channel blockers. Ciprofloxacin, Beta blockers and protease inhibitors may also increase the likelihood of toxicity [25]. When one or more of these drugs is being used by a patient in whom we are performing liposuction on multiple body areas, our approach is to stop the drug 1–2 weeks prior to surgery.

The risk of lidocaine toxicity with cervical and submental liposuction should obviously be low. However, when multiple procedures are being performed with tumescent anesthesia it is important to remember that lidocaine levels may not peak until 12 h later. The authors routinely check their patients on the evening of surgery and are cognizant of the fact that this is when lidocaine toxicity symptoms may manifest. The symptoms of lidocaine toxicity include: nervousness, dysarthria, tinnitus, metallic taste, apprehension, dizziness, double vision, nausea, and vomiting. This can be followed by respiratory depression and seizures. Late manifestations include cardiac toxicity with bradycardia, hypotension, depressed contractility, cardiac conduction, and finally, cardiac collapse.

Epinephrine is an important component of tumescent anesthesia in that its alpha-1 agonist activity causes profound vasoconstriction. This markedly diminishes blood loss and bruising. The epinephrine also decreases the systemic absorption of lidocaine thereby reducing systemic toxicity [26]. A known side effect of epinephrine is tachyarrhythmia secondary to beta-1 agonist activity. In our experience, this is rarely seen in the doses used for submental liposuction. It has been shown that premedicating with the centrally acting alpha 2 agonist Clonidine can reduce the frequency of tachyarrhythmia's [27].

When one is performing liposuction under sedation only, it is important to add bicarbonate to the tumescent solution. Shifting the pH in an alkaline direction will markedly reduce the pain and discomfort that the patient experiences when the relatively acidic lidocaine is injected. The goal is to obtain a bicarbonate concentration of 10 meq/l [28]. For ease of use, an 8.4% solution of sodium bicarbonate is equivalent to 1 meq/ml.

24.7 Liposuction Technique

While standing or sitting the patient is marked with an indelible marker. This is an important step because once tumescent anesthesia has been infused and the patient is in the supine position the patients original landmarks will be obliterated. During marking, it is helpful to outline the mandibular border, the posterior neck margins and areas jowling. If an area does not need suctioning then it is marked in red. If a chin implant is to be performed, this area is outlined on the mandible and the location of the skin incision marked. Digital pictures are then taken in the AP, oblique, and lateral positions (Fig. 24.10). These photos are projected in the operating room for reference during the procedure. With the patient asleep, the face and neck are sterilely prepped and tumescent anesthesia is infused. The author's preferred tumescent solution for work in the face and neck area is: 30 ml of 2% lidocaine with 1.5 ml of 1:1,000 epinephrine in 500 ml of normal saline.

A Wells Johnson (T) pump or an HK Klein (T) pump is used to administer the tumescent solution to the submental region via a 22 gauge spinal needle. A total of 150–200 ml of tumescent solution is infused. The needle enters the skin at three sites. Just under each ear lobe and under the chin. Care is taken to stay above the SMAS and the platysma and out of the external jugular vein. One should also endeavor to avoid a "peau d'orange" appearance of the skin on areas that may be undermined. There are scattered reports of skin sloughing after rhytidectomy that are attributed to infusing too much tumescent too superficially, although we have not seen this problem. The access sites will ultimately be enlarged with a number 11 blade to allow entrance of our microcannulas. These locations allow for efficient and safe liposuction of the neck from multiple directions. Post procedure these access sites are not readily visible. The location of these access sites can easily be incorporated into the incisions for rhytidectomy, submentoplasty, and chin implantation. Following the infusion of tumescent anesthesia, the neck is the re-prepped and draped in a sterile fashion. Ideally, the surgeon should wait 15–20 min prior to initiating liposuction. This allows for maximal vasoconstriction and a slight detumescence of the tissue which facilitates the surgeon's ability to evaluate tissue thickness.

The goal of Type I isolated liposuction of the neck is to restore a more youthful, neck jaw angle. Just as important as removing fat from the neck and the submentum is the sculpting of the mandibular border. To accomplish this one should minimize any fat removal from the body of the mandible and focus on enhancing its shadow by removing fat below this area along the length of the mandible. One must beware however that if too much fat is removed in this area, the underlying submandibular glands and digastric muscles may become visible. Once the tumescent access sites have been enlarged with a number 11 blade a microcannula is introduced into the subcutaneous plane. With the patients neck carefully hyperextended, suctioning is initiated with a back and forth motion (Fig. 24.11). Care is taken to avoid penetration of the platysmal. It is also important to understand where the cannulas suction orifices are located to avoid "rasping" the dermis. To avoid dermal damage with its resultant scarring one must focus on keeping the cannula openings toward the platysma. With each passage of the cannula the surgeon must be sure of which plane the tip of the cannula resides. The depth of the cannula and the amount of fat removed is controlled with the flat portion of the nonworking hand. With increasing pressure against the skin and subcutaneous tissue, the cannula will be more efficient in its fat removal and can be directed deeper.

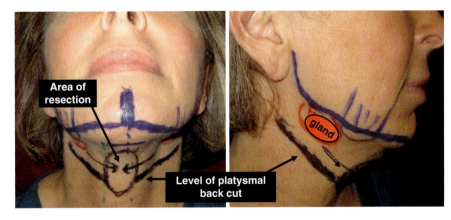

Fig. 24.10 Preoperative markings for submentoplasty demonstrating boundaries such as the mandibular border in *blue* along with the level for a platysmal back-cut if desired. The location of the submandibular gland and maximum jowling is also noted

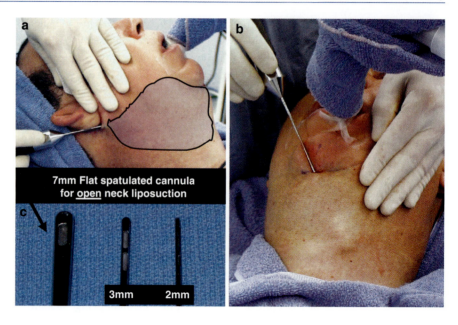

Fig. 24.11 Microcannulas are used for closed liposuction. (**a**, **b**) The three access sites are strategically located under each ear lobe and under the chin. (**c**) Flat spatulated cannula for open neck liposuction. (*Left*) 7 mm. (*Middle*) 3 mm. (*Right*) 2 mm

A smooth surface is developed by suctioning an area from multiple directions in multiple planes. After each pass of the cannula it is directed in a new location. Multiple passes in the same plane will cause irregularities that may not be correctable. The uniformity of the skin surface can be checked visually, and also by feel as one runs ones fingers over the area of interest. Thickness is determined by pinching the skin and subcutaneous layer with the fingers of both hands and comparing one area to another. Another technique is to lift the skin and subcutaneous tissue with the microcannula. Lumpiness will be seen along the length of the cannula if one has not evenly removed fat from this area. The goal is to leave about 5 mm of fat. If fat is removed to the point where the dermis is in contact with the platysma, scarring and retraction are possible long-term sequelae. This is a problem that is not immediately obvious and is very difficult to repair.

Despite the fact that liposuction of subplatysmal fat has been described in the literature we feel that subplatysmal fat removal requires surgical approach through an open submental incision. Clearly, blind liposuction in this area could be hazardous. When suctioning above the mandible in the jowl region, it is important to avoid approaching this area from the submental access site as this will put the facial nerve at risk. In the jowl area, aggressive liposuction is also a reason for marginal mandibular nerve injury. When suctioning the jowl area very little fat needs to be removed and it is easy to create a depression or asymmetry. One can consider using a 10 cc syringe for the source suction in this area and/or a cannula no bigger than 1.75 mm. Typically, only 4–10 ml of fat needs to be removed from each side. Precise measurement of the aspirated fat is easily achieved with this technique and it is more difficult to perform oversuction in the jowl as compared to using traditional aspiration device.

At the completion of the procedure the access sites are closed with a single 5/0 plain gut suture (Ethicon). Reston Foam® 15631 (3M Medical St. Paul Minnesota) is placed over the submental region (Fig. 24.12). It is important to ensure that the underlying skin is smoothly redraped in the neck area prior to dressing placement. Coban® Wrap (3M Medical-Surgical) is then wrapped around the submentum and head for 24 h. On postoperative day one the Coban is removed and a Hopping® neck lift bra is placed. This is worn 24 h each day for the first week and then only at night for the following 2 weeks.

24.8 Summary of Critical Points for Successful Liposuction

1. Proper patient selection is essential.
2. Preoperative markings should be precise.
3. Infiltrate tumescent anesthesia in a uniform manner.

Fig. 24.12 Submental Reston foam® dressing. A pressure head wrap is placed over the foam to add additional compression to close the potential dead space that is often most troublesome from isolated submentoplasty. The dressing is applied in an attempt to decrease the chance for a seroma

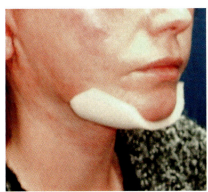
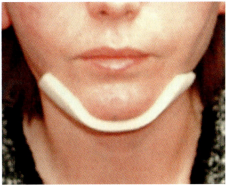

4. Avoid suctioning against the dermis (The cannula holes should be oriented toward the platysma.)
5. Place access sites for maximal cannula overlap and camouflage.
6. Use an appropriate amount of epinephrine in the neck. (The extensive blood supply of the face/neck results in a more rapid loss of vasoconstriction with a resultant bloodier aspirate and potentially an increased likelihood of bruising and seroma formation.)
7. Ensure that the fat is suctioned from multiple directions to decrease the likelihood of contour irregularities.
8. Beware of aggressive suctioning in the region of the marginal mandibular nerve. Consider syringe only suctioning in the region of jowling (4–10 cm^3/side) or, at least limit, the amount of suctioning in the jowl to avoid nerve injury or irregularities.
9. Leave a uniform layer of fat behind.
10. Avoid aggressive suctioning over the mandibular body. One should aggressively suction under this area in order to accentuate the mandibular shadow.

24.9 Chin Implantation

Alloplastic chin implantation is a simple procedure with minimal risk, and is easily reversible. Correcting even mild deficiencies in the chin projection can dramatically improve the patient's appearance. The lack of appropriate chin projection can be congenital or the result of the aging process as mandibular bone begins to resorb. Lack of projection may even be the result of both of these entities. As previously mentioned, the easiest technique to assess whether the patient has adequate anterior projection is to superimpose a line that is perpendicular to the Frankfurt horizontal line. The superimposed line should touch the vermillion border of the lower lip. The chin should ideally just touch this line or be no more than 2 mm posterior to it in females. This technique can also be used to estimate the implant size required preoperatively. Estimates of implant size can be made at the time of surgery using sizers, but patient positioning and tissue distortion from tumescent anesthesia may make intraoperative sizing difficult. Because of this the size of the implant is routinely determined prior to surgery.

The implant is placed through a 1 cm long submental incision if the implant is being placed without neck surgery. The incision must be moved 2–3 mm posterior to the submental crease when augmenting the chin. If the incision is not moved posteriorly the anterior pull of the implant will tend to make the scar visible. Prior to surgery, we determine where the midline of the mentum is and mark it. The authors also outline where we expect the implant to be positioned. Following skin incision electrocautery is used to dissect down to the periosteum of the mandible in the midline. Next, a subperiosteal pocket is created at the lower border of the mandible to the right and left of midline. The pockets should be adequate in length to accommodate the implant while avoiding overdissection so as to not affect implant stability. Care is taken not to injure the mental nerves. This can be achieved by ensuring that the dissection does not extend more than 8 mm above the mandibular border. The periosteal elevator should hug the inferior border of the mandible in the subperiosteal plane to maintain proper position. An Aufricht retractor can be used to help place the implant (Fig. 24.13). The silicone implant is then secured to the fascia at the inferior border of the mandible with a 2-0 Vicryl suture. Prior to securing the

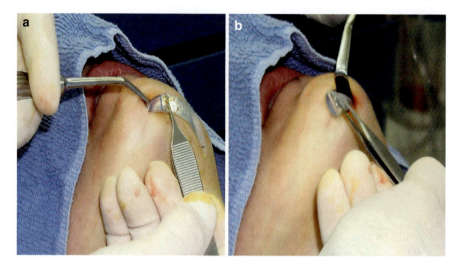

Fig. 24.13 Chin implant placement technique. (**a**) An Aufricht retractor is used facilitate passage of each limb of the chin implant into the subperiosteal tunnel. (**b**) After the first limb is placed the implant is folded to allow placement of the other limb. Care is taken to ensure that the lateral wings do buckle within the tunnel

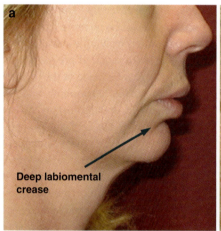
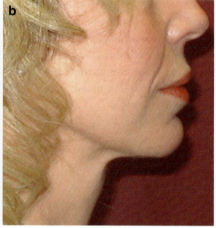

Fig. 24.14 (**a**) Thirty-nine-year-old female who has a Type II AC neck, which implies she is a candidate for an isolated submentoplasty [2] and has a weak mandible (A) and low-anterior hyoid (C). She also has a deep labiomental crease secondary to a deep bite and mandibular hypoplasia. A chin implant would worsen the LM fold. (**b**) Therefore, the patient was treated with a mandibular advancement and isolated submentoplasty to correct perioral rhtyids along with the challenging aesthetic neck problem

implant, it is important to ensure that the lateral wings of the implant have not folded over themselves. Also, it is important to ensure that the increased projection from the implant does not accentuate the depth of the labiomandibular sulcus (Fig. 24.14). If this is a problem one can modify the projection of the implant by shaving off some of its height with a number 15 blade. Mandibular deficiency with a deep bite is a common problem that can lead to a poor aesthetic outcome with a chin implant. Usually this problem requires orthognathic surgery for best results. Once the implant is positioned and secured the wound is closed in two layers with a 4–0 Vicryl deep suture and 5–0 plain gut suture for skin. It should be noted that an intraoral incision can be used for chin implantation but requires cutting the mentalis muscle and an increased risk of morbidity to the mental nerve.

24.10 Submentoplasty

This procedure is designed to treat age-related problems of the neck that cannot be dealt with by liposuction or rhytidectomy alone. It is often combined with rhytidectomy, although it can be very useful as a stand-alone procedure in the correct patient. The goal of submentoplasty is to treat platysmal banding, sculpt subplatysmal fat deposits, and finally, address cutis laxis of the neck. Additionally, ptotic submandibular glands can be treated via the submentoplasty incision, and jowling can be improved somewhat.

24.10.1 Submentoplasty Technique

In all patients, we endeavor to perform the procedure in a minimally invasive fashion. We find that there are very few patients who would require a direct excisional submentoplasty with its associated Z or W Plasty incision [29]. The authors would consider using this approach for the rare elderly male patient with extensive cutis laxis of the neck who is not a candidate medically or psychologically for rhytidectomy or general anesthesia.

During the initial evaluation of the patient, the position of the hyoid and length of the mandible are noted. For those patients who have a low hyoid, which results in an obtuse cervicomental angle, the authors will often recommend a chin implant which can create the illusion of a more acute and pleasing cervicomental angle postoperatively.

Type II (Submentoplasty with or without liposuction) (Fig. 24.15): Prior to making our submentoplasty incision, the neck is infiltrated with approximately 150 ml of tumescent fluid. Ideally, a 15 min waiting period is advised prior to beginning the dissection to allow for maximal vasoconstriction. During the infusion, care is taken to stay within the subcutaneous plane. It is not necessary to infiltrate the subplatysmal fat and this may, in fact, be dangerous. It is essential to leave an even layer of fat attached to the dermis if one wants to avoid unsightly skin irregularities after redraping.

The usual submentoplasty incision is 3 cm in length and is in the submental crease (unless a chin implant is placed). Once the submentoplasty incision is made, an electrocautery with a Colorado needle tip is used to achieve hemostasis and dissect into the plane between the platysma and the subcutaneous fat. Facelift scissors are then used to create a flap of skin with approximately 5 mm of fat attached to the dermis (Fig. 24.16). Closed liposuction is not preformed prior to submentoplasty because control of the thickness of the skin flap can be more precisely controlled using a combination of scissor dissection to elevate the flap and open liposuction under direct visualization. The dissection is extended to the posterior border of the mandible laterally and down to the inferior border of the thyroid cartilage. Care is taken to ensure that the dermis is not exposed or injured and that the undersurface of the flap is smooth. This type of wide undermining eliminates puckering and bunching of the skin and sets the stage for an aesthetic redraping of the skin once the problems with the underlying tissues have been dealt with. Next, we use a flat 7 mm spatulated cannula to liposuction the fat directly over the platysma under direct vision. Again the goal is to leave a smooth surface.

Visualization can be enhanced with a lighted tongue "sweetheart" retractor. The medial edges of the platysma are then identified and grasped with a hemostat or Kelly clamp. The surgeon has the option to resect lax platysma or perform a midline plication. If suture plication is used; the platysma must be healthy and thick or the patient will be at risk for relapse of

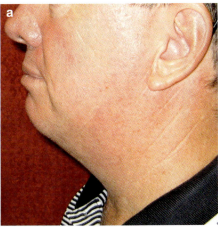 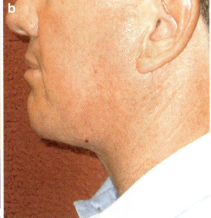

Fig. 24.15 (**a**) Preoperative 40-year-old male. (**b**) One month following an aggressive submentoplasty with subplatysmal fat excision, platysmal resection, and simultaneous chin implant. This is a good example of an obtuse chin neck angle and a diagnosis neck Type II AC

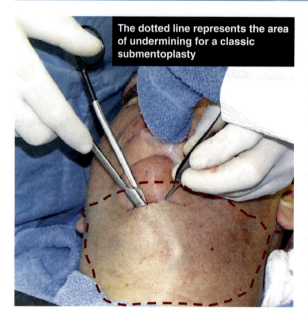

Fig. 24.16 Initial sharp scissor dissection for a submentoplasty from a submental crease incision "prior to" any liposuction in order to leave a uniform thickness (5–7 mm) of fat attached to the undersurface of the skin. A smooth fatty layer protecting the dermis is critical for avoiding fibrous and surface irregularities during liposuction, submentoplasty, or facelifting. The *dotted line* represents the area of undermining for a classic submentoplasty

because of dehiscence of the plication. The electrocautery with a Colorado tip is then used to resect the midline platysma and subplatysmal fat (Fig. 24.17). We make sure not to over-resect fat in this area as this may also lead to a displeasing midline contour postoperatively. It is in this region that the anterior jugular veins can cause problematic bleeding. Therefore, excellent visualization and precise resection of subplatysmal fat is essential. If bleeding is encountered, precise application of cautery or suture ligation will allow the operation to proceed. Once the midline fat has been resected, a decision is made as to how much tension will be present if a simple midline platysmal plication is performed. If tension is deemed excessive, we identify the hyoid and begin to back-cut the platysma at this level with the Colorado tip electrocautery. The incision extends approximately 5–7 cm in length and parallels the inferior border of the mandible. Extreme care is taken to avoid injury to nerves or vessels. Next, the platysma is undermined superiorly along the length of the back-cut. If submandibular gland ptosis is a concern, resection of the superficial lobe of the gland is performed at this time. Once the platysma has been dissected free bilaterally, a corset platysmaplasty can be performed. Beginning inferiorly, the medial platysmaplasty can be performed. The medial platysmal edges are sutured to the hyoid fascia with a 2–0 Monocryl suture (Fig. 24.18). A running suture is then used to further plicate the medial edges of the platysma in a cephalad direction. At the completion of the plication the surface of the platysma must be very smooth

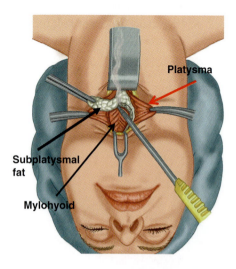

Fig. 24.17 Subplastysmal fat resection via submental incision

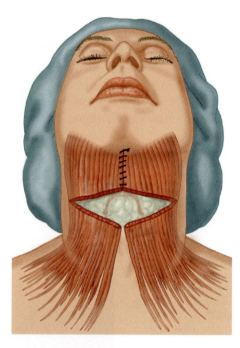

Fig. 24.18 Corset platysmaplasty showing the optional lateral back-cut at the level of the hyoid bone

Fig. 24.19 (*Left*) Preoperative 49-year-old female. (*Right*) Two months following a standard submentoplasty with no liposuction and only direct fat excision along with platysmal back-cutting and anterior advancement with corset plication starting at the hyoid. This is an example of a Type II neck

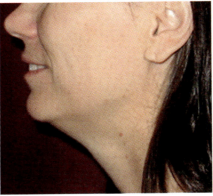
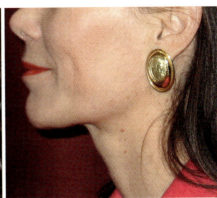

(Fig. 24.19). If a chin implant is to be used to help with deficient chin projection or a low hyoid position, the implant is placed at this time.

When patients present with an obese neck, with or without platysmal banding, we perform a more aggressive submentoplasty. The submentoplasty incision and scissor dissection proceeds in the same manner as described earlier. Again, extreme care is taken to leave a uniform layer of fat attached to the dermis that is approximately 5 mm in thickness. Open liposuction is performed under direct vision and submental fat excised in the midline. Next, lateral division of the platysma is performed at the level of the hyoid, and parallel to the inferior border of the mandible. At this point, instead of performing a corset platysmaplasty a larger amount of platysma is resected superior to this back-cut incision (Fig. 24.20). Patients with heavy difficult necks often have very thin platysma muscle that increases the likelihood of recurrence with only a midline corset plication. A more aggressive resection of the platysma allows properly debulking these heavy necks of sub- and preplatysmal fat that result in a much more refined aesthetic improvement. The deep tissues must be left with a smooth surface. Once the resection is complete, we can "fine tune" or sculpt the surface contour with judicious use of the electrocautery. With this kind of aggressive platysmal resection, it is also helpful to leave a slightly thicker layer of fat on the skin flap (5–7 mm). The technique is challenging but we find it to be a more aesthetically pleasing and durable result in those patients with a thick difficult neck (Fig. 24.21). Using this approach, we no longer worry about the late reappearance of midline paramedian platysmal bands resulting from the breakdown of a plicated

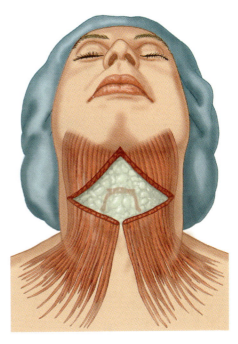

Fig. 24.20 A more aggressive platysmal resection. This technique is useful for heavier necks with extensive platysmal laxity

atretic platysma. Obviously, this type of aggressive resection of the platysma is not appropriate in the patient with a thin neck.

Type III (Rhytidectomy with or without liposuction): In patients with jowling and cutis laxis of the face with a thin neck, we proceed with rhytidectomy and rely on the posterior direction of pull to eliminate laxity in the neck and jowls (Fig. 24.22). When we have decided that cervicofacial liposuction is necessary with the facelift, the liposuction procedure is performed first. This can help to facilitate later flap dissection.

Fig. 24.21 (**a**) Preoperative 58-year-old female. (**b**) Six months following a facelift with aggressive submentoplasty. Her preoperative neck diagnosis would be classified as a Type IV C. Heavy necks like this are some of the most challenging to obtain consistent long-term and dramatic results

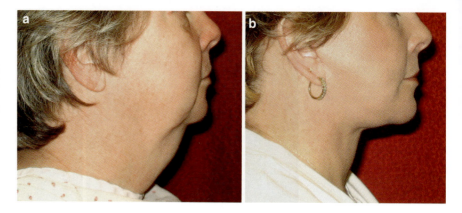

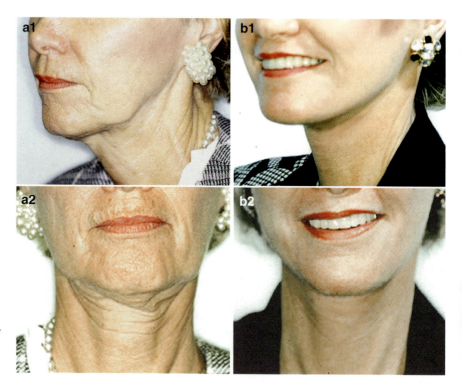

Fig. 24.22 (**a**) Preoperative patient has a classic Type III neck with minimal platysmal banding but severe skin laxity and jowling that responds well to a facelift only. (**b**) Postoperative

Type IV (Rhytidectomy and submentoplasty with or without liposuction): In neck rejuvenation, patients who present with jowling and significantly lax tissue below the mandible, a rhytidectomy will be needed along with a submentoplasty (Fig. 24.23). Some surgeons believe that a submentoplasty is rarely necessary when performing a facelift because moving the SMAS and platysma posteriorly is adequate to improve anterior neck contour. We feel that this leads to early recurrence of neck laxity and platysmal banding. In addition, some surgeons feel that the anterior plication of the platysma may inhibit posterior elevation of the jowl thereby diminishing the efficacy of the facelift (Fig. 24.24). We believe that submentoplasty is virtually always a necessary adjunct to a facelift. Maintaining harmony between the aging face and neck is always an important goal, and we feel that it is the rare patient that will not benefit from directly rejuvenating the neck at the same time that the facelift is being performed. This is especially true if there is heavy subplatysmal fat or major platysmal laxity.

In all postoperative neck rejuvenation patients, care is taken to ensure that the skin is smooth and that folding or wrinkling does not occur when the tailored piece of Reston Foam® is placed. The area is then dressed.

24 Cosmetic Surgical Rejuvenation of the Neck

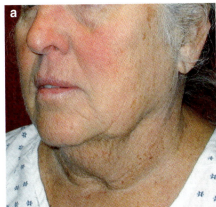
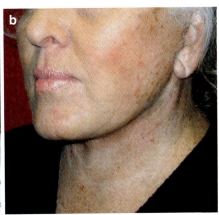

Fig. 24.23 (a) Preoperative 70-year-old female. (b) One month following an aggressive submentoplasty with subplatysmal fat excision, platysmal resection, partial submandibular gland resection, and simultaneous facelift. This is a good example of a grade 4AB

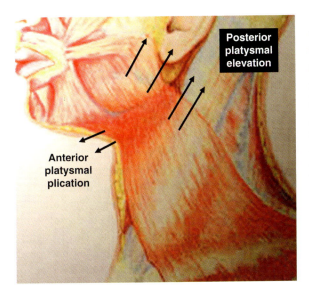

Fig. 24.24 Posterior platysmal and superficial musculoaponeurotic system (SMAS) plication during facelift surgery may have some restrictions when anterior platysmal plication is also performed. While this "hammock" effect may be beneficial overall, elevation particularly in the jowl region may be hampered from the opposing vector effect. Note posterior platysmal elevation

24.11 Dealing with the Visible Submandibular Gland

A visible submandibular bulge after submentoplasty, neck liposuction, or facelift can detract from what would have been an outstanding surgical outcome. One can hopefully anticipate this problem during the preoperative workup. Unfortunately, it is often missed or neglected and not noticed until a few months postoperatively when the patient asks what is this bulge?

Numerous techniques have been described to deal with this situation including Gore-Tex slings used by Conrad et al. [30], Gore-Tex sutures by Ramirez [31], and suspension sutures by Giampapa et al. [32]. More recently, Guyuron and Jackowe [33] described a basket suspension technique for ptotic submandibular glands. The authors have tried many of these techniques including the use of an Alloderm® neck sling and found them not to be durable in our hands. The preferred approach for treating the bulging or ptotic submandibular gland is partial resection of the superficial lobe.

When a submandibular bulge is identified on the preoperative physical exam, one must remember that there are many reasons for a submandibular bulge besides ptosis and benign involutional enlargement. Rarely, bilateral submandibular bulges are due to sialosis (also known as sialadenosis). This is a rare cause of benign, non-neoplastic enlargement of the submandibular glands. It more commonly affects the parotid gland and is most often seen in patients with alcoholic cirrhosis. Also patients with various endocrine disorders such as diabetes and hypothyroidism can develop sialadenosis. One should also remember that a bulge in the submandibular region may represent a malignant process. Although ptotic submandibular glands are often asymmetric, various clues in the patient's history and physical exam should prompt one to proceed with a workup prior to submentoplasty and resection. The typical benign submandibular gland is somewhat moveable, smooth, and firm to touch. A history of rapid change in size or swelling, the presence of pain and changes noted with eating may be helpful. When one is suspicious as to the etiology of the bulge, a fine needle aspiration biopsy may be helpful. The etiology of submandibular lymphadenopathy can also be determined with this technique.

Partial submandibular gland resection is performed through a submental incision after the submentoplasty skin flap has been elevated with facelift scissors. The platysma is elevated laterally beginning at the midline. Excellent visualization with a lighted retractor and a dry operative field are essential. Once an appropriate amount of subplatysmal fat has been removed, the gland is located just lateral to the lateral edge of the anterior digastric muscle. True submandibular gland excess will be obvious at this time and allows for easy location. The submandibular gland should be left alone if no obvious fullness is noted. The gland is covered with a thin layer of cervical fascia and an extended Colorado tip electrocautery is used to incise the fascia. Once the fascia is incised, the pink tissue of the gland is seen. The anatomy of the bilobed submandibular gland as seen through a submental incision is that the superficial lobe wraps around the posterior border of the mylohyoid muscle (Fig. 24.25). During resection, the deep lobe is not seen and only subtotal excision of the superficial lobe is carried out (Fig. 24.26). Typically, the submandibular gland produces only 20% of the saliva in the oral cavity but leaving much of the gland above the mylohyoid helps limit saliva production losses. Long forceps are used to grasp the gland as it is slowly

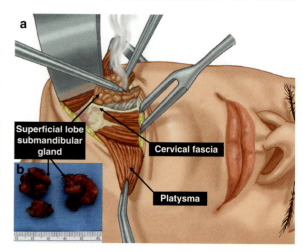

Fig. 24.26 (a) Partial resection of the superficial lobe of the submandibular gland after elevating the platysma laterally. The gland must be approached from the inferior and medial edge to avoid damage to unwanted nerves and vessels. (b) Excised superficial lobe submandibular gland

teased and dissected from its pocket. Resection takes place at the level of the cervical fascia and not within the capsule to protect the surrounding nerves. They include the more superficial marginal mandibular nerve and the deeper hypoglossal and lingual nerves. In a cadaver study by Singer, all nerves were found to be external to the submandibular gland capsule with the exception of the autonomic plexus. The hypoglossal nerve is found posterior to the tendinous junction of the anterior and posterior digastric muscle deep within the visceral layer of the neck. The lingual nerve is located cephalad and medial to the deep lobe. The marginal mandibular nerve is identified approximately 3.7 cm (range 3–4.2 cm) cephalad to the inferior limit of the submandibular gland [34, 35]. The cautery is used to slowly excise the bulging anterior portion of the gland. As one proceeds with resection, the surgeon must remember that the posterolateral portion of the superficial lobe has perforating branches of the submental artery and vein (which arise from the facial artery) that may cause troublesome bleeding. Once the gland is resected, the overlying fascia is closed with a 2–0 Vicryl suture. This may prevent recurrent ptosis and decrease the chance for postoperative hematoma and sialocele. Clearly, one should have expert knowledge of the anatomy and be very comfortable working through a 3 cm incision (Fig. 24.27). Submandibular gland resection is not for the novice submentoplasty surgeon. The potential problems are as follows:

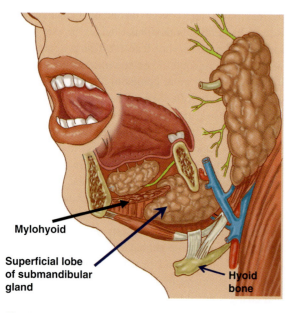

Fig. 24.25 Mylohyoid and superficial lobe of submandibular gland

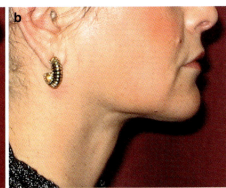

Fig. 24.27 (a) Preoperative 54-year-old female. (b) Six months following an aggressive submentoplasty with subplatysmal fat excision, platysmal resection, small chin implant, and partial submandibular gland resection. Note the slight irregularity where the gland would normally have some residual bulging. Slight over-resection of fat may have contributed to the minor irregularity

1. Difficult to control bleeding from branches of the facial artery
2. Thermal injury or neuropraxia to the marginal mandibular and other nerves in the region
3. The possibility of leaving the patient with xerostomia (low risk)
4. Increased risk of developing a seroma or hematoma
5. Risk of salivary fistula or sialoma (low risk)

24.12 Complications

24.12.1 Over-resection of Fat

Aggressive fat removal with cervical liposuction may result in a pleasing appearance initially but ultimately may result in fibrosis (Fig. 24.28). The term cobra neck deformity has been used to describe the central skeletonized look or hollow mid-submentum that results from over-resection. This deformity can also result from a relative under resection of fat laterally. This is a difficult problem to treat and can potentially result in litigation. We emphasize that it is important to leave at least 4–5 mm of fat on the skin flap and to avoid rasping the dermis with the suction cannula. One must be constantly aware of the orientation of cannula opening and its relationship to the dermis. The use of microcannulas 2–2.5 mm diameter decreases the likelihood of localized over-resection in the neck compared to larger instruments. Ensuring that the cannula is moving to a different location with each pass is essential as is frequent analysis of the thickness of the tissue remaining. The goal in cervicofacial liposuction is to resculpt youthful neck contours while leaving an adequate amount of fat to avoid scarring and unmasking underlying structures such as the submandibular glands, platysmal banding, and digastric muscles.

Once contour irregularities have developed one must decide whether this can be corrected with additional adjacent liposuction or autologous fat grafting. Rarely, it may be necessary to elevate the skin flap to allow for redraping. Residual platysmal banding can be treated with Botulinum toxin Type A. Five unit doses injected into the band at intervals of 2 cm can be helpful [9]. Up to 20 units of Botox is typically required to treat each band. As with any liposuction case, it is much easier to take more out at a later time if needed versus trying to treat fibrosis or a depression due to overzealous liposuction.

24.12.2 Sialocele

The development of a sialocele after cervicofacial liposuction or submentoplasty is rare (<.05%). One would expect to see this more commonly after submandibular gland resection or aggressive facelifts. The sialocele can be a nuisance. Often the patient can swell extensively every time they smell food or get hungry. Immediate enlargement upon eating is diagnostic in most cases to distinguish this straw-colored fluid from a

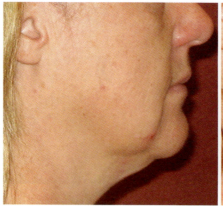 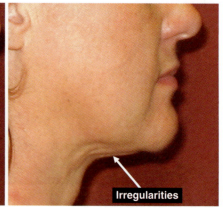

Fig. 24.28 (*Left*) Preoperative. (*Right*) Complication created by liposuction alone when platysmal laxity existed preoperatively. Platysmal bands are noticeable because of the skeletonization over muscle laxity

seroma [36]. They rarely require surgical intervention unless the volume does not decrease or if skin integrity is compromised. The initial treatment is simple needle aspiration and a strategically placed pressure dressing. A sialocele can be differentiated from seroma by the finding of high amylase content although this is rarely required for diagnosis. Repeated aspirations are almost always necessary to resolve the problem. One can also inject Botulinum Toxin Type A, 5 units directly into the gland to hasten sialocele resolution. In addition, scopolamine patches can be applied every 8 h to decrease salivary production. Reassurance is often needed especially if it is from the parotid gland rather than from the submandibular gland, since the parotid produces larger amounts of saliva and may take 1 month to resolve.

24.12.3 Nerve Injury

The most common nerve to be injured from cervicofacial liposuction and or submentoplasty is the marginal mandibular branch of the facial nerve. The injury usually occurs as a result of aggressive suctioning in the region of the jowl or where the nerve crosses the mandibular border. In addition, this injury can occur with aggressive resection of the submandibular gland or platysma resection. Typically, the nerve is extensively arborized in the area of injury, making permanent dysfunction rare. The injury manifests in lower lip depressor dysfunction with associated inability to depress the corner of the mouth and lower lip on that side. The most effective treatment is to inject 5–10 units of botulinum toxin Type A into the contralateral lip depressor. This will provide the patient with symmetry that should last 3–4 months which is the typical time it takes for either the neuropraxia to resolve or the uninjured arborized branches to provide full innervation to the lip depressors. It is reasonable to wait 4–6 weeks prior to using Botox as the resolution of edema may be all that is required to regain function.

24.12.4 Seroma

Any time a skin flap is raised seroma formation is possible. It is estimated to occur at a rate of less than 3% with facial liposuction. Adequate post-operative compression helps to reduce the incidence mechanically. Without a doubt, excessive tissue trauma as seen with overly aggressive liposuction or use of large diameter cannulas increases the risk of seroma formation more than anything else. When submentoplasty is performed, it is essential to ensure that adequate hemostasis has been achieved as the pooling of blood may contribute to this problem. The approach to seroma development is to perform serial needle aspirations that are followed with the placement of compression dressings. Untreated seromas of variable hemoglobin content can lead to fibrosis, unsightly skin retraction with irregularity, and even capsule formation.

24.12.5 Skin Redundancy

This problem is often the result of poor patient selection. As mentioned earlier in this chapter, patients who present with crepe paper-type skin and or excessive laxity are poor candidates for isolated cervicofacial liposuction or submentoplasty. Usually, when there is residual skin laxity it is in the midline. For older men, a reasonable option may include a direct excisional submentoplasty with a Z or W plasty. These men often are not interested in a traditional facelift with its associated downtime and telltale scars. A traditional lower face and neck lift with submentoplasty remains the procedure of choice for significant lower face and neck laxity.

24.12.6 Chronic Pain

Chronic pain is usually not seen after cervical liposuction but can occasionally be seen after submentoplasty. Typically, this will resolve in a few months and can be a result of the tightness of a corset platysmaplasty. The pain also can be a result of irritation of sensory nerves and the character of the pain may help to identify this. Development of a neuroma must also always be ruled out. Medications such as Elavil, Neurontin, or Lyrica may be helpful in dealing with severe chronic neuropathic pain. Fortunately, most postsurgical pain is temporary in the neck.

24.12.7 Post-inflammatory Hyperpigmentation

This is a problem that would be seen more commonly in patients with Fitzpatrick skin Types III or greater. With time, the hyperpigmentation almost always resolves without treatment. One can however speed up the resolution of the hyperpigmentation with the application of prescription grade strengths of hydroquinone (4% or greater) or kojic acid to the affected areas. Use of intense pulsed light or laser therapy to treat post-inflammatory hyperpigmentation is occasionally required.

24.12.8 Infection

Infections after surgical procedures in the head and neck area are rare primarily because of the excellent blood supply. When one suspects infection one should, if possible, obtain a specimen for gram stain along with

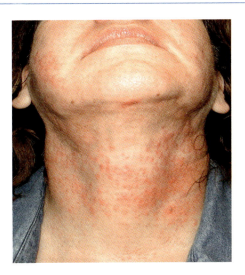

Fig. 24.29 Staph folliculitis after submentoplasty

cultures and sensitivities to guide antibiotic therapy. The most common organisms are typical skin flora, notably *Staphylococcus* and *Streptococcus* (Fig. 24.29). Over the last decade there has also been a shift in the prevalence of methicillin-resistant *Staphylococcus*. Previously, this was hospital-acquired organism whereas now many methicillin-resistant *Staphylococcus aureus* (MRSA) infections are community acquired. The community-acquired MRSA is often sensitive to trimethoprim-sulfamethoxazole and Clindamycin [37]. The initial gold standard treatment for hospital-acquired MRSA remains Vancomycin. Although rare, the patient with severe pain or redness that is disproportionately higher than one would expect or an infection that does not improve with first line treatment should lead the surgeon to suspect the possibility of: Necrotizing fasciitis, atypical mycobacterium, herpetic viral infections, or fungal infections.

24.12.9 Bleeding and Hematomas

Most postoperative hematomas occur within the first 24 h when postoperative pain causes an increase in blood pressure or the patient bends over or valsalvas and increases pressure. The Tumescent anesthesia technique has revolutionized cosmetic surgery in many ways. There is a dramatic reduction in bleeding during procedures with this technique which translates into decreased bruising. The literature does not identify a lower rate of hematoma formation after surgery using tumescent anesthesia versus standard local anesthesia. Reducing the chance of bleeding with surgery begins before the procedure. Uncontrolled hypertension must be corrected. Baker and others have shown that the use of Clonidine preoperatively has lowered the hematoma rate with rhytidectomy. This centrally acting alpha 2 agonist decreases sympathetic out flow and can also cause sedation. It further has been shown to reduce the need for postoperative narcotics [38]. Use of this medication in elderly patients on beta blockers is not recommended. Any history of bleeding problems with prior surgery or within the family should be appropriately investigated. Medications that might affect platelet function or the clotting cascade must be discontinued to allow sufficient time for the return of normal clotting. When performing multiple cosmetic procedures on the same patient it is important to realize that the vasoconstrictive effect of epinephrine will wear off more quickly in the face and neck area as compared to other parts of the body due to the rich blood supply. Because of this a higher concentration of epinephrine is used in the face and neck area. During submentoplasty, the most common area to encounter bleeding is from the anterior jugular veins. Precise suture ligation or cautery performed under direct vision with a very good lighted retractor is critical. When partial submandibular gland resection is performed one can easily develop bleeding from perforators of the submental artery and vein, which are branches of the facial artery and vein. Desperate attempts to control arterial bleeding in this area can increase the risk of injury to the marginal mandibular nerve and lingual nerve. Excellent lighting, exposure and suctioning should facilitate pinpoint cauterization of the vessels. One must always remember to stay calm and simply place gauze packs for pressure to control large areas, so care can be used to isolate each and every significant bleeder. If this is not successful, careful suture ligation should be performed while being mindful of the nearby neural anatomy.

When hematomas occur postoperatively one can consider needle aspiration under local anesthesia if the hematoma is small. Naturally large or rapidly expanding hematomas should be immediately drained surgically. Consider placing a drain at that time even though drains are not used routinely for facial surgery. The literature has not demonstrated that drains decrease the chance of hematoma formation. Close postoperative follow-up in this situation is mandatory. At the time of those postoperative visits one will often see areas of induration in the area where the hematoma was located. This will often respond to external ultrasound and massage. Occasional injections of small doses of Kenalog 10 mg/ml will also help to soften these areas.

24.12.10 Skin Slough

This problem is rare with traditional microcannular liposuction or submentoplasty. Ischemic changes have recently become more common with the use of laser lipolysis. Regardless of the exact wavelength used, too much heat building up below the skin can cause thermal injury. The picture below demonstrates full thickness burn necrosis in a patient who underwent laser-assisted liposuction of the jowls with submentoplasty (Fig. 24.30). The burn likely occurred as a result of not moving the laser fiber continuously and perhaps being too superficial. This type of injury can require local wound care and even skin grafting.

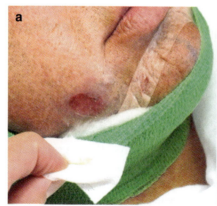
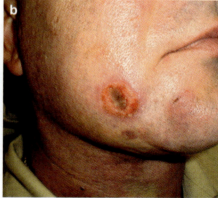

Fig. 24.30 Thermal injury from laser-assisted liposuction. This is a full thickness burn that was treated with local wound care. Avoiding these kinds of injuries requires that the laser fiber be in constant motion, especially when near the dermis

24.13 Conclusions

With our rapidly aging population the number of patients seeking rejuvenation of age-related changes of the neck will undoubtedly increase. While rhytidectomy has traditionally been the cornerstone technique that has been used to achieve this goal, there are many cases where submentoplasty or liposuction is appropriate as stand-alone procedures (Fig. 24.31). When used in the appropriate patient they are truly minimally invasive and yet can provide spectacular results with minimal downtime (Fig. 24.32). Clearly, many patients will benefit from a combination of techniques (Fig. 24.33). To provide an optimal outcome for patients seeking this kind of care, one must be versatile and have "all of the tools in the tool box."

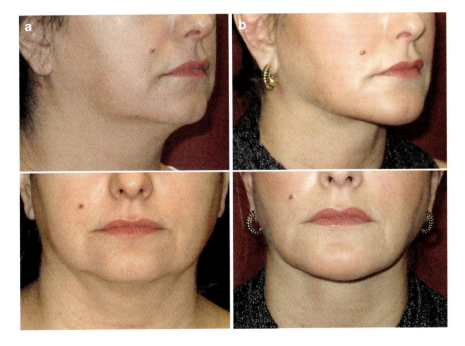

Fig. 24.31 (**a**) Preoperative 40-year-old female. (**b**) One month following an aggressive submentoplasty with subplatysmal fat excision, platysmal resection, and simultaneous facelift. This is a good example of an obtuse chin neck angle grade 4AB

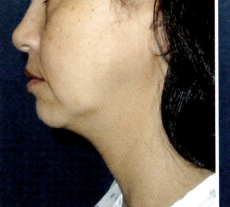
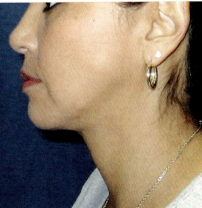

Fig. 24.32 (*Left*) Preoperative 45-year-old Hispanic female. (*Right*) Six months following submentoplasty with back-cutting and anterior platysmal plication along with chin implant placement. She is an example of a type II A neck deformity pre-op. No skin was excised

Fig. 24.33 (**a**) Preoperative 52-year-old female. (**b**) Six months following a facelift with aggressive submentoplasty including partial digastric reduction to compensate for a low hyoid. This good example of a Type IV C neck, which is the most challenging diagnostic situation to treat

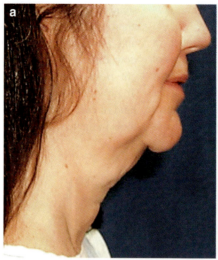 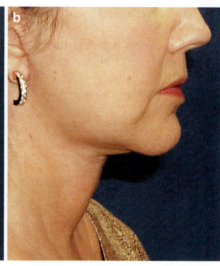

References

1. Bourguet J. La chirugie esthetique de la face: Les rides. Monde Med, 15 Jan 1928.
2. Aufricht G. Surgery for excess skin of the face. In: Transactions of the second international congress of plastic surgery. Edinburgh: E & S Livingston; 1960. pp. 495–502.
3. Connell BF. Neck contour deformities: the art, engineering, anatomic diagnosis, architectural planning, and aesthetics of surgical correction. Clin Plast Surg. 1987;14(4):683–92.
4. Feldman JJ. Corset platysmaplasty. Plast Reconstr Surg. 1990;85(3):333–43.
5. Klein JA. The tumescent technique for liposuction surgery. Am J Cosmet Surg. 1987;4:263–7.
6. Courtiss E. Suction lipectomy of the neck. Plast Reconstr Surg. 1985;76(6):882–9.
7. Hodgkinson DJ. Clinical applications of radiofrequency: nonsurgical skin tightening (thermage). Clin Plast Surg. 2009;36(2):261–8.
8. Goldman A. Laser-assisted liposuction. Clin Plast Surg. 2009;36(2):241–53.
9. Sposito MM. New indications for botulinum toxin type A in cosmetics: mouth and neck. Plast Reconstr Surg. 2002;110:601–11.
10. Park SH, Kim DW, Lee MA, Yoo SC, Rhee SC, Koo SH, et al. Effectiveness of mesotherapy on body contouring. Plast Reconstr Surg. 2008;121(4):179e–85e.
11. Prado A, Andrades P, Danilla S, Leniz P, Castillo P, Gaete F. A prospective, randomized, double blind, controlled clinical trial comparing laser-assisted lipoplasty with suction-assisted lipoplasty. Plast Reconstr Surg. 2006;118(4):1032–45.
12. Matarasso A, Pfeifer TM. Mesotherapy and injection lipolysis. Clin Plast Surg. 2009;36(2):181–92.
13. Gryskiewicz J. Submental suction-assisted lipectomy without platysmaplasty: pushing the skin envelope to avoid a face lift for unsuitable candidates. Plast Reconstr Surg. 2003;112(5):1393–405.
14. Little JW. Treatment of the full obtuse neck (panel discussion). Aesthetic Surg J. 2005;25(4):397.
15. Ellenbogen R, Karlin JV. Visual criteria for success in restoring the youthful neck. Plast Reconstr Surg. 1980;66(6):826–37.
16. Dedo DD. "How I do it" plastic surgery. Practical suggestion on facial plastic surgery. A preoperative classification of the neck for cervicofacial rhytidectomy. Laryngoscope. 1980;90(11 Pt 1):1894–6.
17. de Castro CC. The anatomy of the platysma muscle. Plast Reconstr Surg. 1980;66(5):680–3.
18. Baker DC, Conley J. Avoiding facial nerve injuries in rhytidectomy: anatomical variations and pitfalls. Plast Reconstr Surg. 1979;64(6):781–95.
19. Dingman RO, Grabb WC. Surgical anatomy of the mandibular ramus of the facial nerve based on the dissection of 100 facial halves. Plast Reconstr Surg. 1962;29:266–72.
20. Liebman EP, Webster RC, Gaul JR, Griffin T. The marginal mandibular nerve in rhytidectomy and liposuction surgery. Arch Otolaryngol Head Neck Surg. 1988;104(2):179–81.
21. Larrabee WF, Makielski KH, Henderson JL. Surgical anatomy of the face. Philadelphia: Lippincott Williams & Wilkins; 2004. p. 81–4.
22. Klein JA. Tumescent technique, tumescent anesthesia and microcannular liposuction. St. Louis: Mosby; 2000. p. 4–5.
23. Klein JA. Tumescent technique for regional anesthesia permits lidocaine doses of 35 mg/kg for liposuction. J Dermatol Surg Oncol. 1990;16(3):248–63.
24. Klein JA. Tumescent technique, tumescent anesthesia and microcannular liposuction. St. Louis: Mosby; 2000. p. 30.
25. Klein JA. Tumescent technique, tumescent anesthesia and microcannular liposuction. St. Louis: Mosby; 2000. p. 131–40.
26. Rubin JP, Bierman C, Roscow CE, Arthur GR, Chang Y, Courtiss EH, et al. The tumescent technique: the effect of high tissue pressure and dilute epinephrine on absorption of lidocaine. Plast Reconstr Surg. 1999;103(3):990–6.
27. Hayashi Y, Sumikawa K, Maze M, Yamatodani A, Kamibayashi T, Kuro M, et al. Dexmedetomidine prevents epinephrine – induced arrhythmias through stimulation of central alpha-2 adrenoreceptors in halothane anesthetized dogs. Anesthesiology. 1991;75(1):113–17.
28. Klein JA. Tumescent technique, tumescent anesthesia and microcannular liposuction. St. Louis: Mosby; 2000. p. 126.

29. Bitner JB, Friedman O, Farrior RT, Cook TA. Direct submentoplasty for neck rejuvenation. Arch Facial Plast Surg. 2007;9(3):194–200.
30. Conrad K, Chapkik JS, Reifen E. e-PTFE (Gore-Tex) suspension cervical facial Rhytidectomy. Arch Otolaryngol Head Neck Surg. 1993;119(6):694–8.
31. Ramirez OM. Cervicoplasty: nonexcisional anterior approach. A 10-year follow-up. Plast Reconstr Surg. 2003;111(3): 1342–5.
32. Giampapa VC. Suture suspension technique offers predictable, long lasting neck rejuvenation. Aesthetic Surg J. 2000;20:253.
33. Guyuron B, Jackowe D, Lamphongsai S. Basket submandibular gland suspension. Plast Reconstr Surg. 2008;122(3): 938–43.
34. de Pompe Pina D, Castro Quinta W. Aesthetic resection of the submandibular gland. Plast Reconstr Surg. 1991;88(5): 779–87.
35. Singer DP, Sullivan PK. Submandibular gland I: an anatomic evaluation and surgical approach to submandibular gland resection for facial rejuvenation. Plast Reconstr Surg. 2003;112(4):1150–4.
36. Barron R, Margulis A, Iceksen M, Zeltser R, Eldad A, Nahlieli O. Iatrogenic parotid sialocele following rhytidectomy: diagnosis and treatment. Plast Reconstr Surg. 2001; 108(6):1782–4.
37. Department of Health and Human Services Centers for Disease Control and Prevention. Strategies for clinical management of MRSA in the community: summary of an Experts' Meeting convened by the Centers for Disease Control and Prevention, 2006.
38. Baker DC, Stefani WA, Chiu ES. Reducing the incidence of hematoma requiring surgical evaluation following male rhytidectomy: a 30 year review of 985 cases. Plast Reconstr Surg. 2005;116(7):1973.

Submental Liposuction

Mervin Low

25.1 Introduction

Submental liposuction alone, or as an adjunct to a more formal neck lift with platysmaplasty and/or facelift, is a procedure that can result in significant contour improvement in the submental area. Initially performed in the late 1970s via a lateral approach and a larger cannula, it has since evolved into a procedure performed with smaller cannulas and a submental incision [1, 2]. Liposuction of the mandibular border, jowl, and cheek has also been added to improve the contour of the lower face. Subplatysmal fat, while better excised under direct vision, has also been removed via liposuction.

Submental liposuction is traditionally reserved for younger patients with good skin tone, elasticity, skin contraction, and adherence. The goal of such an operation is to achieve the criteria demonstrated in youthful necks. These criteria have been described as: a distinct inferior mandibular border from mentum to angle with no jowl overhang, a visible subhyoid depression, a visible thyroid cartilage bulge, a visible anterior sternocleidomastoid bulge, a submental-sternocleidomastoid line angle of 90° or a cervicomental angle of 105–120° [3]. The chin neck relationship is also considered in the aesthetic rejuvenation of the lower face. Chin augmentation is oftentimes performed in conjunction with submental liposuction. Individuals who either are not candidates for a facelift or do not desire the extended recovery period of a facelift may achieve improved appearance with submental liposuction alone. In these patients, who are often older in age, midline fullness is the best predictor of a good outcome whereas as thin skin is the best predictor of a poor outcome [4]. The presence of platysmal banding and subplatysmal fat should be noted as these conditions will be inadequately treated by submental liposuction alone.

25.2 Technique

As for all aesthetic plastic surgery procedures, a thorough physical examination of the neck is critical to proper patient selection and the achievement of outstanding results. The examination begins with an assessment of the skin. Crepe paper thin skin is a predictor of a poor outcome unless a concomitant facelift is performed. The presence of multiple, deep horizontal, or oblique creases in the neck predict poor redraping of the skin postoperatively. A snap test demonstrates the tone and elasticity present in the skin. A pinch test revealing an excess amount of skin laxity may dictate an excisional procedure. The apparent cervical skin excess evident after submental liposuction is required for effective contouring of the neck. An assessment of the amount and location of preplatysmal fat is then made. Midline fullness, even more so than age and skin tone, is the best predictor of a good outcome. Generally, a pinch thickness of 1.5–2.0 cm will be evident. Subplatysmal fat is filled with connective tissue and feels firmer than preplatysmal fat. Clenching of the teeth with subsequent contraction of the platysma will help define the presence of preplatysmal fat. The presence of visible platysmal banding with and without animation should be noted. The position of the hyoid-thyroid complex is examined. A low position of the hyoid-thyroid complex often equates to

M. Low
8107, Newport Beach, CA 92658, USA
e-mail: drlow@live.com

a less well-defined cervicomental angle, which may limit the achievement of optimal results following submental liposuction. Asymmetries and submaxillary gland fullness are also noted. Standard preoperative photographs including anterior, lateral, and oblique views should be obtained.

Prior to the initiation of the procedure, appropriate landmarks are outlined in the upright sitting position. This is crucial as landmarks change when in the recumbent position. These landmarks include: the mandibular border, the marginal mandibular nerve, the borders of the sternocleidomastoid muscle, and the thyroid cartilage and the hyoid bone. The localized area of fat is also outlined.

The procedure may be performed under general or local anesthesia. Endotracheal tube placement during general anesthesia may limit the ability to appropriately liposuction the area. Generally, submental liposuction can be performed through a well-placed submental crease incision. Retrolobular incisions are used in those cases where extensive fat removal and/or cross-tunneling is required. A pinch test performed while the cannula is inserted aid in determining the appropriate depth of the cannula. Pretunneling is crucial in this area to determine the appropriate plane of dissection and evacuation. The safe plane is superficial to the platysma muscle. It further aids in the smooth redraping necessary in this area following liposuction. Subdermal suctioning is not recommended as this may result in subdermal vascular plexus injury causing skin loss, surface irregularities, pigmentary changes, and prolonged induration. Small bore (1–3 mm) Mercedes tip cannulas or spatula cannulas with the holes oriented away from the dermis are used. Liposuction performed with the cannula holes directed toward the dermis has also been described [5]. Hyperextension of the neck is a helpful position for this procedure. A gentle to and fro excursion of the cannula is employed. The cannula is passed more frequently over the area of fat deposition with feathering of the edges beyond the area of maximal deposition. Total volumes removed range from 25 to 100 ml or more depending on the size of the neck and amount of fat. Decreased suction power or hand suction can be employed. Constant use of the pinch test to determine the end point or completion of suctioning is vital. A pinch test of less than 1 cm over the entire treated region is usually achieved. Conservative removal of fat will yield excellent results. Less is more in submental liposuction. Over-liposuctioning of fat in this area is disastrous as the remaining inadequate submental fat will result in dermis adhering to the platysma causing unsightly irregularities. This complication is difficult if not impossible to correct. Occasionally, contour irregularities and ridging may occur despite uniform fat aspiration and pinch thickness. Fibrous bands passing from the platysma to the dermis are the usual cause and can be divided using a closed neck dissector or sharp scissor dissection. Layered closure of the incision and the application of a compression garment for at least 7 days complete the procedure.

25.3 Discussion

There have been multiple mechanisms postulated for the generally excellent results obtained following submental liposuction [6]. The results obtained may be related to: amount of fat removed, the creation of multiple tunnels, contractile healing of the multiple tunnels, redraping of skin over liposuctioned areas, and/or the inherent elasticity of the skin. It is likely that a combination of factors is involved in the outcome following submental liposuction.

Complications of submental liposuction include: bleeding and hematoma, infection, hypesthesia, skin loss, hyperpigmentation, prolonged induration, marginal mandibular nerve injury, and perforation of the skin, larynx, trachea, or carotid. Aesthetically, over- or under-resection is possible as is dimpling and contour irregularities. Skin excess or insufficient redraping is also an outcome that is possible is patients inadequately selected for this procedure.

Skin contraction following liposuction is undoubtedly the rate limiting step to an ideal outcome. Traditional suction-assisted lipectomy of the submental area has been demonstrated to produce excellent results in properly chosen patients [4, 7]. Internal ultrasound-assisted liposuction, external ultrasound-assisted liposuction, and power-assisted liposuction have all been employed in the attempt to improve skin contraction and ultimately the aesthetic result [6].

The recent addition of laser-assisted liposuction has added to the adjunctive technological armamentarium available for liposuction surgeon [8]. Laser-assisted lipolysis uses laser energy via a cannula/fiber combination to deliver light energy with subsequent transformation to heat within the adipocyte ultimately causing cell lysis and the liberation of lipids into the extracellular space. The liquefied fat is then usually extracted or aspirated by traditional means. Additional effects of the application of laser energy include: coagulation of vessels within the adipose tissue, coagulation of adipose and dermal collagen, and a reorganization of the reticular dermis with neocollagenesis in the deep dermis and dermal fat junction. These effects clinically translate into less intraoperative blood loss, less postoperative ecchymosis and swelling, more rapid recovery following the procedure, and enhanced skin tightening and skin redraping due to the neocollagenesis. It may also minimize surgeon fatigue while aspirating the fat. The effects on skin tightening are particularly useful in contouring of the submental region. A recent study has elegantly demonstrated objective skin tightening following laser-assisted liposuction using a 1,064 nm wavelength laser [8]. There is also some suggestion that using laser-assisted lipolysis may result in smoother contours with an ultimate decrease in the revision rate [8].

At the time of this writing, multiple differing wavelengths for laser-assisted lipolysis have been FDA approved. These include Nd:Yag and diode lasers of the following wavelengths: 924, 975, 980, 1,064, 1,320, 1,444 nm, and 1,470 nm. The laser energy is applied via 600–1,000 μm optical fibers. Sequencing in laser-assisted lipolysis procedures consists of standard tumescence of the target area followed by laser energy application and then completion aspiration. Some users apply laser energy subsequent to aspiration while others have attempted lasing in revision cases without aspiration. The goal in these cases is to take advantage of the skin tightening effects. The targeted efficacy of each wavelength has been touted and supported by data from each of the respective laser-assisted lipolysis device manufacturers. The most efficacious wavelength in laser-assisted lipolysis is hotly debated and remains to be determined. A recent peer-reviewed article has demonstrated the usefulness of a 1,064 nm wavelength in submental region [9].

25.4 Conclusions

Submental liposuction alone, in carefully selected patients or in conjunction with an additional platysmaplasty or excisional procedure, has been shown to be effective in addressing submental lipodystrophy with improved contours in the lower facial aesthetic subunit (Figs. 25.1–25.4). Careful patient selection,

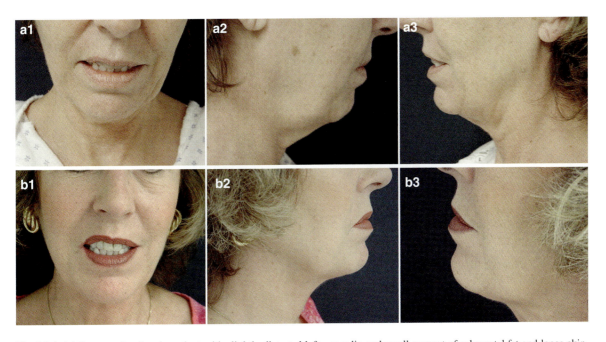

Fig. 25.1 (**a**) Preoperative female patient with slightly distorted left upper lip and small amount of submental fat and loose skin. (**b**) Postoperative (Photos courtesy of Sid J. Mirrafati)

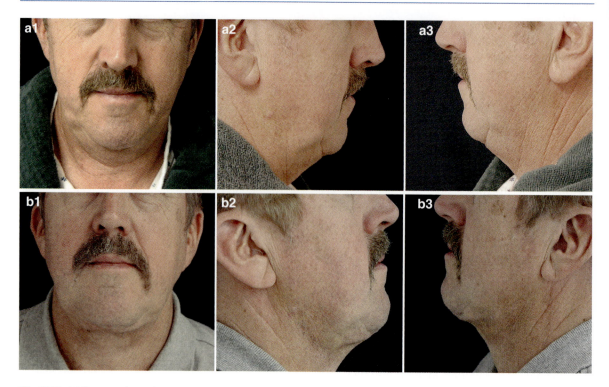

Fig. 25.2 (**a**) Preoperative male patient with large amount of submental fat. (**b**) Postoperative (Photos courtesy of Sid J. Mirrafati)

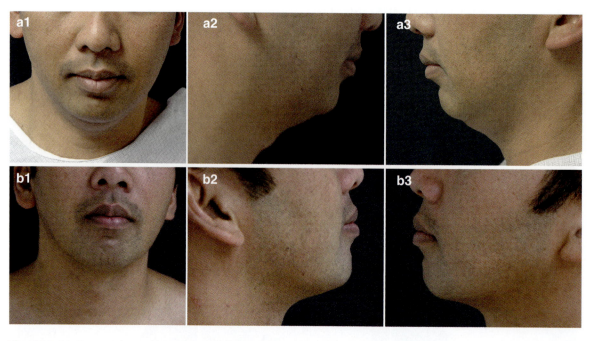

Fig. 25.3 (**a**) Preoperative male patient with small amount of submental fat. (**b**) Postoperative. (Photos courtesy of Sid J. Mirrafati)

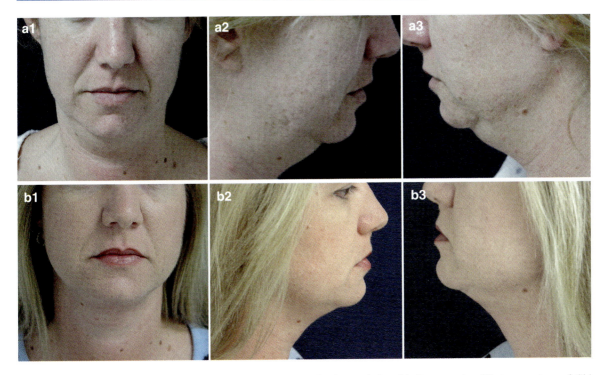

Fig. 25.4 (**a**) Preoperative female patient with large amount of submental fat. (**b**) Postoperative (Photos courtesy of Sid J. Mirrafati)

assessment, and judicious defatting are the keys to success. New technology has been introduced and applied adjunctively while performing submental liposuction. Laser-assisted lipolysis has shown particular promise in minimizing bleeding and downtime while improving the tightening, contouring, and redraping of skin following liposuction.

References

1. Illouz YG. The origins of lipolysis. In: Hetter GP, editor. Lipoplasty: the theory and practice of blunt suction lipectomy. New York: Lippincott Williams & Wilkins; 1984. p. 25.
2. Hetter GP. Lipoplasty of the face and neck. In: Hetter GP, editor. Lipoplasty: the theory and practice of blunt suction lipectomy. New York: Lippincott Williams & Wilkins; 1984. p. 249.
3. Ellenbogen R, Karlin JV. Visual criteria for success in restoring the youthful neck. Plast Reconstr Surg. 1980;66(6): 826–37.
4. Gryskiewicz JM. Submental suction-assisted lipectomy without platysmaplasty: pushing the (skin) envelope to avoid a face lift for unsuitable candidates. Plast Reconstr Surg. 2003;112(5):1393–405.
5. Goodstein WA. Superficial liposculpture of the face and neck. Plast Reconstr Surg. 1996;98(6):988–96.
6. Rohrich RJ, Rios JL, Smith PD, Gutowski KA. Neck rejuvenation revisited. Plast Reconstr Surg. 2006;118(5):1251–63.
7. Courtiss E. Suction lipectomy: a retrospective analysis of 100 patients. Plast Reconstr Surg. 1984;73:780.
8. Goldman A, Gotkin RH. Laser assisted liposuction. Clin Plast Surg. 2009;36(2):241–53.
9. Goldman A. Submental Nd:Yag laser-assisted liposuction. Lasers Surg Med. 2006;38(3):181–4.

Vaser UAL for the Heavy Face

Alberto Di Giuseppe and George Commons

26.1 Introduction

In the last decade, the demand for aesthetic procedures has increased, but for less invasive, less traumatic techniques. Patients look for a faster return to work/life, and mostly they seek a youthful, smooth, non-pulled appearance.

26.2 Technologies

Results with liposuction were generally good, but inconsistent, and with insufficient skin retraction. Earlier generations of ultrasonic devices were potentially too powerful or aggressive for easy, safe, and meticulous head and neck applications. Complications, although minimal, were more threatening.

Vaser technology represents an advanced tool available on the market since 2001, which offers guarantee of safety and quality and allows great results in a simple manner, in expert hands.

Training with Vaser for face and neck is not difficult, but requires technical skills and finesse in working close to the subcutaneous layer with a fine (2.2 mm diameter) titanium probe (Fig. 26.1).

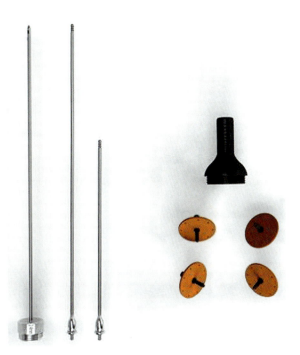

Fig. 26.1 Vaser probes 2.2 mm 10–15 cm. Skin protectors, and 1.8 mm aspiration cannula

26.3 Technique

The probe is always the 2.2 diameter, utilized with 30% continuous mode for fibrous tissue, or 30% Vaser mode. Generally, between 2 or 3 min of application are sufficient to fully undermine each sector of the head and neck area (jowls, chin, mandible, cheeks, etc.). If the neck is heavy with a lot of local fat to be emulsified for facial debulking and contouring, allow another 1 min minimum for the deeper fat layer.

To remove emulsified fat, or to remove infiltrated solution, gentle aspiration with a 1.8 mm cannula at

A. Di Giuseppe (✉)
Via Simeoni, 6, 60122, Ancona, Italy
e-mail: adgplasticsurg@atlavia.it

G. Commons
1515 El Camino Real, Suite C, Palo Alto,
California, 94306, USA
e-mail: gwcommons@gmail.com

low aspiration power is required. Gentle manual shaping and pressure is utilized to help the solution to come out. Tumescence is a temporary status, and in the face and neck fluids are absorbed faster than elsewhere.

Heavy faces occur in many of the potential candidates for Vaser facial contouring. Overweight and obese patients often require a general thinning or softening of the cheeks and lower third of the face (Fig. 26.2).

Figure 26.3 is a patient with an undefined face, fatty cheeks and chin, no mandibular line definition, no orbital cheek sulcus, and no pre-parotid natural depression. This patient underwent a Vaser face contouring of cheeks, jaw line, chin, and nasolabial folds. A total of 400 mL tumescent fluid was infused and 8 min Vaser applied. Seventy five milliliter of fat was aspirated. The result appears natural and well defined.

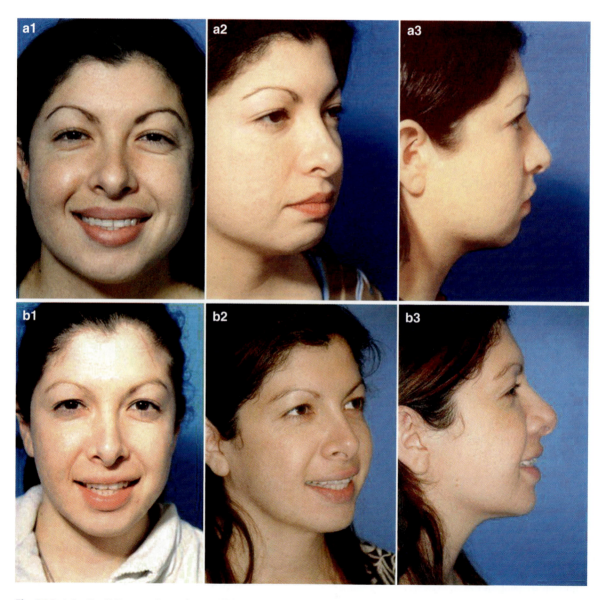

Fig. 26.2 (**a1, a2, a3**) Preoperative patient with a heavy face. (**b1, b2, b3**) Postoperative following Vaser debulking

Fig. 26.3 (**a1, a2**) Preoperative patient with heavy face, cheeks, chin, mandible. (**b1, b2**) Postoperative following Vaser

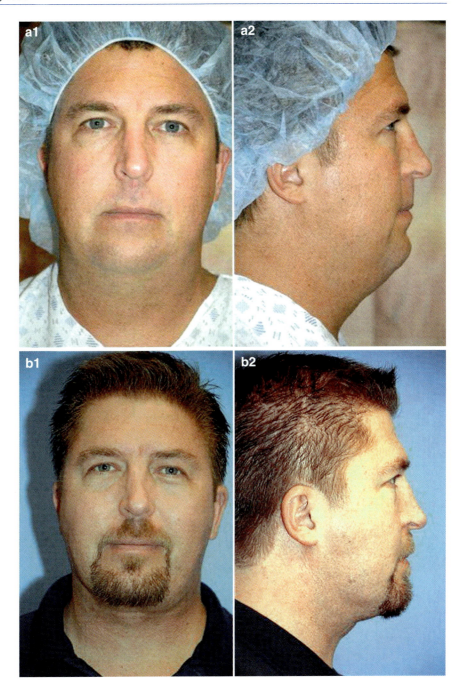

Figure 26.4 is patient with heavy neck and cheeks, mostly obese or overweight, and has no definition at chin and neck due to fat accumulation over platysma muscle. There is a "double" chin and no neck and jaw definition or cheek orbital protrusion. Extensive Vaser emulsification gives a better look, younger and fitter appearance, and more pleasant face. All areas were softened and redraped.

North American population is a mix of different ethnic races, including Hispanic, Afro-Cuban, Latin, Asian, and others. The patient in Fig. 26.5 is a 44-year-old Hispanic overweight woman, unable to

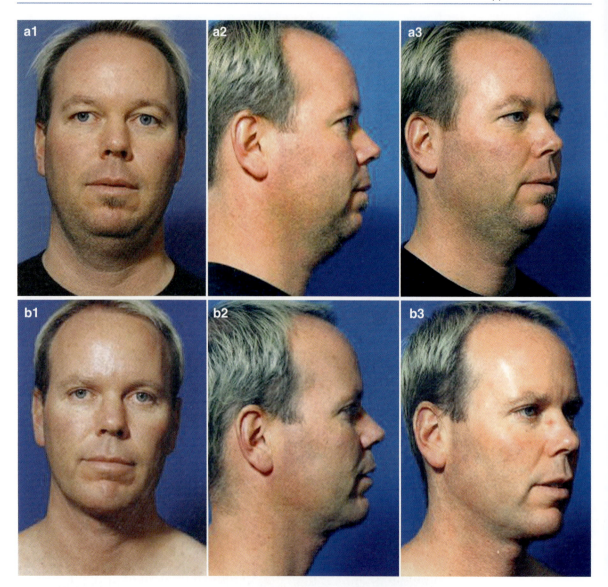

Fig. 26.4 (**a1, a2, a3**) Preoperative patient with heavy face, neck, and cheeks. (**b1, b2, b3**) Postoperative after Vaser of the chin, cheeks, and neck. Note the new mandibular line and submental and chin contouring

improve natural appearance of the face with a hypocaloric regime. With Vaser of the neck, chin, and jaw, the areas were reduced in volume of fat. The skin was fully mobilized in order to redrape nicely. Even the orbital nasal area, cheeks, and pre-parotid areas were softened and redefined.

26.4 Complications

In over 500 cases operated on by two surgeons, there were no significant complications such as nerve deficits, burns, or skin necrosis. The results were pleasing to patient and surgeon. No surgical redo was requested.

Fig. 26.5 (**a1, a2**) Preoperative 44-year-old Mexican-type Spanish "profile," and bulky face. (**b1, b2**) Postoperative following Vaser contouring of the neck, cheeks, and chin

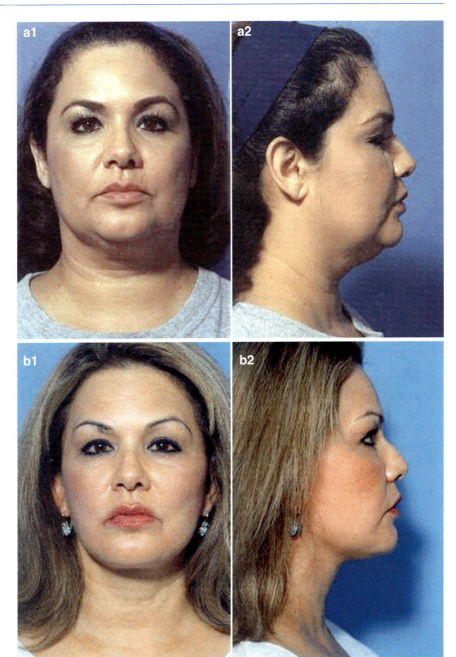

Suture Facelift Techniques

Peter M. Prendergast

27.1 Introduction

In recent years, minimally invasive facial rejuvenation procedures have become more popular. From 1997 to 2008, surgical cosmetic procedures in the USA increased by 180% whereas nonsurgical cosmetic procedures in the same period increased by more than 750% [1]. Patients seek minimally invasive treatments that do not require prolonged recovery periods, are low risk, inexpensive, and provide results that look natural. These include chemodenervation with botulinum toxins, soft tissue augmentation using injectable implants, laser skin resurfacing, and skin "tightening" using a variety of light and radiofrequency-based technologies [2]. Nonsurgical procedures improve hyperdynamic and static wrinkles, volume loss and skin surface imperfections but do not address ptosis of deeper tissues including the malar fat pad and the superficial musculoaponeurotic system (SMAS). Although an open facelift remains the gold standard for sagging skin, fat, and the SMAS in older patients, less invasive measures using various suture systems and designs provide a novel alternative for younger patients with early signs of aging. Suture facelift techniques are used as adjunctive measures during traditional open procedures [3] as a complement to less invasive open techniques [4], or as closed procedures without dissection through minimal incisions or punctures [5]. This chapter will focus on closed suture lifting techniques, commonly referred to as "thread lifts," for the face and neck using various suture materials and designs. These include barbed and non-barbed sutures, coned sutures, and slings using materials such as polypropylene, polytetrafluoroethylene, and polycaproamide sutures.

Although still in its infancy, the practice of suture lifting to improve facial contours, restore appropriate tissue projection, and redefine bony landmarks has been widely adopted. Despite this, published data on safety, efficacy, and long-term results remains scant [6]. Unfortunately, the furor and media-driven hype over suture lifts, touted as "lunchtime facelifts" or "1-hour mini-lifts," often generate unrealistic expectations amongst potentially suitable patients, or sway patients who would best be treated with a conventional rhytidectomy into believing they can achieve similar results with a suture facelift [7]. Nevertheless, these innovative techniques should be embraced rather than discarded so that they can be further studied, improved and refined, and eventually find their rightful place in aesthetic surgery and medicine. In the author's view, suture facelift techniques currently provide a "better alternative" to nonsurgical tissue tightening devices such as radiofrequency and infrared light for patients who would benefit from lifting mild to moderate ptosis, but they do not replace open facelift procedures for those with more severe ptosis or excessive skin laxity (Table 27.1).

27.2 Concept

The goal of any facial rejuvenation procedure is to restore the youthful appearance of the skin and facial features and create contours, proportions, and shapes that are generally perceived as being attractive. These include a gently arching brow in females,

---

P.M. Prendergast
Venus Medical, Heritage House,
Dundrum Office Park, Dundrum, Dublin 14, Ireland
e-mail: peter@venusmed.com

Table 27.1 Advantages of suture lifting techniques

Advantages for the patient	Advantages for the surgeon
• Performed under local anesthesia • Short downtime • Minimal or hidden scars • Provide subtle, natural-looking rejuvenation • Relatively inexpensive • Can be repeated over time	• Short learning curve • Performed in office setting • High patient demand • Useful adjunct to other surgical and nonsurgical procedures

high, defined cheekbones, full cheek anteriorly with smooth lid-cheek junction, and a clearly defined jawline. Several classifications for facial aging have been proposed that describe senescent changes in the upper, middle, and lower thirds of the face as well as the neck [8]. Gravity facilitates the aging process by providing a vertically inferior vector for tissue that has lost elasticity, underlying structural support, or both [9]. Volume changes are usually involutional and are now known to occur both in the underlying bony skeleton [10, 11] as well as the soft tissues. In the forehead and temples, thinning of subcutaneous fat reduces the buffer between skin and the underlying hyperdynamic muscles of facial expression, resulting in horizontal and vertical forehead lines. As periorbital bony support decreases and tissues become lax, the brow drops to a horizontal position below the level of the supraorbital ridge, resulting in dermatochalasis. In the midface, the malar fat pad descends gradually from its normal position over the zygoma. This descent leads to several aging traits. As the fat falls away from the lid–cheek junction, the lower lid appears to lengthen and the infraorbital area above the cheek develops a crescent-shaped hollow or teartrough deformity. The nasolabial fold deepens as the malar fat pad superolateral to it drops. Further inferolateral descent of the malar fat pad accentuates the jowls and flattens the cheek superiorly. In the jowls, fat deposition rather than involution is typical and this reduces jawline definition characteristic of a youthful appearance. Aging in the neck begins with mild skin laxity and hypertrophy of the platysma muscle, which appears as vertical bands. This progresses to prominent sagging platysmal bands and horizontal folds, with varying degrees of submental fat accumulation and submandibular gland ptosis.

The rationale for treatment using suture facelift techniques is to reverse early signs of aging by lifting and suspending tissues that have begun to drop. By repositioning soft tissue in this way, not only are the sagging tissues lifted, but volume is also restored in important areas, such as the midface. Even a lift of 5–10 mm in the midface area restores the beauty triangle by changing the shape of the face from one that is rectangular to a heart-shaped one that is more pleasing and youthful. Suture techniques are not intended to correct more advanced signs of aging where significant skin laxity is present. Similarly, excessive fatty deposits in the face, submental area, and neck are not improved with suture facelift techniques alone, particularly when the overlying skin is tight. These problems require more aggressive measures such as rhytidectomy and lipoplasty.

Closed suture lifting techniques employ sutures of various types and designs to either loop around or "spear" subcutaneous fat or fascia and lift or suspend it in a predetermined vector. The author performs suture lifts under regional and infiltrative local anesthesia only without sedation. These minimally invasive procedures can be performed in an office-based setting, through minimal incisions or punctures, and allow a quick return to normal activities. They offer appropriately selected patients a natural-looking rejuvenation. For the physician, the learning curve is short and several hands-on workshops and preceptor courses are available throughout the world [12].

27.3 Patient Selection

The ideal patient for a suture facelift has mild ptosis of one or more of the following areas: brow, lateral canthus, malar fat pad, jowls, and neck. Even mild ptosis of these areas can produce a sad or sullen look and lifting by a few millimeters will change the overall countenance to a more pleasing one (Fig. 27.1). Visible tear troughs, flattened anterior cheeks, and deepened nasolabial folds are evidence of descent of the malar fat pads and all improve with suture elevation of the fat pads alone. Suture lifting of the face and neck are appropriate when there is interruption in the definition of the jawline and an increase in the cervicomental angle. Most suitable candidates are 30–45 years old, although the author has successfully treated patients

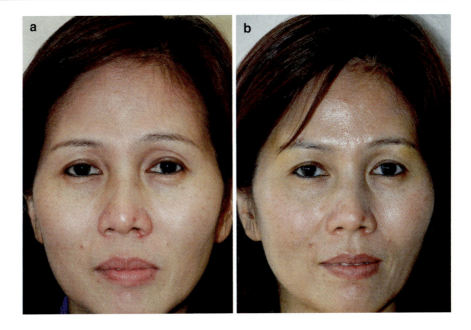

Fig. 27.1 (**a**) Preoperative. (**b**) After suture facelift showing subtle rejuvenation

ranging from 27 to 66 years. Skin laxity should not be excessive and facial volume should be normal or slightly reduced. Expectations should be realistic in terms of both the extent of lifting and the longevity of the results. One maneuver used by the author to determine suitability and likely results achievable from a suture lift is shown in Fig. 27.2. The surgeons' index fingers are placed at the points where the sutures purchase on the subcutaneous tissues and lifted about 10 mm. This degree of lifting is realistic and achievable in most selected cases. Instructions are provided to the patient prior to the procedure (Table 27.2). Following a detailed discussion including all potential risks and complications, a consent form is signed (Table 27.3).

tiny projections called barbs or cogs along their length to grasp tissue; another has tiny cones for the same purpose; and others are non-barbed and designed to simply pass around tissue like a sling. Newer sutures and techniques are emerging as the demand for minimally invasive procedures continues [14]. A classification for suture lifting techniques is presented in Table 27.4. There is a lack of evidence that one technique or system is superior to the others. As such, personal experience, training, and perhaps even marketing influence the decision to adopt one method over another. The author uses absorbable non-barbed sutures for the upper and lower thirds of the face, coned sutures for the midface, and either nonabsorbable or coned sutures for the neck.

27.4 Suture Types and Materials

There are several sutures in use today to lift the face and neck. The wide variation in both suture type and operative technique reflects the origins of suture lifting. There was no one procedure from which all others evolved. Rather, separate inventors and pioneers independently developed their own techniques using different concepts and materials, from countries as disparate as Russia and the USA [13]. Some sutures have

27.4.1 Barbed Sutures

Although the concept of barbed sutures began in 1956 [15], their use for facial rejuvenation was first reported in the 1990s [16]. Barbed sutures are designed with tiny hook-like projections cut into their long axes. The function of the barbs is to grasp tissue, distribute forces along the length of the barbed portion of the suture, and elevate or compress tissue in the direction of the barbs. Over the last decade, several barbed

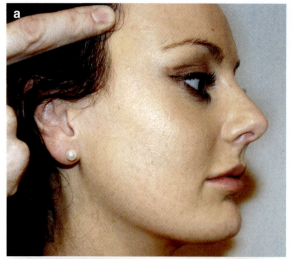
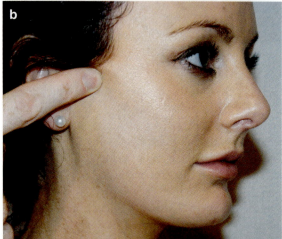
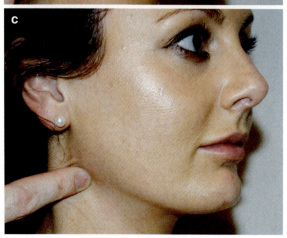

Fig. 27.2 Assessing a patient for a suture lift. The surgeon's finger lifts the tissues 10 mm. (**a**) Temporal lift. (**b**) Lower facelift. (**c**) Neck lift

Table 27.2 Preoperative instructions for suture face and neck lifts

Preoperative instructions: suture lift
1. DO NOT SMOKE for 2 weeks prior to and 2 weeks after surgery. Smoking reduces blood circulation, slows down healing and may increase complications
2. DO NOT TAKE ASPIRIN or products containing aspirin for 2 weeks prior to or following your scheduled surgery. Aspirin affects your blood's ability to clot and could increase your tendency to bleed during surgery or during the postoperative period
3. DO NOT TAKE DIETARY SUPPLEMENTS for 2 weeks before and after surgery. These include vitamins, ginger, Gingko biloba, garlic, ginseng, and fish oils. They may increase your risk of bleeding and bruising during and following surgery
4. DO NOT DRINK ALCOHOL for 5 days prior to surgery. Alcohol may increase your risk of complications such as bruising
5. IF YOU DEVELOP A COLD, COLD SORE, FEVER, OR ANY OTHER ILLNESS PRIOR TO SURGERY PLEASE NOTIFY US
6. WASH HAIR ON THE DAY PRIOR TO SURGERY
7. LEAVE JEWELRY AND VAULABLES AT HOME. Do not wear wigs, hairpins, or hairpieces
8. AVOID WEARING MAKEUP OR FACIAL MOISTURISERS
9. SURGERY TIMES ARE ESTIMATES ONLY. You could be at the clinic longer than indicated
10. HAVE A LIGHT BREAKFAST on the morning of surgery. Your suture lift procedure will be performed under local anesthesia without sedation
I HAVE READ AND FULLY UNDERSTAND THE ABOVE ITEMS 1–10

sutures have been brought to market that vary in length, number of barbs, orientation, and arrangement along the suture, as well as insertion and deployment characteristics.

27.4.1.1 Non-anchored Bidirectional Barbed Sutures

In 1998, Sulamanidze invented a nonabsorbable polypropylene suture with barbs on both halves of the suture converging toward the central portion (Fig. 27.3). Sulamanidze called these sutures Aptos

Table 27.3 Consent for suture lift procedure

What is a suture lift?

A suture lift is a thread lift procedure in which a special thread (e.g., polycaproamide or polypropylene) is passed under the skin, looped around or inserted through fat or other tissue such as the subcutaneous musculoaponeurotic system (SMAS) and retracted back to lift areas of the face or neck. It is minimally invasive, requiring a small incision or puncture, often placed behind the hairline. The procedure is performed under local anesthesia

Suitability for a suture lift

You will be assessed thoroughly beforehand to determine if you are suitable or not. Typically, patients who are suitable have mild drooping or sagging of cheeks, jowls, neck, or brow and are otherwise in good physical and mental health. If you have more severe sagging, a suture lift might not be appropriate, and you will be advised on alternatives

Procedure

A number of markings are made on the treatment area. Then a small incision is placed, usually behind the hairline where it is out of sight, and a stitch is passed under the skin in the fat or under muscle or fascia (layer above muscle). Sometimes a small patch is placed in the incision to secure the sutures. The tissues are gently retracted and the suture is tied, securing the lift. Finally, if present, the skin incision is closed

Special precautions

You should not proceed with this procedure if you are pregnant or breast feeding, or if you are allergic to local anesthetic agents. If you have medical conditions or are on certain medications, such as aspirin, steroids, or warfarin, treatment may be deferred, so you need to give your doctor your complete medical history. You should avoid taking vitamins and herbal supplements such as Gingko billoba and St John's Wort for 2 weeks before treatment

Potential risks and complications of a suture lift procedure

A small cannula (like a needle) is passed under your skin. As such, there is always a small risk of damage to structures under the skin, including the facial nerve, other nerves, and blood vessels, causing facial weakness, numbness, or bleeding. Weakness, although extremely rare, may be permanent. Numbness usually resolves or improves over time You may experience some swelling, bruising, and pain following the procedure. As with any injectable or invasive procedure, you may develop an infection, though the chance is low. You will receive a course of prophylactic antibiotics for 1 week following your treatment

Benefits and outcomes of treatment

It is usual to notice immediate lifting of the treatment area. You may see some "bunching" of skin near the hairline. This is normal and resolves after about 3–4 weeks. There is a small possibility that the procedure will fail if the suture cuts through the fat and tissue under the skin. Adhering to aftercare instructions will lessen this risk. Benefits of a suture lift will last a variable period of time, depending on the individual, and no guarantee of results or longevity of results is given It is usually possible to reverse or repeat the procedure if required

Alternatives to a suture lift procedure

Alternatives to a suture lift procedure include noninvasive skin tightening using infrared light or radiofrequency, other suture lift procedures, a surgical face lift procedure, or indeed no treatment at all

Initial:_____

CONSENT FOR SUTURE LIFT PROCEDURE

Please answer the following questions by ticking the appropriate box

Have you previously undergone a suture lift or facelift procedure?	Yes	No
If yes, specify:_____		
Do you have any known allergies?	Yes	No
If yes, specify:_____		
Are you currently taking any of the following medications: warfarin, aspirin, palvix, steroids?	Yes	No
Are you pregnant or breast feeding?	Yes	No
Have you previously completed a New Patient Data Form at Venus Medical Beauty?	Yes	No

(continued)

Table 27.3 (continued)

Please state if you have any other medical conditions, allergies, or are taking any medications not previously outlined in the New Patient Data Form:

_____
_____
_____
_____
_____

I have read the information on the suture lift procedure outlined on this form and fully understand the nature of treatment, all clinical implications, and potential risks involved. I have had the opportunity to ask questions to my satisfaction. I understand that it is my right to withdraw consent to treatment at any time. I consent to being photographed prior to treatment and understand that this photograph will remain the property of Venus Medical Beauty and may be used for educational or academic purposes. I willingly accept and consent to treatment with the suture lift procedure

Parent signature _____ Date _____

PRINT _____

OFFICIAL USE ONLY

I have explained to the patient the suture lift procedure. I have outlined the expected benefits of treatment, as well as any potential risks, complications, and side effects of treatment. I have given the patient the opportunity to read the literature pertaining to this treatment and clarified any further questions and queries where they existed. I have explained alternatives to treatment, including no treatment

---

Doctor signature _____ Date _____

PRINT _____

Table 27.4 Classification for closed suture lifts

Type	Subtype		Suture
Barbed suture lifts	Bidirectional barbed	Non-anchored	1. Aptos suture (APTOS, Moscow, Russia)
			2. Happy Lift Revitalizing threads (Promoitalia Int Srl, Rome, Italy)
		Anchored	1. Woffles sutures (Singapore)
			2. Articulus (previously Surgical Specialties Corp., Reading, PA)
			3. Happy Lift Double Needle (Promoitalia Int Srl, Rome, Italy)
			4. I-Lift Tensor threads (Argentina)
	Unidirectional barbed		1. Isse Endo Progressive Facelift suture (KMI Inc, Anaheim, CA)
			2. Contour Threads (previously Surgical Specialties Corp., Reading, PA)
			3. Happy Lift™ Anchorage (Promoitalia Int Srl, Rome, Italy)
Non-barbed suture lifts	Subcutaneous lift		1. Curl lift using polypropylene
			2. Malar fat pad sling using ePTFE[a] (Gore-Tex® Inc, Flagstaff, AZ)
	SMAS lift		1. Serdev technique using polycaproamide
Coned suture lifts			1. Silhouette suture (Silhouette Lift, Kolster Methods Inc., Corona, CA)

[a]Expanded polytetrafluoroethylene

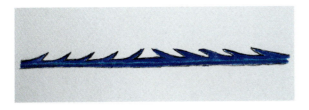

Fig. 27.3 Aptos polypropylene suture with bidirectional barbs

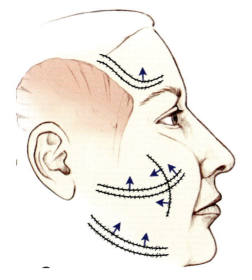

Fig. 27.4 Free-floating Aptos sutures with lifting vectors in the brow, malar fat pad, and jawline

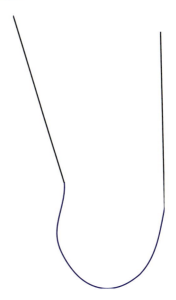

Fig. 27.5 Double Needle Happy Lift suture with bidirectional barbs

threads (APTOS, Moscow, Russia), referring to the "anti-ptosis" procedure they perform. Aptos threads are available in 2–0 and 3–0 sizes and in various lengths. They are inserted into the subcutaneous tissues of the face in predetermined paths by threading them through an 18G spinal needle. Once the needle is removed, the suture remains in place with either end protruding from the skin. The soft tissue is then fashioned around the barbs, as slight traction is applied to each end. This has the effect of bunching up subcutaneous fat along the length of the suture and lifting the tissues in a vector perpendicular to the long axis of the sutures (Fig. 27.4). In this way, the malar fat pad can be made to lift superolaterally and project anteriorly, and the jawline can be made to straighten by lifting the jowls [17, 18]. After manipulating the tissue to create the desired effect, the ends of the suture are trimmed and pushed under the skin.

The Happy Lift Double Needle (Promoitalia International Srl, Rome, Italy) is a newer polypropylene suture with bidirectional barbs arranged convergently. Unlike Aptos threads, there is a straight needle swaged to either end of the suture, obviating the need for a spinal needle for placement (Fig. 27.5). The barbs on Happy Lift threads are forked, presumably to improve purchase on the tissues (Fig. 27.6). There is little information in the literature on the use of these threads.

27.4.1.2 Anchored Bidirectional Barbed Sutures

In 2002, Wu devised a bidirectional barbed polypropylene suture to elevate soft tissue and anchor it to stable temporalis or mastoid fascia [19]. This 60 cm long thread has a 4 cm smooth central portion, a 20 cm section on either side of this with convergent barbs, and a smooth portion measuring 8 cm at either end. This so-called Woffles thread is passed subcutaneously along the chosen vector through an 18G spinal needle via two stab incisions. The needle passes from the inferior incision, through the subcutaneous fat, and bites the deep temporalis or mastoid fascia superiorly.

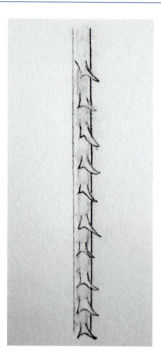

Fig. 27.6 Happy Lift suture with bifid barb morphology

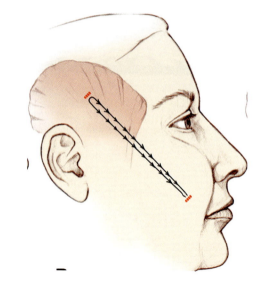

Fig. 27.7 Woffles inverted suture in situ

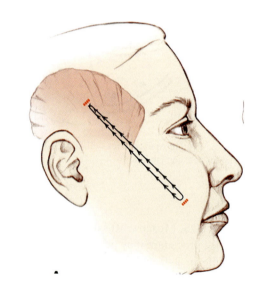

Fig. 27.8 Woffles bidirectional suture in situ

One arm of the thread passes from the inferior to superior incision via the spinal needle as far as the smooth central portion of the thread. The needle is then removed and reinserted through the superior incision to the lower one so the other arm of the thread can be passed in the same way. The needle is removed and the two ends emerging from the superior incision are lifted. This traction lifts the tissues at the smooth end of the thread and fastens the thread ends in the deep fascia via the downward facing barbs (Fig. 27.7). Both ends of the sutures are either cut flush with the fascia or tied to each other above it. Wu has developed second and third versions of this technique by inverting the "V" so that both free ends are in the face (Fig. 27.8), and interlocking two sutures to reduce the likelihood of "cheese-wiring" through the soft tissues at the point of maximal tension.

A second version of the Aptos thread by Sulamanidze employs the same bidirectional barbed suture as the original Aptos thread, but to either end a straight needle is attached. The two needles are lightly fused, enabling a single entry point. After the two needles puncture the skin as one whole, they are broken apart and take two different courses. The point of anchorage using this technique is the point of entry: zygomaticocutaneous ligaments for a midface lift or temporalis fascia for an eyebrow lift.

Ruff, an American plastic surgeon, did extensive work and research on the use of barbed sutures for tissue approximation as well as facial rejuvenation [20]. In 2001, he obtained a patent for his barbed sutures and insertion devices and formed Quill Medical. Working with Surgical Specialties Corporation, Ruff developed and marketed his barbed sutures for facelifting under the name Contour Threads. Although Angiotech has since acquired Quill Medical, and Contour Threads are no longer in distribution, they were used widely [21–23]. One version of Contour Threads, called Articulus, is an anchored bidirectional barbed suture. It consists of a 55 cm clear polypropylene suture with two 17 cm straight needles swaged to the ends. The central 5 cm of the suture is smooth, and adjacent to this there are two 15 cm barbed sections. The barbs are convergent toward the central portion. Each needle is attached to a 10 cm non-barbed section (Fig. 27.9). Placement of the Articulus is via a small incision in the temporal hairline. One of the needles is passed distally through the temporal incision, taking a bite of deep temporal fascia, and exiting in the midface lateral to the nasolabial fold. The second needle follows along a similar vector but exits more inferiorly. The thread ends are then held as the skin and fat pad are "walked up" the barbed suture until their elevated position provides a satisfactory enhancement (Fig. 27.10). The barbs prevent slippage of the elevated tissues whilst the non-barbed central portion of the thread is anchored superiorly to the temporalis fascia. To prevent "cheese-wiring" this portion can be reinforced with a nonabsorbable Gore-Tex® pledget.

I-Lift Tensor Threads, a company based in Argentina and Spain, produce other anchored bidirectional barbed sutures called iLift sutures. These nonabsorbable, clear

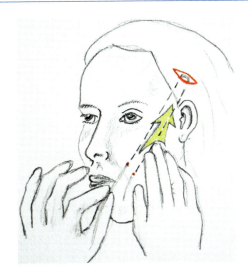

Fig. 27.10 Contouring following the insertion of the Articulus suture. The end of the suture is held as the tissues are pushed up along the barbs. The ends of the suture are then cut flush with the skin

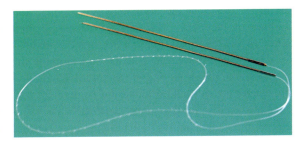

Fig. 27.11 Bidirectional barbed polypropylene sutures with swaged needles from I-Lift Tensor Threads

polypropylene sutures vary in size for face, neck, and brow lifting (Fig. 27.11).

27.4.1.3 Unidirectional Barbed Sutures

The early bidirectional free-floating Aptos sutures, marketed in the USA as FeatherLift, were modified by Isse who designed a unidirectional barbed suture. The Isse Endo Progressive Facelift suture (KMI Inc, Anaheim, Calif), is a polypropylene thread measuring 25 cm with the distal 15 cm bearing 50 unidirectional barbs. Isse describes his technique of closed meloplication using six threads for each malar fat pad [24]. Through a temporal incision, a small area of dissection

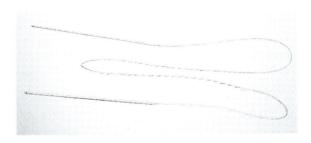

Fig. 27.9 Articulus suture. This is a clear polypropylene suture with two 17 cm straight needles, a smooth 5 cm central portion, two 15 cm barbed sections, and a 10 cm non-barbed portion adjacent to each needle. The barbs converge toward the central portion

is carried toward the zygomatic arch between the superficial and deep temporal fascia. A 20G 16 cm spinal needle is used to thread each barbed suture through the malar fat pad. Once the needle is removed, the sutures are lifted, trimmed, and secured to the deep temporal fascia by tying the smooth ends to a neighboring suture. The upward facing barbs engage the fibrofatty tissue of the malar fat pad and elevate it to a more youthful position. This also reduces the appearance of the tear trough, nasojugal fold, and softens the nasolabial fold.

Contour Threads (Surgical Specialties Corp., Reading, PA) were pioneered by Ruff and patented in 2004. The original and most widely used design is 25 cm, 2–0 polypropylene and contains helicoidally arranged unidirectional barbs along its middle 10 cm. On one end there is a half-circle needle for anchoring to fascia and on the other a 7-in. taperpoint straight needle for thread placement (Fig. 27.12). The straight needle is passed in a serpentine course through small stab incisions in the scalp or behind the ear and exit at the brow, lateral to the nasolabial fold or near the midline of the neck. The straight needle is then removed and the superior end of the thread is secured by suturing it to the fascia. With the patient in the sitting position, the distal end of the suture is held and the tissues are pushed up along the cogs to lift and contour the brow, midface, or neck. Finally, the distal ends of the sutures are cut flush with the skin. Despite being the most widely used barbed suture suspension technique in the USA, there is limited data on their efficacy and longevity [21].

The Happy Lift™ Anchorage sutures (Promoitalia International Srl, Rome, Italy) provide a similar method of suspension to Contour Threads, although

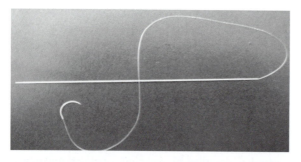

Fig. 27.12 The Contour Thread. A 25 cm, 2–0 polypropylene suture with helicoidally arranged unidirectional barbs along its middle 10 cm. On one end there is a half-circle needle for anchoring to fascia and on the other a 7-in. taperpoint straight needle for thread placement

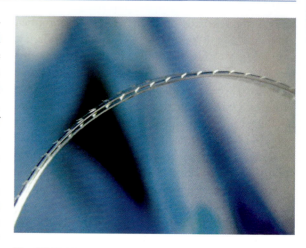

Fig. 27.13 The Happy Lift sutures have ten regularly spaced barbs per 1.6 cm of barbed portion

differences exist. These include a greater barb density on Anchorage sutures (10 barbs/1.6 cm) compared to Contour Threads (7 barbs/1.6 cm) and a different barb-morphology (Fig. 27.13). Happy Lift™ sutures are now also available in both nonabsorbable polypropylene and slowly absorbable polydioxanone.

27.4.2 Non-barbed Sutures

Bukkewitz described the first suture suspension lift for cosmetic enhancement in 1956 [25]. He used a strip of nylon inserted subcutaneously, to retract and improve a ptotic buccolabial fold. Starting in 1966, Guillemain, working with Galland and Clavier, started lifting all areas of the face by passing tendons or nylon into the tissues with a Reverdin needle and in their 1970 publication gave the technique the term "curl lift" [26]. Since then, other materials used to sling and suspend drooping tissues include polypropylene (Prolene), expanded polytetrafluoroethylene (Gore-Tex®), and polycaproamide (Polycon).

27.4.2.1 Nonabsorbable Non-barbed Sutures

Mendez Florez revisited Guillemain's curl lift technique and designed a straight double-bevel needle to pass the polypropylene suture into the tissues (Fig. 27.14) [26]. A small puncture is made in the cheek or brow and another one behind the hairline. The straight needle

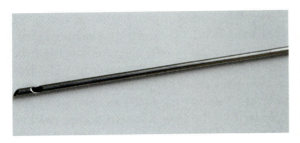

Fig. 27.14 Double-bevel needle used for curl lift

Erol and Hernandez-Perez described simplified suture suspension techniques to elevate the brow using nylon and polypropylene, respectively [27, 28]. Small punctures are made at the hairline and at the level of the brow to allow passage of the sutures in the subcutaneous plane using a needle (Fig. 27.15). In Erol's technique, the brow is suspended in the elevated position it assumes when the patient lies supine. Following infiltration of lidocaine 2% with 1:200,000 adrenaline, four stab incisions are made using a #11 blade, two directly above the lateral brow and two at the temporal hairline. A 4-0 nylon suture is passed from the medial to lateral brow incisions and the needle is then cut from the suture. Then an angiocatheter is passed subcutaneously from the lateral hairline incision to lateral brow incision and the end of the suture is passed through the eye of the catheter. The angiocatheter is withdrawn, bringing the suture out through the lateral hairline incision. The same maneuver is performed for the medial end so that both ends are exiting from the hairline incisions. Finally, the angiocatheter is passed from the medial to lateral incisions to bring the suture to the

passes through the lower incision and exits via the one in the scalp to receive one end of the thread. Then the thread is retracted back into the wound to a point just cephalad to the inferior puncture. Here, the needle is rotated 180° and tunneled once again toward the scalp incision, just parallel to the first passage. The other end of the thread exits and the two ends are lifted and tied. This is a simple, quick technique to lift subcutaneous fat but the smooth inelastic polypropylene suture tends to cut through the soft tissue at the point of lifting and results are short-lived.

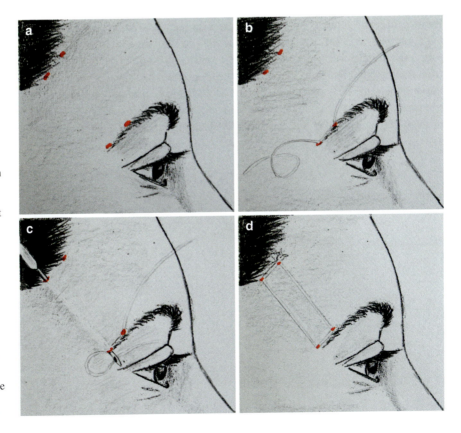

Fig. 27.15 Brow suspension using a simple suture. (**a**) Two stab incisions are made at the lateral brow and two at the temporal hairline. (**b**) A suture is passed from the medial brow incision to the lateral one and the needle is cut from the suture. (**c**) An angiocatheter is passed subcutaneously to bring the suture end to the lateral temporal incision. (**d**) The same maneuver is repeated so that a loop is created and both suture ends exit at the medial hairline incisions. The suture is tied to suspend the brow in an elevated position

medial incision. A knot is made to hold the eyebrow in position so that it does not drop inferiorly when the patient stands upright. Hernandez-Perez uses 3–0 polypropylene and a Keith needle to lift the brow in a similar manner and proposes that the loose tissues of the lateral brow, the undermining effect of the Keith needle, and the postoperative fibrosis that occurs along the sutures are enough to hold the brow in place without cheese-wiring. These brow lift procedures require superficial passage of needles, just under the skin, to avoid injuring the temporal division of the facial nerve where it passes about 2 cm above the lateral brow.

For midface rejuvenation, permanent sutures or slings elevate the malar fat pad without the need for long incisions, undermining, or dissection [3]. Sasaki describes his technique using either permanent CV-3 expanded polytetrafluoroethylene (Gore-Tex Inc, Flagstaff, AZ) or 4–0 clear Prolene sutures. The suture system used consists of a CV-3 Gore-Tex suture, a 3–0 braided Vicryl suture, a 3×8 mm Gore-Tex anchor graft, a second 4×4 mm anchor graft, two 10 cm Keith needles, and a 4–0 dyed Prolene guide suture (Fig. 27.16). Two stab incisions using a #11 blade are made along the nasolabial fold and a 1.5 cm incision is made in the temple 1 cm above the hairline. The first Keith needle with suture slings attached passes through the upper incision near the nasolabial fold and travels subcutaneously, through the malar fat pad, and exits from the temporal incision. The second needle passes through the same incision at the nasolabial fold but in a course parallel to the first needle and also exits through the incision behind the hairline. Then the braided Vicryl suture is used like a gigli saw to cut through any dermal attachments at the nasolabial puncture site before the Gore-Tex sling and anchor graft are pulled under the skin through the puncture. The dyed Prolene suture is used to guide the anchor graft into place, or to retrieve the graft if it does not lie correctly. Once the Gore-Tex sling is in place and the malar fat pad is suspended adequately, the Vicryl and guide sutures are removed and the Gore-Tex ends are secured by passing them through the second 4×4 mm anchor graft and suturing them to the deep temporal fascia using a French-eye needle (Fig. 27.17). This technique can also be performed during open procedures, or with some dissection along the deep temporal fascia to create a pocket anteriorly past the brow [29]. Yousif describes his technique using expanded polytetrafluoroethylene (Gore-Tex MycroMesh, W.L. Gore and Associates, Flagstaff, AZ) to lift the malar fat pad in a vertical vector, although this is a true sling and not a suture and is performed as an open procedure [30].

The Aptos Needle, invented by Sulamanidze, consists of a smooth non-barbed polypropylene suture attached to the middle of a double-pointed needle (Fig. 27.18) [16]. Midface elevation is achieved using the suture to loop around the tissues to lift them in different superior vectors. The double-point allows passage of the needle in a loop without the need to completely exit the skin so that the suture remains in the same plane throughout its course. A single incision need only be made and the sutures are anchored to the periosteum of the lateral or inferior orbital rim (Fig. 27.19). A similar longer Aptos Needle is used to

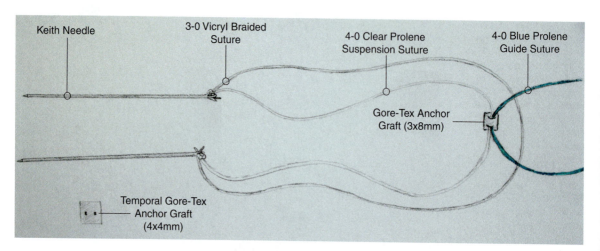

Fig. 27.16 Sasaki's suture suspension system for elevation of the malar fat pad

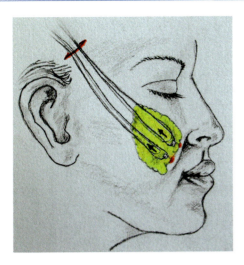

Fig. 27.17 Elevation of the malar fat pad using polypropylene slings with Gore-Tex anchor grafts

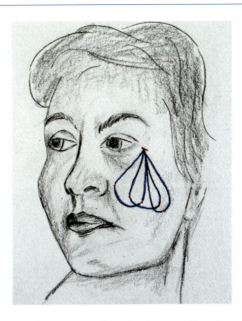

Fig. 27.19 Suture suspension using Aptos needles. The sutures are passed like slings around the tissues of the midface and anchored to periosteum on the infraorbital rim

27.4.2.2 Absorbable Non-barbed Sutures

Serdev, a Bulgarian cosmetic surgeon, improved upon Guillemain's original and Mendez-Florez's revised curl lift techniques by using slowly absorbable non-barbed semi-elastic polycaproamide sutures to lift moveable tissues and secure them to stable structures such as deep fascia or periosteum [32–34]. Using curved suture-passing needles (Fig. 27.20), the braided, antimicrobial sutures are passed through the platysma of the neck, the SMAS of the mid and lower face, the malar fat pad, and the superficial temporal fascia of the upper face. These tissues are gently lifted and suspended by passing the suture ends under the mastoid fascia, periosteum, or deep temporal fascia. These suspension techniques improve the cervicomental angle and definition of the jawline, reduce the appearance of jowls, elevate the malar fat pad, and lift the corner of the eyes and tail of the brow (Fig. 27.21). There are certain advantages of Serdev's techniques. The propensity of the sutures to "cheese-wire" through the tissues is less because the SMAS, and not just subcutaneous fat, is lifted. The braided sutures also yield somewhat to movement due to their elasticity. Using special needles, the sutures are anchored to deep fascia or periosteum through tiny punctures only, obviating the

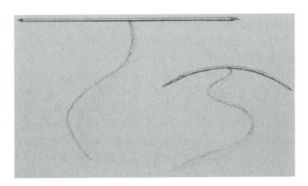

Fig. 27.18 Aptos needles are designed to pass through tissues without the need to exit completely. This keeps the suture in the same plane throughout its course

rejuvenate the neck. For this, an incision is made in the retroauricular area and a 2–0 Prolene suture is placed in the mastoid fascia as a holding suture. By passing the long Aptos Needle from one retroauricular incision to the contralateral side, without completely exiting the skin as above, the suture is brought from one side to the other subcutaneously and functions as a sling. Each end of the suture is tied to the holding sutures, securing them to the mastoid fascia. More than one suture can be placed in this way until the tissues are lifted and the cervicomental angle is restored. Giampapa described a similar suture suspension technique to improve the cervicomental angle using Prolene in combination with liposuction and partial platysmaplasty through a submental incision [31].

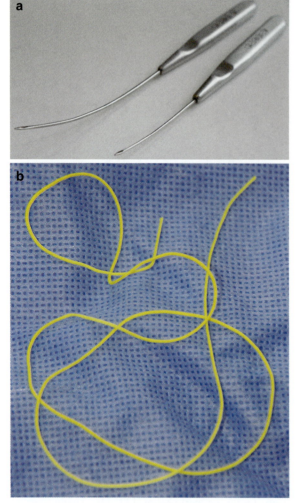

Fig. 27.20 (a) Curved suture passing needles for percutaneous superficial musculoaponeurotic system (SMAS) lifting techniques. (b) Braided anti-microbial slowly absorbable polycaproamide sutures are used to lift and anchor moveable tissues to stable ones

need for incisions or skin closure. The polycaproamide sutures absorb over 2–3 years, an obvious advantage for suture lifting where subsequent procedures are likely as the aging process continues. These simple but effective suture suspension techniques will now be described for the upper, mid, lower face, and neck.

Upper Face

The suture facelift technique in the temporal area provides a subtle but important rejuvenation of the upper face by lifting the tail of the eyebrow, the lateral canthus, and the upper cheek (Fig. 27.22). In the periorbital area, elevation of soft tissues by 1–3 mm provides noticeable rejuvenation (Figs. 27.23 and 27.24). Markings are made at the proposed incision points. The first is along a line drawn perpendicular to the tail of the eyebrow, just behind the temporal hairline. A second point is made just behind the hairline 4–5 cm inferior to the first point. Two further points are made superior to the first points, along the desired vector lines of lift. One of these points should be along the superior temporal crest line where the deep temporal fascia attaches to periosteum. The hair is tied or retracted to expose the skin at the marked points. After skin preparation and sterile draping, local anesthesia using lidocaine 1–2% with 1:200,000 adrenaline is injected along the proposed path of the suture subcutaneously between the lower two points, on the periosteum between the upper two points, and under the superficial temporal fascia and above the deep temporal fascia between each upper and lower point. The superficial temporal fascia is a continuation of the galea over the frontalis muscle and the SMAS of the middle and lower thirds of the face. Stab incisions using a #11 blade are made at the marked points. The curved needle is passed from the upper medial incision to the lower medial incision, under the superficial temporal fascia but above the deep temporal fascia. To find this plane, lift a tuft of hair above the path of the needle and pass the needle deeply. There should be a thick layer of tissue covering the needle following passage, but it should not be so deep that the patient's head rocks when the needle is moved. This indicates that the needle has passed under the deep temporal fascia. Once the needle tip exits the inferior point, a USP #2 polycaproamide sutures is passed through the eye of the needle and the needle is withdrawn. Next, the needle is passed in the superficial subcutaneous plane from the lower lateral incision to the lower medial incision and the suture end is threaded through the needle's eye and brought to the lower lateral incision. The suture is above the superficial temporal fascia along this line. Then the suture is brought from the lower lateral to the upper lateral incision under the superficial temporal fascia as before. Finally, the needle is passed into the upper medial incision, taking a bite of periosteum and deep temporal fascia along the superior temporal fusion line, and exits from the upper lateral

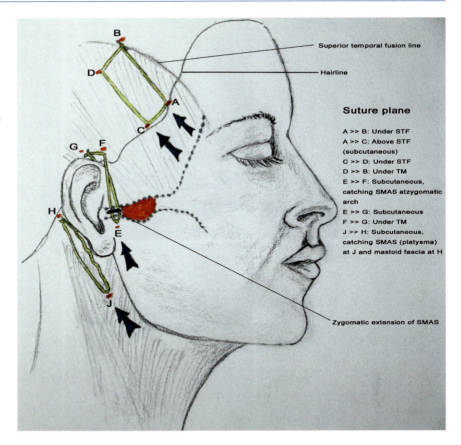

Fig. 27.21 Suture lift of superficial musculoaponeurotic system (SMAS [moveable]) to deep fascia or periosteum (non-moveable) through minimal incision (*red dots*). The red area shows area of zygomatic arch over which the facial nerve passes (0.8–3.5 cm from external acoustic meatus). *STF* superficial temporal fascia, *TM* temporalis muscle, *ZES* zygomatic extension of SMAS

Superior temporal fusion line
Hairline

Suture plane

A >> B: Under STF
A >> C: Above STF (subcutaneous)
C >> D: Under STF
D >> B: Under TM
E >> F: Subcutaneous, catching SMAS at zygomatic arch
E >> G: Subcutaneous
F >> G: Under TM
J >> H: Subcutaneous, catching SMAS (platysma) at J and mastoid fascia at H

Zygomatic extension of SMAS

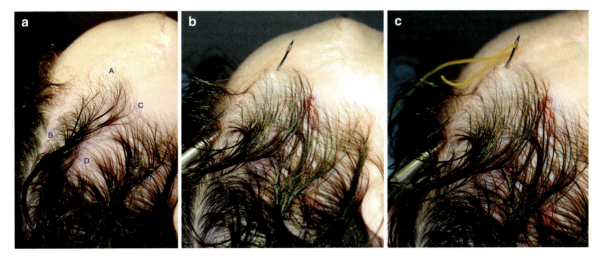

Fig. 27.22 Upper face (temporal) SMAS lift using slowly absorbable polycaproamide sutures. The superficial musculoaponeurotic system (SMAS) is called the superficial temporal fascia (STF) in the temporal area and the galea aponeurotica medial to this over the forehead. (**a**) Four points are marked as shown and stab incisions using a #11 blade are made. One of the superior incisions (*B*) is made along the superior temporal crest line. (**b**) The curved needle is passed under the STF (above the deep temporal fascia) from point *B* to *A*. (**c**) A USP#2 or #4 polycaproamide suture is passed through the eye of the needle and the suture is brought back from point *A* to *B*. (**d**) The needle is passed from point *C* to *A* in the superficial subcutaneous plane (above STF) and the suture end is threaded through. (**e**) The suture is brought to point *D* under STF as before. (**f**) Now both ends of the suture are exiting at the upper incisions. (**g**) The needle is passed deep into point *B* until it reaches periosteum. (**h**) A deep bite is taken, underneath the deep temporal fascia, and the needle receives the suture end at point *D*. (**i**) The needle is retracted so that both ends exit at point *B*. The sutures are gently lifted and tied. This lifts the STF, tail of the brow, and upper face. The suture is cut and buried by applying traction to the puncture site with the tip of an artery forceps

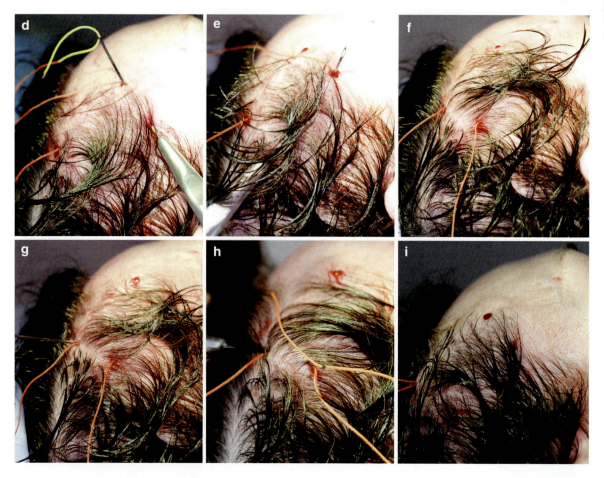

Fig. 27.22 (continued)

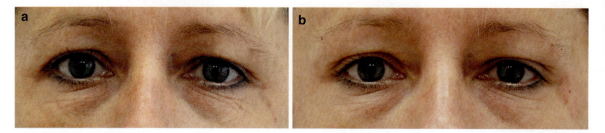

Fig. 27.23 (**a**) Preoperative. (**b**) After temporal superficial musculoaponeurotic system (SMAS) lift using absorbable sutures. Even a 1–2 mm lift makes the eyes look less tired

incision. The suture is brought from this incision to the upper medial one so that both ends exit from the same incision. The suture ends are lifted gently to elevate the superficial temporal fascia (temporal SMAS) along the hairline, and elevate the tail of the brow and upper face. The suture is tied and the incision points, if inverted or tethered down, are released using the tip of a mosquito. The incisions heal quickly by secondary intention. A small amount of bunching of skin is usual along the hairline but this

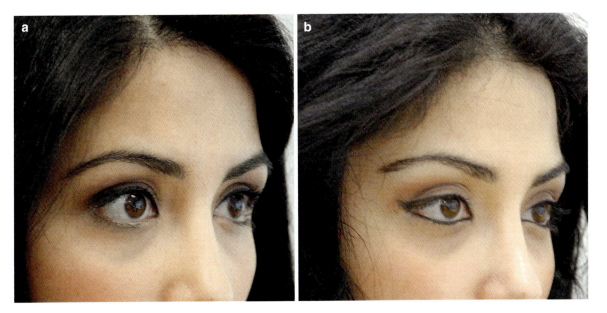

Fig. 27.24 (a) Preoperative. (b) After temporal superficial musculoaponeurotic system (SMAS) lift to lift the tail of the brow in a younger patient

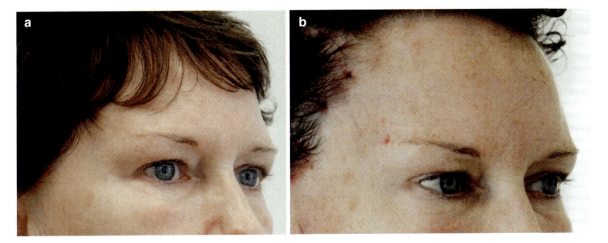

Fig. 27.25 (a) Preoperative. (b) Immediately after temporal superficial musculoaponeurotic system (SMAS) lift

contracts and disappears in 1–2 weeks. This technique provides an instant rejuvenation, particularly around the eyes (Fig. 27.25).

Midface

Traditional rhytidectomy procedures that include resection, retraction, or plication of the SMAS often do not achieve optimal elevation of the malar fat pad and midface. The triangular malar fat pad is oriented with its base along the nasolabial fold and apex over the zygoma. It is superficial to the medial part of the SMAS and adherent to the overlying skin. Retracting the SMAS in this region does not elevate the malar fat pad and may deepen the nasolabial fold. Repositioning the malar fat pad using the suture suspension technique restores the beauty triangle of the face, softens the nasolabial fold, and reduces the lower lid length (Fig. 27.26). The vector of lift to achieve this is superolateral. Three punctures are made: two in the temporal hairline over the temporal

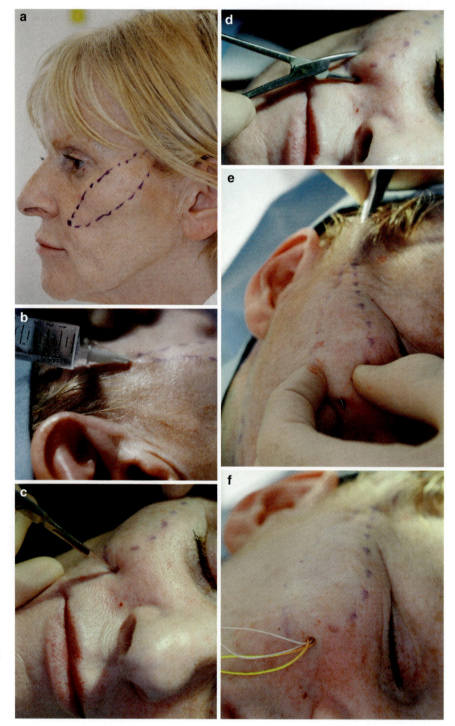

Fig. 27.26 Closed suture suspension of the malar fat pad. (**a**) A point is marked just lateral to the nasolabial fold and two points in the temporal hairline. The markings represent the proposed course of the suture to lift the malar fat pad in a superolateral vector. (**b**) Lidocaine with epinephrine is infiltrated subcutaneously along the marked lines. (**c**) Using a #11 blade, stab incisions are made at the three points. (**d**) The dermis is fully penetrated at the inferior incision to minimize dimpling of the skin. (**e**) The curved needle is passed along the lower line from the posterior temporal incision and exits at the incision lateral to the nasolabial fold. (**f**) A USP#4 polycaproamide suture, together with a 3–0 Vicryl suture, are passed through the eye of the needle and withdrawn to the temporal incision. (**g**) The needle is passed from the anterior temporal incision along the other line and receives the ends of the sutures. (**h**) The needle and sutures are withdrawn, creating a loop around the malar fat pad. (**i**) The Vicryl suture is grasped and a sawing motion is used to cut through any dermal attachments at the inferior puncture until the skin is smooth. The Vicryl suture is then removed. (**j**) The needle is passed between the temporal incisions, below the deep temporal fascia, and the polycaproamide sutures are brought through one incision. (**k**) The sutures are lifted gently to elevate the malar fat pad, and tied. The punctures are allowed to heal by secondary intention. A Steristrip or 6–0 suture is used to seal the puncture at the nasolabial fold

Fig. 27.26 (continued)

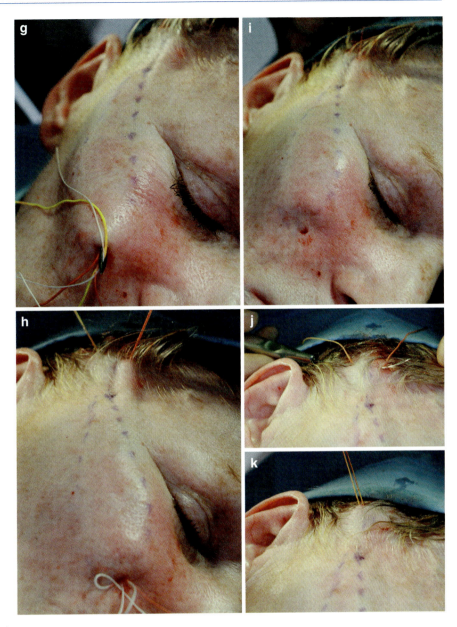

fascia and one just lateral to the nasolabial fold. An artery forceps is inserted into the incision at the nasolabial fold to make sure the incision has passed thoroughly through the dermis. Using the curved needles, a USP#2 or USP#4 polycaproamide suture is passed from the nasolabial fold incision to the temporal incisions, forming a sling around the malar fat pad. A braided suture such as Vicryl can be passed together with the polycaproamide suture. This second suture is used to cut through the dermis or other connections to the skin that might cause a depression or dimple at the nasolabial fold incision. Once the skin is smooth at the site of lifting, the Vicryl suture is removed and the remaining suspension suture sits in place. The suture is then anchored beneath the deep temporal fascia using the curved needles. As well as lifting the malar fat pad superiorly, it projects anteriorly and improves infraorbital volume loss (Fig. 27.27).

Lower Face

Descent of the lower face and jowls obscures jawline definition and changes the shape of the face from a desirable inverted triangle or heart-shape to

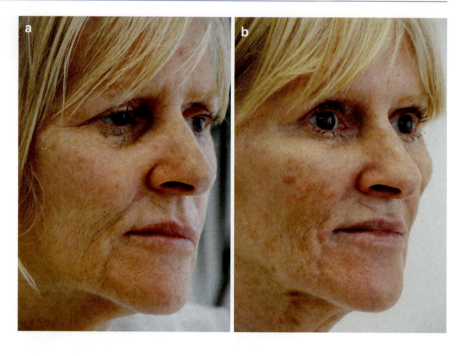

Fig. 27.27 (a) Preoperative. (b) After suture lift of the malar fat pad. Note the anterior projection of the cheek and improvement in tear trough hollows. A temporal superficial musculoaponeurotic system (SMAS) lift has also improved dermatochalasis of the lateral brow

an undesirable rectangular one (Fig. 27.28). To lift the jowls, the zygomatic extension of the SMAS is lifted using an absorbable non-barbed suture and anchored to temporalis fascia above the ear. Three points are marked: two above the ear in the hairline and one just below the zygomatic arch in front of the lobule of the ear. Lidocaine with adrenaline is infiltrated in the subcutaneous plane between the three points, and deeper on the periosteum between the upper two points. Stab incisions using a #11 blade are made at the three points. The tip of an artery forceps is used to puncture through the entirety of the dermis at the lower point to reduce the likelihood of dimpling. A curved needle is passed subcutaneously from the upper anterior incision downward toward the lower incision. At the level of the zygomatic arch, a slightly deeper bite is taken to catch the SMAS. It is important to stay within 8 mm from the external acoustic meatus at this level to avoid injury to the facial nerve. The nerve always passes over the zygomatic arch between 8 mm and 3.5 cm from the external acoustic meatus and usually about 2.5 cm from it [35]. After biting SMAS, the needle comes superficially and exits through the lower incision and the suture is passed through the eye of the needle. The needle is withdrawn and a similar maneuver is made in order to pass the suture from the lower incision to the upper lateral incision. The needle is then passed deeply into the upper lateral incision to catch the periosteum under the temporal fascia and exits from the upper medial incision to receive the suture end. In the correct position under this deep fascia, any movement of the needle should rock the patient's head. The suture end is brought through to the upper lateral incision where the two ends can be lifted gently and tied. The lifting of the zygomatic extension of the SMAS as well as the attached overlying skin should smooth the jawline and even lift part of the neck (Fig. 27.29). Any dimpling or inversion of skin at the puncture sites is released using the tip of an artery forceps. Some bunching in front of the ear is normal and resolves spontaneously in 1–2 weeks.

Neck

Mild to moderate ptosis of the neck can be treated using suture lifting alone, or in combination with lipoplasty to remove fat under the chin, along the jawline and in the jowls (Fig. 27.30). The suture suspension technique using absorbable sutures is simple and quick. After infiltrative local anesthesia, two skin punctures are made: one behind the ear over the mastoid and one in the upper neck over the anterior border of the sternocleidomastoid muscle. The needle is passed through the upper point, deeply at first to include the mastoid fascia or periosteum, and advanced in a sinusoidal path superficially under the skin toward the lower point. Before exiting from the lower incision, a deeper bite is taken to catch the posterior border of platysma. A USP# 2 polycaproamide suture is threaded through the needle and brought back to the retroauricular incision. Another pass is made, taking a parallel course to the first pass, and the end of the suture is passed from the lower to upper incision so that both ends of the suture exit behind the ear. The sutures are retracted enough to lift the platysma and improve the contour of the neck, and tied. If there is dimpling of the skin at the lower puncture, an artery forceps tip is passed into the incision and gently lifted until the dimple is softened. Bunching of skin along the length of the suture improves without intervention.

27.4.3 Coned Sutures

Isse designed a polypropylene suture with regularly spaced knots along its length and small floating cones made of poly-L-lactic acid. He modified his earlier

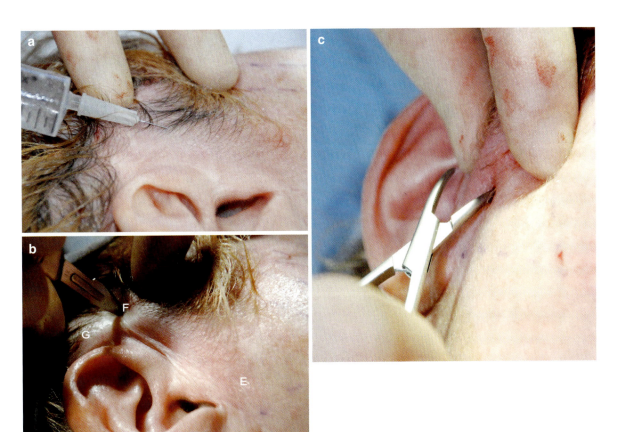

Fig. 27.28 Lower superficial musculoaponeurotic system (SMAS) suture facelift. (**a**) Local anesthesia is infiltrated subcutaneously in front of the ear and under the temporal fascia above the ear. (**b**) Three stab incisions are made at points *E*, *F*, and *G*. (**c**) An artery forceps is used to penetrate the full thickness of the dermis at point *E*. (**d**) The curved needle is passed in the subcutaneous plane from point *F* toward point *E*. At the lower border of the zygomatic arch a deeper bite is taken to catch the zygomatic extension of SMAS. (**e**) The needle is advanced superficially and exits at point *E*. A USP#2 or USP#4 polycaproamide suture is threaded through the eye of the needle. (**f**) The needle is withdrawn. (**g**) The needle is passed subcutaneously from incision *G* to point *E* and receives the distal end of the suture. (**h**) The needle is withdrawn so that a sling around the SMAS is created. (**i**) To anchor the suture superiorly, the needle is passed under the deep temporal fascia above the ear from point *G* to point *F*. Moving the needle in this plane should move the patient's whole head. (**j**) The suture end is passed through the tip of the needle and the needle is withdrawn. (**k**) Both ends exit from the incision *G*. Lifting the sutures lifts the patient's jowls and even neck as the SMAS is suspended. The suture is tied. (**l**) The incisions are lifted to bury the knot

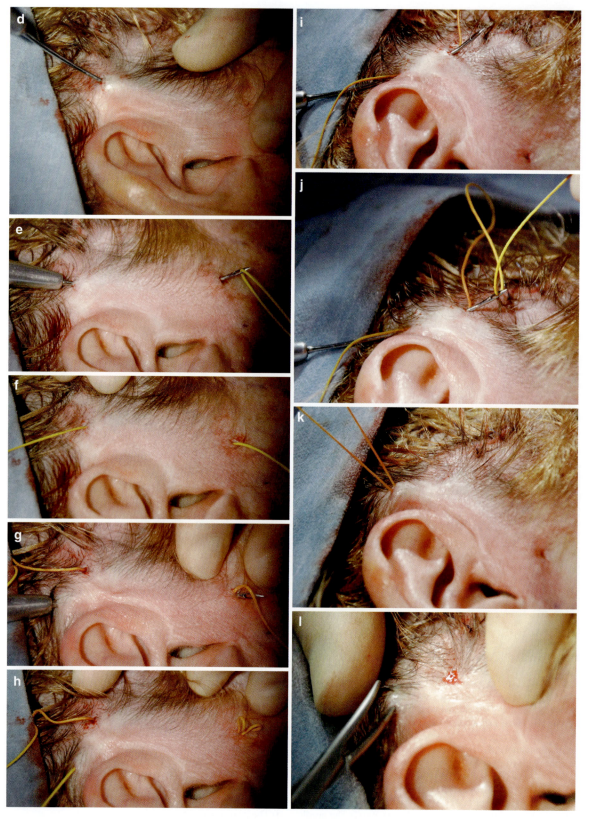

Fig. 27.28 (continued)

27 Suture Facelift Techniques

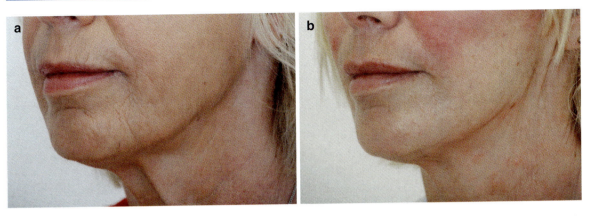

Fig. 27.29 (a) Preoperative. (b) After lower suture facelift. There is an improvement in the jawline as well as the platysmal bands of the neck

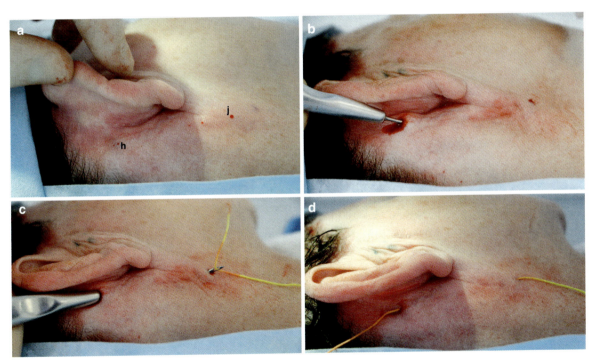

Fig. 27.30 Neck lift using suture suspension technique. (a) Local anesthetic is infiltrated superficially along lines h to j. An incision using a #11 blade is made behind the ear (h) and over the anterior border of the sternocleidomastoid muscle (j). (b) A curved needle is passed from incision h toward incision j. Just before exiting at j, the needle takes a deeper bite to catch the platysma muscle (SMAS). (c) The needle exits and a USP#2 polycaproamide absorbable suture is passed through the tip. (d) The needle is retracted through point h. (e) The needle is advanced again through the same puncture, taking a serpentine course through the superficial tissues, and exits at the distal incision to receive the end of the suture. (f) The needle is retracted again so that both suture ends exit at the retroauricular incision. (g) Retracting the sutures lifts the neck and improves the cervicomental angle. If there is a dimple at the inferior incision, this is released with an artery forceps. (h) The sutures are tied and cut. Slight bunching along the length of the suture is normal and resolves spontaneously in 2–3 weeks

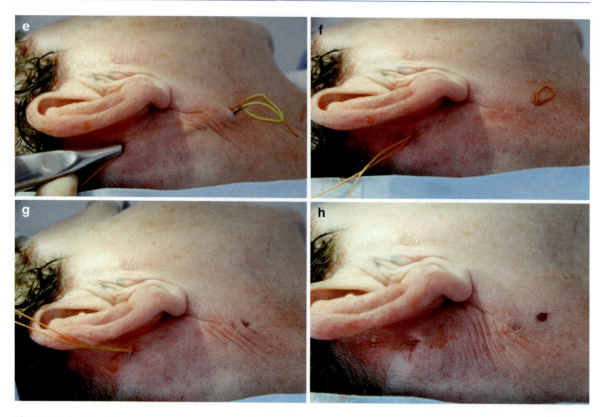

Fig. 27.30 (continued)

barbed polypropylene suture for several reasons. Firstly, he felt a suture with knots would be stronger than a suture designed with cuts to create barbs, since the tensions applied to the barbs are prone to linear shredding where the barbs meet the body of the suture. Secondly, the cones are made of a material that incites an inflammatory response and stimulates collagen to secure the sutures over time. Finally, Isse believed the biomechanics of the cone design would be inherently stronger than most barbed sutures. Isse's suture is currently marketed as the Silhouette Suture (Silhouette Lift, Kolster Methods Inc., Corona, CA). This is presented as a clear 3–0 polypropylene suture with 10 cones and multiple knots to prevent slippage of the cones and to hold them equidistant from each other within the tissues. A newer dyed polypropylene Silhouette Suture is also available containing 6 cones. The cones are made of poly-L-lactic acid and are absorbed over 8–10 months. There is a 20.3 cm 20G straight needle swaged to the distal end of the suture and a 26 mm half-circle needle to the proximal end (Fig. 27.31). Included

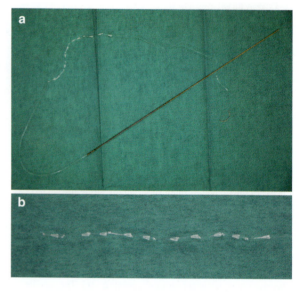

Fig. 27.31 (**a**) Silhouette suture. A straight needle is swaged to one end of the polypropylene suture and a half-circle needle to the other. There are knots and cones along its length. (**b**) Absorbable poly-L-lactic acid cones

with Silhouette Sutures are 2×0.5 cm polypropylene mesh patches for anchorage to deep fascia. These coned sutures are particularly useful for midface and neck rejuvenation and can be performed under local anesthesia through minimal incisions [36]. There is evidence that coned sutures offer a more secure and stable lifting than most popular barbed sutures and are more resistant to structural damage in human tissues [37]. The author uses Silhouette Sutures alone or in combination with non-barbed absorbable sutures for midface, lower face, and neck lifting. The technique of midface and neck lifting using Silhouette Sutures is described below.

27.4.3.1 Midface

The patient is marked in the sitting position (Fig. 27.32). A line is drawn from the lobule of the ear to the modiolus. Sutures should not cross this line as animation and movement at the mandible may lead to disruption. The proposed path for the sutures is marked along the sides of the face. These markings reflect the appropriate lifting vectors, which are superior and superolateral. The inferior points mark the exit sites for the needles and start about 1 cm lateral to the nasolabial fold with 1.5 cm between each point. The vector lines converge in the temporal area, behind the hairline, where a 3 cm mark is

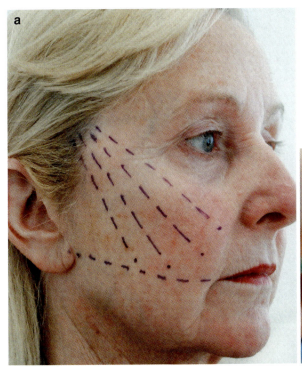

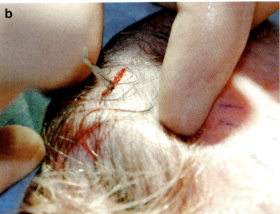

Fig. 27.32 Silhouette suture midface lift. (**a**) The patient is marked in the sitting position. The inferior points start about 1 cm lateral to the nasolabial fold. Subsequent points are spaced 1.5 cm apart. (**b**) A 2–3 cm incision is made in the temporal area behind the hairline where the vector lines converge. (**c**) The superficial temporal fascia is grasped and opened. (**d**) The shiny white deep temporal fascia is exposed. (**e**) A 1×1.5 cm piece of polypropylene mesh is cut and placed in the wound on the deep temporal fascia. (**f**) The mesh is sutured to the deep temporal fascia using a 4–0 nonabsorbable suture (**g**) The Silhouette suture is placed over the face to measure how many cones will span the malar fat pad and midface without extending into the upper face. This determines how many cones, if any, should be cut from the distal end of the suture after placement. (**h**) The straight needle is passed just superficial to the superficial temporal fascia (STF) at the temporal incision, and through the subcutaneous fat of the cheek to exit at the first of the marked points. The STF splits into two leaves just inferior to the hairline and the temporal branch of the facial nerve travels through its layers. Staying superficial to the STF avoids inadvertent injury to the nerve. (**i**) The Silhouette suture is slowly pulled through the midface until the cones emerge from the inferior puncture. A number of cones can be cut from the suture at this time. (**j**) The suture is then cut distal to one of the knots and retracted to lift the malar fat pad. Each suture is tied to a neighboring one, and anchored to the deep temporal fascia and mesh, before closure in two layers

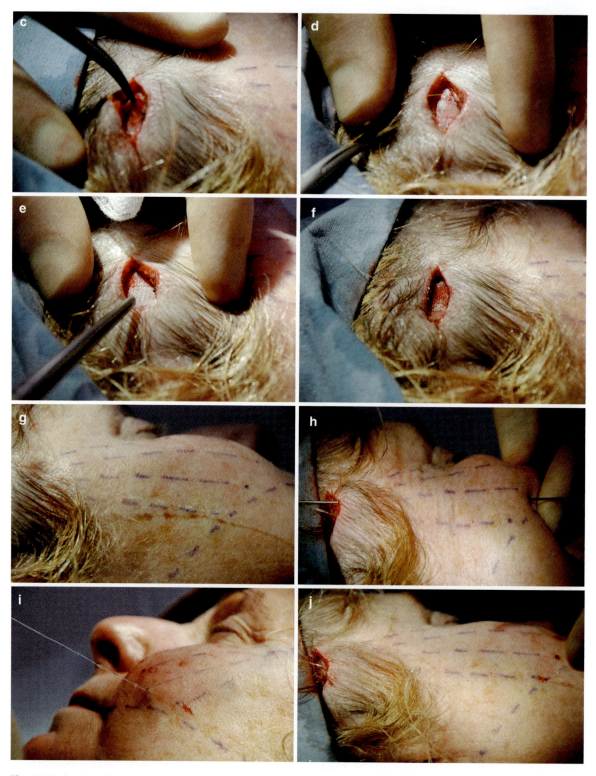

Fig. 27.32 (continued)

made for the incision site. After skin preparation and sterile draping, the marked areas are infiltrated with 2% lidocaine with 1:200,000 epinephrine. A 3 cm incision is made in the temporal area and diathermy is used for hemostasis. The superficial temporal fascia is exposed, grasped, and opened, exposing the shiny, white deep temporal fascia. A small 1.5×0.5 cm patch of polypropylene mesh is placed on the deep temporal fascia and sutured in place. The first Silhouette suture is measured externally over the cheek to determine how many cones are needed to run the length of the malar area. If all of the cones are left on the suture, some of the proximal ones may be visible under the thin skin of the temple area, or they may catch on the superficial temporal fascia when the suture is retracted. The author usually cuts three to four cones from the distal end of the suture after they exit at the inferior points. Cones are usually not removed if a Silhouette Suture with 6 cones is used. The suture is passed in the deep subcutaneous plane from the temporal incision, along the marked path, to the exit points. To do this, the straight needle enters the tissues just above the superficial temporal fascia under direct vision at the upper incision. The nondominant hand gently grasps the tissues over the needle as it passes through the temple and then malar fat pad, maintaining the same depth throughout. If the suture passes too superficially it may catch the dermis and result in irregularities. If it passes too deeply it risks injury to facial nerve branches, particularly the frontal branch as it passes between the layers of the superficial temporal fascia lateral to the eye. The needle should exit the skin at the inferiorly marked points perpendicularly to avoid catching the dermis. The straight needle is pulled through until the cones begin to emerge from the skin. At this point, one or more cones can be cut from the suture as outlined above, making sure not to pull through any cones that are to remain on the suture. The suture is cut just distal to one of the knots and retracted proximally to visualize the lifting effect on the tissues. The proximal half-circle needle is passed through the superficial temporal fascia at the incision and then the needle is passed through both the deep temporal fascia and the anchored polypropylene mesh. The suture is not tied until all other sutures have been passed. Usually a total of four sutures are placed on each side of the midface. Once all of the sutures are in place, the half-circle needles are cut from the proximal ends and each suture is gently lifted and tied to its neighboring suture. The temporal incision is closed in two layers. A gentle lift is sufficient to elevate the malar fat pad and even jowls and provide pleasing results (Fig. 27.33).

27.4.3.2 Neck

The coned Silhouette sutures are also used to lift mild to moderate ptosis of the neck (Fig. 27.34). If ptosis is coupled with significant submental and submandibular fatty deposits, lipoplasty combined with the Silhouette lift is more appropriate [34]. The author commonly uses ultrasound-assisted lipoplasty (VASER) combined with Silhouette sutures for this purpose. For the Silhouette suture lift, markings are made from behind the ear, along the neck under the line of the mandible to a point just proximal to the midline. Alternatively, this line can continue across the midline to a point just distal to it. A 1 cm retroauricular incision is made and the first suture is passed in the subcutaneous fat along the line of marking, and exits at the distal point. The author prefers to continue across the midline, so that the suture acts as a sling to support and lift the midline and improve the cervicomental angle. To bring the suture across the midline, the needle should first exit from a point just proximal to the midline. Before the needle exits completely from the skin, with the proximal end of the needle still under the skin, the needle is turned around so that the proximal end of the needle with the suture attached is now advancing toward the midline. It is advanced to a point just distal to the midline where a stab incision with a #11 blade is made to allow the blunt end of the straight needle to emerge. Once the suture is seen, it is cut from the needle and the needle is removed from the site. The suture end is pulled until the most distal knot on the suture is just visible. The suture is cut just distal to the knot and the proximal end of the suture at the retroauricular incision is gently retracted. The coned portion of the suture passes across the midline and provides a lifting along its length as well as a suspension of the submental area. Usually two sutures are passed on either side of the neck. The proximal ends of the sutures are secured to the mastoid fascia using the half-circle needles and tied to one another. The incision is then closed.

27.5 Postoperative Care

Although suture facelift techniques are minimally invasive and performed through small incisions or punctures, postoperative care is important. The closed techniques described in this chapter do not involve dissection or undermining. The relatively atraumatic insertion of sutures, although advantageous in terms of downtime, means there is less inflammation and fibrosis around the sutures, which can dislodge or migrate or potentially become disrupted in the tissues. Careless handling of the face or neck following a suture lift can disrupt the sutures or result in cheese-wiring of the tissues through the sutures. Ideally, the treatment area should be taped and a head garment should be worn for 3–4 days to immobilize the tissues (Fig. 27.35). Patients should be instructed to avoid excessive facial animation, chewing gum and laughing for a week, and to be gentle when handling the face or neck for 4–6 weeks following the procedure.

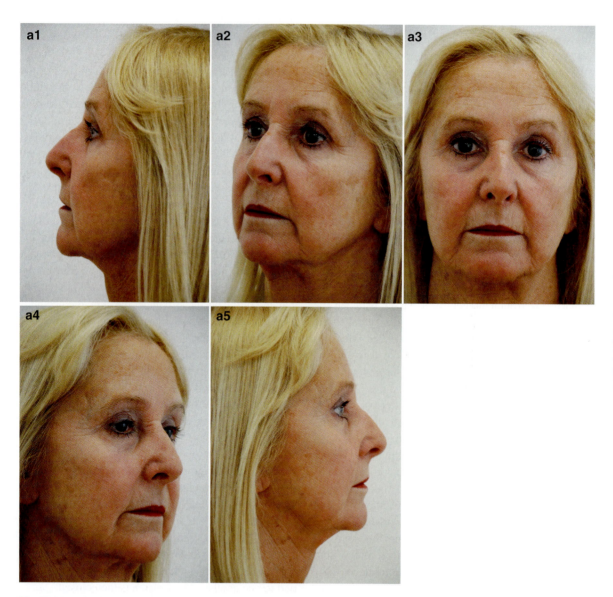

Fig. 27.33 (**a1-a5**) Preoperative. (**b1-b5**) After midface and lower face lift using Silhouette and polycaproamide sutures, respectively

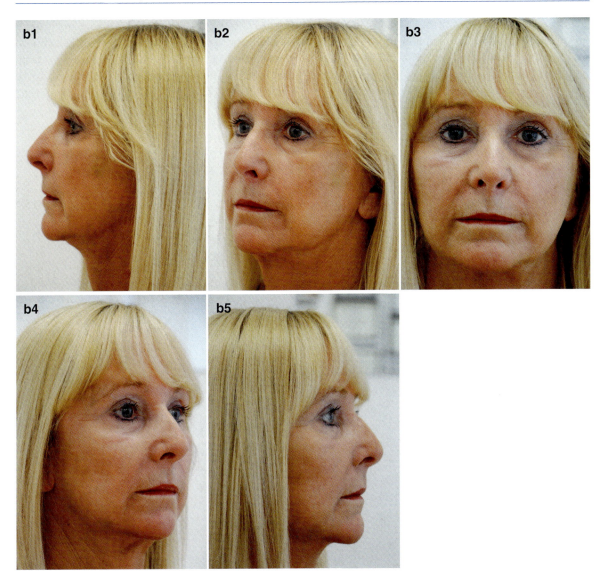

Fig. 27.33 (continued)

This includes cleansing or applying makeup upward along the vector of lifting rather than downward against the sutures. Following the procedure, the author administers cephalexin for 5 days and tramadol for 3 days as needed if simple analgesia is insufficient to control discomfort. Normal sequelae following suture lifts include edema, ecchymosis, and point tenderness over the suture ends. To reduce swelling, the patient is advised to use cold packs and sleep with the head elevated for a few days. A clear instruction leaflet should be provided, including a contact telephone number in case the patient has any concerns following the procedure (Table 27.5). A follow-up appointment is arranged in 1 week, at which time sutures, if present, are removed.

27.6 Complications

Patients tolerate suture lift procedures well under infiltrative local anesthesia with complementary regional nerve blocks, if required. These methods are preferred as they eliminate unnecessary risk associated with intravenous sedation or general anesthesia. Mild edema, ecchymosis, tenderness, and transient bunching of overlying skin are common following suture lifts. Complications include infection, bleeding, palpability, visibility, skin irregularities, migration, extrusion, prolonged pain, nerve injury, and asymmetries (Figs. 27.36 and 27.37) [38–40]. These complications should be prevented by proper placement of appropriate sutures using sterile techniques. If they do occur, they often resolve spontaneously or can easily be treated (Table 27.6).

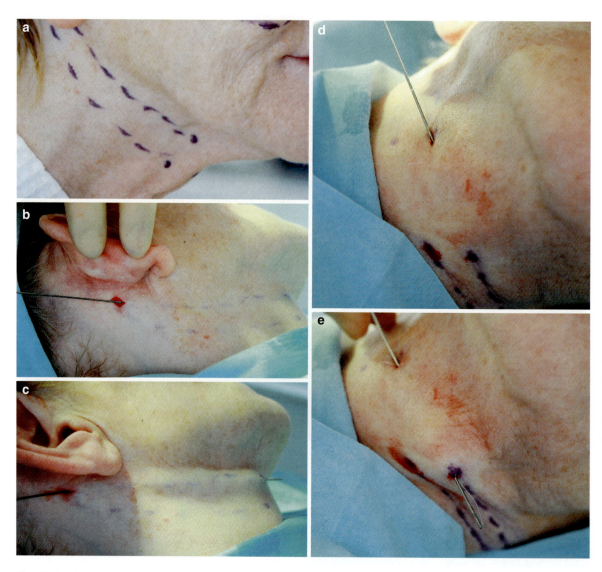

Fig. 27.34 Coned (Silhouette) suture lift of the neck. (**a**) Markings are made behind the ear and along the neck under the mandible to a point about 2 cm proximal to the midline. A second point is marked 2 cm distal to the midline. (**b**) After local infiltration of lidocaine with epinephrine along the marked points, a 1 cm retroauricular incision is made and the Silhouette needle is passed subcutaneously toward the midline. (**c**) The needle exits at the first point proximal to the midline. (**d**) The needle is redirected so the blunt end advances across the midline toward the point on the contralateral side. (**e**) A stab incision is made to allow the blunt end to emerge with suture attached. The suture is cut. (**f**) The end of the suture is grasped and pulled through until the first knot is visible. The suture is cut again just distal to the knot. (**g**) The half-circle needle is used to pass the proximal end through the mastoid fascia for anchorage. (**h**) A second suture is passed in the same way parallel to the first one. Both sutures are retracted to lift the neck, and tied to one another. The retroauricular incision is closed with interrupted sutures

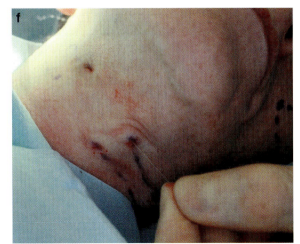
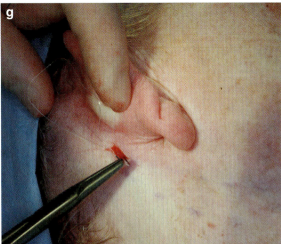
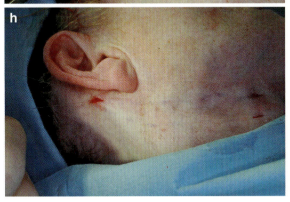

Fig. 27.34 (continued)

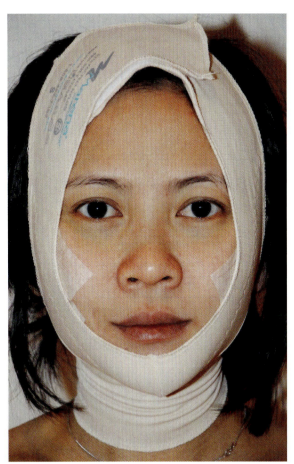

Fig. 27.35 Tape and head garment are used to immobilize the tissues for 3–4 days following a suture lift

27.7 Conclusions

There has been a dramatic increase in patient demand for nonsurgical cosmetic procedures in the last decade. Suture facelift techniques offer a quick, safe, and effective rejuvenation by elevating soft tissues and restoring the youthful contours of the face and neck. The aim is to lift tissues that have dropped, restore the beauty triangle by creating a heart-shaped face, and improve definition of the jawline and neck. Patients who benefit from suture facelift techniques have mild tissue laxity or ptosis and realistic expectations. The results are usually subtle and natural and often make the patient appear a few years younger. The author combines suture facelift techniques with other nonsurgical procedures such as botulinum toxins, fillers, and cheek and lip enhancement (Fig. 27.38). Combined approaches using different sutures and methods in the same patient is also appropriate and may provide superior results than one method alone. Longevity of results following a suture facelift is variable and depends on several factors, including the sutures used, the lifting technique,

Table 27.5 Postoperative instructions

Postoperative instructions: suture lift
IF YOU EXPERIENCE EXCESSIVE PAIN OR BLEEDING, FULLNESS OR SPREADING REDNESS IN TREATMENT AREAS, OR FEVER, PLEASE CALL US IMMEDIATELY 1. Do not massage or rub vigorously the treatment area for at least 4 weeks; this could disrupt the sutures under the skin 2. Wear the head garment 24 h/day for 3 days and then in bed at night for a further 1 week 3. Continue to refrain from smoking for at least 2 weeks during the healing process. Smoking affects blood supply and nourishment to skin and soft tissues 4. Complete the prescribed course of antibiotics 5. Be gentle when brushing your hair until your stitches are removed 6. There may be some "bunching" of skin near the hairline following the lift. This will soften out over 1–4 weeks, depending on skin quality 7. You may experience a tighter sensation over your face where skin has been retracted. Some of this tightness will lessen over 1–2 weeks as the skin relaxes into its new position 8. You may experience some swelling, bruising, or tenderness over the first week but this will subside and fade over time. If you notice increasing redness, swelling, and tenderness a few days after the procedure that was not there before, call our clinic. This may be a sign of infection, which is uncommon 9. If you received skin stitches you will need to return to the clinic after 5–7 days for removal I HAVE READ AND FULLY UNDERSTAND THE ABOVE ITEMS 1–9 Patient Signature _____ Date _____

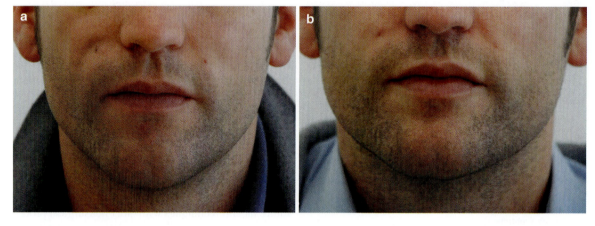

Fig. 27.36 (**a**) Dimpling of skin at the right nasolabial fold incision following a suture suspension lift. (**b**) After subcision using an 18 gauge needle to release dermal attachments

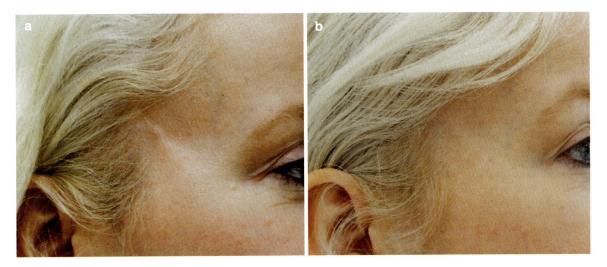

Fig. 27.37 (**a**) Palpable and visible cones in the temple following a Silhouette suture lift. (**b**) Spontaneous improvement after 2 months without intervention. Cutting a few cones from the distal end of the suture after placement will prevent this problem

Table 27.6 Complications of suture facelift techniques

Complication	Prevention	Management
Skin irregularities and dimpling	1. Avoid superficial placement of suture in dermis 2. Release dermis with artery forceps during procedure	1. Conservative, massage 2. Subcision 3. Remove suture and redo procedure
Palpability or visibility	1. Avoid patients with thin, translucent skin 2. Place sutures in deep subcutaneous plane, or deeper	1. Conservative, massage if absorbable 2. Remove if barbed, non-absorbable
Migration or extrusion	1. Use anchored sutures 2. Bury sutures when appropriate	1. Trim sutures 2. Remove sutures completely
Prolonged pain or nerve injury	1. Use absorbable sutures 2. Avoid path of facial nerve	1. Remove sutures 2. Analgesia
Asymmetries	1. Proper marking 2. Equal tension bilaterally	1. Add or remove sutures to restore symmetry
Infection	1. Ensure sterile technique 2. Prophylactic antibiotics 3. Keep hair out of punctures and incisions	1. Antibiotics 2. Remove sutures
Bleeding or hematoma	1. Use lidocaine with epinephrine for infiltrative local anesthesia 2. Use diathermy for temporal incisions 3. Discontinue antiplatelets, vitamins, and herbal supplements before procedure	1. Pressure hemostasis 2. Conservative for ecchymosis and hematoma 3. Drainage for large hematoma (rare)

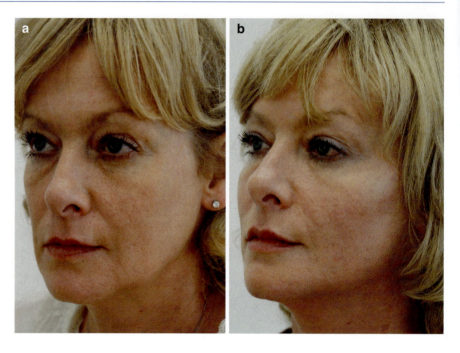

Fig. 27.38 (a) Preoperative. (b) After suture facelift combined with cheekbone and lip enhancement using temporary fillers

the patient's tissues, and the aftercare. For a stable lift the author prefers to employ techniques that lift the SMAS rather than just the subcutaneous fat, and to use coned sutures to elevate the fibrofatty malar fat pad. To improve healing, patients must stop smoking for at least 2 weeks before and after the procedure, wear a head garment for 3 days, and handle the face and neck carefully for 6 weeks. Once the patient understands what can be achieved with suture facelift techniques, the limitations, and the value of combination procedures for optimum results, the likelihood of success and satisfaction for both patient and surgeon is high.

References

1. The American Society for Aesthetic Plastic Surgery. Cosmetic surgery national databank statistics 2008; ASAPS website, www.surgery.org
2. Hodgkinson DJ. Clinical applications of radiofrequency: nonsurgical skin tightening (Thermage). Clin Plast Surg. 2009;36(2):261–8.
3. Sasaki G, Cohen AT. Meloplication of the malar fat pads by percutaneous cable-suture technique for midface rejuvenation: outcome study (392 cases, 6 years' experience). Plast Reconstr Surg. 2002;110(2):635–54.
4. Paul MD. Barbed sutures for aesthetic facial plastic surgery: indications and techniques. Clin Plast Surg. 2008;35(3): 451–61.
5. Hochman M. Midface barbed suture lift. Facial Plast Surg Clin North Am. 2007;15(2):201–7.
6. Villa MT, White LE, Alam M, Yoo S, Walton RL. Barbed sutures: a review of the literature. Plast Reconstr Surg. 2008;121(3):102e–8e.
7. Teitelbaum S. Enthusiasm versus data: how does an aesthetic procedure become "hot"? Aesthetic Surg J. 2006;26(1): 51–3.
8. Shiffman MA. Facial aging: a clinical classification. In: Shiffman MA, Mirrafati SJ, Lam SM, editors. Simplified facial rejuvenation. New York: Springer; 2008. p. 65–7.
9. Vleggaar D, Fitzgerald R. Dermatological implications of skeletal aging: a focus on supraperiosteal volumization for perioral rejuvenation. J Drugs Dermatol. 2008;7(3): 209–20.
10. Mendelson BC, Hartley W, Scott M, McNab A, Granzow JW. Age-related changes of the orbit and midcheek and the implications for facial rejuvenation. Aesthetic Plast Surg. 2007;31(5):419–23.
11. Kahn DM, Shaw RB. Aging of the bony orbit: a three-dimensional computed tomographic study. Aesthetic Surg J. 2008;28(3):258–64.
12. Master course in suture facelift techniques: European College of Aesthetic Medicine (ECAM). www.ecamedicine.com
13. Kress DW. The history of barbed suture suspension: applications, and visions for the future. In: Shiffman MA, Mirrafati SJ, Lam SM, editors. Simplified facial rejuvenation. New York: Springer; 2008. p. 247–56.
14. Bisaccia E, Kadry R, Rogachefsky A, Saap L, Scarborough DA. Midface lift using a minimally invasive technique and

a novel absorbable suture. Dermatol Surg. 2009;35(7): 1073–8.
15. Alcamo JH. Surgical suture. US patent 3,123,077; 1964.
16. Sulamanidze MA, Sulamanidze GM. Flabby, ageing face. A new approach. II Congress on aesthetic and restorative surgery, Moscow, 1998:15.
17. Sulamanidze M, Sulamanidze G. APTOS suture lifting methods: 10 years of experience. Clin Plast Surg. 2009; 36(2):281–306.
18. Sulamanidze M, Fournier PF, Paikidze TG, Sulamanidze G. Removal of facial soft tissue ptosis with special threads. Dermatol Surg. 2002;28(5):367–71.
19. Wu W. Barbed sutures in facial rejuvenation. Aesthetic Surg J. 2004;24(6):582–7.
20. Ruff G. Techniques and uses for absorbable barbed sutures. Aesthetic Surg J. 2006;26(5):620–8.
21. Garvey PB, Ricciardelli EJ, Gampper T. Outcomes in threadlift for facial rejuvenation. Ann Plast Surg. 2009;62(5): 482–5.
22. Kaminer MS, Bogart M, Choi C, Wee S. Long-term efficacy of anchored barbed sutures in the face and neck. Dermatol Surg. 2008;34(8):1041–7.
23. DeLorenzi CL. Barbed sutures: rationale and technique. Aesthetic Surg J. 2006;26(2):223–9.
24. Lee S, Isse N. Barbed polypropylene sutures for midface elevation: early results. Arch Facial Plast Surg. 2005;7(1): 55–61.
25. Bukkewitz H. Die Nade Tecnik der subcutanen Gewebsrafung einer schnittlosen Korrekturmethode bei kosmetischen Brust und Gesichtoperationen. Zentralbl Chir. 1956;81(29): 1185–92.
26. Fournier PF. The curl lift: a rediscovered technique. In: Shiffman MA, Mirrafati SJ, Lam SM, Cueteaux CG, editors. Simplified facial rejuvenation. Berlin: Springer; 2008. p. 285–91.
27. Erol ÖO, Sozer SO, Velidedeoglu HV. Brow suspension, a minimally invasive technique in facial rejuvenation. Plast Reconstr Surg. 2002;109(7):2521–32.
28. Hernandez-Perez E, Khawaja HA. A percutaneous approach to eyebrow lift: the Salvadorean option. Dermatol Surg. 2003;29(8):852–5.
29. Keller GS, Namazie A, Blackwell K, Rawnsley J, Khan S. Elevation of the malar fat pad with a percutaneous technique. Arch Facial Plast Surg. 2002;4(1):20–5.
30. Yousif NJ, Matloub H, Summers AN. The midface sling: a new technique to rejuvenate the midface. Plast Reconstr Surg. 2002;110(6):1541–53.
31. Giampapa VC, DiBernardo BE. Neck recontouring with suture suspension and liposuction: an alternative for the early rhytidectomy candidate. Aesthetic Plast Surg. 1995; 19(3):217–23.
32. Serdev NP. Ambulatory temporal SMAS lift by minimal hidden incisions. Int J Cosmet Surg. 2001;1(2):20–7.
33. Serdev NP. Lower SMAS-platysma facelift using hidden retro-lobular approach. Int J Cosmet Surg. 2001;1(3):13–9.
34. Serdev NP. Serdev suture method for ambulatory medial SMAS facelift. Int J Cosmet Surg. 2002;2(4):1550–62.
35. Zide BM. The facial nerve: cranial nerve VII. In: Zide BM, Jelks GW, editors. Surgical anatomy around the orbit. The system of zones. Philadelphia: Lippincott Williams & Wilkins; 2006. p. 19–41.
36. Gamboa GM, Vasconez LO. Suture suspension technique for midface and neck rejuvenation. Ann Plast Surg. 2009; 62(5):478–81.
37. Sasaki GH, Komorowska-Timek ED, Bennett DC, Gabriel A. An objective comparison of holding, slippage, and pull-out tensions for eight suspension sutures in the malar fat pads of fresh-frozen human cadavers. Aesthetic Surg J. 2008;28(4): 387–96.
38. Lee CJ, Park JH, You SH, Hwang JH, Choi SH, Kim CH. Dysesthesia and fasciculation: unusual complications following facelift with cog threads. Dermatol Surg. 2007;33(2): 253–5.
39. Silva-Siwady JG, Diaz-Garza C, Ocampo-Candiani J. A case of Aptos thread migration and partial expulsion. Dermatol Surg. 2005;31(3):356–8.
40. Helling ER, Okpaku A, Wang PTH, Levine RA. Complications of facial suspension sutures. Aesthetic Surg J. 2007; 27(2): 155–61.

Bio-Lifting and Bio-Resurfacing

28

Pier Antonio Bacci

28.1 Introduction

Throughout history, men and women have always had the desire to improve their appearance beginning with improving the state of the skin, so that we could say that "Aesthetic surgery of the skin is as old as humankind" [1]. In primitive societies, shells and details stones were used for engraving and to smooth the skin. Egyptians used a cream of sulfur and resorcine to smooth the skin, and thanks to animal oils and alabaster, regeneration of skin was improved. In the Papyrus of Edwin Smith (1700 BC) and in the Papyrus of Ebers (1600 BC) magic prescriptions are found for the hair or for the cutaneous lesions. In Mesopotamia, the Babylonians became experienced in surgery as noted in the code of Hammurabi (2000 BC), in China medicine and Chinese surgery blossomed as noted in the "Canon of the Medicine" (2600 BC). In the "Rig Veda" (1500 BC), the Indian surgeons pointed out their particular interest in the reconstruction of the nose cut off in thieves. In ancient Greece, physician developed care of the skin and the hair with ancient physicians specialized in the art of cutaneous exfoliation. The Renaissance Europeans studied exfoliation of the skin through translating ancient Greek manuscripts giving a greater development to aesthetics in dermatology, medicine, and surgery.

Today, there is a tendency to confuse aesthetic surgery with plastic surgery that evolved after the First World War from dentistry and adopting techniques from ancient dermatology and general surgery. Plastic surgery is surgery for the recovery of form and function, while aesthetic surgery is more like dermatologic surgery and is surgery of the physical aspect and the desires to be better looking. Aesthetic surgery overlaps many disciplines and is not within any specific specialization.

28.2 Patient Desires

One of the principle objectives of aesthetic medicine and surgery is the rejuvenation of the face, where the years and the various pathologies have left the signs of tissue and metabolic alteration as wrinkles, loss of elasticity and skin tone, alterations of the hair, and the aesthetic pathologies tied to alterations of the quantity and quality of the fat tissue.

Alterations of the basal activities of cells and vital systems constitute signals sent by those structures, so that dysfunction of the regulation of metabolic exchanges constitutes the beginning of chronic and degenerative pathologies as well as the processes of aging. Maintaining the state of health from aesthetic pathologies belongs to "Medicine for the health and the comfort of the patient" through maintenance of the functional harmony of the whole body and of the patient's own image.

28.3 Aging of the Face

The observation of an aged face asks for a careful reflection both on the trials that have provoked the various modifications and on the nature of the same alterations.

P.A. Bacci
Via Monte Falco n. 31, 52100 Arezzo, Italy
e-mail: baccipa@ntc.it

Reprinted with Permission of Springer, Berlin and revised

In aging, the face suffers changes in the principal structures: the bony skeleton, the adipose tissue, and the musculocutaneous system.

According to the rules of universal proportions [2], the face can be separated into three equal segments: the first one from the joining of the hair to the eyebrow, the second from the glabella to the subnasal furrow, and the third one from this line to the chin.

Aging provokes a slow but continuous resorption of the bony structure with reduction of mass so that an unbalance is provoked between bony mass and cutaneous tissue so that there is too much skin and subcutaneous tissue in comparison to its content. Such disproportion is most evident in the inferior part of the face from the retraction of the jaw and reduction of the dental structure.

Dzubow [3] noted that aging provokes alterations and degeneration (Fig. 28.1). The continuous hormonal and circulatory modifications induced from the style of life, particularly by the improper feeding, sedentariness, and smoking provoke alterations in the metabolism of all the tissues ending in the reduction of the quantity of water and subcutaneous adipose tissue (typical of the young face) as well as the muscular and cutaneous vascularization that their structural and metabolic reduction provokes. All these modifications provoke a change in the muscular structure that manifests in the reduction of the fibers with reduction of the tone and of tropism with consequent decrease in glide for the gravity of the tissues.

At the same time and in the same way, there is a decrease of the metabolic and vascular activities of the skin and subcutaneous tissue that provoke reduction of the structure and the cutaneous tone, where we have a less soluble and more rigid collagen, a fragmented elastic net, and regression of the microcirculation with reduction of the "cells to veil," that is of that lymphoadipose and microvascular system that surrounds and nourishes the same microcirculatory system. All of this provokes reduction and atrophy of the skin and the systems of support with consequent low glide in gravity. It is this low glide of the tissues, caused by the gravity and altered metabolism that increases the initial vascular, metabolic, and aesthetic alterations of the face (Fig. 28.2).

The process of aging of the face is from a series of mechanical, physics, and physiological chemical alterations induced by the stress of life that reduces the metabolic activities and vascular function that activates those alterations of chronic degenerations characterized by cutaneous excess, reduction of fat and the glide of the fat tissue, and atrophy of the skin.

Changes usually induced by feeding, smoke, hormones, and intestinal dysfunctions alter the equilibrium of the interstitial matrix with increase of free radicals, alteration of the systems of oxyreduction, alteration of the metalloproteasis, alteration of the production of collagen, reduction of the microarterial circulation, increase of the microlymphatic stasis, and finally activation of the processes that will bring degeneration of aging characterized by the fibrosis [4, 5]. Various degenerative changes due to gravity and loss of glide of the tissues evolve into the typical alterations of the aging (Fig. 28.3).

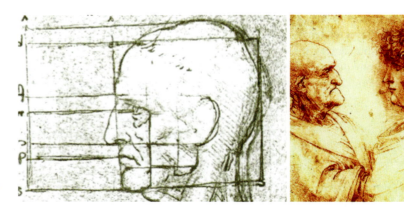

Fig. 28.1 Aging of the face with alteration of tissues that change the proportions

Fig. 28.2 Jowling is a sign of aging of the face with prolapse of tissue

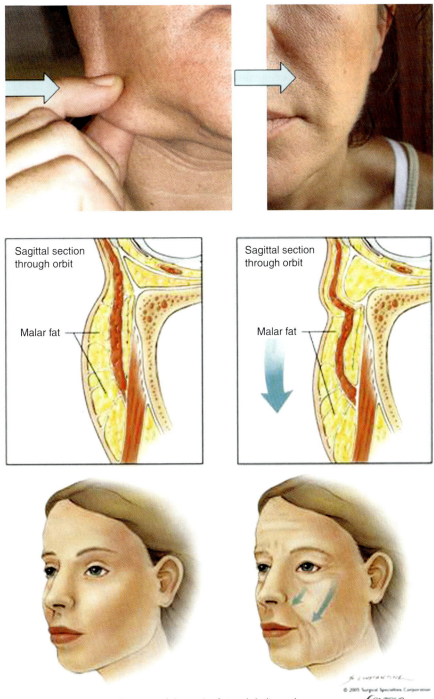

Fig. 28.3 Prolapse of tissue causes the formation of lower eyelid bulge. (Courtesy of Contour Threads)

Descent of the malar fat pad during aging

The process of evolution of the suborbicularis adipose bulge is typical. While cutaneous excess of the superior eyelid with relative adipose bulge depend, mostly, upon the yielding of the frontal structures and from reduction of the eyebrow fat, in the lower eyelid the yielding of the malar structure with reduction of the adipose tissue and its prolapse stretches the ligament and suborbicular septum provoking formation of the bulge and the cutaneous excess.

While the tissues droop, there are some morphological alterations (in the temporal and spatial position) both of the microvascular systems of nutrition and purification of the tissues of the neurological and metabolic systems, that provoke signals and the production of the structural substances, among which are collagen and elastin. It is this association of metabolic alterations with the mechanical alterations induced by the droop of the tissues that is key to the interpretation of these changes [6].

Bringing the tissues to a more juvenile, more pleasant, and less severe appearance to the face reduces the annoying wrinkles and cutaneous excess folds (Fig. 28.4). Bringing the tissues to their best position means slowing down the processes of aging and improving oxygenation, decreasing the lymphatic stasis and the tissue toxicity, reducing free radicals and the oxidative alterations, reducing the alterations of the metalloproteasis as well as the process of fibrosis. It means to return the normal function to the extracellular matrix.

According to the type and degree of aging of the face, different treatments can be used such as surgical or dermatologic cosmetic treatments. A fundamental rule is to make a basic classification to plan the most correct therapeutic procedure (Table 28.1).

Table 28.1 Process of aging face and tissues

1. Prolapse and skin excess
(a) Correct by traditional surgery or surgery using threads
2. Reduction or glide in low adipose tissue with reduction of volume of tissues with juvenile cutaneous turgidity
(a) Correct with fillers or autogenous fat tissue to increase the volume and to offer the good fundamental hormonal substances activating the metabolism
3. Alteration of the skin structure with loss of substances and consequential aging
(a) Correct by nutritional dermoelectroporation and local mechanical, physical, and chemical treatments

1. Prolapse and excess of skin
   (a) When the face has cutaneous excess, surgical treatment must be used to allow tissue recovery and elimination of the cutaneous excess. Traditional lifting, in its various modifications, provides a new position of the deep tissues with duplication and fixation of the superficial muscular aponeurotic system (SMAS) to guarantee a more lasting result, but not eternal. Aesthetic surgery results in about 5 years (between 3 and 8 years according to the type of skin, of the age,

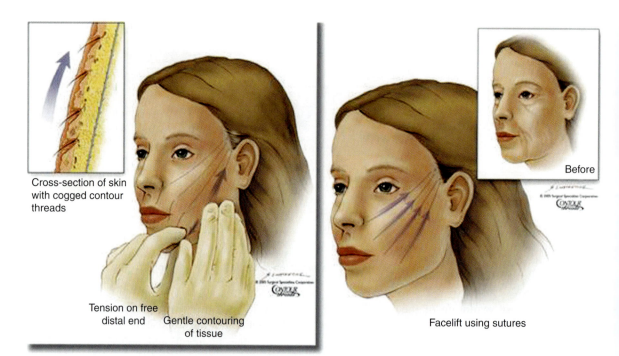

Fig. 28.4 Threads can be used to lift up tissues, contour the face, and recover new metabolism. (Courtesy of Contour Threads)

and of the style of life) of improvement. In selected patients the mini-invasive solution using surgical barbed or non-barbed threads can give good results but they should give a new good position of the skin reducing all processes of aging. These soft methods are indicated as the most diffuse and suitable treatments particularly for the non-advanced phases and for preventive indications with their mini-invasiveness in multiple sessions and with almost no complications or scars.

2. Reduction of volume
   (a) When there is no true skin excess but the aesthetic pathology is characterized by reduction of the skin structure with reduction or regression of the adipose and the connective tissues, surgery is not suitable and can only be of help in particular cases.
   (b) The elective treatment is the use of substances to fill and thereby increasing the volume and to redraw the contours of the face. The principal fillers are found in the family of the hyaluronic acid that has the principal characteristic to be absorbable and practically without complications. Except for particular cases, it is best to avoid nonabsorbable fillers because of their complications. When necessary to use nonabsorbable fillers it is better to use solid prosthesis, such as solid silicone or Gore-Tex.
3. Skin aging
   (a) In the case of patients without skin excess or reduction of the volume, but with underlying irregularity and degeneration of the cutaneous structure (the true cutaneous aging) it is necessary to adopt some protocol of noninvasive dermatologic cosmetic treatment that reduces the skin irregularities and improve the external aspect that favors a resumption of the microcirculation, of the oxygenation, and of the production of a physiological connective tissues [7–10].

When there is prolapse of the tissues, the angles of the mouth go down and, often, there may be formation of white saliva at the angles that interferes with the patient's life of relationships. Aesthetic treatment allows the patient to reach the desire to maintain his own dignity and role in society.

28.4 T3 Bioresurfacing

Old age causes modifications, both physical and functional, of the organisms that, in the past, were considered as a sad and disheartening decadence of the bodily harmony and the human activities. From such feeling was born the instinctive impulse for the man to fight against the senile phenomenon.

In the case of patients with neither cutaneous excess nor reduction of the volumes, but have underlying cutaneous aging with irregularity and degeneration of the dermoepidermal structure, dermatologic cosmetic and noninvasive protocols of treatment are used to reduce these irregularities and improve the external aspect favoring improvement of the metabolism. The author has named such protocol " T3 - Bioresurfacing," meaning an attempt to rejuvenate the skin by stimulating the natural physiological regeneration with a triad of integrated treatments.

"Bioresurfacing" uses an integrated protocol by different methods to regulate the activity of the skin:

1. Endermologie – LPG®: Physical therapy finalized to vascularize and to drain the lymph
2. Young-Peel: This phase is used to regulate and to stimulate the skin
   (a) Scrub-Peel: To regulate and to eliminate the horny layer of the skin
   (b) Trans-Peel: To introduce substances and to stimulate the cellular activities
3. Photodynamic treatment: To bring energy and to activate the cellular functions

The integration of these methods has produced interesting results with limited complications and interruption of the working activity.

28.4.1 Endermologie LPG System®

LPG-System represents a true revolution in the field of physical therapy and aesthetics, both in the idea and in the practical application. It deals with patented equipment that uses air in the phases of aspiration and compression and a head with two rolls that allows traction on the tissues to perform some maneuvers and has physiotherapeutic applications. Such treatments allow the morphological and functional reconstitution of the connective and the adipose tissue [11–14].

The LPG System acts on the skin and on the subcutaneous tissue to improve the connective tissue, the fat tissue, and the arteriolar, venous, and lymphatic microcirculation, and the blood flow containing the hormones (Fig. 28.5). With LPG, the therapist can increase the therapeutic results by use of the "palper-roller" characterized by movements of compression and tissue rotation allowing the return of the elasticity of the tissues. This allows better function by producing stimulation of metabolism and vascularization and, secondarily, the effect of lymphatic drainage and purification of the tissues [15, 16]. The application of the different possibilities of treatment obtains the best results as can be seen in different histological biopsies (Fig. 28.6).

Physical methodology by Endermologie System uses Lipomassage to care tissues of the body and Lift massage to care tissues of the face, a strategy based on the stimulation of particular skin receptors finalized to the stimulation of the fibroblasts and interstitial matrix.

28.4.2 Young-Peel Method

This dermatologic cosmetic treatment is finalized to regulate the cutaneous irregularities, as results of acne or cutaneous atrophy, and to introduce nutritional substances avoiding the use of needles. For this purpose, it uses an association of superficial microdermabrasion (Scrub-Peel) and transdermal electric introduction of substances.

28.4.2.1 Superficial Microdermabrasion (Scrub-Peel)

Dermabrasion has been one of the most important weapons in the hands of the dermatologists surgeon

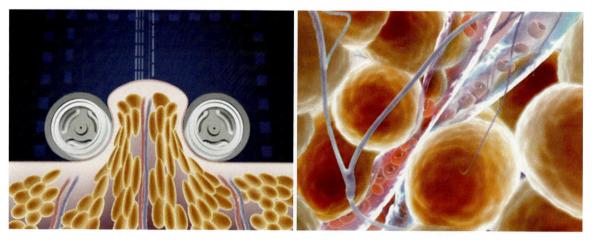

Fig. 28.5 Endermologie LPG system is the revolution in physical therapy. Vascularization and metabolism can be activated

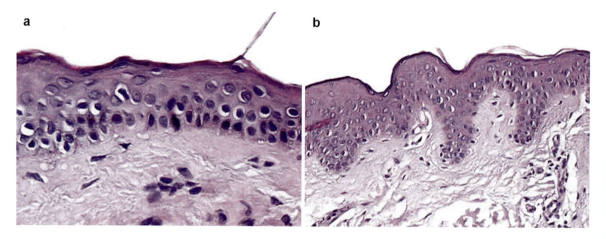

Fig. 28.6 New metabolism of the tissue in papillary dermal layer after dermatologic cosmetic treatment. (**a**) Before. (**b**) After

[17–19]. It is generally used to remove the epidermis and some layers of the dermis according to the irregularities needed to be treated. The author uses it only for the treatment of the horny layer.

In aesthetic pathologies characterized by skin irregularities and dystrophies, such as acne, wrinkles, stretch marks, and sagging of the skin, the treatment of transdermal introduction of substances is preceded by a surface microdermabrasion treatment performed by a system using corundum powder crystals (aluminum oxide in a sterile, disposable package) that produces removal of the corneous layer with simultaneous vascularization of the tissue by mechanical stimulation (light suction–light pressure–dermabrasion).

A particular ultrasonic probe can be used vibrating at 25,000 Hz (Bright – Skin by Eporex® Method) [20] to remove the superficial layer and to prepare the skin to the introduction of the substances containing elastin, collagen, and amino acids. The same protocol is used for the treatment of cellulite. The treatment is integrated into the protocol.

28.4.2.2 Transdermal Introduction of Substances (Trans Peel)

The skin has an exchange function with the outside environment, which is also used as a means of pharmacological introduction [21–24]. Endermal diffusion is a passive phenomenon, in fact the skin behaves like a passive membrane. Penetration of the substances takes place in two stages characterized by:

- Dormancy stage, in which the dermal layer is charged, usually electrically
- Flow stage, in which the flow becomes constant

Dermoelectroporation treatment is a method that enable absorption using an equipment that generate electric pulses allowing the opening of special "electric gates" promoting the passage of substances of adequate size. The apparatus used for medical and aesthetic purposes is Transderm Ionto® by Mattioli Engineering. Dermoelectroporation treatment is applied by a discharge given by an electric inductor charged at a controlled current value and then discharged with a typical kind of reversible exponential voltage wave [25–30].

The reason why the method works well only after dermabrasion of the horny layer is because the high voltage in the classical electroporation produces partly poration of the horny layer and partly poration of the dermis (with the residual energy after having perforated the horny layer).

Dermoelectroporation eliminates the need of the high voltage because the horny layer is eliminated with the dermabrasion and so the voltage to go through the dermis is lower. It works like the high voltage electroporation, however, replacing the dangerous and hardly controllable effect of the high voltage on the horny layer with the safer dermabrasion. The lesser energy is used only in order to open watery channels in the dermis. As the intradermal or subcutaneous use of collagen, hyaluronic, or elastin is the natural trial of regeneration or production plotted here, while it is being known as the plotted regeneration, can be stimulated using the substances of base that constitute the precursors of such substances.

All of this has opened a new frontier in the antiaging protocols of regeneration and rejuvenation reducing the use of needles and bloodier methodologies. Immediately after microdermabrasion, active substances such as collagen, hyaluronic acid, amino acids, and elastin or their precursors are introduced by means of dermoelectroporation treatment.

28.4.3 Photodynamic Treatment

Photorejuvenation using Intensive Pulsed Light (IPL) is an evolution of the laser since it does not send forth a wavelength coherent light that strikes water or other elements with direct surgical action, but it uses a photon as a flash that strikes particular photodermoreceptors that are stimulated or altered. Suitable mainly to affect hemoglobin and dark colors, it has shown an ability to transfer energy to the tissues that directly stimulates the principal vital reactions of the extracellular matrix and the new production of physiological collagen [31–33].

IPL is used at the end of the session of Transderm (crystals microdermabrasion and Dermoelectroporation) or Eporex™ System (Ultrasonic scrub and iontotransfer) where it guarantees the transfer of a quantity of such energy to favor the use of the introduced substances and the activation of the tissue reactions of the matrix. Energy's quantity is produced in the form of heat that allows important microarteriolar vascularization that favors the oxygenation of skin that is found in a state of microcirculatory suffering, particularly in the people who smoke or use the estrogen-progestin pill or drugs.

The author prefers to use a wavelength around the 640–690 nm in association with a lower wavelength (530–580 nm) nm in most cases. Normally, in the patients with Fitzpatrick, 5–6 IPL is not used. The scheme for the use of IPL in Bioresurfacing is:

1. Endermologie treatment
2. Scrub peel
3. Intensive pulsed light
   - 640 nm × 23–27 J/cm^2
   - 560 nm × 24–28 J/cm^2
4. Sessions at 15, 21, and 30 days

When it is necessary, the result can be increased using a non-ablative diode laser 532 by a rotating scanner for stimulating new connective structure and new cellular metabolism [34, 35] (Fig. 28.6).

28.5 T3-Bioresurfacing: Protocol of Treatment

The treatment is used for the cutaneous improvement of the skin irregularities and for the signs of aging by stimulating the production of new collagen and stimulating the extracellular matrix. Different sessions at 15, 21, and 30 days are performed.

1. Physiotherapeutic phase with lymphatic drainage, skin vascularization, and connective stimulation using Lift Massage Endermologie® LPG System.
2. Scrub-peel using superficial microdermabrasion with crystals of corundum to smooth the skin and to open the horny layer followed by introduction of precursor substances of collagen, elastin, and hyaluronic acid using dermoelectroporation connected to the instrument "Ultrapeel Transderm®" or "Eporex System®" that allows opening of the pores that are the watery channels.
3. Energy administration by Intensive Pulsed Light offered by an instrument Quantum® IPL with an energy of 532–695 nm, or rotating diode laser scanner 532 nm (by Italian laser Eufoton®) that allows stimulation of the cellular function and the extracellular matrix.

At the end, an antiherpetic cream or lenitive substances can be applied for therapy or cosmetic action.

Bioresurfacing allows the patient to use makeup about 20 min after the procedure. Particularly in winter, the patient uses a nighttime cream based with phytic acid and vitamin C (Stand By 5% Vitamin C® cream), to alternate sometimes with a mix of retinoic acid (0.0025%) and lower part of cortisone cream in low dosage. Such protocol will not produce immediate visual effects from the surgery or from the use of fillers but it will favor a slow but continuous improvement of the aspect and the tropism of the skin with progressive rejuvenation of the face.

28.6 Biolifting

In patients without true cutaneous excess and tissue prolapse and where the aesthetic pathology is characterized by a reduction of the "structure" and of the "tropism" of the skin with reduction or regression of the adipose and the connective tissue, surgery is not always suitable and is not the first indicated treatment, even if it can be sometimes of help. These cases, as a rule, represent the large majority of the patients 25–40 years of age. These patients do not have an indication for the traditional surgery with traction and excision of the tissues. They are patients with "nasogenial wrinkles" that begin to become "nasogenial folds" and, especially in hyperactive subjects, where the crows' feet and the peribuccal irregularities are in association with the true and deep wrinkles. As a rule, these patients are found in the central phase of their social evolution and working activity. They normally request lesser treatments and above all wish to improve without changing. The treatment of choice is dermosurgical, mini-invasive treatments, and the use of substances of fillers to increase the volume and to redraw the contours of the face.

The substances that the author prefers are the traditional "Fillers" that have the characteristic to be natural and to be reabsorbed in different periods of time, but always absorbable substances. These substances belong to two major groups: the family of collagen and that of hyaluronic acid. The collagen was initially derived from tendons of ox and horse that required testing for the dangers of allergies and complications. Today, such risks are reduced and we have a new pork collagen not requiring test and with good results on the time (Evolence®).

Hyaluronic acid can also be used. It has the principal characteristic to be natural (not from animal derivation), absorbable, and does not have complications. Non-linked hyaluronic acid constitutes a substance of great use in ophthalmology and orthopedics. The non-linked form has a duration of few days when inserted in the dermal layer and does not behave as a filler, but as substance of stimulation for the production of the physiological collagen, particularly if associated with precursors of collagen, elastin, or hyaluronic acid.

In the linked form, named "cross-linked," it is hooked to benzyl alcohol and has a more complex form so that it is reabsorbed more slowly. According to the concentration and of the type of application it can last from 2 to 8 months.

As a rule, these products do not give true complications in comparison to the non-absorbable substances. The author believes that we must avoid the complications of non-absorbable substances. It is better to use solid prosthesis such as solid silicone or Gore-Tex.

"Biolifting" is a treatment that has the tendency to restructure the skin and to increase the lost volume in the process of aging, this strategy use chemical substances in association to particular laser introduced into the tissues "Endo Light Lift" and a new revolutionary methodology to increase energy in the tissues "Biodermogenesi®."

28.6.1 Method

In synergy with treatments of Bioresurfacing, a protocol of treatment can be performed that allows the stimulation of the tissues and increases the volume with new harmony of the contours of the face. In this sense of "tissue fullness" and of "good hydration" it will give a juvenile aspect to the face. Only using absorbable substances such as hyaluronic acid in different concentrations, increases the length of time it will last.

Different forms of revitalizing substances or fillers containing hyaluronic acid can be used. These products contain a low quantity of proteins that limit the production of free radicals, reduce inflammation, and therefore allow the increase of the length of time the product lasts. This method improves the quality of the skin, reduces the wrinkles, and improves the expression of the eyes harmonizing the external aspect [36].

28.6.1.1 Superficial Layer

Non-linked hyaluronic acid is introduced by mesotherapy (drop by drop), by lines in the dermoepidermal layer, or in superficial intradermal layer. Good results can be obtained in the treatment of the neck, acne, and in superficial irregularities of the skin. Restylane Vital® (Q-Med® company) is normally used for this use.

28.6.1.2 Middle Layer

Linked hyaluronic acid is used in low concentration, introduced drop by drop in the middle dermal layer. Good results are obtained for the treatment of the middle wrinkles and in the cutaneous restructuring. Typical areas are nasogenial folds where we can use normally Restylane® (Q-Med® company) or Teosyal 27 or 30 (by Swiss company Teoxane®), that contain reticulated hyaluronic acid.

28.6.1.3 Deep Layer

Linked hyaluronic acid used in high concentration is introduced into the deep dermal layer or into a submuscular layer in the treatment of the zygomatic area (where it improves the contours). Particularly, in submuscular area, the author prefers hyaluronic acid Sub-Q (Q-Med® company) or pork collagen (Evolence™), in association with barbed threads too.

28.6.1.4 Threads of Support

Prolapse of the tissues (tissue ptosis) causes contortion of the morphological anatomy and of the functional anatomy of the microstructures with alteration of the metabolic functions of the extracellular matrix with consequent formation of local lipo-lymphedema. Morphological alterations of the microvessels cause deceleration and lymphatic stasis that alters of the systems of oxidative reduction and increases the free radicals with metabolic damage to the extracellular matrix that activates the process of oxidative stress with microedema, formation of lipo peroxidation, mitochondrial and metalloproteasis damage, alteration of the collagen, inflammatory and chronic evolution toward the pathological fibrosis. Reposition of the tissue provides new metabolism and a new life for the same tissues (Fig. 28.7).

When an initial yielding of the skin results in irregularities and cutaneous depressions, (not yet requiring lifting or mini-lifting), the application of surgical threads can be added. Surgical unidirectional barbed

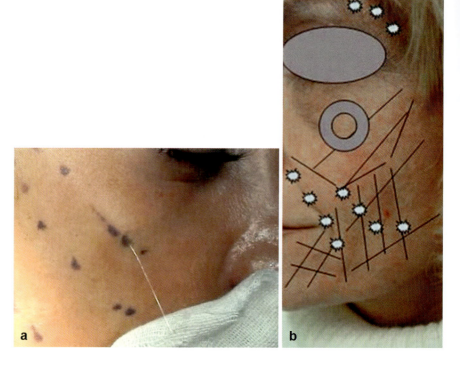

Fig. 28.7 T-3 biolifting. (**a**) Surgical suspension threads. (**b**) Fillers when necessary

thread, absorbable or nonabsorbable, can be used. Using a particular and personal instrument too, the author uses the American Quill™ barbed threads or semielastic barbed French threads Spring Threads™. This method gives rapid improvement without complications giving a more juvenile aspect of the face and lengthens the lifetime of the substances reducing the free radicals and the vascular and metabolic alterations, thanks to the spatial new position of the tissues [37].

28.7 Endo Light Lift

When it is necessary to stimulate tissues, we must use a revolutionary endodermal laser, as for the treatment for capillaries. A sophisticated small laser 808 or 980 nanometrics is connected to a microfiber of 100 or 200 μm that succeeds in entering without incisions under the skin to create some energetic grates and to stimulate a new collagen restructuring the tissues. Using this minimally invasive methodology, named "Endo Light Lift™" (by Eufoton® laser), initial cutaneous excess and initial adipose palpebral bag can be treated [38] (Fig. 28.8). Using this method an endo tissue net of laser light can be created to increase the cellular activity without complications or allergic risks.

The introduction of the microfiber into the tissues improves the quality of water and blood, increases temperature and cellular activity, and finally increases the tropism of the skin.

28.8 Biodermogenesi™

This new method is aimed to treat either for aesthetics or for the structural aspect of the skin with stretch marks. The evolution of this method provides a strategy to improve the youth of the face in association with Endo Light Lift also. Particularly, this method, named Biodermogenesi™ Face (by Expo Italia™), is used with a little special oval or bell-shaped handful, which creates a slight vacuum permitting a slight blood afflux in the treated area and a new mitotic cellular activity thanks to a special generator of bio-compatible magnetic fields [39].

The persisting migration of the ions contributes to raise the derma and hypoderm temperature of 2°, 3°, enough to permit an increasing of the cellular mitosis, until the 300% more compared to the physiological reproductive cycles on the treated patient (Van't Hoff law), which, furthermore, is an important reactivation of the primary functions of the fibroblast, thanks to the afflux of blood and oxygen, consequence of the vacuuming action, so that we assist to a hyperemia of the surface, normally absent in the aging face's tissue. So the synergy produced permit for the first time to expand one more time the derma and nourish the cells and provide oxygen to the tissue, encouraging a progressive renovation of the capillary calibre. Biodermogenesi is based on the application of a screened electrode, which does not permit a direct energy transition to the treated skin, to which will be projected inside a huge energy quantity with variable frequency that will alternate moments of positive valence to moments of negative valence.

During this phase, the sodium and potassium move to the inside of the cellular membrane bringing nutritional factors. At the end of this phase, we have the presence of Na+ and K+ almost exclusively to the inside of the cells; in this case, they are extremely rich and well nourished, thanks to the increasing of the pumping of these two elements, normally in charge of bringing inside the membrane, the nutritional cellular factors. Thanks to this application, the phenomenon of the cell's enrichment can be accelerated that is essential to access the following mitosis. When the distribution of the negative signal is terminated, the sodium and potassium ions are brought to the outside of the cellular membrane allowing the toxins elimination of the cutaneous cells, essential to encourage a better cellular mitosis.

The regenerative process of the Biodermogenesi™ is determined with the production of collagen and elastic fibers in order to permit a stability of the obtained result (Fig. 28.9). The elastic collagen starts to take its

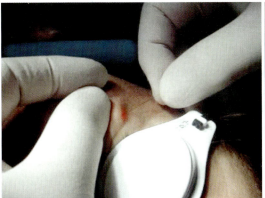
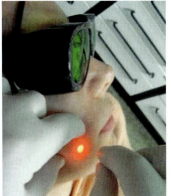

Fig. 28.8 Endo Light Lift™ laser Eufoton 808–904 nm, 5.8 W, and 5 shots at 40/50 ms

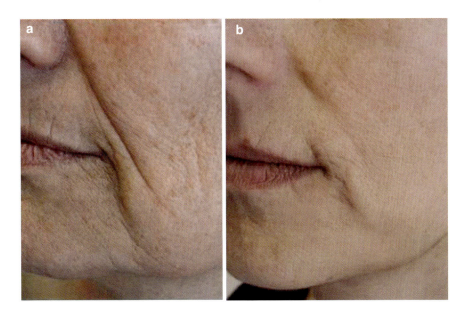

Fig. 28.9 Biodermogenesi and compressive microvibration. (**a**) Pretreatment patient. (**b**) Posttreatment

specific action inside the skin which gives the correct support that permits the blood supply of capillary and re-activate the fibroblast.

28.9 Bio-Lifting: Protocol of Treatment

Typical indications for Biolifting are the treatment of wrinkles and harmonization of the face. The session is minimally invasive and practically without risks. At the end of the session, the patient may use makeup. The author suggests this protocol of treatment:

- When is necessary: Filler or soft lift with barbed threads
- Endo Light Lift: One session of treatment, to create a grate of subdermal laser light in midface, eye brown, and submental area, any 3–4 weeks for 3–4 sessions for years (we suggest in winter).
- After 15 days from Endo Light Lift: We suggest a session of Biodermogenesi Face to increase the effect of laser therapy.
- Maintenance: We suggest 1 session any 3–4 weeks of Biodermogenesi Face in association to LiftMassage LPG™ to maintain the result.

28.10 Conclusions

Bioresurfacing and Biolifting are dermocosmetic treatment used to rescue the signs of aging and to improve the youthfulness of the face and neck, but not to reduce the age. If used well, these strategies offer good results without complications for the patients. It is necessary to have correct indications and interview the patient prior to treatment in order to have the best results and the satisfaction of the patient.

References

1. Coleman PW, Hanke CW. Storia della chirurgia estetica dermatologica. In: Coleman PW, Hanke CW, Alt TH, Asken S, editors. Chirurgia estetica dermatologica. Rome: Verduci; 1999. p. 1–6 (Original book: Coleman PW, Hanke CW, Alt TH, Asken S., editors. Cosmetic surgery of the skin, St Louis: Mosby Year Book; 1997).
2. Dzubov L. L'invecchiamento del volto. In: Coleman PW, Hanke CW, Alt TH, Asken S, editors. Chirurgia estetica dermatologica. Rome: Verduci; 1999. p. 7–17 (Original book: Coleman PW, Hanke CW, Alt TH, Asken S, editors. Cosmetic surgery of the skin. St Louis: Mosby Year Book; 1997).
3. Bacci PA. Le celluliti. Arezzo: Alberti; 2000. p. 17–73.
4. Albergati FG, Bacci PA, Mancini S. La matrice extracellulare. Arezzo: Minelli; 2005. p. 71–301.
5. Goldman M, Bacci PA, Hexsel D, Liebaschoff G. Cellulite: pathophysiology and treatment. New York: Taylor & Francis; 2006. p. 7–75.
6. Ball P, Knuppen R, Haupt M, Breuer H. Interactions between estrogens and catecholamines. 3. Studies on the methylation of catechol estrogens, catecholamines and other catechols by the catechol-O-methyltransferases of human liver. J Clin Endocrinol Metab. 1972;34(4):736–46.
7. Bjorntorp P. Fat cell distribution and metabolism. Ann N Y Acad Sci. 1987;499 (Human Obesity):66–72.
8. Krotkiewski M, Björontorp P, Sjöström L, Smith U. Impact of bosity on metabolism in men and women. Importance of regional adipose tissue distribution. J Clin Invest. 1983;72(3):1150–1162.
9. Bacci PA. Chirurgia estetica minimamente invasiva con hilos tensors. Caracas: Amolca; 2007.
10. Adcock D, Paulsen S, Shack RB, et al. Analysis of the cutaneous and systemic effects of endermologie in the porcine model. Aesthetic Surg J. 1998;18(6):414–22.
11. Fodor PB, Watson J, Shaw W, et al. Physiological effects of Endermologie: a preliminary report. Aesthetic Surg J. 1999; 19(1):1–7.
12. Moretti E, Schapira A, Kaplan G, Alonso E. Estudo macro e microsópico da fáscia superficial em membros inferiores: um concieto diferente sobre a cellulite. Mesoter Atual. 1997; Buneos Aires.
13. Bacci PA. La fascia superficiale. In: Bacci PA, editor. Le celluliti. Arezzo: Alberti; 2000.
14. Foeldi M. Symposium ueber die sogenannte Zellulitis, Feldberg, 1983.
15. Adcock D. et al. Analysis of the effects of deep mechanical massage in the porcine model. Plast. Reconstr. Surg. 2001 Jul., 108(1): 233–40.
16. Revuz J. et al. Clinical and histological effects of the Lift6® device used on facial skin ageing. Nouv. Dermatol. 2002; 21: 335–342.
17. Dzubow LM. Dermabrasion. J Dermatol Surg Oncol. 1994; 20(5):302.
18. Benedetto AV, Griffin TD, Benedetto EA, Humeniuk HM. Dermabrasion: therapy and prophylaxis of the photoaged face. J Am Acad Dermatol. 1992;27(3):439–47.
19. Bacci PA. Il trattamento eporex. In: Bacci PA, editor. Chirurgia estetica mini-invasiva con fili di sostegno. Arezzo: Minelli; 2006. p. 151–7.
20. Suhonen M, Bouwstra JA, Urtti A. Chemical enhancement of percutaneous absorption in relation to stratum corneum structural alteration. J Control Release. 1999; 59(2):149–61.
21. Prausnitz MR, Bose VG, Langer R, Weaver JC. Electroporation of mammalian skin: a mechanism to enhance transdermal drug delivery. Proc Natl Acad Sci. 1993;90(22):10504–8.
22. Hadgraft J, Guy R. Transdermal drug delivery, development issues and research initiatives. New York: Marcel Dekker; 1989.

23. Lombry C, Dujardin N, Préat V. Transdermal delivery of macromolecules using skin electroporation. Pharm Res. 2000;17(1):32–7.
24. Tezel A, Sens A, Mitragotri S. Incorporation of lipophilic pathways into the porous pathway model for describing skin permeabilization during low-frequency sonophoresis. J Control Release. 2002;83(1):183–8.
25. Kontturi K, Murtomaki L. Mechanistic model for transdermal transport including iontophoresis. J Control Release. 1996;41:177–85.
26. Bacci PA. La dermoelettroporazione: osservazioni cliniche. In: Archivio Mattioli Engineering, Firenze, 2002.
27. Curri S. Microcircolazione. Inverni della beffa, 1986.
28. Pacini S, Peruzzi B, Gulisano MS, et al. Transdermal delivery of heparin by means of alternate current skin electroporation. Ital J Anat Embryol. 2004;109(1): 223.
29. Pacini S, Peruzzi B, Gulisano M, Bernabei, et al. Analisi microscopica, qualitativa e quantitativa del trasporto transdermico di farmaci e macromolecole biologiche mediante un nuovo tipo di dermoelettroporazione. In: La Flebologia in Pratica. Alberti: Arezzo; 2004.
30. Maimon T. Stimulated optical radiation in ruby. Nature. 1960;187:483.
31. Anderson RR, Parrisch JA. Selective photothermolysis: precise microsurgery by selective absorption of pulsed radiation. Science. 1983;220(4596):524–7.
32. Garden JM, Tan OT, Parrish JA. The pulsed dye laser: its use at 577 nm wavelength. J Dermatol Surg Oncol. 1987;13(2): 134–8.
33. Marangoni O, Longo L. Lasers in phlebology. Bagnara arsa (Udine): Edizioni goliardiche; 2006.
34. Marangoni O, Longo L. Leg telangectasias resistant to the sclerotherapy, comparison between laser 532, 808, 980 nm. Lasers Med Sci. 2003;18 Suppl 2. 30–33.
35. Bacci PA. Biolifting. In: Bacci PA, editor. Cirurgia estetica minimamente invasiva. Caracas: Amolca; 2008. p. 91–124.
36. Bacci PA. I fili di sostegno. In: Bacci PA, Mancini S, editors. Chirurgia estetica mini-invasiva con fili di sostegno. Minelli: Arezzo; 2006. p. 40–150.
37. Bacci PA. Biolifting. In: Bacci PA, editor. Cirurgia estetica minimamente invasiva. Caracas: Amolca; 2008. p. 124–7.
38. Bacci PA. The biodermogenesi for stretch marks and face. International congress of aesthetic Medicine, Warsaw, 2008.
39. Bacci PA. Dell'avanzato R. Biodermogensei e laserdermogenesi. Nouve strategie per le smagliature. Biodermogenesis and laserdemogenesis: new strategy about stretch marks. X International Congress of Aesthetic Medicine, Milano, 9–11/10/2008, pp. 20–21.

Standard Facelifting

Shoib Allan Myint

29.1 Introduction

Traditional face-lifting techniques consisted of only elevation and redraping of the facial skin [1]. Since then, there has evolved many different surgical variations including the more recent minimally invasive procedures involving less dissection and more simplified anatomical approach [2]. This paradigm shift in the surgical approach to face-lifting has been predicated on the demand of the patient population wanting less morbidity and faster recovery. As we understand more of the facial dynamics and facial anatomy, cosmetic facial plastic surgeons are staying in the cutting edge of constantly searching for more innovative and improved methods to perform this very successful cosmetic procedure. In trying to understand the demands of the patient, surgeons must realize that sometimes less is better. This chapter will lay down the basic fundamentals of face-lifting technique via skin flap, addressing the SMAS with redraping.

29.2 Technique

Some relative contraindications for rhytidectomy include (1) smoking and/or alcohol abuse; (2) collagen vascular disorders; (3) poor nutritional status; (4) anticoagulation bleeding disorder; (5) use of Accutane, high-dose steroids, or immunosuppressants; and (6) poor medical condition (e.g., uncontrolled hypertension, poorly controlled diabetes, significant chronic airway disease (CAD), significant chronic obstructive pulmonary disease (COPD).

The surgeon should first and foremost understand the patient's needs. Place a mirror in front and ask them what about their face bothers them, and what specific areas in the face they want addressed. This initial patient evaluation is of paramount importance. Unrealistic desires can lead to a surgery, which fails to please them. Make note of the quality of the skin, the amount of redundant tissue, presence or absence of platysmal bands, and the amount of submental fat. Evaluation of the chin and neck directly affects the surgery performed in this area. If submental fat and skin laxity is present, submental liposuction or lipectomy is performed. The skin dissection in this case should not extend to the central neck and submental area. If there is significant laxity and submental fat then the dissection extends further into the neck (Fig. 29.1) with possible lipectomy and platysmal plication.

In addition to the surgical evaluation preoperatively, it is important to discuss the importance of smoking and medication usage with the patient. Smoking can lead to flap necrosis secondary to vasoconstriction. It is imperative the patient stops smoking. If they continue, it is imperative to tell them to stop 2 weeks before and 2 weeks after the surgery. Any medications that inhibit platelets or coagulation must be stopped 1–2 weeks prior to surgery. These include, but not limited to, NSAIDS, aspirin, Warfarin (coumadin), and clopidogrel (Plavix). All these medications can increase the risk of hematoma under the skin flap, which can potentially lead to flap necrosis.

S.A. Myint
Ophthalmic Plastic and Reconstructive Surgery
and Orbital Diseases and Eye and Facial Plastic
Surgery of Las Vegas,
7955 West Sahara Ave. Suite 101, Las Vegas,
NV 89117, USA
e-mail: shoibmyint@gmail.com

With the patient sitting up, the incision is marked both in front of the ear continuing behind the ear (Fig. 29.2). If the patient presents with significant cervical skin laxity, a retroauricular skin flap may be necessary for optimal results [3]. Marking should be performed prior to administering the anesthetic. If there are platysmal bands, they should be marked to facilitate finding the medial borders during the plication procedure. If significant submental fat is present, the lateral extent of this compartment should be marked to guide submental liposuction or direct lipectomy.

Once the markings are completed, intravenous (IV) sedation is utilized depending on the preference of the surgeon. For surgeons starting to do face-lifts for the first time, it is recommended to use IV sedation instead of straight local injection. An equal mixture of 1% lidocaine with epinephrine and 75% bupivicaine is injected along all incision lines. When significant submental fat is present, either liposuction from a submental incision or direct lipectomy is performed at this time. A 2.5 cm submental incision allows direct visualization of the fat and eventually the edges of the platysmal muscle. A subcutaneous dissection is performed in the previously marked submental area. Approximately, 5 mm of subcutaneous fat is left attached to the skin flap which prevents adherence to the underlying tissues. Preplatysmal fat is removed. The edges of the platysma muscle can be visualized and plicated if significant platysmal bands are present (Fig. 29.3). The medial edges are plicated with multiple 4–0 permanent sutures. Skin

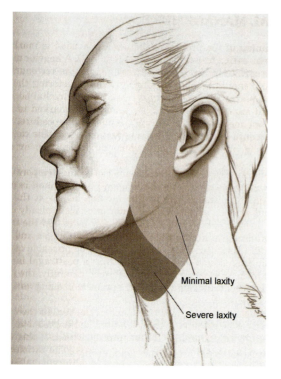

Fig. 29.1 Extent of subcutaneous skin dissection for minimal and severe laxity of the neck skin

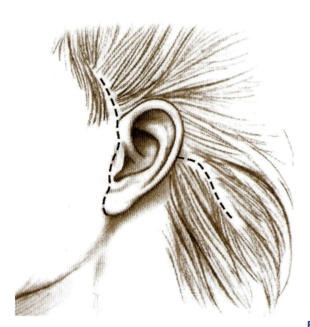

Fig. 29.2 Typical incision for rhytidectomy

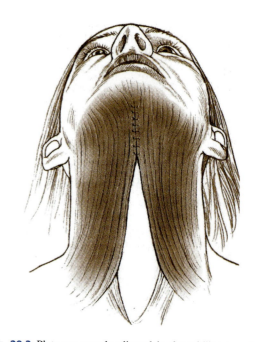

Fig. 29.3 Platysma muscle plicated in the midline to reduce banding in the neck

closure is usually performed with running 6–0 nylon or plain gut. Skin excision here is usually not performed unless there is significant amount of excess submental skin.

Once the neck is addressed, the face-lift incision can be performed. The incision is kept parallel with the hair follicles to avoid hair loss. In the temporal region, blunt dissection avoids damaging the hair follicles and stays superficial to the frontal branch of the facial nerve which runs along the superficial temporal fascia (Fig. 29.4). The limit of the subcutaneous dissection is half way between the ear and the lateral canthus.

Anterior to the ear, a subcutaneous skin flap is created approximately 3–8 cm in length. Behind the ear the skin overlying the mastoid process is quite adherent to the skin and careful dissection is done to overcome this. As the dissection proceeds inferiorly in the neck, it is important to maintain a superficial dissection plane between the subcutaneous tissue and the superficial musculature. The greater auricular nerve becomes extremely superficial as it crosses the body of the sternocleidomastoid muscle 6.5 cm below the external auditory canal. Deep dissection in this area can severe the nerve.

Once the flaps have been raised, various techniques can be used to treat the superficial musculoaponeurotic system (SMAS). The goal of the SMAS modification is to provide deeper support and tightening for the areas of the jowls, nasojugal fold, nasolabial fold, and neck. SMAS modification can impart longevity to the procedure and allows less tension to be applied directly to the skin, giving a more natural appearance. One has an option to do SMAS plication, SMAS imbrication, or deep SMAS dissection. The SMAS plication is the simplest of the three techniques. The SMAS is sutured to itself in several locations without excising any tissue. When the SMAS is grasped near the anterior mandibular ramus and the platysma is grasped in the neck, the entire complex can be repositioned in a posterolateral direction. A nonabsorbable suture such as 4–0 is used for the plication. Three primary areas of the SMAS are tightened (Fig. 29.5). The first and most superior suture addresses the nasolabial fold. The next suture repositions the jowls and nasojugal fold. The final suture helps elevate the neck. Several interrupted or mattress sutures are used in each location (Figs. 29.6 and 29.7).

SMAS imbrication involves excising an ellipse of the SMAS and suturing the edges together. A safe area of the excision lies between the zygomatic arch and the angle of the mandible. The facial nerve is deep to the

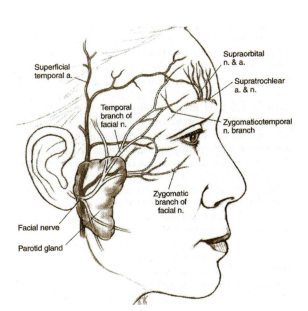

Fig. 29.4 Anatomy of the temporoparietal fascia, facial nerve, and deep fascia

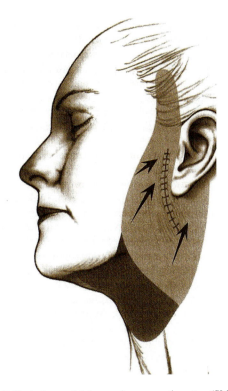

Fig. 29.5 Typical superficial musculoaponeurotic system (SMAS) incision and direction of the SMAS elevation

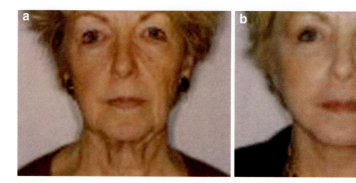

Fig. 29.6 (a) Preoperative. (b) Postoperative after face-lift with platysmal plication and SMS plication

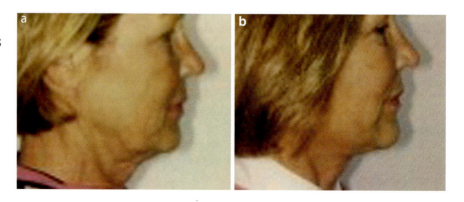

Fig. 29.7 (a) Preoperative. (b) Postoperative following face-lift, neck-lift, and SMAS plication

SMAS in this area. The marginal mandibular nerve is at risk if the excision extends over the angle of the mandible. The excision starts just below the zygomatic arch and extends 1.5 cm anterior to the tragus. Excision is performed toward the angle of the mandible. The greater the tissue laxity the wider the dissection. Sutures are placed in the same area as the plication. One additional suture is placed grasping the platysma below the ear and elevates it superiorly and slightly posteriorly, attaching it to the fascia overlying the mastoid process.

During a deep SMAS dissection, a shorter skin flap is created. Again, the safe area of the SMAS dissection is between the inferior border of the zygoma and the angle of the mandible. Dissection continues medially to the area of the malar eminence. Redundant SMAS is excised, elevated, and sutured as described previously. Because a smaller skin flap is created, this technique is more dependent on SMAS repositioning for optimum result. This type of approach is more appropriate for those patients with prominent jowls and nasojugal folds.

Once the SMAS is repositioned, the skin can be redraped in a natural appearing posterior and slightly superior direction. Very little tension is applied to prevent significant scarring. Prior to skin excision, cardinal staples are placed to provide support for the skin flap with minimal tension. The first is placed at the anterosuperior border of the ear where the ear meets the scalp. When the ideal angle is determined, the point of overlap is marked. A linear incision is made to the point of overlap, and the flap is secured to the fixation point with a single staple. The second cardinal staple is positioned at the most anterior portion of the occipital incision in the retroauricular sulcus. The skin of the neck is elevated posteriorly and superiorly to reduce the rhytids in the neck.

Subcutaneous sutures are then placed to close the remainder of the occipital region. The skin must be trimmed and closed meticulously. In the preauricular area, it is critical the skin is closed without tension to minimize scarring. Additionally, the tragus can be pulled forward opening the ear and producing an unnatural postsurgical appearance. A running nonabsorbable suture such as 6–0 nylon can be used here. Only a small amount of skin is typically excised in the temporal area. This temporal incision is mainly to prevent a "dog ear" when closing the flap. In contrast, in the occipital area, a larger amount of skin can be excised. This allows tightening the skin of the neck. This area can tolerate moderate tension. Absorbable sutures such as 4–0 Vicryl can be used for subcutaneous closure. Closure of the skin in this area can be done with surgical staples. Closure from posterior to anterior direction can minimize the development of "dog ear" deformity. The ear lobe sits approximately 12–15° posterior to the long axis of the ear. Excessive skin removal in this area of the ear lobe can displace it anterior or inferior. If desired, the ear lobe may be secured in position with a single interrupted 6–0 vicryl suture. This suture subcutaneously attaches the most inferomedial portion of the ear lobe to the underlying SMAS tissue.

29.3 Postoperative Care

The use of drains is controversial. If desired a Jackson-Pratt drain can be placed through a small stab incision in the occipital portion of the flap and passed into the neck. It can be removed in the first postoperative day. ABD and Kerlex dressing can be applied. It should not be so tight as to cause pain or place pressure on the flaps. Excessive pressure can lead to flap necrosis. The dressing is removed in 24 h. Sutures are removed in 1 week and staples at 7–10 days. Patients can be placed on a Medrol Dose pack if there is no contraindication. This can help with postoperative edema.

29.4 Complications

Complications following rhytidectomy can be devastating, particularly because of the elective nature of this procedure [4]. As with all surgical procedures, complication prevention is paramount. Proper patient selection, mastery of pertinent anatomy, attention to meticulous surgical technique, and conscientious postoperative care are all important factors in preventing face-lift surgery complications.

Complications may include (1) hematoma, (2) nerve injuries, (3) infection, (4) skin flap necrosis, (5) hypertrophic scarring, (6) alopecia and hairline/earlobe deformities, and (7) parotid gland pseudocyst. With emerging so-called minimally invasive procedures such as thread lifts, new complications have been reported, including Stensen's duct laceration and suture visibility and extrusion.

29.4.1 Hematoma

Major hematomas are a true emergency. Immediate surgical drainage is necessary to avoid flap necrosis. Often no discrete bleeding vessel is identified during surgical exploration. Direct evacuation of minor hematomas is preferred if the hematoma is detected early and is easily reachable through an existing incision. Otherwise, minor hematomas may be treated with serial needle aspirations and pressure dressing. Antibiotic prophylaxis is suggested.

29.4.2 Nerve Injury

If a motor nerve is knowingly transected, immediate microscopic neurorrhaphy is indicated. If nerve injury is noted postoperatively, institute expectant management. Eliminate anesthetic effect. Transient paralysis is more likely than permanent paralysis.

29.4.3 Infection

Major infections requiring intravenous antibiotics are rare. The predominant organisms causing infection are staphylococci. Patients with minor hematomas may warrant oral antibiotic prophylaxis.

29.4.4 Skin Flap Necrosis

Treat partial-thickness injury with moist surgical bandage, occlusive ointments, or both. These injuries may result in normal healing, hypertrophic scar formation, or abnormal pigmentation. Treat full-thickness injury with conservative debridement and healing by secondary intention.

29.4.5 Hypertrophic Scarring

This condition may be treated with intralesional corticosteroid injections or silicone topical therapy (e.g., Cica-Care, Kelo-cote gel). Perform scar revision only after complete wound maturation.

29.4.6 Alopecia and Hairline/Earlobe Deformities

Transient traumatic alopecia is likely to normalize in 3 months. Permanent alopecia may be corrected with local flaps or micrografts and minigrafts. Observe earlobe distortion for spontaneous improvement. Surgical correction with local advancement flaps may be used for persistent deformity.

29.4.7 Parotid Gland Pseudocyst

Treat this condition with frequent needle aspirations and suction drain insertion.

29.5 Discussion

The different approaches to face-lifting presented here can achieve the desired results for any cosmetic surgeon if the "rules" are followed carefully. First and foremost patient selection is critical, knowing who to do the surgery on is very important. However, knowing which patients not to do the surgery on is an art. The selection criteria will prevent unnecessary patient drama postoperatively. Making sure the patient is fully and completely comfortable with all the risks, complications, and benefits explained in consultation will again prevent further confusion and frustration. Having meticulous surgical technique and fully understanding the facial anatomy is crucial in avoiding serious complications. Keeping the patient comfortable in the postoperative period with appropriate medicine and communication skills will keep the surgeon above and beyond the complication arena.

29.6 Conclusions

Even though we have entered an age in medicine where noninvasive technology is competing, and potentially outdoing our traditional surgical modalities, there has always been and always will be a place for surgical intervention in the right population of patients. If proper channels are utilized, the results can be spectacular with high patient satisfaction. Our success as surgeons depend on patient satisfaction, so the surgical intervention of face-lifting should address the primary concerns of our patients, not the physicians, taking into account safety, morbidity, and efficacy. We should always stay true to our mission as cosmetic surgeons: unparallel personalized service (UPS).

References

1. Passot R. La chirugie esthetique des rides du visage. Presse Méd. 1919;27:258–62.
2. Baker DC. Minimal Incision rytidectomy (short scar facelift) with lateral SMA Sectomy. Aesthetic Surg J. 2001;21: 68–79.
3. Gladstone GJ, Myint S, Black EH, Brazzo BG, Nesi FA. Oculoplastic surgery atlas: cosmetic facial surgery. New York: Springer; 2005.
4. Becker FF, Castellano RD. Safety of face-lifts in the older patient. Arch Facial Plast Surg. 2004;6(5):311–4.

30
Suspension of the Retaining Ligaments and Platysma in Facelift: From "Fake-Lift" to "Facelift"

Keizo Fukuta

30.1 Introduction

Facelift is a procedure to pull sagging tissue of face by means of excising skin in front of the ear so as to conceal postoperative scar. Excision of skin is a means; it is not a purpose. The goal of facelift is to correct bulges and grooves which develop due to sagging deformity in an aging face and to restore smooth facial contour.

Sagging of soft tissue is more evident in the central zone of the face where the tissue is more mobile for facial expression than in the lateral cheek near the ear. It is, therefore, anticipated that facelift procedure should correct the aging deformity of the central facial zone. Skin excision in the preauricular region can stretch the soft tissue in the lateral cheek, but it cannot provide sufficient lift to the medial face. To achieve expected stretch in the central face, it is essential to manage the subcutaneous musculoaponeurotic system (SMAS) and retaining ligaments. Facelift procedure with treatment of SMAS and retaining ligaments only provide one-dimensional pull. However, the aging deformity occurs in two or three dimensions. The facelift may not be adequate enough to restore bulges and grooves in selective cases. For those situations, liposuction and lipofilling are to be applied.

30.2 The Role of Facelift Procedure in Facial Rejuvenation

Different areas of the face show different signs of aging (Figs. 30.1 and 30.2). Up to now, surgeons have developed many procedures to treat each area; for example, forehead lift for the forehead, upper blepharoplasty for upper eyelid, lower blepharoplasty for lower eyelid, and facelift for lateral cheek and neck. Each procedure treats aging deformity of limited area. The facelift does not rejuvenate the

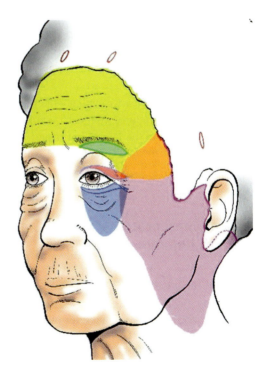

Fig. 30.1 Different surgical procedures are available to treat the forehead, upper eyelid, lower eyelid, midface, cheek, and neck separately

K. Fukuta
Verite Clinic Ginza, New Ginza Building 3rd floor,
5-5-7 Ginza Chuo-ku, Tokyo, 104-0061, Japan
e-mail: fukuta@veriteclinic.com

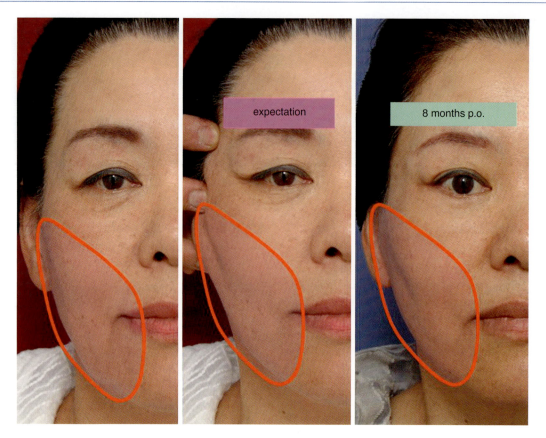

Fig. 30.2 (*Left*) Facelift procedure to correct sagging deformity in the preoperative lateral cheek marked in a *red circle*. The effect of the facelift must be evaluated regarding a change in shape within the *red circle*. (*Middle*) Patient's *expectation* for the facelift. (*Right*) Actual outcome 8 months after facelift, lower blepharoplasty, and upper blepharoplasty

whole face. Therefore, when we evaluate the surgical outcome of facelift procedure, we must examine correction of the contour in the lateral lower part of the face, particularly on the jowl, marionette line and nasolabial fold.

30.3 Anatomic Location of the Retaining Ligaments

The skin and subcutaneous fat of the face adhere to the underlying deep structure such as the parotid gland, deep temporalis fascia, masseter muscle, and facial skeleton (Fig. 30.3). The strength of adherence is not uniform all over the face. The retaining ligaments, which are present in limited areas, anchor the skin to the deep tissue [1–3]. Those ligaments originate from the deep structure, penetrate the SMAS, and insert into the dermis with many ramifications. Therefore, the ligaments provide with strong adhesion between the skin and SMAS and also between SMAS and deep structure. The parotid cutaneous ligaments connect the preauricular skin to the parotid fascia along the anterior margin of the parotid gland. The zygomatic ligaments adhere to the zygomatic body from just lateral to the zygomatic major muscle, extending medially across the zygoma and maxilla in relation to the origin of the zygomatic minor muscle and levator labii superioris muscle. The masseteric ligaments are the vertical septum-like structure which conjoins with the masseteric fascia at the anterior border of the masseter muscle and attaches to the mandibular ramus and body along the anterior margin of the masseter muscle. The mandibular ligament anchors to the anterior third of the mandibular body. The orbital retaining ligament adheres to the inferior orbital rim.

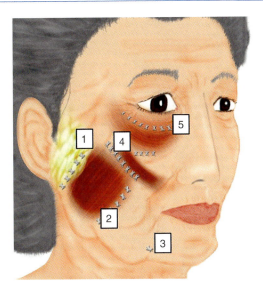

Fig. 30.3 Anatomical location of the retaining ligaments. (*1*) Parotid cutaneous ligaments. (*2*) Masseteric ligaments. (*3*) Mandibular ligament. (*4*) Zygomatic ligaments. (*5*) Orbital retaining ligaments

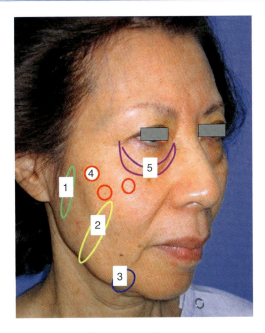

Fig. 30.4 Bulges and grooves develop with aging on the skin surface in accordance with presence of the retaining ligaments. (*1*) Parotid cutaneous ligaments. (*2*) Masseteric ligaments. (*3*) Mandibular ligament. (*4*) Zygomatic ligaments. (*5*) Orbital retaining ligaments. Bulges develop at the area bounded by the different retaining ligaments

30.4 Role of the Retaining Ligaments in Aging Face

During the process of aging, the skin and subcutaneous fat lose the firmness and become difficult to maintain their shape while resisting against the gravity (Figs. 30.3–30.5). The adherence of the skin to the underlying structure is not uniform in strength, as the retaining ligaments attach the skin to the facial skeleton or fascia in limited areas. The skin over those ligaments shows minimal displacement under the influence of gravitation. The skin adjacent to the retaining ligaments loosely adheres to the deep tissues and shows greater ptosis.

In the upright position, the skin between the retaining ligaments, due to the lack of strength of the retaining ligaments slides down due to the gravity. The retaining ligaments hold the soft tissue falling down from the above. This creates depressions or grooves at the skin over the retaining ligaments and bulges in the neighboring area.

The jowl deformity is a bulge along the mandibular border, which develops due to sagging of the soft tissue between the masseteric ligaments and mandibular ligament. The lower border of jowl overlies the mandibular ligament. The malar pouch is a bulge due to ptosis of the soft tissue between the orbital retaining ligaments and zygomatic ligaments. The mid-cheek groove overlies the zygomatic ligaments [3]. Thus, the face develops multiple grooves (concavities) and bulges (convexities) on the surface with aging.

30.5 Role of the Retaining Ligaments on Facelift

The purpose of the facelift procedure is to pull up the sagging skin and subcutaneous fat and to change a facial contour with bulges and grooves into a smooth one (Figs. 30.5–30.7). The aging sign of the face is more prominent in the central portion of the face than in the lateral part. The facelift is a procedure which excises the skin in front of the ear; thereby the operation can stretch the facial skin in the lateral cheek with greater tension. Because the skin is an elastic tissue, the traction power of facelift, which is applied to the lateral edge of skin flap, is less efficient in the central part of the face. It is considered that lifting of the central tissue

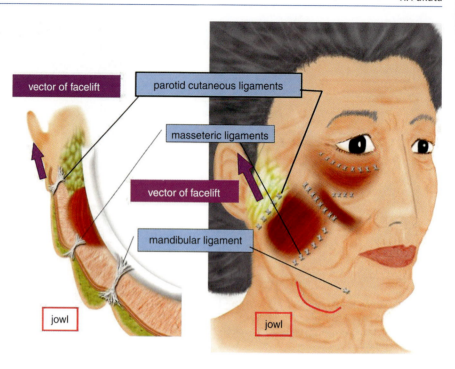

Fig. 30.5 Jowl deformity is a bulge of skin and fat between the masseteric ligaments and mandibular ligaments

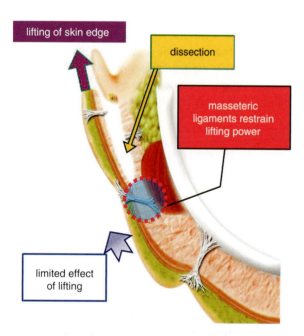

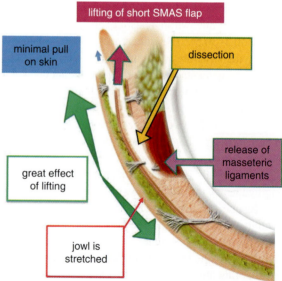

Fig. 30.6 The lift procedure with limited subSMAS dissection. The masseteric ligaments that are *left* intact block a lifting power applied to the skin along the preauricular incision

Fig. 30.7 Extensive subSMAS dissection releases the masseteric ligaments. The traction applied at the preauricular tissue stretches the medial cheek including the jowl

is more effective if traction is applied to the tissue in the more medial region away from the ear. The lateral edge of the SMAS flap is closer to the central face zone than the lateral edge of the skin flap. The use of SMAS allows for traction of more anterior tissue than the preauricular skin incision line. Since the SMAS is strongly anchored to the underlying tissue by the retaining ligaments, the ligaments restrain the traction power when the lateral margin of the SMAS is pulled, unless the retaining ligaments are released [4, 5]. It is, therefore, essential to release the zygomatic ligaments and masseteric ligaments in order to transmit the lifting power to the medial tissue [4, 6, 7].

In order to provide stronger lift effect to the central facial zone, traction should be applied to the medial tissue. Therefore, the lateral edge of SMAS flap should be made medially apart from the ear. The use of a short SMAS flap elevated over the masseteric muscle is more effective when compared with the long SMAS flap elevated in the preauricular area [6].

The retaining ligaments are distinctive fibrous band which has strong adhesion to SMAS and skin. Suspension of masseteric ligaments and zygomatic ligaments is a theoretically appropriate technique to provide strong lift in the medial face [8]. The author has found that practically this procedure is not worth adapting because it is complicated and time consuming. First, this treatment requires the ligation of each ligament before it is cut to secure the ends. Second, suspension of each end might produce a dimple if excess traction is applied. In case dimples occur, loosening of suspension or release of subcutaneous fibrous tissue is necessary. The author has no longer used direct suspension of masseteric ligaments. Currently, the zygomatic ligaments are used for suspension.

30.6 Correction of Bulges and Grooves Caused by Aging

It is said that facial skin sags with aging. What is sagging? With aging, skin and subcutaneous fat lose the firmness and they become vulnerable to gravity. The skin is stretched and expands its surface are. Although the cheek skin shows downward ptosis in the upright position, the skin surface area does not expand only in the vertical direction, but also in the horizontal direction. In sum, the stretching takes place in two dimensions. The expansion does not appear uniformly over the whole face. The skin over the insertion of the retaining ligaments develops minimal expansion. The skin surrounded by the retaining ligaments expands to a certain degree in two dimensions, which causes bulging out. As a result of aging process, multiple protrusions develop over the facial skin just like a buttoned-up sofa. In addition, subcutaneous fat lose the volume with aging. As the volume reduction occurs unevenly over the facial surface, greater diminution of fat causes depression evidently in certain areas. Thus, aging change of surface contour of the face takes place not in one dimension but in three dimensions; expansion of skin surface area and change in fat thickness. Although release of restraining effect of the retaining ligaments and use of short SMAS flap provide greater stretch to the skin in the medial face, this lift is limited in one direction only and is not sufficient to correct the three-dimensional deformity. To achieve improvement in three-dimensional deformity, liposuction and lipofilling are indispensable.

30.7 Presurgical Planning of Facelift

It is helpful to pull the skin in front of the ear with hands to see a possible result from facelift operation (Fig. 30.8). This simple simulation helps a surgeon to determine the direction of lift, whether it should be in superoposterior direction or should be in more vertical direction. It is also useful to examine the facial contour while pulling the preauricular skin, and evaluate whether there is a need for volume reduction or volume filling. If volume reduction is found to be necessary, liposuction should be employed at the same time of facelift. In the consultation while lifting the preauricular skin, the area where bulge remains is marked for liposuction procedure. In addition, while pulling the preauricular skin, depressed areas are determined and marked for lipofilling. Fat injection is commonly applied to the nasolabial fold, marionette line, cheek depression anterior to the masseteric muscle, upper midface, temple, lips, and chin. To determine adequate fat volume needed for lipo-injection, it is useful to fill the area planned for lipofilling with local anesthetic solution.

30.8 Facelift Procedure with Release and Suspension of the Retaining Ligaments and SMAS

30.8.1 Design of Skin Incision

Short scar technique is currently used. An interiorly mild, curved incision is made for about 4 cm in the hair-bearing skin in the temporal region (Figs. 30.9 and 30.10). The incision continues in the preauricular area, corners around the ear lobe and is terminated in the retroauricular groove. The author used to place the incision along the posterior margin of the tragus (retrotragal incision). It was found that the retrotragal incision hides the scar but produces deformity of tragus, in spite of careful tailor of the skin to cover the tragus cartilage (Fig. 30.11). At present, an incision is used along the groove in front of the tragus. This pretragal incision causes no deformity of tragus and the resultant scar is well accepted by patients, although it is visible. A short horizontal incision is placed along the sideburn. Trimming of a triangular skin below this horizontal incision helps to reduce superior displacement of the sideburn and temporal hairline.

This design of incision line is not used for all cases. For those who have a remarkable skin redundancy, for

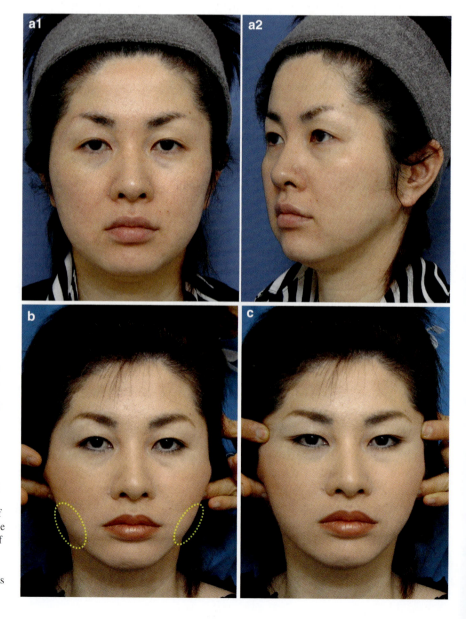

Fig. 30.8 (**a**) Preoperative patient. (**b**) Presurgical simulation. Traction of the preauricular skin demonstrates a remaining bulge in the lower cheek indicated in *yellow dot line*. Liposuction is planned to treat this bulging area. (**c**) Presurgical simulation. Traction of the preauricular and temporal regions demonstrates the lateral pull of the lateral canthus, making the eyes look very sharp. The patient disliked this appearance. (**d**) Presurgical simulation of forehead lift shows a possible improvement of heaviness of the upper eyelids. (**e**) Six months after facelift with release of retaining ligaments and liposuction

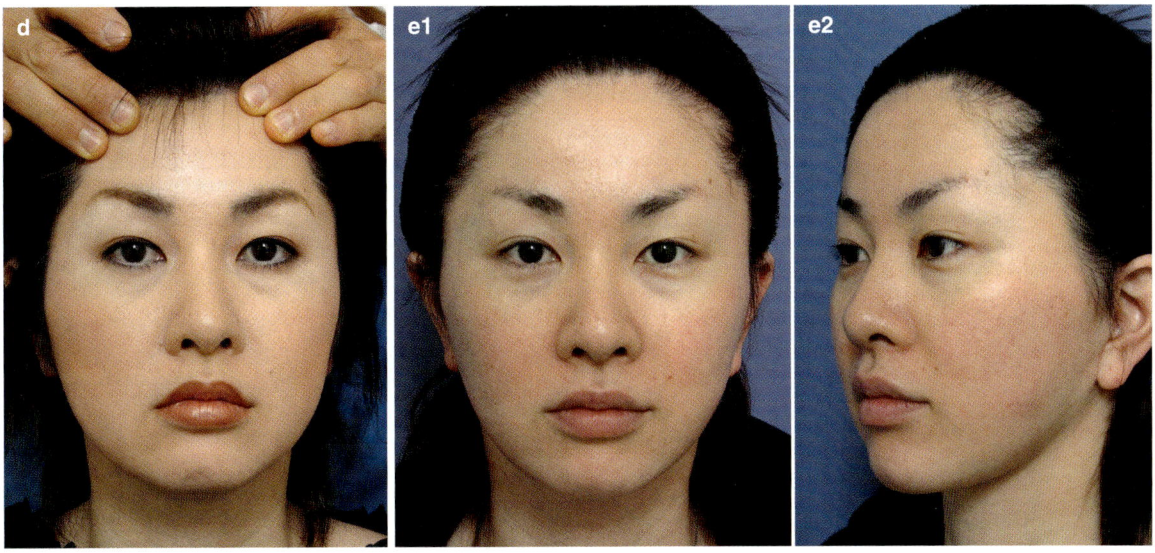

Fig. 30.8 (continued)

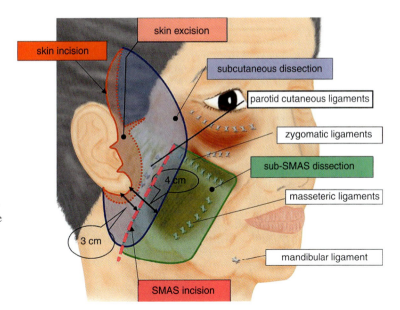

Fig. 30.9 The lateral margin of muscle portion of SMAS and platysma is present at approximately 3 cm from the ear lobe. Through a short scar incision, the subcutaneous dissection is performed for 4 cm from the ear lobe. An incision is made in the SMAS and platysma at 3 cm from the ear. The subSMAS and subplatysma dissection continues beyond the anterior margin of the masseteric muscle in order to release all the masseteric ligaments

example, elderly patients or those who undergo the secondary facelift, the author chooses a hairline incision in the temporal area instead of an incision inside the hair-bearing skin (Fig. 30.10). For those who have vertical wrinkles in the neck or excess skin in the neck or those who request particularly for tightening of neck, the retroauricular incision is extended into the posterior hairline. An incision is made in the postauricular non-hair-bearing skin to bridge between the postauricular groove and occipital hairline. Care has to be taken so as to hide this scar by the ear when viewed from side. In pushing the ear down to the head, the outline of the helical margin is drawn on the postauricular skin. An incision in the postauricular non-hair-bearing skin has to be made within this outline of the ear. Afterward, the incision continues along the occipital hairline.

30.8.2 Dissection

The lateral margin of platysma and muscular portion of SMAS is located at, approximately, 3 cm from the ear lobe (Figs. 30.9, 30.10, and 30.12). The subcutaneous dissection is made up to 4 cm from the ear lobe. An incision is made in the SMAS and platysma at 3 cm from the ear lobe. Deep cut has a risk of facial nerve injury. After

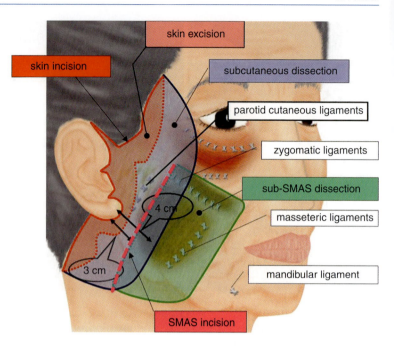

Fig. 30.10 Long scar incision is used in selected cases such as remarkable skin redundancy and sagging neck. A skin incision is made along the temporal hairline and occipital hairline. The medial extent of subcutaneous dissection and subSMAS dissection is same as that for the short scar procedure

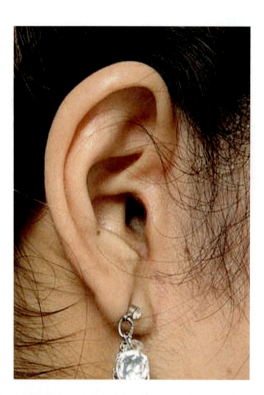

Fig. 30.11 Retrotragal incision. Postoperative scar along the posterior border of tragus is not visible but the tragus has lost the projection and the contour of the tragus has become dull

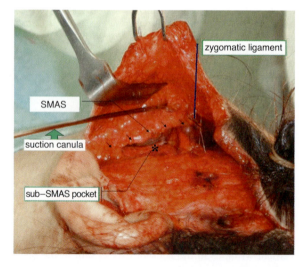

Fig. 30.12 *Small arrows* indicate the lateral margin of SMAS flap that is 3 cm from the ear lobe. *Mark indicates the sub-SMAS pocket. A suture ligation was placed on the cut end of the zygomatic ligament of the skin side. A 16 gauge liposuction cannula is inserted in the subcutaneous layer superficial to the SMAS

the muscular layer of SMAS and platysma is cut with care, blunt tip scissors are used to open the incision. Once the tip of the scissors enters the subSMAS and subplatysma space, the deep dissection continues forward with the spreading maneuver. The dissection is relatively easy because the attachment of SMAS and platysma on the underlying tissue is loose. When the deep dissection approaches to the anterior margin of masseteric muscle, the spreading procedure encounters resistance due to the presence of the masseteric ligaments. After identifying the masseteric ligaments, the ligaments are cut. This dissection continues from the mandibular border inferiorly to the neck and also superiorly. When extending the deep dissection superiorly, the distinctive fibrous band of zygomatic ligament is encountered. The ligament is cut after ligating the ligament in the skin side with 4–0 nylon suture. The further dissection in the superomedial area exposes the zygomatic major muscle. The dissection continues in the inferomedial direction following the lateral margin of the muscle up to the cross point of the lateral margin of the zygomatic major muscle and anterior margin of the masseteric muscle. At this point, a strong ligament band is found. The deep dissection is completed when this thick ligament is cut. At this point, the subSMAS dissection releases all the masseteric ligaments and lateral row of the zygomatic ligaments, which allow us to pull the medial portion of the skin and SMAS with traction of the SMAS flap.

30.8.3 Liposuction

Subcutaneous liposuction before surgical dissection of facelift may make the following subcutaneous dissection easy (Figs. 30.12 and 30.13). This method has a risk to injure the SMAS tissue and make the SMAS flap too weak to be used for suspension. Therefore, liposuction is performed after the subSMAS dissection is completed. A 16 gauge cannula is inserted into the subcutaneous fat layer above the SMAS under direction vision. The liposuction is performed in the bulging area according to the presurgical marking.

30.8.4 Treatment of Crow's Feet and Sagging Lower Eyelid

The subcutaneous dissection from the temporal incision toward the lateral canthal region reveals the lateral

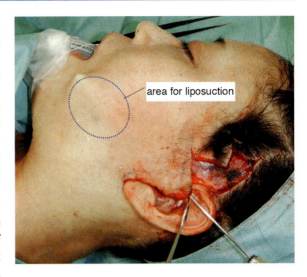

Fig. 30.13 Liposuction is performed in the subcutaneous layer within the area marked at the presurgical plan

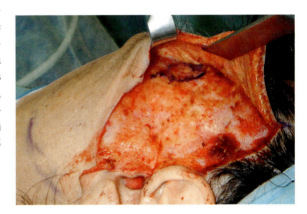

Fig. 30.14 The subcutaneous dissection exposes the orbicularis oculi muscle. To treat crow's feet, the lateral portion of the orbicularis oculi muscle marked in blue is excised

margin of orbicularis oculi muscle (Fig. 30.14). In order to reduce the wrinkles in the lateral canthal area (crow's feet), the orbicularis oculi muscle is excised in a fan shape in the lateral quadrant from 45° angle superiorly to 45° angle inferiorly.

The bulge of lower eyelid can be treated in this approach. Horizontal tightening of orbicularis oculi muscle on the lower eyelid can be performed with facelift dissection. After making an incision in the orbicularis oculi muscle, the dissection is carried out under the muscle. The orbicularis oculi muscle is elevated off from the periosteum of the zygomatic body and inferior orbital rim. This dissection is in the supraperiosteal (sub-muscular) plane. After completing the dissection to the medial corner of inferior orbital rim, the lateral edge of the orbicularis oculi muscle flap is pulled laterally and sutured to the periosteum of the lateral orbital rim and deep temporal fascia. It is important to suspend the muscle fibers closer to the lateral canthal tendon, related to the preseptal portion of the orbicularis oculi muscle in order to restore tight tension band in the lower eyelid (Fig. 30.15).

30.8.5 Suspension

The vector of the lift is determined in the presurgical planning as described (Figs. 30.16 and 30.17). The lateral margin of the SMAS is pulled in the direction according to the vector decided preoperatively, commonly in the superolateral direction. The 1 cm long SMAS cuff that is attached to the medial skin flap is

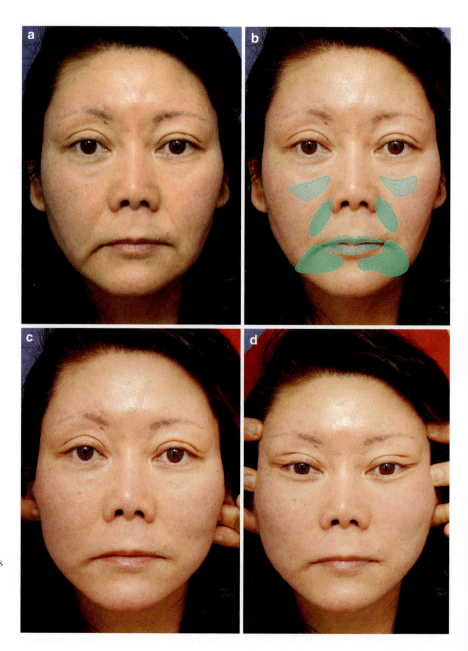

Fig. 30.15 (a) Preoperative patient. (b) The areas to be treated by lipofilling are shown in *green*. (c) Presurgical simulation. Traction of the preauricular skin. (d) Presurgical simulation. Traction of the preauricular and temporal regions demonstrates the lateral pull of the lateral canthus and tightening of lower eyelid. (e) One year after facelift with release of retaining ligaments and lipofilling. The patient shows correction of hollow cheek and jowl deformity. The lower eyelid shows tightening and reduction of bulge

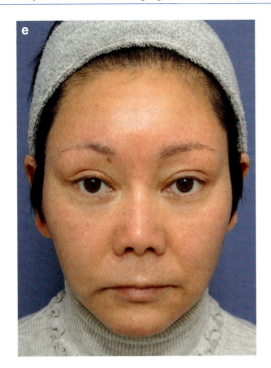

Fig. 30.15 (continued)

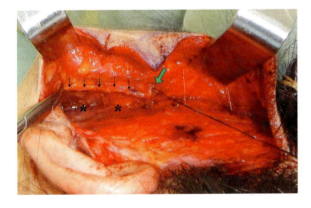

Fig. 30.16 Before suspension of 1 cm long cuff of SMAS (*small arrows*) and zygomatic ligament (*a large arrow*). **Marks show the subSMAS pocket

sutured to the SMAS over the parotid in the preauricular region. The SMAS over the parotid is relatively immobile and provides a good platform to suspension. The most medial zygomatic ligament is suspended to the periosteum of the zygomatic body using the ligation suture if it has been tied with suture before cutting. The zygomatic ligaments in more lateral position are then suspended to the zygomatic arch or temporal fascia. The lateral margin of the platysma is anchored

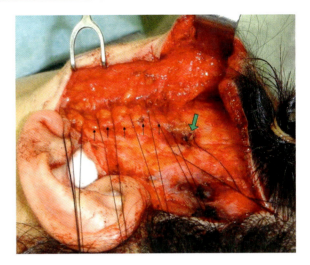

Fig. 30.17 The lateral margin of SMAS flap (*small arrows*) is sutured to the SMAS over the parotid gland. The zygomatic ligament (*large arrow*) is sutured to superficial temporalis fascia

to the mastoid fascia. At this point, the skin of the medial face has been lifted and fixed; therefore, further traction of the margin of the skin flap in front of the ear has no more effect to lift the medial face. At the completion of SMAS suspension, dents or grooves may be evident on the skin surface along the attachment of the cuff of the SMAS and platysma to the skin. The excess skin is then trimmed along the incision and the skin is approximated under the tension which is just enough to smooth out the dents or grooves. At first, the wound is closed in the preauricular region. A triangular piece of skin is trimmed below the horizontal incision at the sideburn, minimizing upward displacement of the sideburn. In case of short scar facelift, where the postauricular incision is terminated in the postauricular groove, excess skin is produced and appears behind the ear lobe. Wound closure in the postauricular groove may develop a dog ear or gathers, although it was tailored with meticulous care. The deformity may fade away in 3 months; otherwise it needs to be corrected with skin trimming 3 months after the facelift procedure.

30.8.6 Lipofilling

Lipofilling is performed after completing the skin closure. Although a common donor site for fat harvest is the lower abdomen, the flank or medial thigh can be chosen at the patient's request. The fat is harvested with liposuction maneuver and centrifuged for 3 min at 3,000 rpm. The fluid in the lower layer is discarded. The remaining fat layer is collected and used for injection. An 18 gauge cannula with blunt tip is used for injection. It is considered that only 30% of injected fat remains and the rest is absorbed; therefore, it is reasonable to inject the fat three times as much as the volume required to correct the depression. The necessary volume is determined at the beginning of operation in simulation with injection of local anesthetic solution. For the correction of nasolabial fold, marionette line and mid-cheek groove, subcision (subcutaneous dissection with 18 gauge sharp tip needle) is employed. The pocket space created with subcision is filled with fat. Additional volume is injected under the subcision pocket. For other area, such as lips, lateral cheek, upper midface, temple and chin, the fat is injected in the subcutaneous layer without dissection.

30.9 Clinical Cases

In the past, the author used the small SMAS flap with minimal subSMAS release, which is limited over the parotid. This procedure released the parotid cutaneous ligaments under the SMAS, but it left the masseteric ligaments and zygomatic ligaments intact. The author also had experience with the lateral SMASectomy and the lateral SMAS plication. Neither of these techniques released the masseteric ligaments off the SMAS. The review of the patients who underwent those three types of procedures showed that the early result was excellent. The facial contour line along the mandible was straight, with no evidence of jowl. However, the jowl recurred in 1–3 months. Although the relapsed deformity was not more than the preoperative situation in some cases, it looked almost the same as the preoperative one in others (Figs. 30.18 and 30.19).

Review of the patients who underwent the current operation with release of the retaining ligaments and suspension of the short SMAS and platysma flap showed less or no recurrence of jowl deformity (Figs. 30.20 and 30.21).

It was found that suspension of the orbicularis oculi muscle in the lateral canthus area was useful to improve the bulging of the preseptal portion of lower eyelid without removal of orbital fat (Fig. 30.15). It is important to choose a proper portion of the muscle and right fixation point to achieve good improvement in the lower eyelid.

For Caucasian patients, the midface lift via the temporal approach, which mobilizes the midface soft tissue toward the zygomatic body, is useful. This results in enhancement of the malar protuberance. Most of Oriental patients do not like this change. In addition, traction of the tissue in the temple into the superolateral direction tends to exaggerate the appearance of

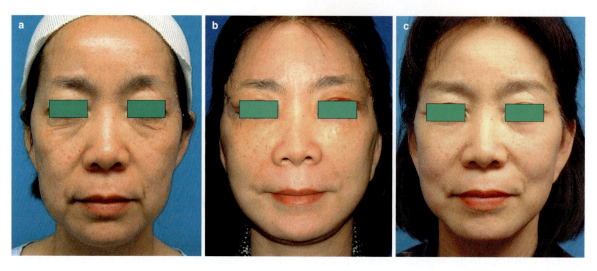

Fig. 30.18 (**a**) Preoperative patient. (**b**) One week after facelift with SMAS flap. (**c**) Three months after facelift with SMAS flap

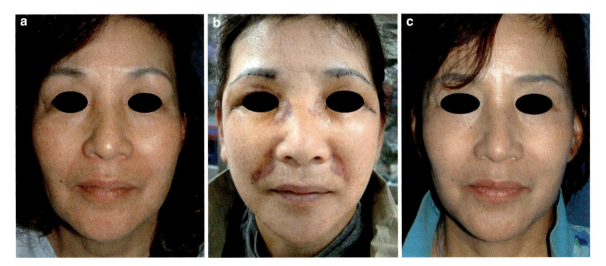

Fig. 30.19 (**a**) Preoperative patient. (**b**) One week after facelift with lateral SMASectomy. (**c**) Three months after facelift with lateral SMASectomy

Mongoloid slant of Oriental eye. Although a few patients requests for this change in the lateral canthal area, it is a rare demand. Thus the facelift procedure using an approach from the temporal and preauricular incision is not effective to correct the nasolabial fold, although the release of retaining ligaments and suspension of deep tissue are involved. Lipofilling combined, particularly, with subcision is very useful to improve the nasolabial fold. The vertical direction is considered appropriate for the midface lift in Orientals. This should be performed via the lower eyelid incision. Volume augmentation of the upper midface is valuable in selective cases.

30.9.1 Case 1

A 42-year-old female presented with mild jowl deformity and heavy appearance in the upper eyelid (Fig. 30.8). Her facial contour appeared to be square rather than triangular. In the preoperative planning, traction of the preauricular skin with fingers demonstrated a possible result from the short scar facelift, changing the square facial contour into a triangular one. The simulation showed budging in the lateral cheek in spite of the strong pull. In order to trim down the bulge, which would remain after facelift alone, it was decided to use liposuction combined with facelift. The simulation of facelift with temporal lift made the lateral canthus look sharper. The patient did not wish to have a temporal lift. The simulation of the brow lift, in which the vector of traction was applied mainly in the lateral portion of the eyebrow, showed improvement of heavy impression in the upper eyelid.

The patient underwent the short scar facelift. The incision was made in the hair-bearing skin in the temporal region and terminated in the postauricular groove. After release of the retaining ligaments with subSMS dissection, the subcutaneous fat was liposuctioned with a 16 gauge cannula in the lower lateral cheek in accordance with the presurgical marking. Additional liposuction was carried out in the submental area. Since her forehead was narrow, the endoscpic brow lift was performed, retracting the lateral part of eyebrow. A 1 cm cuff of SMAS and zygomatic ligaments were used for suspension.

Six months after surgery, the patient showed improvement of heavy upper eyelid with mild elevation of eyebrow. Her face obtained a triangular contour and her face line showed reduction of bulge better than the one shown in the presurgical simulation. The improvement of neck contour was also evident.

30.9.2 Case 2

A 59-year-old female presented with a history of having had skin excision along the temporal hairline and incisional upper blepharoplasty (Fig. 30.15). A hollow in the lower cheek anterior to the masseteric muscle, jowl

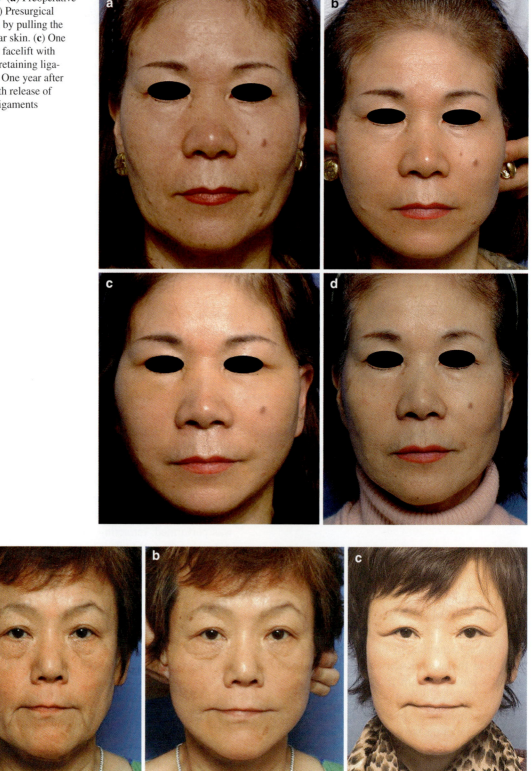

Fig. 30.20 (**a**) Preoperative patient. (**b**) Presurgical simulation by pulling the preauricular skin. (**c**) One week after facelift with release of retaining ligaments. (**d**) One year after facelift with release of retaining ligaments

Fig. 30.21 (**a**) Preoperative patient. (**b**) Presurgical simulation by pulling the preauricular skin. (**c**) Six months following facelift with release of retaining ligaments

deformity, and marionette lines were evident. The nasolabial fold was relatively mild. The neck showed no significant aging deformity. In the presurgical planning, the preauricular skin was pulled with fingers, which showed the improvement of depression in the lower cheek and jowl. The patient requested for the lift of the lateral canthal area. The simulation of facelift and temporal lift showed significant pulled appearance of lateral canthal area in the superolateral direction and also the tightening of the lower eyelid and correction of its protrusion. After comparing with two types of simulation, the patient chose to have the temporal lift and facelift. It was anticipated that lift procedure would correct the cheek hollow without filling. The lipofilling was planned in upper midface, marionette line, nasolabial fold, and lips.

The incision was made along the temporal hairline and in the preauricular area. After the subcutaneous dissection from the temporal incision, the lateral quadrant of orbicularis oculi muscle was excised. The suborbicularis dissection and muscle suspension at the lateral corner was performed for tightening of the lower eyelid with no removal of the orbital fat. The subSMAS dissection released the lateral row of the zygomatic ligaments and all the masseteric ligaments. The lipofilling was carried out after suspension of SMAS and zygomatic ligaments and skin closure. The subcision was used in the nasolabial folds and marionette lines prior to fat injection. In the temporal region, excess skin was trimmed and closed under minimal tension just enough to eliminate possible dents resulting from orbicularis muscle suspension at the lateral canthal area. No deep dissection or deep suspension was used in the temporal area.

One year after surgery, the patient showed correction of hollow cheek and jowl deformity. Although the nasolabial fold had improved, the marionette line showed little improvement. The lower eyelid revealed tightening and reduction of bulge.

References

1. Furnas DW. The retaining ligaments of the cheek. Plast Reconstr Surg. 1989;83:11–6.
2. Mendelson BC, Muzaffar AR, Adams Jr WP. Surgical anatomy of the midcheek and malar mounds. Plast Reconstr Surg. 2002;110:885–96.
3. Muzaffar AR, Mendelson BC, Adams Jr WP. Surgical anatomy of the ligamentous attachments of the lower lid and lateral canthus. Plast Reconstr Surg. 2002;110:873–84.
4. Mentz III HA, Ruiz-Razura A, Patronella CK, Newall G. Facelift: measurement of superficial muscular aponeurotic system advancement with and without zygomaticus major muscle release. Aesthetic Plast Surg. 2005;29:353–62.
5. Mendelson BC. Surgery of the superficial musculoaponeurotic system: principles of release, vectors, and fixation. Plast Reconstr Surg. 2001;107:1545–52.
6. Hamra ST. A study of the long-term effect of malar fat repositioning in face lift surgery: short-term success but long-term failure. Plast Reconstr Surg. 2002;110:940–51.
7. Barton Jr FE, Hunt J. The high-superficial musculoaponeurotic system technique in facial rejuvenation: an update. Plast Reconstr Surg. 2003;112:1910–17.
8. Ozdemir R, Kilinc H, Unlu RE, Uysal AC, Sensoz O, Baran CN. Anatomicohistologic study of the retaining ligaments of the face and use in face lift: retaining ligament correction and SMAS plication. Plast Reconstr Surg. 2002;110:v 1134–47.

Personal Technique of Facelifting in Office Under Sedation

Anthony Erian

31.1 Introduction

The author refers to a facelift as facial rejuvenation since the word facelift is confusing to both the patient and surgeon. It is also a misnomer, and dividing the face could be difficult as some muscles, like platysma, have a wide origin.

In today's modern surgery, one tends to combine one surgical procedure and one nonsurgical procedure at the same time so it is more appropriate to refer to the whole procedure as rejuvenation.

31.2 Consultation

This is a vital part of the operation. The patient must see you personally, not counselors or representatives, as they might increase the expectations to unrealistic levels which might come back to "bite" you. Always have a chaperone with you who you might need as a witness in the future. She or he will also be a silent evaluator of the patient. Normally, the author has a nurse and my fellow, who are usually familiar with the methods. The Consultation Form is used (Table 31.1).

At consultation, the patient must be asked "what is it that brings you here?" It is preferable to ask her this question with a mirror in her hand, and listen intently before examining her. The consultation goes in chronological order, so you methodically focus on her face and exclude any problem that might interfere with the surgical management. It is essential to document all the areas that you can fix/improve by surgery, and others that might not achieve a good result.

The elements of the face are examined:

1. Skin being the largest organ in the body, it deserves special attention and also influences the outcome. Getting the skin in its best possible form is very important.
2. The bone structure. It is important to assess the skeletal deformities that can influence the result, especially the chin, as a receding chin might need some form of augmentation as it seems to affect the result especially, from the profile, and the opposite is true.

31.3 Counseling, Imaging and Preoperative Preparation

After an initial consultation, the patient is invited again for a further consultation with the team and a psychologist to ascertain the mental state and frame of mind that can be missed in the initial consultation. This seems to lower litigation and prepare the patient more fully.

In the same visit, imaging is sometimes done, especially in profile surgery, rhinoplasty, or chin or cheek implants, after the patient signs a form that they understood is only image simulation.

The lab work necessary for the procedure is done and any special tests the anesthetist may wish to be done.

The patient is given the consent form and the pre- and postoperative instructions at this stage (Table 31.2).

A. Erian
Pear Tree Cottage, Cambridge Road,
Wimpole 43, SG8 5QD Cambridge, United Kingdom
e-mail: plasticsurgeon@anthonyerian.com

Table 31.1 Consultation report

CONSULTATION REPORT
Consultation Date ....
Ref by ....
Tel. No. ....
Patient's Details:
Forename/s ....
Surname ....
Address ....
Date of Birth ....
Sex ....
Tel. No. ....
Patient's GP:
Name ....
Address ....
....
....
Procedure/Interest..
....
....
....
History of Present Complaint..
....
....
....
....
Previous Surgery and Medical Illness..
....
....
....
....
Previous Mental Problems...
....
Family History:
Husband/Wife ....
Children ....
Work ....
Social ....
Family/Friends ....
....

Table 31.1 (continued)

Patient's Hope and Expectations of Surgery..
....
....
....
....
....
....
....
....

General History:

   Smoking ....

   Drinking ....

   Pill ....

Drugs/Medications..
....
....

Allergies...

Previous Anesthetic..

Examination and General Description..
....
....

Specific Description of Relevant Areas...
....
....

General Examination:

   BP ....

   HS ....

   Pulse ....

   CVS ....

   Chest ....

   Abdomen ....

Opinion/Comments..
....
....
....
....
....

Patient is: (A) Good Candidate

                          (B) Suitable with Reservations

                          (C) Poor Candidate and Surgery not indicated

(continued)

Table 31.1 (continued)

CONSULTATION REPORT
Operation Recommended: ....
....
....
....
....
....
Clinic .... No. of nights ....
Type Anesthetic ....
Date .... Time to Report....................................
Last Food/Liquid...
Special Instructions to Patient...
....
....
....
....
....
Signature..
I agree to your contacting my GP and for him to provide you with details of my medical history.
Signed..
Date..
I do not wish you to contact my GP
Signed..
Date..

31.3.1 Consent

The patient is admitted to the hospital or clinic after a routine check up with the nurse (Table 31.2). The author goes and signs the consent with the patient. Always have a chaperone as a witness, who also signs the form. The author answers any questions the patient might want to ask or missed at consultation.

31.3.2 Photography

At this stage the author takes a lot of digital photographs. Eight views are preferred (1) anterior, (2) two lateral, (3) two anterolateral,(4) neck, (5) eyes, and (6) one on animation. The background is blue and the distance is constant, using a macro lens help to achieve clear and consistent results.

Another preoperative photo is taken after marking the patient.

31.3.3 Preoperative Markings

It is important to mark the patient while awake so she/he is aware of the position of scars and decides whether the scar is pretragal or posttragal. The extent of postauricular scar depends on the state of the neck and extent of dissection in the neck. Superiorly, the scar is inside the hairline as long as the superior flap migrates and rotates.

The extent of dissection is marked in the neck depending on the amount of submental fat and laxity of anterior fibers of platysma.

31.3.4 Preoperative Preparation on the Operating Table

It is important for the patient to be comfortable on the table. The patient is placed on a head ring that is soft

Table 31.2 Pre- and postoperative instructions

FACELIFT
BEFORE SURGERY
Your procedure will be performed under twilight anesthesia (intravenous sedation)
1. For your comfort, please bring a pair of sunglasses, headscarf, or hat to wear after surgery
2. No makeup or lotions on your face prior to surgery. No vitamin E for a week prior to surgery
3. If you bleach, tint, color, or perm your hair, then please do so not later than 1 week prior to surgery. It will be at least 6 weeks before you can have this done again
4. DO NOT CUT YOUR HAIR before surgery in order for incisions to be covered postoperatively
NEXT MORNING
1. Please write down your questions so that the Surgeon and staff may prepare you well to go home
2. You will be seen by the Surgeon in the treatment room where your bandages will be changed and your dressings checked
AFTER SURGERY (THIS INFORMATION SHOULD BE ADHERED TO, TO ENSURE A SAFE RECOVERY)
1. You may experience some swelling of the face and you may also have bruising on the neck and chest. This is normal and should disappear within 2 weeks. You can apply ice compresses to exposed areas for the first 48 h
2. Consume a soft diet for 3 days after surgery
3. You may wash your hair 3 days after surgery
4. When sleeping, LIE ON YOUR BACK with your head at approximately a 45° angle for seven nights after surgery to help minimize any swelling. This can be accomplished with two pillows under your head and one under your shoulders
5. Limit activities such as bending, straining, and lifting. Avoid excessive neck turning movements and heavy physical exertion for the first month. Avoid also any movements that will give you the feeling of pulling or tightness along the incision line. We do not want you to stretch your incisions. No hot baths for 1 week
6. Should you have pain not relieved by your prescribed medications, please call. Do not take aspirin for up to 1 week postoperatively
7. If you are bleeding through your bandages, do contact the surgeon or the hospital immediately
8. No alcohol should be taken for 1 week after surgery
9. Protect your skin always with a daily sunblock
10. You may have a facial, hair coloring, perms after 6 weeks. Enjoy!

and stable. The hair is combed back and parted where the incisions are planned. The skin is cleaned with iodine. Two probes are inserted for use of the nerve stimulator in order to monitor the temporal and mandibular branches of the facial nerve, especially when the dissection is subplatysmal. The area of surgery should be properly exposed, so the neck, face, and temporal regions are draped appropriately.

31.3.5 Anesthesia: Intravenous Sedation

See Chap. 6.

31.3.6 Nerve Mapping

Before operating and infusing local infiltration, the vital nerves that might be encountered during surgery are mapped. The following are the ones the author maps.

1. Temporal branch: below a line drawn from 0.5 cm below the tragus to 2 cm above lateral eyebrow and above zygoma 4 cm from lateral canthus.
2. Mandibular branch 2 cm posterior to oral commissure.
3. Posterior auricular nerve 6.5 cm below external auditory canal.
4. Also map the extent of the dissection and the areas that might need fat transfer in the midface, or for direction of pull if threads are used during open surgery.

31.3.7 Infiltration

The infiltration fluid is simple to constitute:

1. Saline, 250 ml at normal temperature
2. Lignocaine, 20 ml, 1%
3. Pure adrenaline, 1:1,000

Chloromycetin eye ointment or chloramphenicol drops is used in the eyes.

A spinal needle with a 10 ml syringe is used to infiltrate preferably LuerLock.

The neck is infiltrated first according to markings. Being left-handed, the author starts on the right face. The preauricular subcutaneous tissue is injected to the level of the markings, and beyond, in the temporal region, the injections are placed deeper above the galia as the dissection changes planes. Retroauricular injections are placed carefully to cover the whole extent of the operative field using about 125 ml per side. One side is infiltrated at a time.

31.3.8 Instrumentation

Very few instruments are used to perform this operation but some of the specialist tools make the operation a lot easier. The main instruments are:

1. A nice pair of forceps and scissors that fit the hand and are sharp and flat at the tip. This helps to get into the plane of dissection.
2. Two skin hooks and two cats paws.
3. One fiberoptic retractor with suction at the end to check the flaps for bleeding.
4. Nerve stimulator (Fig. 31.1).
5. Prolene, monocryl sutures, and staples for the skin.
6. Vaselene gauze.
7. Cotton bandage and dressings.
8. Bandage, 4 in.
9. Elastoplast roll, 1 in.
10. The author's special cannulas for liposuction of the neck.

31.4 Procedure

The author always starts with liposuction to the neck. This is performed with the patient in neutral position. A small 2 mm cannula (Fig. 31.2) is introduced in the midline. The author uses the Mercedes variety to start with to take the maximum volume out.

Remember your other hand must help you assist with position of the cannulas at all times. Other longer flat cannulas are then introduced to remove the rest. A layer of fat must be left behind to drape over the tissue. A second incision is performed under the ear lobe to get the jowl area and the rest of the fat in the neck. Using the pinch technique will assist in determining the correct amount to be removed and also ensure the smoothness of the surface.

The facelift incision begins in the temporal scalp, approximately 4–5 cm above the ear and 5 cm behind the hair line, curves parallel to the hairline toward the superior root of the helix just in front to avoid a bridle scar, continues caudally into a natural skin crease or intratragal until passes under the lobe of the ear. The posterior incision is outlined on the posterior surface

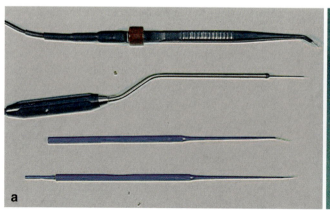
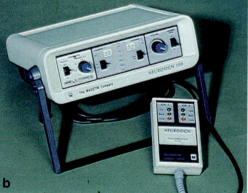

Fig. 31.1 (a) Nerve stimulator. (b) Machine for nerve stimulation which can also give a print out

of the concha, slightly higher as it tends to migrate downward; the rest of the incision is inside the hairline, occipitally. A retractor is used.

Subcutaneously, the dissection is started in the retroauricular area (Fig. 31.3). The correct plane of dissection is identified. There are three layers of fat; supraplatysmal, subcutaneous, and a fine layer in between. The author chooses the supraplatysmal plane as this is the most bloodless. The assistant retracts with cats paws; dissection should be meticulous and bloodless. It is easier to start posteriorly toward the occipital end as this is the softest part. Dissection in the neck proceeds toward "Erbs" point avoiding the superficial nerves, mainly the posterior auricular. Dissection then continues toward the neck (Figs. 31.4 and 31.5) for about 7 cm then stops. A gauze swab is placed in the wound, and dissection started on the front.

An incision is made with a scalpel in the front either pre- or postauricular. Treat the skin delicately and establish a plane of dissection superficial to avoid any

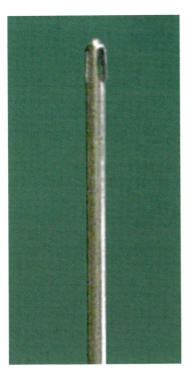

Fig. 31.2 Cannula, 2 mm

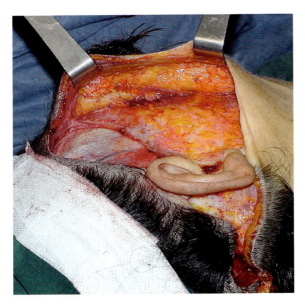

Fig. 31.3 Extensive subcutaneous undermining. The facelift incision begins in the temporal scalp

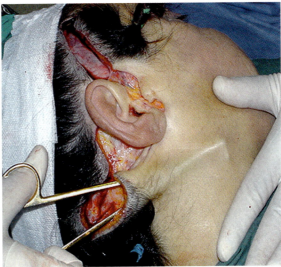

Fig. 31.4 Technique of scissor dissection to avoid injury of auricular and cervical nerves

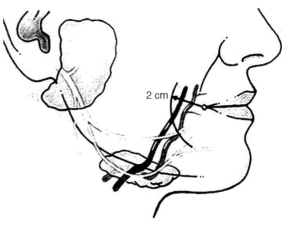

Fig. 31.5 Mapping of mandibular branch

nerves (Figs. 31.6 and 31.7). In the temporal region, a deeper plane is established and the transitional zone is the zone of Morano where the vessels and nerves are situated.

In the front, dissect until the mid-cheek is reached where a fiberoptic retractor is used. Undermining must extend beyond the area of redundancy. In general, the dissection extends within 1 cm of the lateral orbital rim, across the malar region to nasolabial folds and inferiorly to the thyroid cartilage. It is important to release the zygomatic ligament and the mandibular ligament so you can get a better traction and a better jaw line.

31.5 The SMAS

The superficial musculoaponeurotic system (SMAS) is a fibromuscular fascial extension of the platysmal muscle that arises superiorly from the fascia over the zygomatic arch and is continuous in the inferior cheek with the platysmal muscle. The facial nerve lies deep to the SMAS and innervates the mimetic muscles of the forehead and mid-face from the ventral aspect of the muscles.

The SMAS fascia is a fanlike fascia that envelops the face and provides a suspensory sheet which distributes forces of facial expression. The SMAS is continuous with the platysma muscle inferiorly and the superficial temporal fascia superiorly, and it is superficial to the parotomasseteric fascia. The SMAS connects to the fascial musculature in the nasolabial, perioral, and periorbital regions.

The anatomy of the SMAS/platysma must be studied in detail before embarking on this. The SMAS dissection begins transversely one finger breadth below the zygomatic arch (Figs. 31.8 and 31.9), then a vertical incision is made 0.5 cm anterior to the tragus extending downward beyond the mandibular angle to connect with the lateral margins of the platysma muscle. They are both dissected in continuity (Fig. 31.10). The dissection is extended to the anterior border of the parotid gland after elevating it from the parotid fascia.

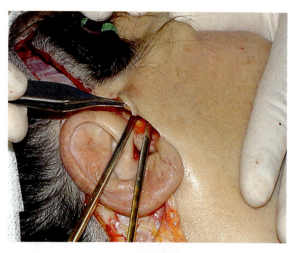

Fig. 31.6 Dissection below the zygomatic arch can reach anterior eminence

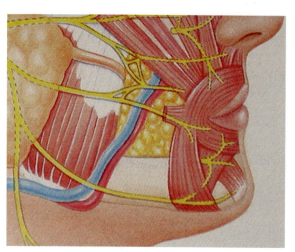

Fig. 31.7 Zygomatic and buccal branches

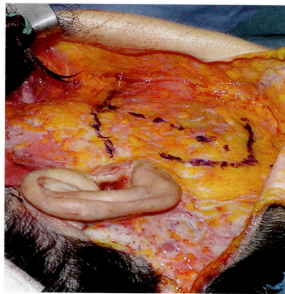

Fig. 31.8 Markings of SMAS elevation

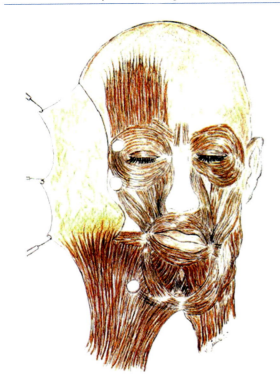

Fig. 31.9 Extension of SMAS

At this time, it must be decided if limited SMAS or an extended (one where the dissection is continued to the zygomatic major muscle) dissection will be done. The whole flap can then be rotated into a cephal posterior direction (Fig. 31.11) where smoothness of the jowl soon appears. The author also prefers a cephalad direction. The excess is then removed and sutured with interrupted nonabsorbable sutures.

In the neck, the anterior fibers of the platysma are dealt with separately via a submental incision. The author uses the plication method with or without excision of the redundant muscle subject to the severity.

The author also sometimes inserts the threads (Figs. 31.12 and 31.13) to help with raising the cheeks and further improvement to the midface.

Before closure, the size of the ear and lobe is checked and if more the 6 cm, a v-shaped flap is rotated and excised from the lobe of the ear, which gives it a more youthful appearance.

For closure, four anchor points are used: (1) just above the ear in the temporal region, (2) retroauricular, (3) the lower margin of the lobe, and (4) two sutures are inserted to stabilize the retrotragal flap. The excess is removed by carefully tailoring round the wound, and stopping about 1 in. higher than the lower end of the

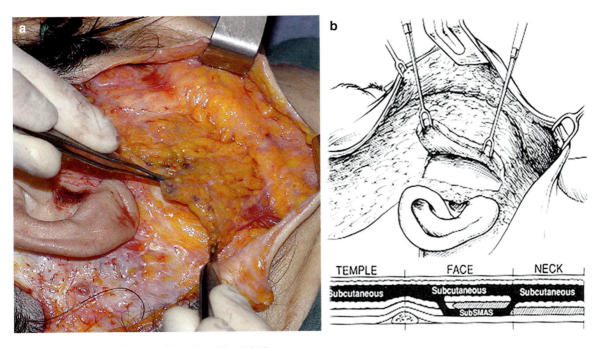

Fig. 31.10 SubSMAS dissection (elevation of the SMAS)

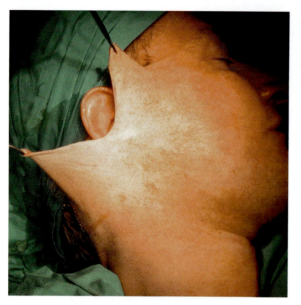

Fig. 31.11 Direction of advancement of the flaps

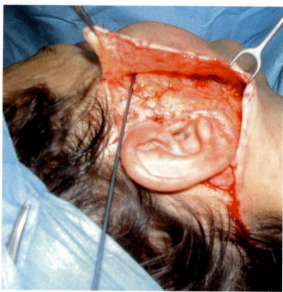

Fig. 31.13 Direction of inserting the needle + threads to elevate the cheeks

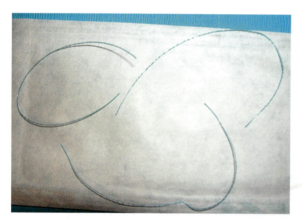

Fig. 31.12 Cogged threads

lobe, then making a snug fit around the lobe as scars tend to migrate downward and drag the ear lobe down. Subcutaneous sutures should be inserted to remove tension which is important to the final result. Staples are inserted in the posterior hair-bearing area and the temporal wound. The rest are sutured with fine 4/0 Monocryl. Subcuticular sutures are preferred in front of the ear.

31.6 Dressings

Vaseline gauze is applied to the wounds, followed by 4×4 dressings, cotton wool is applied, and a 4 in. crepe bandage is meticulously applied and secured with 1 in. elastoplast.

31.7 Results

Final results are shown in Figs. 31.14–31.16.

Fig. 31.14 (a) Preoperative. (b) Postoperative

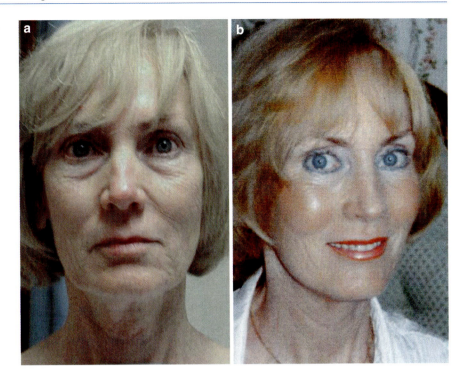

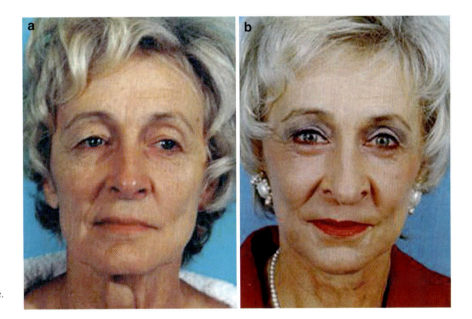

Fig. 31.15 (a) Preoperative. (b) Postoperative

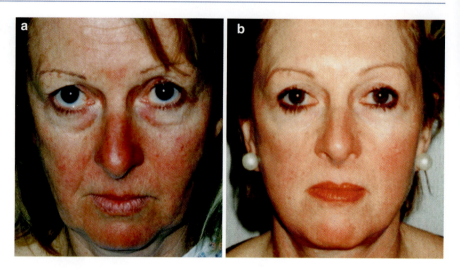

Fig. 31.16 (a) Preoperative. (b) Postoperative

References

Adamson PA, Dahiya R, Litner J. Midface effects of the deep-plane vs the superficial musculoaponeurotic system plication face-lift. Arch Facial Plast Surg. 2007;9(1):9–11.

Baker DC. Lateral SMASectomy, plication and short scar facelifts: indications and techniques. Clin Plast Surg. 2008;35(4):533–50.

Berry MG, Davies D. Platysma-SMAS plication facelift. J Plast Reconstr Aesthet Surg. 2010;63(5):793–800.

Caplin DA, Perlyn CA. Rejuvenation of the aging neck: current principles, techniques, and newer modifications. Facial Plast Surg Clin North Am. 2009;17(4):589–601.

Gassner HG, Rafii A, Young A, Murakami C, Moe KS, Larrabee Jr WF. Surgical anatomy of the face: implications for modern face-lift techniques. Arch Facial Plast Surg. 2008; 10(1):9–19.

Jones BM, Grover R. Reducing complications in cervicofacial rhytidectomy by tumescent infiltration: a comparative trial evaluating 678 consecutive face lifts. Plast Reconstr Surg. 2004;113(1):398–403.

Mendelson BC, Freeman ME, Wu W, Huggins RJ. Surgical anatomy of the lower face: the premasseter space, the jowl, and the labiomandibular fold. Aesthetic Plast Surg. 2008; 32(2):185–95.

Mentz III HA, Ruiz-Razura A, Patronella CK, Newall G. Facelift: measurement of superficial muscular aponeurotic system advancement with and without zygomaticus major muscle release. Aesthetic Plast Surg. 2005;29(5):V 353–62.

Prado A, Andrades P, Fuentes P, Eulufi A, Cuadra A. The use of intra-SMAS absorbable barbed sutures to reinforce a high-vector pull during rhytidectomy. Plast Reconstr Surg. 2008;122(6):215e–6e.

Schaverien MV, Pessa JE, Saint-Cyr M, Rohrich RJ. The arterial and venous anatomies of the lateral face lift flap and the SMAS. Plast Reconstr Surg. 2009;123(5):1581–7.

Sundine MJ, Kretsis V, Connell BF. Longevity of SMAS facial rejuvenation and support. Plast Reconstr Surg. 2010; 126(1):229–37.

Trussler AP, Stephan P, Hatef D, Schaverien M, Meade R, Barton FE. The frontal branch of the facial nerve across the zygomatic arch: anatomical relevance of the high-SMAS technique. Plast Reconstr Surg. 2010;125(4):1221–9.

van der Lei B, Cromheecke M, Hofer SO. The purse-string reinforced SMASectomy short scar facelift. Aesthetic Surg J. 2009;29(3):180–8.

Waterhouse N, Vesely M, Bulstrode NW. Modified lateral SMASectomy. Plast Reconstr Surg. 2007;119(3):1021–6.

Design and Management of the Anterior Hairline Temporal Incision and Skin Take Out in the Vertical Facelift and Lateral Brow Lift Procedures

Mary E. Lester, Richard C. Hagerty, and J. Clayton Crantford

32.1 Introduction

A substantial amount of skin can be presented to the temporal area with the vertical facelift and lateral subcutaneous brow lift. The challenge is to excise as much skin as needed while maintaining hair follicles, minimizing scars, and eliminating unsightly anterior gathering of the skin. The significant advantage of the anterior hairline incision lies in the amount of vertical lift that can be provided to the lateral brow. There is a large amount of skin that can be removed from this area while continuing to allow the growth of hair anterior to the incision. This combination results in a natural-appearing vertical pull on the lateral face and less obvious scarring than previous techniques. The major criticism, and rightly so, is the possibility of unacceptable scarring.

Proper planning of the incision and skin excision can minimize the problems of scarring in the temporal area by paying attention to vector points in the hairline. The rationale for this procedure is based on the position of the hairline and the underlying anatomy and the orientation of the hair follicles [1, 2].

The purpose of this chapter is to address the scarring issue and present a surgical strategy to possibly decrease the negative ramifications of the anterior temporal hairline incisions. The senior author has routinely used this technique over the past 5 years in over 200 cases. His experience over 1 year is presented with 41 patients (Table 32.1).

32.2 Technique

It is important to first examine the patient from the frontal view and delineate the leading point for skin excision. The leading point should be placed 0.5 cm posterior to the hairline, just inferior to the receding hairline of the temporal area. The more skin that needs to be removed, the more lateral the leading point is placed in the temporal hairline. It is critical to preserve at least 2 cm between the eyebrow and the hairline (Fig. 32.1). This may mean removing hair-bearing skin. The scar must not be obvious from the frontal view, so the more laterally it is placed, the less conspicuous it will be.

The incision is further planned by placing a 4 cm line at about a 45° angle from the lead point into the receding hairline. The skin is incised at a 45° angle to preserve hair follicles. The rest of the temporal incision in the preauricular area is made with a W-plasty type incision incorporating hair follicles with the excised skin (Fig. 32.1). A limited incision can be carried around the lobule to the posterior auricular space depending on the amount of neck lift needed. The majority of the improvement in neck appearance is from the vertical pull for the neck lift. Very little neck skin is pulled in a diagonal vector as described below. Next, a subcutaneous lateral brow dissection is performed extending superiorly to the forehead over the temporalis muscle, medially to the lateral canthal

M.E. Lester (✉)
University of Florida, 100286, Gainesville, FL 32610, USA
e-mail: medmlester@yahoo.com

R.C. Hagerty
Medical University of South Carolina, 261 Calhoun St., Suite 200, Charleston, SC 29401, USA
e-mail: dukehagerty@aol.com

J.C. Crantford
Medical University of South Carolina, 375 Hoff Ave.,
Charleston, SC 29407, USA
e-mail: crantfo@musc.edu

Table 32.1 Experience with 41 patients

Average age	58 years	
Age range	34–79 years	
Follow-up average	138 days	
Comorbidities		
None	19 patients	46%
HTN	6 patients	14%
Depression	5 patients	12%
Hypothyroidism	4 patients	10%
GERD	3 patients	7%
Osetoarthritis	2 patients	5%
Bipolar	1 patient	2%
Emphysema	1 patient	2%
Osteoporosis	1 patient	2%
Seizure disorder	1 patient	2%
Tobacco use	0 patients	0%
Complications		
None	41 patients	

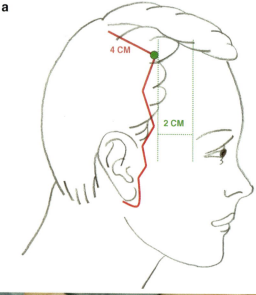

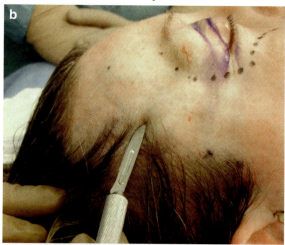

Fig. 32.1 (a) Leading point is shown as a *green circle* at least 2 cm from the lateral brow. A 4 cm incision (*red line* A) is into the temporal receding hairline and W-plasty incision along temporal hairline to lobule. (b) Beveled angle of scalpel to skin that preserves hair follicles

tendon, and inferiorly to the zygoma (Fig. 32.2). Once this elevation and the facelift subcutaneous dissection are complete, the skin is excised in a tailor-tacking fashion with the placement of key sutures and rotation of forehead skin. The first key suture involves proper placement of the lateral canthal tendon (Fig. 32.3). The lateral canthal tendon should be placed with superior and lateral tension, placing it higher than the medial canthal tendon. The next key suture ensures the vertical pull of the check and neck lift and is placed near the root of the helix. The excess skin or dogear of the forehead is excised by rotating the skin medial to lateral. This is accomplished by removing a Burrow's triangle of skin in the receding hair line along the most lateral position of the temporal incision (Fig. 32.4).

Rotating the skin from the medial incision to the lateral incision closes the Burrow's triangle. The length of the medial incision is significantly longer than the recipient lateral incision. This discrepancy necessitates a bunching or imbrication of the medial incision to accommodate closure, which is completed differentially down the lateral superior (cephalad) suture line to minimize bunching anteriorly (Fig. 32.5). This imbrication principle is similarly applied in a large breast reduction, where the skin on the inferior aspect of the breast incision is bunched to minimize the length of the scar into the axilla. The corresponding W-plasty incisions can be made in a tailor-tacking fashion and the incisions are closed with deep interrupted sutures of 5–0 Monocryl and either running 5–0 Prolene or interrupted 4–0 silk figure-of-eight sutures along the entire length (Fig. 32.6).

32.3 Complications

No scar revision was necessary and no complications were reported with the surgery. All patients were satisfied with the results of their surgery.

32.4 Discussion

Virtually all patients are candidates for this procedure, with only exception being the patients who have no hair follicle skin in this area, including balding men

32 Design and Management of the Anterior Hairline Temporal Incision

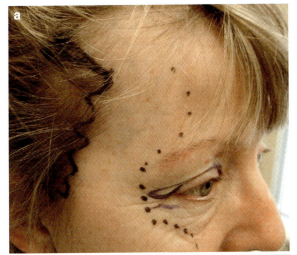

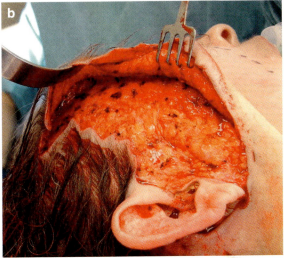

Fig. 32.2 (**a**) Area between temporal incision and *dotted line* shows planned subcutaneous dissection. (**b**) Skin flaps undermined in the subcutaneous plane and canthal tendon is seen

with significant recessive hairlines. Thin hair itself is not a contraindication because the skin of the scalp heals fairly well. The procedure described has been limited to patients with Fitzpatrick I through IV. Patients with thicker skin may also have thicker scars.

The thickness of the hair, the natural hairline, skin quality, and the amount of brow ptosis all need to be evaluated prior to surgery. In a patient with better skin elasticity and better skin health, less skin excision is necessary. Conversely, the more damaged the skin and the less elasticity, the more skin needs to be removed to support the brow laterally as well as to obtain the vertical lift laterally.

Proper management of temporal skin excision is important particularly when doing a vertical facelift because this is a critical area for support of the

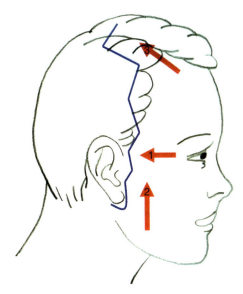

Fig. 32.3 *Arrows* delineate the direction of tension along the three key areas. First the canthal tendon is set. Second the vertical pull of the facelift with the key suture placed in the preauricular area. Third the rotation of the forehead skin from medial to lateral eliminates a dog ear

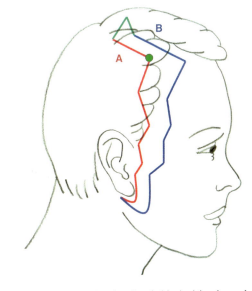

Fig. 32.4 The Burrow's triangle of skin incision is marked in *green* that is superolateral to line A. Line B is then drawn longer and parallel to *line A*

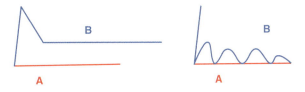

Fig. 32.5 Differential line lengths, excision of Burrow's triangle, and imbrication technique

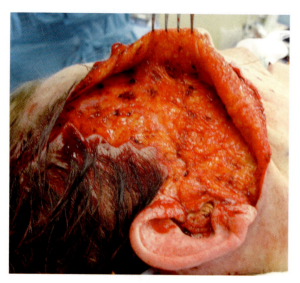

Fig. 32.6 Tailor-tacking technique of W-plasty incision and figure-of-eight sutures with the first key suture setting the height of the canthal tendon

facelift [3–7]. The more skin we are able to excise, the more options we have in what we can do with supporting the brow and the cheek areas. The design described significantly reduces, if not eliminates, the bunching at the anterior part of the brow. Basically, this bunching is displaced laterally over a much bigger area, thereby reducing the consequences. Because of the thinness of the skin, scarring is rarely a problem. Because of the design, hair follicles are preserved where they are most needed and the aesthetic quality of the hairline is retained (Figs. 32.7–32.10).

32.5 Conclusions

Over the past 10 years, the authors have progressed from the classic hair excision to the vertical with the aggressive temporal excision as described earlier by the senior author [8]. The significant advantage of the vertical lift is the natural vector pull of the facelift is respected, which gives a much more natural look to the patient. The initial disadvantage was the anterior scar line across the hairline, which was originally described as a straight line. The revision rate was unacceptable. Replacing the straight-line closure with multiple Z-plasty flaps and a beveled cut helped reduce scarring [4].

The excess tissue in the apex of the temporal area, however, continued to be an issue because of the significant amount of excess skin that gathered there, which resulted in an unattractive three-dimensional quality. A potential solution to this problem brought about the design as presented. Essentially, the gathering of tissue is redistributed now laterally across the naturally occurring recessive hairline, allowing more temporal skin removal.

In addition, over the past years a subcutaneous lateral brow dissection to the vertical facelift has been added, which significantly helps to permanently improve the position of the brow laterally. The dissection extends subcutaneously to the forehead region, over the temporalis muscle, inferiorly to the lateral eyebrow, and anteriorly to the zygomatic arch. The lateral brow lift can be combined with a central lift [9], a canthopexy [10], and/or the vertical facelift when indicated. Surgical dissection between the lateral canthal ligament and the tendon allows for increased tension on the lateral canthal ligament with superior repositioning of the lateral canthus itself. The increase in our ability to remove more skin in the temple area results in more tension on the lateral canthal ligament, resulting in lateral and superior rotation of the lateral canthus.

Management of the temporal incision line is important for the long-term appearance of the scar as well as for proper positioning of the lateral canthus, brow, and hairline. The authors' approach utilizing W-plasty technique, proper design, and dissection is very successful. Modification over the years has resulted in this approach, which is reproducible, safe, and effective. While the anterior hairline scar is not eliminated, it is reduced enough to make the vertical lift worthwhile.

32 Design and Management of the Anterior Hairline Temporal Incision

Fig. 32.7 (**a**) Preoperative patient. (**b**) Postoperative

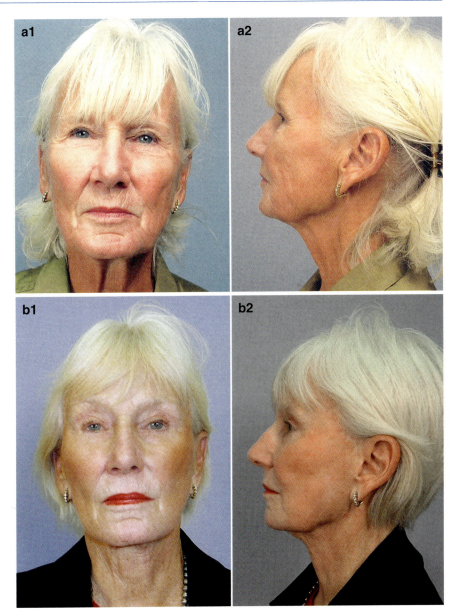

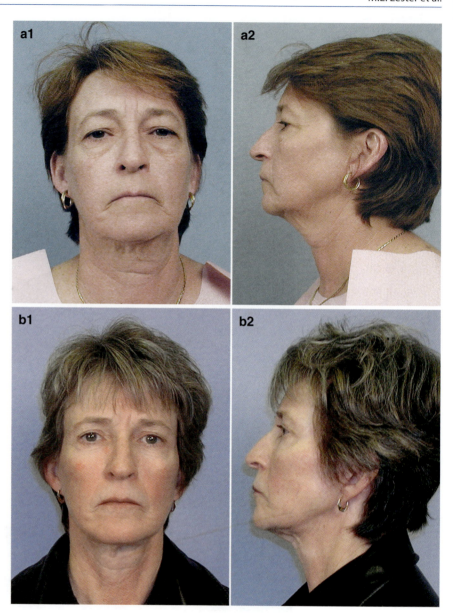

Fig. 32.8 (**a**) Preoperative patient. (**b**) Postoperative

32 Design and Management of the Anterior Hairline Temporal Incision

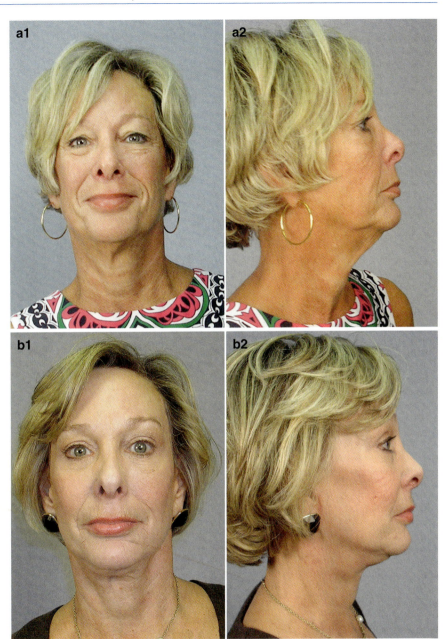

Fig. 32.9 (**a**) Preoperative patient. (**b**) Postoperative

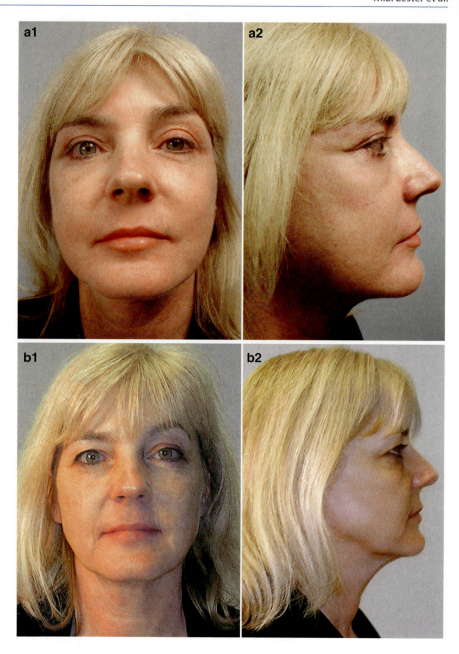

Fig. 32.10 (**a**) Preoperative patient. (**b**) Postoperative

References

1. Baker DC, Conley J. Avoiding facial nerve injuries in rhytidectomy: anatomical variations and pitfalls. Plast Reconstr Surg. 1979;64(6):781–95.
2. Mowlavi A, Majzoub RK, Cooney DS, Wilhelmi BJ, Guyuron B. Follicular anatomy of the anterior temporal hairline and implications for rhytidectomy. Plast Reconstr Surg. 2007;119(6):1891–5.
3. Hagerty RC, Scioscia PJ. The medial SMAS lift with aggressive temporal skin take out. Plast Reconstr Surg. 1998;101(6):1650–6.
4. Hagerty RC, Mittelstaedt SJ, O'Neill P, Harvey TS. Lateral canthopexy using the hollow needle technique. Plast Reconstr Surg. 2006;117(4):1289–91.
5. McCord CD, Doxanas MT. Browplasty and browpexy: an adjunct to blepharoplasty. Plast Reconstr Surg. 1990;86(2):248–54.

6. Knize DM. Limited incision forehead lift for eyebrow elevation to enhance upper blepharoplasty. Plast Reconstr Surg. 2001;108(2):564–7.
7. Miller TA. Continuing medical education examination–facial aesthetic surgery: lateral subcutaneous brow lift. Aesthetic Surg J. 2003;23(3):205–10.
8. Baker DC. Minimal invasive rhytidectomy (short-scar facelift) with lateral SMASectomy. Aesthetic Surg J. 2001;21(1):68–79.
9. Mitz V. Current face lifting procedure: an attempt at evaluation. Ann Plast Surg. 1986;17(3):184–93.
10. Hagerty RC. Central suspension technique at the midface. Plast Reconstr Surg. 1995;96(3):728–30.

Short-Scar Facelift with Extended SMAS/Platysma Dissection and Limited Skin Undermining

Hamid Massiha

33.1 Introduction

Short-scar cervicofacial rhytidectomy is an excellent approach to facial rejuvenation [1]. While it achieves fully advanced results as much as any extended scar facelift, it also achieves this result with a much shorter incision and lesser skin undermining that in turn decreases complications [1].

Historically, one of the earliest facelift publications [2] described use of a short preauricular incision and only very limited skin undermining. During the decades that followed, surgeons decided to undermine skin farther to achieve better results by removing more of the excess skin. Obviously this resulted in excess skin at the end part of excisions resulting in dog ears. The attempt to remove dog ears involved incisions at the temple and occipital area as conventional face-lift scars with often ill effects at temporal hair growth and anatomy and adverse alterations in hair line and its growth pattern in the occipital area. Some European surgeons had started to use short incisions with the elimination of occipital scar, but still using temporal scars [3]. In 1993, I started basic additions to this technique to make it usable in the majority of aging deformities even in patients in their seventies. Understanding these alterations will help the plastic surgeon to better utilize the technical detail that is to follow more efficiently.

H. Massiha
Department of Plastic Surgery, Louisiana State University, School of Medicine, 3939 Horima Blvd., Suite 216, Metairie, LA 70006, USA
e-mail: massihamd@aol.com

33.2 Author's Addition and Deletion to Short-Scar Technique

1. Elimination of temporal incision. At the present status of my technique there are no incisions at the hair-bearing areas of the scalp. Addition of incision at the sideburn area makes this change very easy to achieve.
2. Extended SMAS/Platysma dissection while keeping skin dissection to a minimum.
3. Skin undermining to a minimal and to the as needed level. Thus when SMAS is lifted and fixed at the appropriate level on the cheek and preauricular area, the skin of the neck, jowls, and neck line area is pulled up while still attached to the SMAS/platysma. The attachments of skin with SMAS/platysma are very firm due to fibrotic band that arises from SMAS/platysma and penetrates dermis [3]. This fact helps the skin move up together with the SMAS.

The benefits of this approach are:

1. Tension on skin per se is less.
2. Circulation to the skin is preserved better by not dissecting it.
3. The vectors of lift are different for SMAS and skin. Since SMAS is more pliable than skin and excision of it in any direction does not cause visible scarring the vectors could be fashioned to achieve the most natural aesthetic outcome. But, skin excision vectors could be fastened in such a way that while being aesthetically pleasing, the scars could be kept short and well hidden [1].
4. Posteroanterior vectors of lift at the postauricular and mastoid area.

In advanced cases where extension of incision to the postauricular crease is inevitable, posteroanterior vectors could help to keep the incision line deep in the postauricular crease. In the meantime, this will help tighten and reduce the posterior neck skin redundancy in advanced cases [1].

These innovations and some minor ones, to be discussed, in technique of the procedure have made this a rock solid technique. Even in repeat facelifts where patients already have temporal and occipital scars, I often do a short-scar technique and do not disturb or use old scars unless there are deformities that necessitate intervention.

33.3 Surgical Technique of Short-Scar Facelift

33.3.1 Marking

The patient is marked in sitting position in the holding area preoperatively. The marking gives a chance to the surgeon to refresh his memory with the particular individual characteristic of each patient's facial structures and degree of lift to correct it. I usually mark the approximate skin dissection area and SMAS/platysma area and incision line (Figs. 33.1 and 33.2).

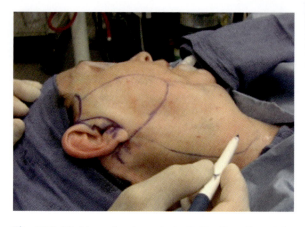

Fig. 33.2 Markings showing extent of skin dissection at the cheek area and SMAS/platysma dissection to the lower neck, down the midline of the neck if needed. Sternocleidomastoid muscle is marked as the posterior limit of dissection

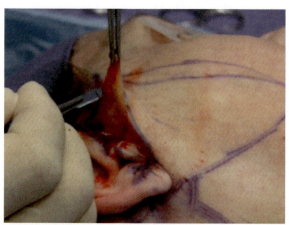

Fig. 33.3 Skin dissection is started using a scalpel to make a thin flap and then continued with Rees/Aston scissors. Notice that a strip of skin resection at the preauricular area facilitates skin and SMAS dissection

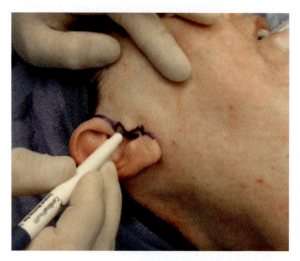

Fig. 33.1 Markings are drawn showing that the incision line follows the anatomical creases (e.g., w-plasty idea). Incisions that are placed at the apex of the tragus will heal well enough making the scar virtually invisible

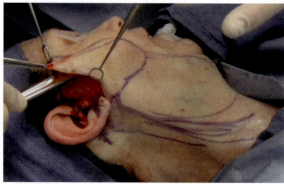

Fig. 33.4 Skin dissection is continued anteriorly in direction of the nose, nasolabial fold, and corners of the mouth

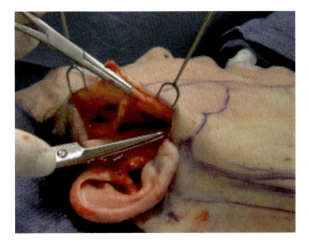

Fig. 33.5 SMAS dissection is being started. This dissection will extend anteriorly and inferiorly at the jaw line area when dissection reaches the platysma muscle. Dissection is extremely easy and can be done bluntly to prevent nerve damage

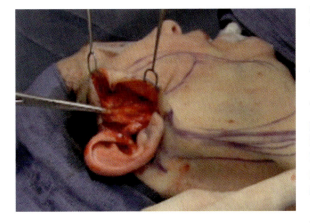

Fig. 33.6 SMAS/platysma dissection is necessary at the completion to release the platysma connections at the highest parts of the anterior edge of the SCMM to gain mobility of the flap

Fig. 33.7 The traction on the now mobile SMAS/platysma unit pulls the skin upward in unison with the platysma. This is due to strong connections between the skin and SMAS/platysma

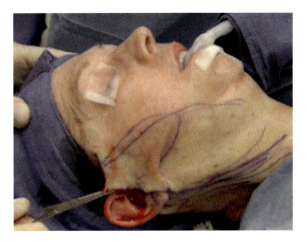

Fig. 33.8 When skin is draped over the pulled SMAS, the spot where skin dissection over the SMAS/platysma is stopped is seen like a demarcation area. Also notice how vertical the vector of the traction is

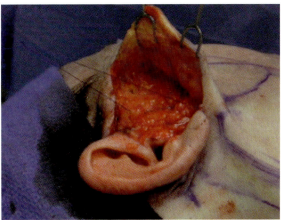

Fig. 33.9 Sutures are placed to actually lift the SMAS and consequently platysma and overlying skin upward resulting in extreme correction in the vertical neck and jaw line

33.3.2 Anesthesia

This surgery could easily be done with local anesthesia preferably with MAC anesthesia with local infiltration. If it is being done in patients with moderate aging deformity less extensive undermining may suffice. The author uses a mixture of 50 ml of lidocaine 0.5% 50 ml of Marcaine 0.25% + 1 ml of epinephrine 1/1,000 (50 ml per side).

In advanced cases or cases that are combined with other procedures, general anesthesia with local infiltration is chosen. In any case, both sides are infiltrated at the beginning of surgery.

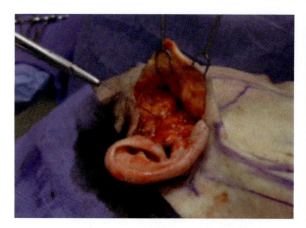

Fig. 33.10 Multiple interrupted sutures are placed on the SMAS in a direction that will assure a smooth skin contour

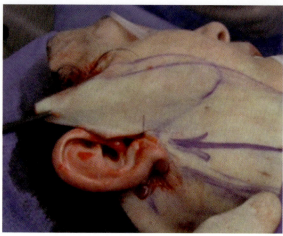

Fig. 33.12 Skin is pulled upward at an angle close to 90°. Removal of the dog ears at the sideburn area is easier than that of the posterior auricular area. The more vertical the vector, the less skin redundancy will be behind the ear

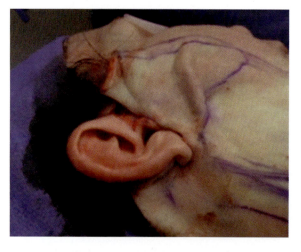

Fig. 33.11 SMAS repair is complete. Now there is a lot of redundant skin to be excised. Notice the demarcation of the dissected and nondissected skin

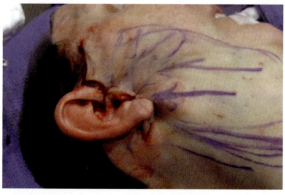

Fig. 33.13 Guide sutures are placed and excess skin is removed. Still there is some skin redundancy behind the ear lobule to be dealt with

There are at least two reasons for this approach:

1. While injecting the second side, the first side will blanch enough to start incisions right away. This will save time and by the time first side is finished, second side is well blanched, provided the surgeon is moving on and doesn't take more than 60–70 min to do the first side.
2. In cases where sedation is being given, most of the pain of the injection subsides in the beginning of the case and deep sedation may be avoided for the rest of the procedure.

33.4 Technique of Short-Scar Facelift with Extended SMAS/Platysma Dissection and Repair
(Fig. 33.1–33.16)

The incision is made at the sideburn and carried to preauricular area. Traveling through natural lines above the tragus then in front or at apex of the tragus – not behind it – it dips under the tragus and contours at the lobular crease and stops just under the ear lobule to facilitate dissection. A piece of skin is removed from the preauricular area [4].

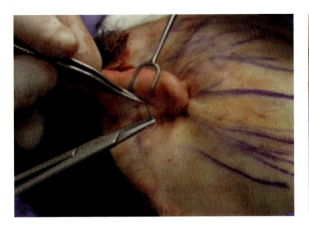

Fig. 33.14 Deep sutures between dermis and mastoid fascia are important. They prevent ear lobule migration inferiorly and also are helpful in tucking down the pleated areas

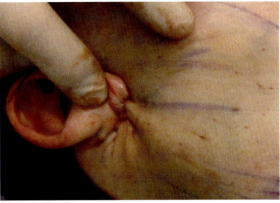

Fig. 33.16 Short posterior auricular scar even in advanced cases. If needed, incisions could be extended as far as necessary superiorly

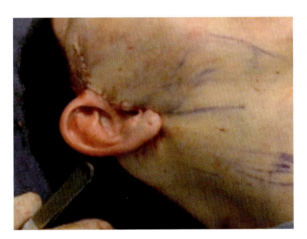

Fig. 33.15 At completion of the operation there is a smooth natural-looking face and neck. Different degrees of pleating may occur that usually subside in time. Pleating usually is more noticeable at the side done first

Skin dissection is done several centimeters anteriorly and inferiorly. Then, the SMAS is identified and dissected. If the skin flap is thin, finding the SMAS is easier; otherwise, SMAS may be included in a thick flap and difficult to find.

The SMAS is dissected with direct vision anteriorly and inferiorly. When dissection reaches to platysma level dissection is very easy,so blunt dissection will suffice. I use facelift scissors and only spread with no cutting. However, any blunt dissection device could be used to mobilize the SMAS/platysma adequately. It is necessary to release attachments of platysma from anterior edge of sternocleidomastoid muscle (SCMM) usually several centimeters at its most superior portion. At this time, pulling on the SMAS on proper direction should show immediate improvement in neck and jaw line area. If mobility is restricted you should identify the attachment band and release it until you are happy with the correction. There is not a set where the SMAS should be attached. It should be placed in an angle where the best correction is achieved. Usually my first suture is placed at the angle between the sideburn and the preauricular area and subsequent sutures are placed at the zygomatic arch and preauricular area. The bunching of SMAS at the zygomatic area may be kept to enhance the cheek area. If it is not needed, it could be trimmed off. We recommend use of 3–0 PDS sutures on SH needle for SMAS repair.

At the end of the SMAS lift, the surgeon will notice that the skin has moved up as folds of redundancy and are ready to be excised. Redundant skin is excised with moderate tension after placement of guide sutures at the points

1. Below the tragus.
2. Above the tragus.
3. Immediately behind the ear lobule.
4. At the angle between sideburn incision and preauricular incisions. Excision of skin at sideburn area and preauricular area are usually uneventful and easily done.

Difficulty often is at the area under and behind the ear lobule that may need some finesse. In this part, directly superior and posteroanterior vectors are helpful. At this area, namely under and behind the ear lobe, solid dermal to deep fascia suturing is a helpful step. These sutures take the stress from the ear lobule and will prevent the scar from migrating inferiorly, pulling, and deformity of ear lobule postoperatively. To combat the redundant skin problem at the postauricular area, first and foremost is attention to keep the incision very limited around the ear lobule at the start of the case. This, like any dog-ear situation like eyelid surgery [5] will reduce the dog ear.

Irregularities at the postauricular crease are often present and improve by time. Skin repair is then done with running subcuticular sutures (4–0 Monocryl or PDS sutures on a PS2 needle).

33.4.1 Dressings

Steri-strips are placed on the incision line and at the jowl and upper neck area to reduce tension on the skin and help healing. No drains are used. A Kerlex wrap is used and covered with a 3 inch ace bandage postoperatively. The dressing is removed the next day and a chin strap is applied. The patient can resume activities as soon as he or she desires.

33.5 Advantages of the Short-Scar Facelift

1. Obviously the less incisions, the less scarring and the less scar-related problem.
2. Preserving integrity of natural hair lines in sideburn area and occipital hairline area. Sideburn incisions not only help to reduce the dog ear at upper part of incisions, but also prevent raising sideburn higher and giving bald sideburn areas. In postauricular/occipital area, the interruption of hair line which used to be tell tale of facelift (with or without hair loss) is fully avoided. Bald spots at temporal area due to hair loss or scar widening is also avoided.
3. Limited skin undermining and doing the lift mainly with a composite flap of skin SMAS/Platysma has its own advantages, e.g., preserving better circulation and innervation to the skin. In short term this will help the healing process and minimize chances of skin necrosis and in long term may prevent premature aging and loss of collagen and elastin due to poor circulation or denervation of the skin.
4. Since the fat compartments at perioral area and jowls are mainly between skin and platysma [6], lifting these two structures in unison will lift these fat pads in a natural-looking fashion.
5. Platysma bands: The author seldom uses a midline incision under the chin or does anything else at the midneck to deal with platysma bands. It seems that dissecting under the platysma either damages bands or the firm lift on those bands then bows superiorly, causing the correction, no matter what the reason is, and it does correct the bands in most cases with no additional interventions of these bands. It could be asserted that both these factors jointly are effective for this favorable outcome.

33.6 Disadvantages

Difficulty in removing skin in the postauricular area is the only drawback that the author has found. Excess skin in sideburn area is well manageable even if it may mean extending incisions in pretragal area of temple (preferably in a w-plasty manner). This redundancy and subsequent pleating behind the ears, although it subsides later, has to be discussed with the patients before surgery. Patients that accept and expect even a negative point in the surgery are more prone to be happy like a member of the surgical team.

References

1. Massiha H. Short scar face lift with extended SMAS platysma dissection and lifting and limited skin undermining. Plast Reconstr Surg. 2003;112(2):663–9.
2. Lexer E. Zur gesichtsplastik. Arch Klin Chir. 1910;92:749.
3. Ansari P. S-lift: a sensational method of face-lift. Presented at the 25th annual meeting of the American Society for Aesthetic Plastic Surgery, Los Angeles, 15 May 1992.
4. Rees TD. Aesthetic plastic surgery. Philadelphia: W.B. Saunders; 1980.
5. Massiha H. Combined skin and skin-muscle flap technique in lower blepharoplasty: a 10-year experience. Ann Plast Surg. 1990;25(6):467–76.
6. Skoog T. Plastic surgery: new methods and refinements. Philadelphia: W.B. Saunders; 1974.

Extent of SMAS Advancement in Facelift with or without Zygomaticus Major Muscle Release

34

Henry A. Mentz III

34.1 Introduction

There are many forms of face lifting techniques that have evolved since the earliest skin excisions performed more than a century ago. The most substantial addition to the myriad of techniques has been incorporation of SMAS advancement and the lifting and anchoring of midface soft tissue. While skin excisions serve to tighten skin and reduce wrinkles, skin does not function well as a supportive structure. Furthermore, using skin to support midface soft tissues like heavy jowls can result in stretch artifact. These unnatural lines are represented by sweeping lines to the nose, mouth, and chin, contrary to relaxed skin tension lines. As a result, many surgeons advocate vertical lifting and anchoring of midface soft tissue apart from the skin lift portion. Separating the lift of skin from soft tissue allows more substantial elevation of midface cheek and jowl fat without elevation of the temporal hairline. It also allows independent lift and tension for each layer and therefore allowing the surgeon to customize the lift. Patients who may have more soft tissue descent and less skin laxity can be treated with more SMAS lift than skin tightening and vice versa.

SMAS lifting began initially with deep layer undermining, advocated in 1974 by Skoog. More precise anatomic descriptions began with Mitz and Peyronie in 1976, who used cadaveric dissections to define this midplane layer as the superficial musculoaponeurotic system or SMAS. Many modifications either kept SMAS and skin together or divided the layers [19–24] to allow separation of lifting directions or vectors. Hamra introduced deep layer lifting in 1992 and many adaptations and modifications followed. Hamra's composite lift had limited skin undermining, wide midface SMAS elevation with orbicularis repositioning, but required more substantial elevation of the temporal hairline since the skin lift followed the SMAS lift. Furnas and Stuzin provided valuable research by outlining the anatomy of the frontal branch of the facial nerve and the SMAS retaining ligaments. With release of the zygomatic and masseteric cutaneous retaining ligaments the SMAS flap was far more mobile and could be lifted more substantially. These releases allow for movement of the SMAS flap, thus enhanced movement of the cheek and jowl midface soft tissue mass. With an increase in SMAS elevation, most recommended dividing the layers of skin and SMAS to reduce the lift of hairline. More medial elevation has been advocated using malar fat pad suspension [25, 26]. Lateral elevation can be improved with release of the temporoparietal mesentery [27] and the neck platysma [20]. Liposuction or direct fat excision of the jowl can reduce fullness low in the cheek ([28–31]). Direct excision is more the standard now.

When patients have more extensive jowling, then maximal movement of the SMAS medially becomes necessary for correction. SMAS flap release can define the extent of movement medially and laterally. For example, when the SMAS is dissected and retaining ligaments released, the attached flap rotates on the pivot point at or near the zygomaticus major muscle (ZMM) resulting in substantial SMAS lift at the ear and minimal lift at the attached pivot point near the cheek. In order to achieve more substantial movement of the SMAS flap medially, a release of the flap from

H.A. Mentz III
The Aesthetic Center for Plastic Surgery, 4400 Post OAk pkwy, 2260 Houston, TX 77027, USA
e-mail: lupeacps@yahoo.com

the ZMM can allow more movement of the midface SMAS. This converts the SMAS flap from a rotation flap to an advancement flap resulting is more movement at the cheek and jowl. Careful preoperative examination and operative planning is necessary for optimal results.

34.2 Strategy and Selection of SMAS Flap

The surgeon begins with comprehensive patient assessment (Figs. 34.1–34.6). Initially, interview of the individual and specific needs and goals can provide direction and focus for the rejuvenation. Examination should include evaluation of the four specific types of facial aging, skin quality, skin laxity, soft tissue laxity, and soft tissue atrophy. A plan should be created to address each entity. Skin quality concerns should be addressed with topical agents, facials, microdermabrasions, lasers, and pulsed light. Skin laxity should be evaluated for the correct skin incision and direction of lift to provide wrinkle reduction with minimal distortion to the anatomy of the hairline, ear, and mouth. Soft tissue atrophy should be assessed for each area and amount of fill. Fine needle fillers can be used for fine lines and fat grafts and implants may be used for volume restoration. Finally, soft tissue laxity or descent should be evaluated and measured preoperatively for SMAS lift planning. The extent of descent can be measured by gently lifting the cheek or jowl into the desired position and determining the advancement.

The most substantial jowl descent is the midpoint between the retaining ligaments at the anterior edge of parotid gland and the retaining ligaments at the nares and mentum. It is between these fixed points that the SMAS is unattached and sags most. Minor looseness can be corrected with minimal techniques and more extensive jowling will have the need for more substantial lifting techniques. In evaluating the movement of jowl soft tissue, less than 10 mm of movement to correct jowl laxity can be corrected with skin tightening and SMAS plication. Ten to fifteen millimeters of laxity requires release of the retaining ligaments and unfurling of the sagging SMAS with a high or low SMAS elevation and fixation (Fig. 34.2). When 15–20 mm of laxity is present, then a retaining ligament release plus more medial ZMM release of the SMAS is required to unfurl and elevate the flap (Fig. 34.3). And finally, greater than 20 mm may necessitate release of retaining ligaments, ZMM release, and thinning of the jowls under direct vision.

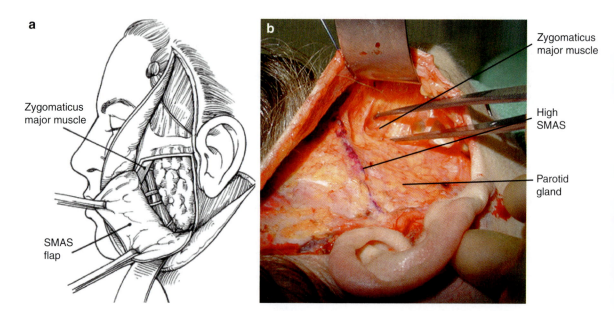

Fig. 34.1 (**a**) Technique of SMAS flap elevation. (**b**) Flap elevation to the zygomaticus major muscle

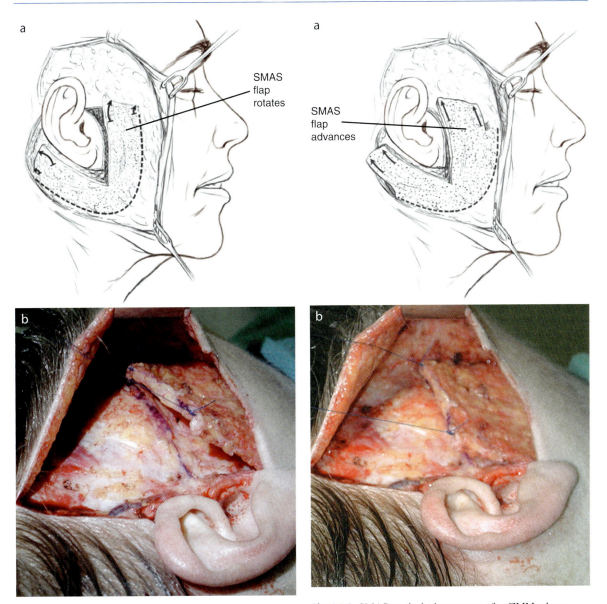

Fig. 34.2 Rotational advancement pivots around the ZMM origin

Fig. 34.3 SMAS vertical advancement after ZMM release

34.3 SMAS Flap Study

The retaining ligaments of the face support facial soft tissue in normal anatomic position [1]. However, gravitational changes occur with age and fat descends into the plane between the superficial and deep facial fascia. Face lift procedures are designed to lift these sagging tissues. The choice of flap design may have some impact on the direction and extent of the lift. The nature of this lift was studied in 22 rhytidectomy SMAS flaps and measurements of the vertical advancement were compared using two different SMAS patterns. Elevation and fixation of the SMAS was accomplished under the same conditions, and by the same surgeon. A high SMAS elevation was performed after skin and retaining ligaments were released. The ligaments at the lateral edge of the

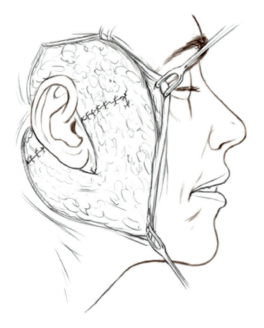

Fig. 34.4 Final result after SMAS elevation and fixation

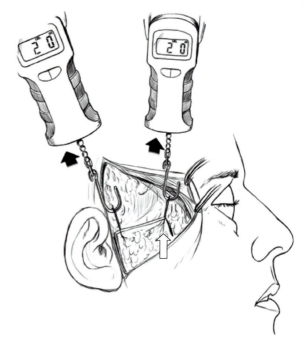

Fig. 34.6 *White arrow* is the medial edge of the flap at the Zygomaticus major muscle

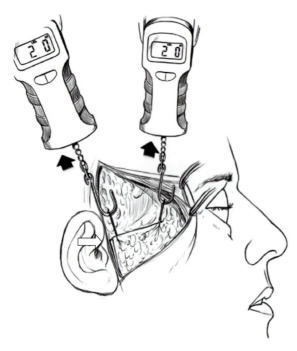

Fig. 34.5 Anatomical points to measure the advancement lift. *White arrow* is the superior lateral edge of the SMAS flap

ZMM were also released. SMAS flap movement was measured with precise and equal tension at two points on the cheek SMAS flap, medially and laterally. Then, a second measurement was obtained after placing a back cut on the SMAS at the lateral edge of the ZMM. The flap was again weighted with the exact tension medially and laterally. The result was a substantial additional flap shift after this simple and quick maneuver. The most significant change was the movement medially, or most specifically on the jowl. The comparison of vertical SMAS flap advancement is shown in Table 34.1. An improvement in lateral flap shift with identical tension was demonstrated in 18 of 22 flaps with an average improvement in flap shift gain of 3.5 mm. Most importantly, a significant gain in flap shift was obtained with identical tension on the medial portion of the flap. This was demonstrated in 22 of 22 flaps with an average improvement in medial flap shift gain of 14.04 mm. This additional medial flap shift improved substantially the shelving of the malar soft tissue onto the malar eminence and lifted the jowl far more effectively. There were no complications from these measurements in a 16 month follow-up period. This demonstrates and quantifies an increased medial SMAS advancement shift with this maneuver and therefore improves the cosmetic appearance of the jowls and the midface.

34 Extent of SMAS Advancement in Facelift with or without Zygomaticus Major Muscle Release

Table 34.1 Comparative measurements of vertical flap advancement

Number	Surgery date	Age	Gender	Side	Lateral flap advancement	After ZMM release	Difference (in mm)	Medial flap advancement	After ZMM release	Difference (in mm)
1	12/18	45	Female	Left	29	32	+3	20	25	+5
2	12/18	45	Female	Right	29	32	+3	6	25	+19
3	12/19	57	Female	Right	32	39	+7	14	33	+19
4	12/19	57	Female	Left	28	40	+12	33	41	+8
5	12/26	53	Female	Right	25	25	+0	5	29	+24
6	12/26	53	Female	Left	25	30	+5	17	29	+12
7	12/30	59	Female	Right	28	29	+1	24	4	+10
8	12/30	59	Female	Left	26	27	+1	13	25	+12
9	12/30	54	Female	Right	11	24	+13	15	21	+6
10	12/30	54	Female	Left	25	8	+3	19	25	+6
11	12/31	58	Female	Right	36	37	+1	16	39	+23
12	12/31	58	Female	Left	28	28	+0	15	25	+10
13	01/02	60	Female	Right	42	46	+4	40	55	+15
14	01/02	60	Female	Left	34	34	+0	29	40	+11
15	01/06	54	Female	Right	16	22	+6	2	32	+30
16	01/06	54	Female	Left	28	29	+1	18	30	+12
17	01/08	57	Female	Right	31	33	+2	16	30	+14
18	01/08	57	Female	Left	21	23	+2	7	26	+19
19	01/13	60	Male	Right	34	34	+0	21	39	+18
20	01/13	60	Male	Left	19	24	+5	20	33	+13
21	01/15	59	Male	Right	17	26	+9	15	27	+12
22	01/15	59	Male	Left	15	15	+0	13	24	+11
Average					26.3	29.8	3.5	17.1	29.8	+14.04

The medial SMAS movement increased an average of 14.04 mm after the ZMM release, allowing more movement of the SMAS at the jowl. The photographs above illustrate the results in patients before and after these measurements

34.4 Discussion

The present strategies for midface rejuvenation include skin quality refinement, skin tightening, soft tissue repositioning, and volume restoration. In soft tissue repositioning, various patterns have emerged for SMAS release, elevation, and anchoring. This review considered only two of these patterns, comparing a high SMAS elevation, two layer dissection, multivector suspension to the same with an additional back cut in the SMAS flap over the zygomaticus major muscle.

The release of these structures tethering ptotic midfacial tissue may improve the vertical movement of soft tissue and allow for better repositioning. This study quantifies the measurement of the SMAS vertical advancement flap before and after release from the zygomaticus major muscle. The large improvement in the medial movement of an additional 14 mm under the same tension resulting from the release of the zygomaticus major muscle validate this small surgical maneuver and has not been associated with any particular negative effect. SMAS excess at the zygomatic arch may be overlapped for additional augmentation of the arch. Resecting the excess SMAS in the zygomatic area provides restoration without the appearance of skeletal change if desired. In special cases of extreme malar deficiency, the SMAS excess can be folded and tucked into a pocket over the ZMM and malar eminence. There are many other patterns to be investigated and quantified. These maneuvers are important in improving midface soft tissue repositioning without relying on excessive skin tension and can be utilized to provide additional contour shaping when necessary.

34.5 Conclusions

The aim of today's facial aesthetic surgery is to rejuvenate the aging face in an anatomic and physiologic way. Special attention must be given to obtain consistency and to improve longevity of results. For correction of the aging process, various techniques have evolved that have been used with both advantages and disadvantages [2–6].

The evolution of midface soft tissue contouring in rhytidectomy has progressed significantly [7–18] (Figs. 34.7–34.14). Cheek skin was initially used as a supportive structure and tightened sufficiently to unfurl wrinkles and to flatten sagging soft tissues [10]. Since skin stretched and aging contours reappeared, cheek fat was then contoured through excision and later through tightening with SMAS plication [11, 12]. The composite lift incorporated elevation of the SMAS attached to the skin flap and repositioned skin and soft tissue for restoration. After detailed description of the SMAS retaining ligaments, release of tethering ligaments allowed for improved repositioning [13–18]. Next, separation of the SMAS and skin allowed for more vertical SMAS lift with less temporal hairline shift and splitting the SMAS created bidirectional SMAS movement for better midface vertical elevation and improved platysma suspension.

Multiple strategies have evolved to maximize midface soft tissue repositioning. In order to maximize SMAS lifting, various authors have advocated more aggressive elevation and release of the retaining ligaments. A back cut over the zygomaticus major muscle substantially improves the vertical elevation and repositioning of the medial SMAS. Midface restoration may be best utilized by an advancement rotation flap because of improved vertical advancement, especially medially, for longer lasting results and better shelving of the medial cheek portion of the SMAS flap. Since there is more even mobilization of the flap and the cheek is elevated to a similar distance as the preparotid fat, the tension appears to be more even throughout the flap and may have less distortion with time. Without the ZMM release the axis of rotation is near the ZMM origin and sometimes the SMAS can appear very tight over the parotid and still loose in the midface. Release of the zygomaticus major muscle allows for more significant movement of the medial SMAS, by providing more midface soft tissue elevation. This single maneuver aids in cheek and jowl elevation and preserves midface soft tissue. The surgeon should have an adequate comfort level with the described anatomy and fit the procedure to the patient's needs and recovery time.

Restoration of the midface has become one of the great challenges of facial rejuvenation, in part because of the success of improved brow and neck lifting techniques, leaving the midface sometimes with less than anticipated results. Also, adjacent structures like the lower lid and ear create limitations in midface lifting, since overzealous elevation can create deformity and distortion of these structures, like ectropion, scleral show, and a pixie ear. Undue tension on the skin can create increased postoperative morbidity, a tight or wind-blown appearance, and with time the possibility of lateral lines of relaxation. There are other limitations. Lifting the ptotic cheek fat with repositioning and suspension is limited by medial flap movement and failure results in recurrent nasal labial folds, jowling and tear troughs. Challenges still lie in the selection of the most advantageous flap design for a specific set of contour abnormalities. The utilization of multiple flap patterns and strategies may provide a more tailored and elegant result.

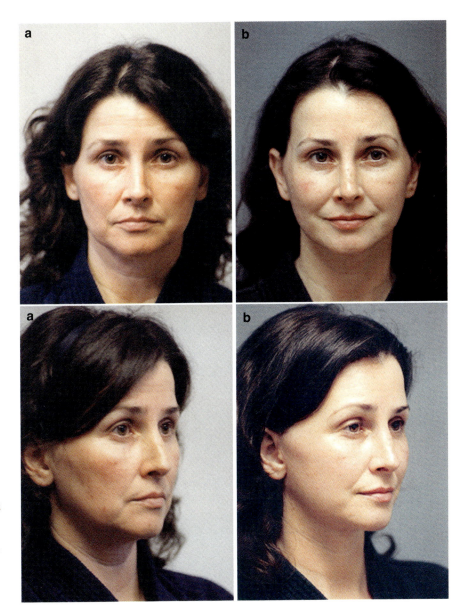

Fig. 34.7 Endoscopic browlift, facelift with SMAS pattern of high SMAS, excised excess, no platysma or ZMM SMAS release, and neck lift with minimal cervical scissor lipectomy. (**a**) Preoperative. (**b**) Postoperative

Fig. 34.7 (continued)

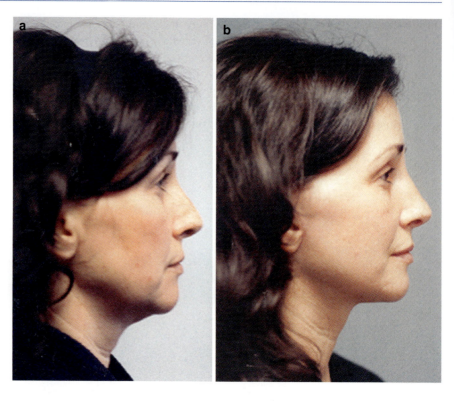

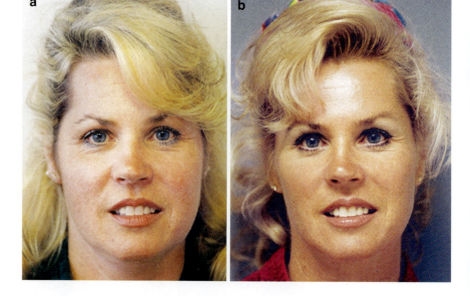

Fig. 34.8 Facelift with SMAS pattern of high SMAS, excised excess, no platysma or ZMM SMAS release, and neck lift with moderate cervical scissor lipectomy and platysmaplasty. (**a**) Preoperative. (**b**) Postoperative

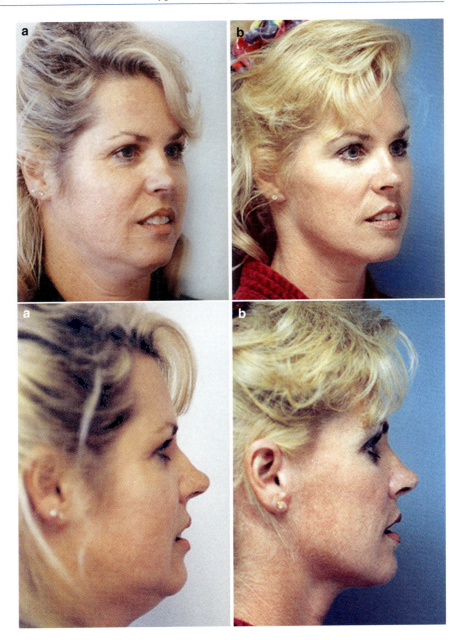

Fig. 34.8 (continued)

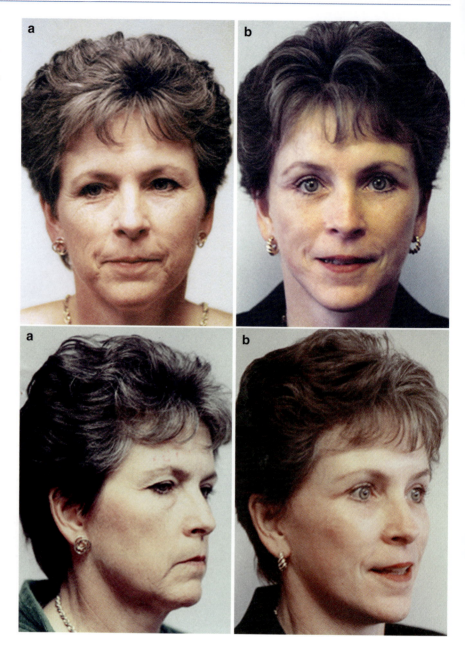

Fig. 34.9 Endoscopic browlift, upper and lower blepharoplasty, facelift with SMAS pattern of high SMAS, excised excess, with ZMM SMAS backcut and no platysma backcut, and neck lift with minimal cervical scissor lipectomy and platysmaplasty.
(**a**) Preoperative.
(**b**) Postoperative

Fig. 34.9 (continued)

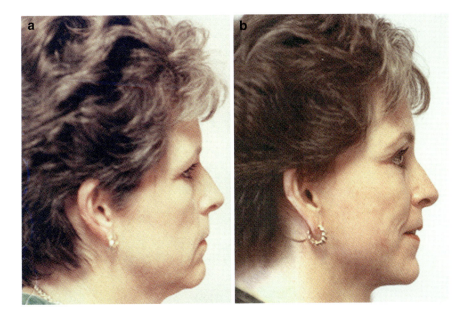

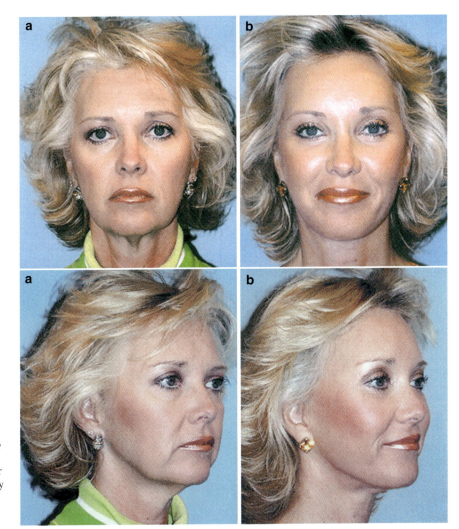

Fig. 34.10 Endoscopic browlift, upper and lower blepharoplasty with right suture canthopexy, facelift with SMAS pattern of high SMAS, excised excess, with ZMM SMAS backcut and no platysma backcut, neck lift with minimal cervical scissor lipectomy and platysmaplasty and fat graft to the cheek.
(**a**) Preoperative.
(**b**) Postoperative

Fig. 34.10 (continued)

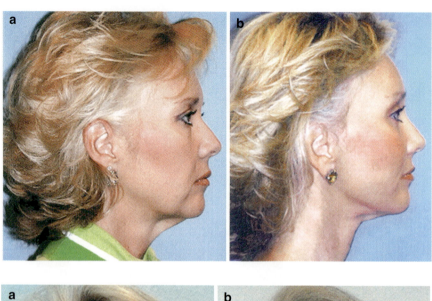

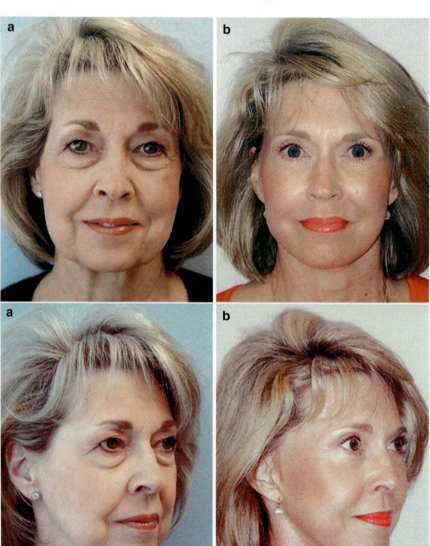

Fig. 34.11 Upper and lower blepharoplasty with bilateral suture canthopexy, facelift with SMAS pattern of high SMAS, excised excess, with ZMM SMAS backcut and lateral platysma backcut, neck lift with minimal cervical scissor lipectomy and platysmaplasty and fat graft to the cheek, nasolabial fold, and prejowl.
(**a**) Preoperative.
(**b**) Postoperative

Fig. 34.11 (continued)

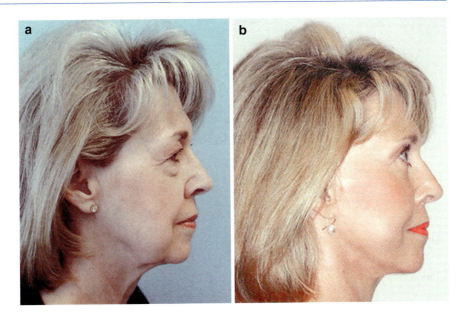

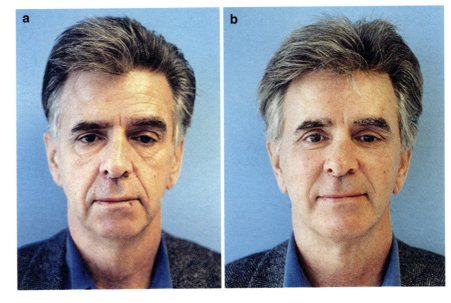

Fig. 34.12 Upper and lower blepharoplasty with bilateral suture canthopexy, facelift with SMAS pattern of high SMAS, arch excess tucked over ZMM into malar area, with ZMM SMAS backcut and lateral platysma backcut, neck lift with minimal cervical scissor lipectomy and platysmaplasty, fat graft to the cheek, nasolabial fold, and prejowl, and chin augmentation.
(**a**) Preoperative.
(**b**) Postoperative

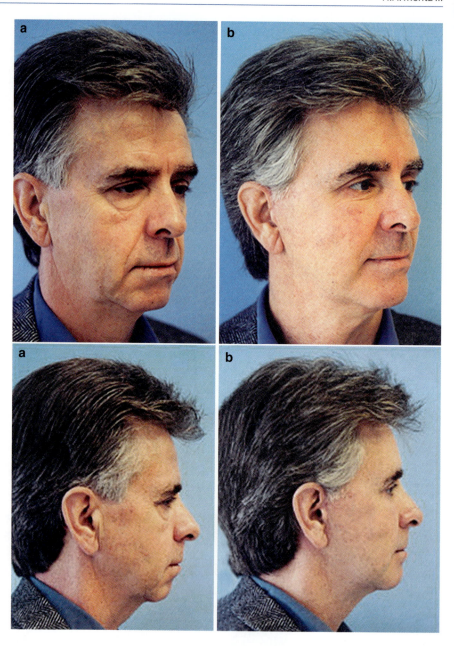

Fig. 34.12 (continued)

Fig. 34.13 Endoscopic browlift, upper and lower blepharoplasty with bilateral suture canthopexy, facelift with SMAS pattern of high SMAS, arch excess tucked over ZMM into malar area, with ZMM SMAS backcut and lateral platysma backcut, neck lift with minimal cervical scissor lipectomy and platysmaplasty, fat graft to the cheek, nasolabial fold, prejowl, and chin.
(**a**) Preoperative.
(**b**) Postoperative

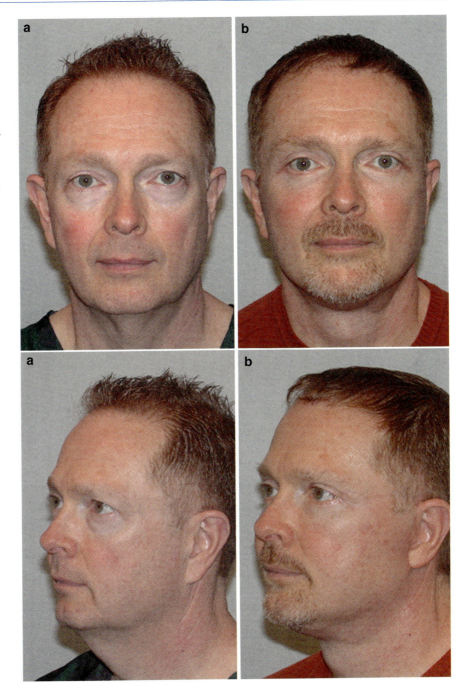

Fig. 34.13 (continued)

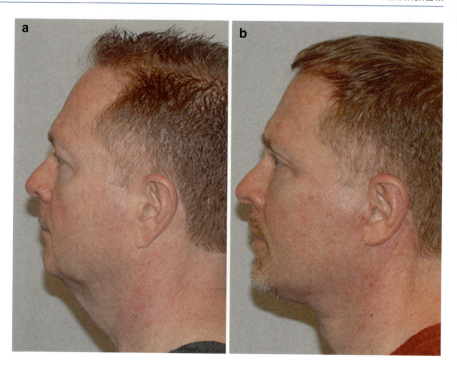

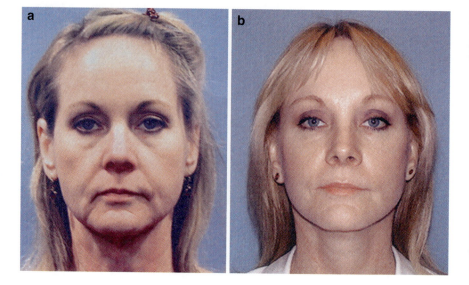

Fig. 34.14 Endoscopic browlift, lower blepharoplasty with bilateral suture canthopexy, facelift with SMAS pattern of high SMAS, excess excised, with ZMM SMAS backcut, neck lift with no lipectomy, platysmaplasty, fat graft to the cheek, nasolabial fold, prejowl, and corner of the mouth lift. (**a**) Preoperative. (**b**) Postoperative

Fig. 34.14 (continued)

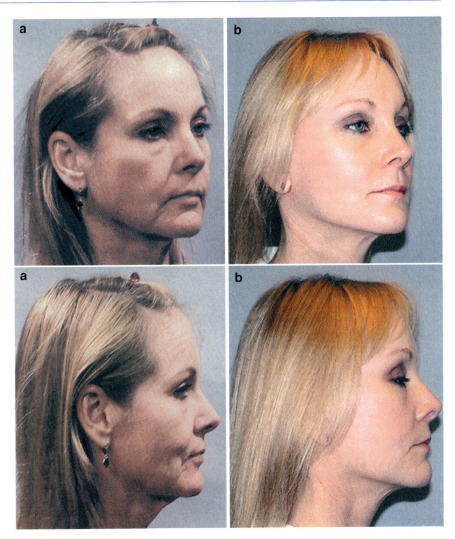

References

1. Mentz H, Ruiz-Razura A, Patronella C, Newall G. Facelift: measurement of superficial muscular aponeurotic system advancement with and without zygomaticus major muscle release. Aesthetic Plast Surg. 2005;29(5):353–62.
2. Mentz H. Multilayer rhytidectomy. In: Evans G, editor. Operative plastic surgery. New York: McGraw Hill; 2000. p. 143–62.
3. Marten TJ. Facelift. Planning and technique. Clin Plast Surg. 1997;24(2):269–308.
4. Massiha H. Short scar face lift with extended SMAS platysma dissection, lifting and limited skin undermining. Plast Reconstr Surg. 2003;112(2):663–9.
5. Saulis A, Lautenschlager E, Mustoe TA. Biomechanical and viscoelastic properties of skin, SMAS, and composite flaps as they pertain to rhytidectomy. Plast Reconstr Surg. 2002;110(2):590–8.
6. Ivy E, Lorenc Z, Aston S. Is there a difference? A prospective study comparing lateral and standard SMAS face lifts with extended SMAS and composite rhytidectomies. Plast Reconstr Surg. 1996;98(7):1135–43.
7. Stuzin JM, Baker TJ, Gordon HL, Baker TM. Extended SMAS dissection as an approach to midface rejuvenation. Clin Plast Surg. 1995;22(2):295–311.
8. Connell BF, Semlacher RA. Contemporary deep layer facial rejuvenation. Plast Reconstr Surg. 1997;100(6):1513–23.
9. Baker TJ, Stuzin JM. Personal technique of face lifting. Plast Reconstr Surg. 1997;100(2):502–8.
10. Baker DC. Lateral SMASectomy. Plast Reconstr Surg. 1997;100(2):509–13.
11. Stuzin J, Baker TJ, Baker TM. Refinements in face lifting: enhanced facial contour using vicryl mesh incorporated into SMAS fixation. Plast Reconstr Surg. 2000;105(1):290–301.
12. Furnas D. The retaining ligaments of the check. Plast Reconstr Surg. 1989;83(1):11–6.

13. Hamra ST. The deep-plane rhytidectomy. Plast Reconstr Surg. 1990;86(1):53–61.
14. Mendelson BC. Extended sub SMAS dissection and cheek elevation. Clin Plast Surg. 1995;22(2):325–39.
15. Hamra ST. Composite rhytidectomy. St. Louis: Quality Medical Publishing; 1993.
16. Stuzin JM, Baker TJ, Gordon HL. The relationship of the superficial and deep facial fascias: relevance to rhytidectomy and aging. Plast Reconstr Surg. 1992;89(3):441–9.
17. Hagerty RC. Central suspension technique of the mid-face. Plast Reconstr Surg. 1995;96(3):728–30.
18. Teimourian B, Delia S, Wahrman A. The multiplane face lift. Plast Reconstr Surg. 1994;93(1):78–85.
19. Owsley JQ Jr. Platysma-fascial rhytidectomy: a preliminary report. Plast Reconstr Surg. 1977;60(6):843–50.
20. Owsley JQ Jr. SMAS-platysma face lift. Plast Reconstr Surg. 1983;71(4):573–6.
21. Owsley JQ Jr. Re.: Vilain: Dallas platysmaplasty (letter). Ann Plast Surg. 1985;14:98.
22. Hamra ST. The tri-plane facelift dissection. Ann Plast Surg. 1984;12:268.
23. Lemmon ML. Superficial fascia rhytidectomy. A restoration of the SMAS with control of the cervicomental angle. Clin Plast Surg. 1983;10:449.
24. McKinney P, Tresley GE. The "maxi-SMAS": management of the platysma bands in rhytidectomy. Ann Plast Srug. 1984;12:260.
25. Anderson RD, Lo MW. Endoscopic malar/midface suspension procedure. Plast Reconst Surg. 1998;102:2196.
26. Mentz, Newall. Endoscopic Facelifting Techniques, Malar Suspension. Annual Meeting of the International College of Surgeons, Cancun, Mexico, 1999.
27. Stuzin, Wagstrom, Kawamoto, Wolfe. Anatomy of the frontal branch of the facial nerve: the significance of the temporal fat pad. Plast Reconst Surg. 1989;83:265–71.
28. Illouz YG, Fournier P. Illouz's technique: collapsing surgery and body sculpture. Paris, 1983.
29. Hetter GP. Facial lipolysis. In: Hetter GP, editor. Liposysis: the theory and practice of blunt suction lipectomy. Boston, MA: Little Brown & Co.; 1984.
30. Lewis CM. Lipoplasty of the neck. Plast Reconstr Surg. 1985;76(2):248–57.
31. Teimourian B. Face and neck suction-assisted lipectomy associated with rhytidectomy. Plast Reconstr Surg. 1983;72(5):627–33.

The Safe Facelift Using Bony Anatomic Landmarks to Elevate the SMAS

Bradon J. Wilhelmi and Yuron Hazani

35.1 Introduction

Traditional facelift surgery relies on the tightening of skin and subcutaneous tissue in order to restore a youthful appearance to the aging face. In 1976, Mitz and Peyronie [1] provided a detailed anatomic description of the superficial musculoaponeurotic system (SMAS) as a distinct layer deep to the subcutaneous tissue. Years before the SMAS was formally described, Skoog [2] used the SMAS for plication and flap suspension in his facelift procedures. In recent years, the use of the SMAS has been described in a multitude of facelift techniques. Some prefer plication or imbrication of the SMAS layer. Others advocate the sub-SMAS biplanar approach with deep or extended SMAS dissection.

Modifications to the limited SMAS dissection may achieve the goal of improved facial contouring with long-lasting effects. Nonetheless, the risk of facial nerve injury is greater with the inclusion of SMAS elevation anterior to the parotid gland as compared with a standard SMAS dissection. Given the proximity of the facial nerve to the plane of dissection, surface anatomic landmarks are necessary to predict the location of the nerve as it courses deep to the SMAS layer.

The safe facelift technique addresses these needs and provides the surgeon with bony anatomic landmarks to elevate the SMAS. While soft tissue landmarks can vary significantly among patients and even change position with aging, the use of facial bony prominences can serve as a more reliable method. Prior to utilizing the anatomic landmarks for elevating the SMAS, a thorough understanding of the pertinent anatomy is necessary.

35.2 Anatomic Considerations

The soft tissue of the face is arranged in multiple consistent layers with retaining ligaments that anchor the soft tissue to the facial skeleton. Structures within each layer maintain their anatomic location while the thickness of each layer can change as the dissection proceeds medially. The six distinct layers are, skin, subcutaneous fat, superficial facial fascia (SMAS), mimetic muscles, deep facial fascia (parotidomasseteric fascia), and the plane of the facial nerve, buccal fat pad, parotid duct, and the facial artery and vein.

35.2.1 The Facial Nerve

The facial nerve originates in the pons between the cranial nerves VI and VIII (Table 35.1) [3–8]. The facial nerve leaves the calvarium, passing through the facial canal of the temporal bone to exit from the stylomastoid foramen. The main trunk of the facial nerve courses 0.5–1.5 cm before entering the posterior aspect of the parotid gland. The critical landmarks which can be used to identify the main trunk of the facial nerve include 1 cm below the conchal cartilaginous pointer, and 6–8 mm below the tympanomastoid

B.J. Wilhelmi (✉)
Plastic Surgery Division, Department of Surgery,
University of Louisville, 2nd floor ACB Building,
550 South Jackson Street, Louisville,
KY 50202, USA
e-mail: bjwilh01@louisville.edu

Y. Hazani
Aesthetic Surgery Fellow Harvard,
Massachusetts General Hospital,
Boston, MA, USA

sulcus, where it crosses the styloid process and the anterior to posterior belly of the digastric muscle.

The facial nerve enters the parotid gland and splits it into superficial and deep lobes. Within the parotid gland, the nerve divides into an upper and lower portion. Further divisions and intercommunications result in five major branches that emerge through the anterior border of the parotid gland. These are the frontal, zygomatic, buccal, marginal mandibular, and cervical branches.

The frontal branch courses cranially and over the zygomatic arch in a consistent course from 0.5 cm below the tragus to 1.5 cm above the lateral brow. Stuzin et al. defined the location of the frontal branch in three-dimensional planes on the underside of the temporoparietal fascia (superficial temporal fascia). In the temporal region, the frontal branch innervates the frontalis, lateral orbicularis oculi, corrugator supercilii, and procerus muscles.

The buccal, zygomatic, and marginal branches exit the anterior edge of the parotid gland and proceed along the superficial layer of the masseter, immediately below the deep facial fascia. The zygomatic branch extends toward the zygomaticus major muscle and provides motor innervation to the upper third of the muscle belly. Some fibers cross over the anterior aspect of the zygomaticus major muscle and arborize within the orbicularis oculi muscle.

The buccal branch courses over the buccal fat pad and join the plane of the parotid duct, and the facial artery and vein. A rich plexiform of nerve connections between the buccal and zygomatic branches innervates the mimetic muscles of the buccal region. These include muscles responsible for movement of the cheeks, nostrils, nasolabial fold, upper lip, and oral commisures.

Along the inferior border of the mandible, the marginal mandibular branch crosses over the facial vessels and proceeds toward the major lip depressors and mentalis muscle. The cervical branch emerges from the caudal edge of the parotid gland and courses in a longitudinal vector. In the neck, it is deep to the platysma and the deep cervical fascia. The cervical branch innervates the platysma muscle (Table 35.1).

35.2.2 The SMAS Layer

The SMAS is a strictly superficial anatomical structure of the face derived from the primitive platysma, and does not possess any bony insertions. It is composed of

Table 35.1 The anatomy of the facial nerve branches and the specific innervated muscles and resultant muscle action

Facial nerve branch	Muscle	Action
Temporal	Anterior auricular	Pulls ear forward
	Superior auricular	Raises ear
	Frontalis	Moves scalp forward
	Corrugator supercilii	Pulls eyebrow medially and downward
	Procerus	Pulls medial eyebrow downward
Temporal and zygomatic	Orbicularis oculi	Closes eyelids
Zygomatic and buccal	Zygomaticus major	Elevates corners of the mouth
Buccal	Zygomaticus minor	Elevates upper lip
	Levator labii superioris	Elevates upper lip and midportion nasolabial fold
	Levator labii superioris alaeque nasi	Elevates medial nasolabial fold and nasal ala
	Risorius	Aids smile with lateral pull
	Buccinators	Pulls corner of mouth backward and compresses cheek
	Levator anguli oris	Pulls angles of mouth upward and forward midline
	Orbicularis oris	Closes and compresses lips
	Nasalis	
	Dilator naris	Flares nostrils
	Compressor naris	Compresses nostrils
Buccal and marginal mandibular	Depressor anguli oris	Pulls corners of mouth downward
Marginal mandibular	Depressor labii inferioris	Pulls down lower lip
	Mentalis	Pulls skin of chin upward
Cervical	Platysma	Pulls down corners of mouth

May and Schaitkin [11]

a fibrofatty tissue layer of collagen and elastic fibers interdispersed with fat cells and some muscle. It is continuous with the posterior portion of the frontalis muscle and the temporoparietal fascia in the upper face, the platysma muscle inferiorly in the neck, and the risorius and triangularis in the cheek. Retaining ligaments support the SMAS layer by anchoring it to the deep facial fascia and prevent its descent. Weakening of these ligaments account for the stigmata of the aged face including, formation of jowls, descent of the malar fat pad, and deepening of the nasolabial fold.

35.3 Indications

While all facelift procedures carry a certain risk, great caution is needed when a sub-SMAS dissection is undertaken. The surgeon must always be aware of the inherent danger of each technique and dissect in safe planes to avoid an inadvertent nerve injury. The safe facelift technique is particularly suitable for procedures that involved a sub-SMAS dissection that end at the anterior border of the parotid gland to avoid injury to the facial nerve branches. These include the standard SMAS facelift and the lateral SMASectomy facelift with plication.

The extended SMAS, lamellar high SMAS, deep plane, and foundation facelift procedures are more aggressive in their attempt to address the problems of midface descent and nasolabial fold deepening. Nonetheless, these extensive SMAS elevation techniques anterior to the parotid gland place the facial nerve branches in great jeopardy. Additionally, the superficial fascia tends to thin out as it is dissected more anteriorly, making the SMAS prone to tears. Particular concern is raised when the sub-SMAS dissection proceeds along the lateral border of the zygomaticus major and along the inferior border of the mandible. For these danger zones of the face, the safe technique relies on additional landmarks that can predict the location of the nerve at its most vulnerable points.

35.4 Technique

Given its clinical significance, anatomic landmarks are first used to predict the location of the anterior border of the parotid gland. The inferior lateral orbital rim and the masseteric tuberosity are identified preoperatively. The anterior edge of the parotid gland is found along the oblique vector between these landmarks. On average, the anterior edge of the parotid gland is approximately 3.9 cm from the tragus along the transverse vector of the zygomatic arch [9] (Fig. 35.1). Subcutaneous dissection proceeds anteriorly to elevate skin posterior to the lateral canthus. As the facial nerve courses through the parotid gland, it is relatively safe and protected by the substance of the gland. Elevation of the SMAS anterior to the parotid gland as identified by the anatomic landmarks is discouraged as it places the facial nerve at greater risk to injury.

The patient is marked in the preoperative area with the surgeon's preferred technique. Local anesthesia with sedation is my preferred anesthesia method for a facelift procedure. The facial and neck skin is infiltrated with 0.25% lidocaine with 1:100,000 epinephrine mixed with 0.25% Marcaine and 1:100,000 epinephrine. The pre and postauricular skin is incised and the skin flaps are elevated superficial to the SMAS in the anterior direction to the vertical vector of the lateral canthus. As the facial nerve courses through the parotid

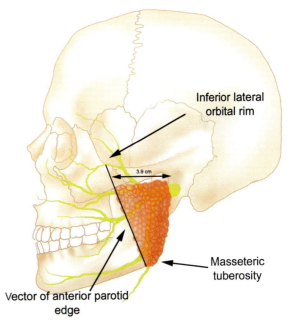

Fig. 35.1 The facial nerve enters the parotid gland and splits it into superficial and deep lobes. Therefore, during the course of the facial nerve through the parotid gland, it is safe from injury. The branches of the nerve can be injured as they exit the anterior edge of the parotid gland. The anterior edge of the parotid gland can be predicted along an oblique course from the inferior lateral orbital rim (3.9 cm from the tragus) to the palpable masseteric tuberosity (Modified from Wilhelmi et al. [9])

gland, it is relatively safe and protected by the substance of the gland during this subcutaneous dissection.

If temple skin tightening is required, the author prefers the presideburn incision to avoid widening temporal hairline to lateral canthal space, which can look unnatural. In performing a presideburn incision, incising the skin perpendicular to the hair follicles allows for hair growth through the skin. It is critical to elevate the temple skin flap in the plane superficial to the temporal parietal fascia to avoid the facial nerve frontal branches, which are found immediately beneath this fascia. The anterior incision is then continued inferiorly and curved into the natural crease toward the helical root (Fig. 35.2). The incision can be continued in the retrotragal position; however, defatting of the flap (tragal area) at inset and defatting of the tragal area will be required to recreate the thin skin normally found over the tragus. In continuing the incision around the ear lobe, a 2 mm cuff of facial skin should be preserved to avoid the pixie ear deformity. Postauricularly, the incision is placed 2 mm posterior to the postauricular sulcus. As this incision is extended postauricularly, the superior margin of the postauricular incision can be made directly posterior to the helical root to minimize risk of postauricular skin flap necrosis (Fig. 35.3). When continuing the postauricular incision into the hairline the scar can be hidden better if the incision is made into the hair in a lazy S fashion, initially along the hairline and then horizontally into the junction between the thick and thin hair, again perpendicular to the hair follicles. When platysmal resection is anticipated the cervical skin elevation can be completed with the additional exposure through a submental incision. This submental incision should be placed 5 mm posterior to the natural submental crease to avoid creation of witches chin or exaggerated indentation in the crease with resultant protruding chin pad.

Then the SMAS is marked inferiorly along the zygomatic arch 3.9 cm from the tragus and along the oblique vector in the direction of the masseteric tuberosity, corresponding to the anterior edge of the parotid, to avoid injury to the midfacial branches of the facial nerve, where they exit the parotid (Fig. 35.4). Then, the SMAS is infiltrated with local anesthesia along the proposed plane of dissection. The SMAS elevation is performed in the posterior to anterior direction starting at the tragus. The SMAS is then elevated along the inferior border of the Zygomatic Arch to avoid the Facial nerve frontal branches. Above the zygomatic arch the frontal branches become more superficial and at risk for injury. The SMAS is elevated anteriorly and inferiorly up to the oblique vector corresponding to the parotid anterior edge. Cessation of SMAS elevation at the 3.9 cm location reduces the risk for facial nerve injury to the midfacial nerve branches that course through the parotid gland. SMAS dissection continued past the anterior edge of the parotid gland risks injury

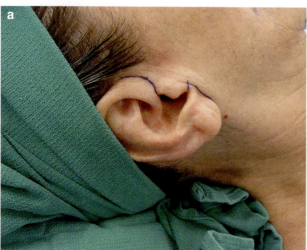
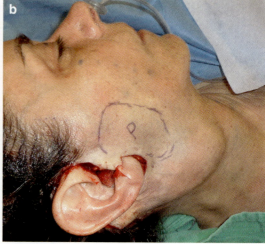

Fig. 35.2 (**a**) The anterior incision is continued inferiorly and curved into the natural crease toward the helical root. The incision can be continued in the retrotragal position; however, defatting of the flap (tragal area) at inset and defatting of the tragal area will be required to recreate the thin skin normally found over the tragus. (**b**) In continuing the incision around the ear lobe, a 2 mm cuff of facial skin should be preserved to avoid the pixie ear deformity

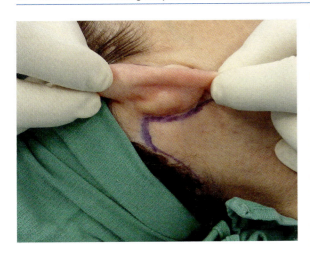

Fig. 35.3 Postauricularly, the incision is placed 2 mm posterior to the postauricular sulcus. As this incision is extended postauricularly, the superior margin of the postauricular incision can be made directly posterior to the helical root to minimize risk of postauricular skin flap necrosis. When continuing the postauricular incision into the hairline the scar can be hidden better if the incision is made into the hair in a lazy S fashion, initially along the hairline and then horizontally into the junction between the thick and thin hair, again perpendicular to the hair follicles

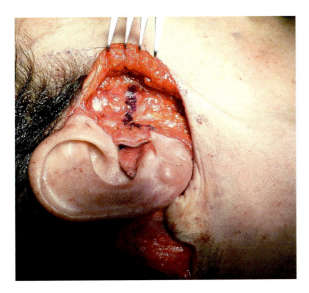

Fig. 35.4 Then the SMAS is marked inferiorly along the zygomatic arch 3.9 cm from the tragus and along the oblique vector in the direction of the masseteric tuberosity, corresponding to the anterior edge of the parotid, to avoid injury to the midfacial branches of the facial nerve, where they exit the parotid

to the facial nerve midfacial branches. Another landmark for cessation of SMAS elevation is the SMAS fat pad, found along the superior aspect of the anterior parotid edge. The SMAS is elevated in continuity with the platysma. SMAS elevation should not be performed in the area where the facial artery courses over the mandible, as the marginal mandibular facial nerve branches become superficial in this location and are at risk. Then the SMAS is advanced posteriorly and superiorly and plicated from zygomatic arch to the mastoid area. The skin is then carefully pulled along a horizontal vector posteriorly. Initial sutures are placed at the cephaloauricular sulcus and anterior superior postauricular region. The excess skin is removed carefully to avoid excessive tension on the wound edges, which could result in widened scars. Drains are not routinely used. The sutures can be removed within a week. Pressure garment is encouraged for 2 weeks.

Modifications to the traditional SMAS dissection attempt to improve the nasolabial prominence by elevation of the malar soft tissue ptosis. In the extended SMAS facelift, it is advocated to release SMAS fibers spanning the upper lateral border of the zygomatic major muscle followed by continued dissection medial to this muscle. Release and subsequent medial dissection increases the risk of facial nerve injury, particularly the zygomatic branch fibers to the orbicularis oculi muscle. Again, bony anatomic landmarks are used to predict the location of this danger zone. The upper extent of the lateral border of the zygomaticus major muscle is located in relation to an oblique line extending from the mental protuberance to the inferior lateral orbital rim. On average, the lateral border of the zygomaticus major muscle is 0.4 cm lateral and parallel to this line.

Techniques attempting to release the SMAS anterior to the parotid gland along the mandibular border place the marginal mandibular at great risk. During a sub-SMAS cheek dissection, the marginal mandibular branch can be found in the buccal space, emerging from the parotid gland and coursing along the inferior border of the mandible. The most vulnerable point is the region where the nerve courses over the anterior facial artery and vein. Since the marginal branch is just deep to a thin platysma-SMAS layer, any effort to control bleeding from an injured facial vessel can cause irreversible damage to the nerve. We advocate the use of distance ratios to predict the location of the nerve as it crosses over the facial artery. The distance between the masseteric tuberosity and the mental protuberance is measured. At approximately one-fourth of the distance from the masseteric tuberosity, the marginal mandibular branch is predicted to cross the facial artery on its way to innervate the depressor anguli oris and mentalis muscles.

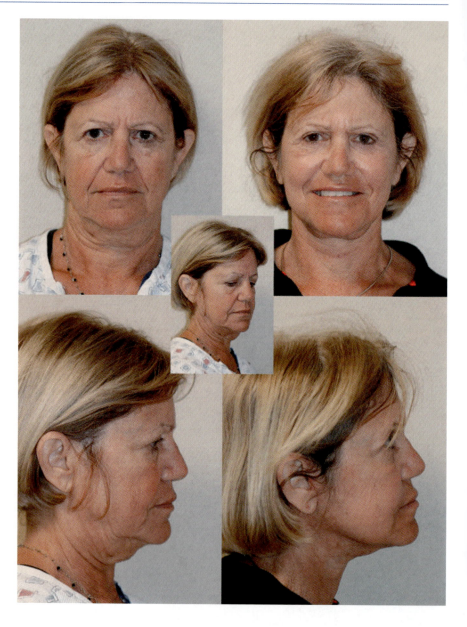

Fig. 35.5 (*Left* and *center*) Preoperative patient with tired appearance of her eyes, face, and neck. (*Right*) Postoperative following a safe facelift with pre and postauricular incisions and submental approach in conjunction with upper and lower blepharoplasty procedures. Note a dramatic improvement in her neck contour and jowl line

The goal of the safe facelift is to provide the patient with a natural look postoperatively and to avoid the appearance of an operated face (Fig. 35.5).

35.5 Discussion

Biochemical studies have demonstrated an advantage to the addition of SMAS tightening to the facelift procedure. Har-Shai [10] studied the viscoelastic properties of the SMAS and found that it had less slackening effect compared with preauricular skin, which would explain the lasting effect of with the use of the SMAS. Several different SMAS tightening procedures have been described. There has certainly been considerable controversy over which tightening procedure provides the best aesthetic outcome. A prospective study compared the lateral, standard, and extended SMAS and composite rhytidectomies and found no discernable difference between these procedures. Although most plastic surgeons agree that treatment of the SMAS should be a component of the facelift, there is still a controversy over which is the best operation.

Regardless of what technique of SMAS dissection is performed with facelift procedure, it is important to avoid injury to the facial nerve branches. Therefore, knowledge of the facial nerve anatomy is paramount. Davis et al. [3] described six different facial nerve patterns after 350 facial half dissections. These branches are susceptible to injury once they emerge from the anterior edge of the parotid gland. Several anatomic studies of the facial nerve have been performed to minimize the risk of injury of the structure with facial procedures. In the course of the facial nerve branches to their target muscles, there are three danger zones where these branches are susceptible to injury: the frontal branches, the marginal mandibular branches, and the midfacial branches.

Pitanguy et al. [5] described the frontal branch of the facial nerve as having a consistent course from 0.5 cm below the tragus to 1.5 cm above the lateral eyebrow. Ishikawa described the safe zone for prevention of injury to the frontal branch to be 4 cm above and 7 cm posterior to the lateral canthus. The frontal branch has also been found to have multiple rami in another cadaver study by Gosain et al. [6]. The most important anatomic study was performed by Stuzin et al. [7], who defined the location of the frontal branch in three-dimensional planes located on the undersurface of the temporoparietal fascia above the zygomatic arch. Therefore, when dissecting in the area cephalic to the zygomatic arch, it is critical to be subcutaneous to the superficial temporal fascia or deep to the superficial layer of the deep temporal fascia to avoid injuring the frontal branch.

The marginal mandibular branch was extensively studied by Dingman and Grabb [4] in 100 cadaver dissections. They found that, posterior to the facial artery, the marginal mandibular nerve passed above the inferior border of the mandible in 81% of their dissections. Anterior to the facial artery, 100% of the marginal branches were located superior to the inferior mandibular edge. Based on our observations, the facial artery is on average 3 cm anterior to the masseteric tuberosity along the mandible, or approximately one-fourth of the distance between the masseteric tuberosity and the mental midline.

In the midface, knowing the location of the anterior edge of the parotid gland, where the buccal and zygomatic branches exit, can minimize the risk of these midfacial branches. The sub-SMAS fat pad can also aid in identifying the location of the anterior edge of the parotid gland. If the SMAS is not freed just anterior to the parotid, it does not move freely because of the resistance of the parotidocutaneous ligaments. Use of the masseteric tuberosity and the inferior lateral orbital rim as surface anatomic landmarks can predict the location of the anterior edge and facilitate safe release of the parotidocutaneous ligaments. In addition, our anatomic landmarks can provide the surgeon with the safe zone of the SMAS dissection, where the facial nerve is protected within the parotid gland and at minimal risk for injury.

35.6 Complications

35.6.1 Hematoma

As with any facelift procedure, bleeding is the most common complication. Blood pressure control is the single most important preventive measure. Other significant factors that can reduce the risk of bleeding and result in a safer procedure are avoidance of medications interfering with clotting or coagulation. Preoperative preparation and proper anesthesia can aid with preventing vomiting, coughing, pain, or any event resulting in a Valsalva-like maneuver.

35.6.2 Nerve Injury

The great auricular nerve is the most common symptomatic nerve injury after a facelift. Transection of this large sensory nerve can result in permanent numbness to the lower half of the ear and sometimes in a painful neuroma. A more dreaded complication is an inadvertent injury to a branch of the facial nerve. The buccal and zygomatic branches are injured more often than the frontal and marginal mandibular branches. Fortunately, the zygomatic and buccal branches interconnect freely superficial to the buccal fat pad. Consequently, the nerve palsy is usually less noticeable and paralysis is not permanent in most cases. Injury to these branches can cause the upper lip and oral commisure to sag.

Although, the frontal and marginal mandibular branches are less likely to be injured during a facelift, the clinical outcome of these injuries can be devastating. Paralysis of the frontal branch affects the forehead of the involved side with ptosis of the brow. The marginal mandibular branch innervates the major depressors of the lip. Therefore, paralysis of this nerve results in an inability to show the lower teeth with grimacing. At rest, the corner of the mouth will elevate due to the unopposed pull of the innervated zygomaticus major.

Treatment of facial nerve injury can be controversial, but ideally, primary microsurgical repair is advocated when nerve transection is noticed in the operating room. For patients who present with palsy in the postoperative period, several options are available. Since neuroprexia is the most likely cause of facial palsy after a facelift, most symptoms will improve after a 6 months period of observation. If nerve function does not return after a year of conservative management, patients may benefit from chemical (Botox) or surgical denervation of the contralateral side. This is particularly applicable for frontal nerve palsy patients. Other approaches include static sling procedures or ipsilateral nerve transfers. Dynamic facial reanimation procedures can restore spontaneous motion to affected side of the face; however, these are complex operations requiring a surgical team skilled with the microsurgical technique.

35.7 Conclusions

In elevating the SMAS with a facelift, the facial nerve branches are prone to injury anterior to the parotid gland. The safe facelift technique is based on surface anatomic landmarks to predict the location of the anterior edge of the parotid gland and avoid inadvertent injury to these branches. The facial nerve branches can be predicted to exit the anterior edge of the parotid gland 3.9 cm anterior to the tragus along a transverse axis of the zygomatic arch. Moreover, the anterior edge of the parotid gland can be predicted to be near the oblique vector from the inferior lateral orbital wall to the masseteric tuberosity. Based on our safe approach to facelift surgery, a sub-SMAS dissection anterior to the parotid gland is discouraged given the inherent risk of a more aggressive dissection.

References

1. Mitz V, Peyronie M. The superficial musculo-aponeurotic system (SMAS) in the parotid and cheek area. Plast Reconstr Surg. 1976;58(1):80–8.
2. Skoog T. Plastic surgery: new methods and refinements. Philadelphia: W.B. Saunders; 1974.
3. Davis RA, Anson BJ, Budinger JM, Kurth LR. Surgical anatomy of the facial nerve and parotid gland based upon a study of 350 cervicofacial halves. Surg Gynecol Obstet. 1956;102(4):385–412.
4. Dingman RO, Grabb WC. Surgical anatomy of the mandibular ramus of the facial nerve based on the dissection of 100 facial halves. Plast Reconstr Surg Transpl Bull. 1962;29:266–72.
5. Pitanguy I, Ramos AS. The frontal branch of the facial nerve: the importance of its variations in face lifting. Plast Reconstr Surg. 1966;38(4):352–6.
6. Gosain AK, Sewall SR, Yousif NJ. The temporal branch of the facial nerve: how reliably can we predict its path? Plast Reconstr Surg. 1997;99(5):1224–33.
7. Stuzin JM, Wagstrom L, Kawamoto HK, Wolfe SA. Anatomy of the frontal branch of the facial nerve: the significance of the temporal fat pad. Plast Reconstr Surg. 1989;83(2):265–71.
8. Stuzin JM, Baker TJ, Gordon HL. The relationship of the superficial and deep facial fascias: relevance to rhytidectomy and aging. Plast Reconstr Surg. 1992;89(3):441–9.
9. Wilhelmi BJ, Mowlavi A, Neumeister MW. The safe face lift with bony anatomic landmarks to elevate the SMAS. Plast Reconstr Surg. 2003;111(5):1723–6.
10. Har-Shai Y, Bodner SR, Egozy-Golan D, Lindenbaum ES, Ben-Izhak O, Mitz V, et al. Viscoelastic properties of the superficial musculoaponeurotic system (SMAS): a microscopic and mechanical study. Aesthetic Plast Surg. 1997;21(4):219–24.
11. May M, Schaitkin BM. The facial nerve. 2nd ed. New York: Thieme Medical Publishers; 2000. p. 97.

Recommended Reading

Baker DC, Conley J. Avoiding facial nerve injuries in rhytidectomy. Anatomical variations and pitfalls. Plast Reconstr Surg. 1979;64(6):781–95.
Gonyon Jr DL, Barton Jr FE. The aging face: rhytidectomy and adjunctive procedures. SRPS. 2005;10(11):7.
Hazani R, Mowlavi A, Wilhelmi BJ. Facelift anatomic landmarks to avoid injury to the marginal mandibular nerve. Aesth Surg J. 2011;31(3):286–9.
Mathes SJ, Hentz VR. Plastic surgery, vol. II. Philadelphia: Elsevier; 2005. p. 159–297.
Mowlavi A, Wilhelmi BJ. The extended SMAS facelift: identifying the lateral zygomaticus major muscle border using bony anatomic landmarks. Ann Plast Surg. 2004;52(4):353–7.
Nahai F. The art of aesthetic surgery: principles & techniques, vol. II. St. Louis: Quality Medical Publishing; 2005.
Owsley JQ, Agarwal CA. Safely navigating around the facial nerve in three dimensions. Clin Plast Surg. 2008;35(4):469–77.
Seckel BR. Facial danger zones: avoiding nerve injury in facial plastic surgery. St. Louis: Quality Medical Publishing; 1994.
Thorne CH. Facelift. In: Thorne CD, editor. Grabb & Smith's plastic surgery. Philadelphia: Lippincott-Williams & Wilkins; 2007.

Anatomicohistologic Study of the Retaining Ligaments of the Face with Retaining Ligament Correction and SMAS Plication in Facelift

Ragip Ozdemir

36.1 Introduction

Aging changes are first noticed in visible regions. The most important one of these regions is probably the facial region. The fact that the first aging changes appear in the facial region often bothers people. Plastic surgeons are striving to bring back the changing regions of the face to their normal anatomic positions. To this end, new technical definitions have been and are still being developed through varying researches.

Plastic surgery strives to obtain a harmony between exterior view and soul by camouflaging the exterior changes. In order to understand the impacts of aging, one should first understand the anatomy of the facial soft tissue and the changes aging brings. Facial bones and fat, muscle tissue, fascia, and positions of the retaining ligaments and the skin flap gives this multiple stratified form its shape.

36.2 Surgical and Functional Anatomy of the Face

When the skin is anatomically picked up, a homogeneous facial fat tissue is to be seen. This stratum forms the subcutaneous tissue and covers the whole face over SMAS (subcutaneous musculoaponeurotic system). In the medial plane it is the nasolobial fold anterior to the lips that diffuses to the zygomatic arch superiorly and ends in the orbicularis oris becoming a fascia over the lips. It thickens with fat and septae and forms the cheek. This tissue is called the facial fat layer. This layer detaches from then SMAS and forms the fat pad anteriorly by imprisoning the cheek fat tissue. In this region the facial portion sticks to the epidermis densely and is resistant to separation. Orbicularis oculi reaches superficial to the preorbital piece in the zygomatic arch medially [1–7].

The SMAS is to be found under the facial fat layer although it differentiates anatomically and histologically from this layer. It leaves the platysma in a muscular form and has a fibrous form on the parotid (Fig. 36.1). The SMAS goes from platysma to depressor anguli oris, the superficial fragment of orbicularis oris. It lays under the facial fat layer while reaching to superior and unites with the preorbital piece of the orbicularis oculi. From this point SMAS leaves the facial fat layer, reaches to superolateral, and unites with the subcutan tissue 1cm. under the zygomatic arch. Temporoparietal fascia unites with the superficial folium of deep temporal fascia 1 cm above arch. Above arch, there is facial fat layer in subcutan fat tissue as septas. SMAS is bound to the lower tissues and muscles with fibrous fascias. It binds the zygomaticus major in the superolateral of the nasolobial fold and unites with the superficial piece of orbicularis oris. SMAS is bound to the bone with some ligaments. The most important one of these ligaments is zygomatic ligament and it lays 4 cm inferolateral to the inferior orbital rim. It is connected closely to the facial nerve. Additionally the ligamentous connections right under the orbital rim supports the SMAS [4, 8–24].

In the study conducted by Har-Shai et al., it was found that the SMAS was a composite fibrofatty layer consisting of collagen and elastic fibers interspersed with fat cells, and a considerable number

R. Ozdemir
Faculty of Medicine, Division of Plastic and Reconstructive Surgery, Suleyman Demirel University, Mehmet Tonge Mahallesi, 225. Cadde, No:5, Isparta, Turkey
e-mail: ragipoya@hotmail.com

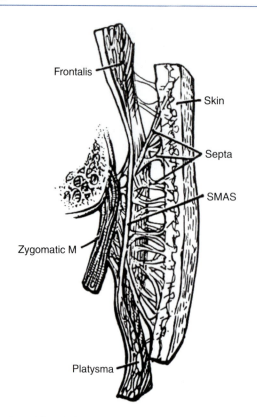

Fig. 36.1 The relation of SMAS and skin and the lower tissues

of elastic fibers were in close relationship to the collagen fibers, microscopically. Mechanical tests displayed definite viscoelastic properties of skin and SMAS, with the viscoelastic properties of the SMAS being less [21].

36.2.1 Parotidomasseteric Fascia

Parotidomasseteric fascia is a thin transparent layer between SMAS and facial nerve. This form lays over the parotis and becomes the superficial cervical fascia. Marginal mandibular nerve can be seen in this layer. In temporal region and scalp it continues as innominate and subgaleal fascia. In temporal region it lays between superficial temporal fascia and deep temporal fascia. It is seen between Scalp, galea, and pericranium. Galea, frontal muscle, temporoparietal fascia, SMAS, orbicularis oculi, and platysma can be considered as monolayer similar to subgaleal fascia, innominate fascia, parotidomasseteric fascia, and superficial fascia [1, 4, 5, 9–11, 14, 16, 20, 21].

36.2.2 Temporal Fascia

It originates inferiorly in the superior temporal line and continues to the zygomatic arch. When we go from superficial plane to deep, first comes dermis and temporoparietal fascia under subcutan tissue. This fascia continues with epicranial aponevrose which includes the frontal muscle in the frontal region. In addition, this fascia is also known as the superficial folium of temporal fascia. Under this fascia, there is innominate fascia. According to some sources, this form is the soft fat tissue which lays between superficial and deep temporal fascia. Under this fascia, we see the deep part of the temporal fascia. In this region, facial nerve goes through the low level superficial of deep temporal fascia. There is temporal muscle under the deep temporal fascia. Deep and superficial foliums unite over the zygomatic arch and take one form [4–6, 10, 12, 18–20, 25].

36.2.3 Deep Cervical Fascia

From superficial to deep, there are skin, percutaneous and platysma. The form which lays under the platysma is called cervical fascia and it continues as a part of Parotidomasseteric fascia [1, 19, 20, 26].

36.2.4 Malar: Buccal Fat Pad

Malar fat pad is a subcutaneous form which belongs to the second layer of the face. It lays in the superficial layer of SMAS like Zygomaticus minor and major muscles. It can be elevated with Malar fat pad, skin flap, or SMAS. Buccal fat goes along superficial with the buccal branches of facial nerve, anterior to the pad masseter musclepad (Fig. 36.2). There is buccinator muscle deeper in the Fat pad. Buccal fat pad can be found with sub-SMAS decession or by eliminating the buccinator muscle in the mouth [1, 3–5, 10, 12–14, 16, 24, 27].

36.2.5 Facial Mimetic Muscles

Frailinger classifies the facial muscles as four layers.
  Layer 1: Depressor anguli oris, zygomatic minor, orbicularis oculi.

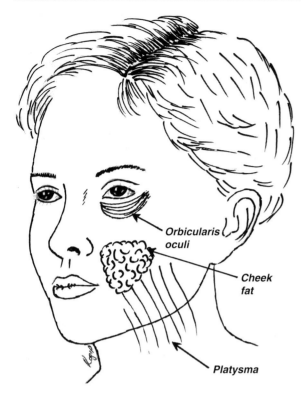

Fig. 36.2 The localization of facial fat pad

Layer 2: Depressor labii inferioris, risorius, platysma, zygomatic major, levator labii superioris alaeque nasi.
Layer 3: Orbicularis oris, levator labii superior.
Layer 4: Mentalis, levator anguli oris, buccinator.

The muscles in the first three layers are deeply innervated, and the ones in the fourth layer are superficially innervated [19, 20].

36.2.6 Facial Nerve

The most traumatic branches of the facial nerve in face-lift surgery are buccal and marginal mandibular branches. However, temporal facial nerve plays a big role in this section. Temporal branch is 2.3(±)0.6 mm deeper than subcutaneous face-lift decession plane and 5 cm. away from the parotis edge. It is the most superficial branch. Nerve is under the superficial temporal fascia with temporal artery. There are two branches 3–4 cm posterior to the line drawn from lateral canthal region to tragus and temporal facial nerve is the terminal branch that is least communicated to the other branches. Buccal and zygomatic facial branches have the ability of cross innervation with a range of 70–90%, although they are more traumatic due to being much communicated. Zygomatic branch consists of two ramus as superficial and buccal. Its superficial branch goes superficial of the zygomatic major muscle and its lower branch goes deep in the muscle. Buccal branch crosses the masseter in the form of two ramus. Buccal and zygomatic branches are 2 cm. ahead of the parotis. Zygomatic branch has a relation with zygomatic ligament, buccal branch with masseteric cutaneous ligament, and marginal mandibular branch with mandibular ligament. Marginal mandibular branch is specific and leaves the parotis at the angle of mandibular 1cm underneath. It goes under Platysma, anterior to the facial vein. In the airy dissection the nerve was identified 1–4 cm. under the bottom edge of mandibula. All the way, it is related to the mandibular ligament [2, 4, 16, 18, 26, 29].

36.2.7 Retaining Ligaments

The definition of the retaining ligaments of the face was first described by Mc Gregor with the zygomatic cutaneous ligament (McGregor's Patch). As a result of the studies made by Furnas, Anterior platysma cutaneous ligament, Platysma auricular ligament, and Mandibular ligament were defined. Stuzin et al. and Mendelson defined the masseteric cutaneous ligament. Apart from their anatomical studies, they also defined their own techniques for the repositioning of the aging face. The fixation of the retaining ligaments are today advocated and applied by Stuzin and Mendelson [8–11, 29, 30].

The descending part in the cheek and midface region is composed of fat tissue in between the septa of the facial fat layer. The structures supporting the cheek are named as the retaining ligaments of the face, preventing the descent conservatively [31].

- Zygomatic cutaneous ligament (McGregor's patch)
- Platysma auricular ligament (Preauricular parotid cutaneous ligament)
- Masseteric cutaneous ligament (Parotidomasseteric cutaneous ligament)
- Anterior platysmacutaneous ligament
- Mandibular ligament

These ligaments go toward the fibrous form and stick to dermis as a part of the facial compartment (Fig. 36.3) [1, 3–5, 8–12, 26, 31, 33–35].

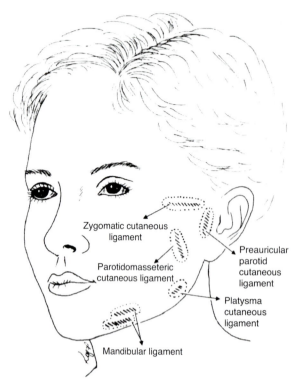

Fig. 36.3 The localization of the midface retaining ligaments [32]

was a vertical septum that extended between the investing masseteric fascia and the overlying SMAS, and the septum varied in density and strength, being strongest superiorly in the region of the junction between the zygomatic arch and the body of the zygoma [12]. Greenberg noted the presence of a small buccal branch of the facial nerve and a branch of the transverse facial artery in the midportion of this patch. McGregor described the ligament as the area of fibrous attachment between the anterior edge of the parotid fascia and the dermis of the cheek skin [34].

Zygomatic Cutaneous Ligament is located 5–9 mm posterior to the zygomaticus minor muscle and inferior to the zygomatic arch, 4.2–4.8 cm in front of the tragus with a length of 1.8–3.4 cm and a width of 2.9–3.4 cm in men. It is 3.9–4.5 cm in front of the tragus, with a length of 1.6–3.0 cm and a width of 2.7–3.3 mm in women. A small branch of the zygomatic branch of the facial nerve and a branch of the transverse facial artery were identified traveling in the company of the middle portions of the ligament. The extent of the ligament ranged from 7 to 10 mm (Fig. 36.4), between skin and zygoma, which was histologically identified by using Masson trichrome stain (Fig. 36.5) [32].

36.3 Anatomicohistologic Study of the Retaining Ligaments of the Face

36.3.1 Zygomatic Cutaneous Ligament (McGregor's Patch)

Furnas has described the zygomatic ligaments as the stout fibers that originate at or near the inferior border of the anterior zygomatic arch, behind the insertion of the zygomaticus minor muscle, and they insert in the skin serving as an anchoring point. These fibers are located 4.5 cm in front of the tragus with a 3 mm width and 0.5 mm thickness. Anterior to this first bundle may be a second bundle. Interspersed around these two bundles will be several smaller bundles. Typically, an artery and a sensory nerve course to the skin in the company of these bundles. The ligaments are approximately 6–8 mm in length, traveling directly from the zygomatic bone to the dermis [31, 33, 36]. Owsley stated that in the region of the anterior border of the masseter, there

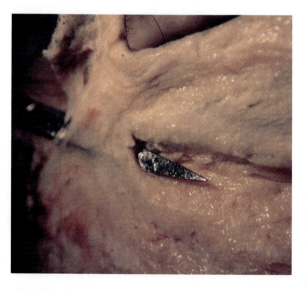

Fig. 36.4 View of the zygomatic cutaneous ligament in the cadaver dissection [32]

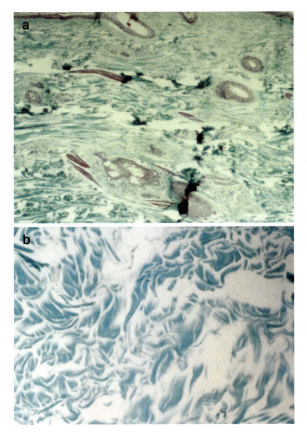

Fig. 36.5 From the dermis (**a**), extending to the periosteum (**b**), significant collagenized connective tissue formation (Mason trichrome: ×10) [32]

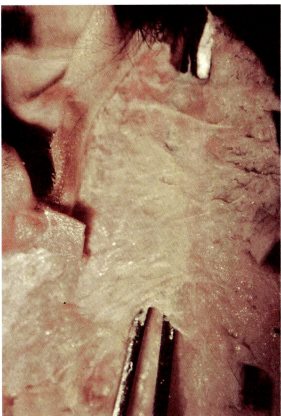

Fig. 36.6 Preauricular parotid cutaneous ligament in the cadaver dissection [32]

36.3.2 Preauricular Parotid Cutaneous Ligament

Furnas stated that the posterior border of the platysma receded into an intricate fascial condensation that often attached intimately to the overlying skin, providing firm anchorage between the platysma and the dermis of the inferior auricular region, and some cutaneous branches of the great auricular nerve were often seen on the surface of the ligament or interwoven with the fibers underlying the parotid fascia [31, 33].

The preauricular parotid cutaneous ligament is localized in the anteroinferior Auricular region, vertical preauricularly, with a length of 2.7–3.1 cm and a width of 2.3–2.8 mm in men and with a length of 2.4–2.8 cm and a width of 1.9–2.5 mm in women. During the dissections, a cutaneous nerve was identified in the ligament (Fig. 36.6). The presence of the ligament extending between skin and parotid fascia macroscopically was supported by histologic examination using Masson trichrome stain (Fig. 36.7) [32].

36.3.3 Parotidomasseteric Cutaneous Ligament

Stuzin et al. emphasized the fibrous structure extending between masseter and skin, with a vertical orientation and neighboring with the zygomatic branch of the facial nerve, and stressed the necessity of caution in this region of dissection [8, 9]. Mendelson explained the inverted L orientation of the cheek ligaments and noted the parotidomasseteric ligament extending between the masseteric fascia and the skin [10, 11]. The direction of the ligament is not completely vertical but is somewhat oblique, with localization in the distal portion of the parotid gland and the middle of the

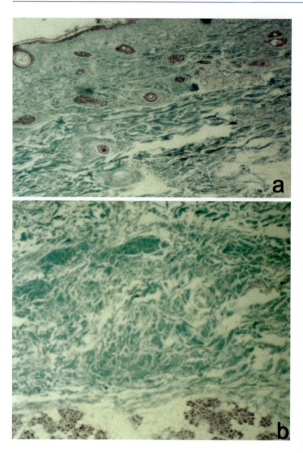

Fig. 36.7 From the dermis (**a**), extending to the salivary gland (**b**), significant collagenized connective tissue formation (Mason trichrome: ×10) [32]

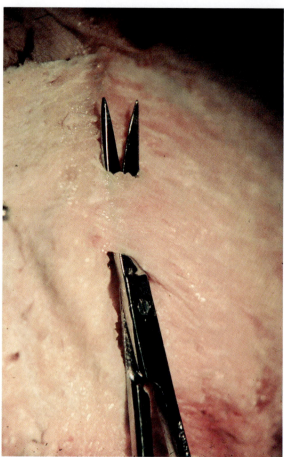

Fig. 36.8 Parotidomasseteric cutaneous ligament in the cadaver dissection [32]

masseter muscle, indicating variations not only in cadavers but also in patients. The zygomatic branch of the facial nerve is observed in close proximity to the ligament, in which neither an artery nor a nerve was identified. The length of the ligament is 1.8–2.7 cm and the width is 1.2–1.8 mm in men and 1.6–2.4 cm and 1.1–1.5 mm in women, respectively (Fig. 36.8). The extension of the ligament between skin and parotidomasseteric fascia is determined with Masson trichrome staining of the histologic specimens (Fig. 36.9) [32].

36.3.4 Platysma Cutaneous Ligament

Furnas observed that the aponeurotic connections were sometimes seen between the anterior platysma and the skin of the middle and anterior cheek, which were the bands of condensed connective tissue that pass obliquely forward from the platysma to the dermis [31, 33, 34]. In many of the cadavers and the patients, the ligament was observed to be in a septal form rather than in a significant ligamentous form. The observed connection is localized between the mandibular body and angle superiorly (Fig. 36.10). The extension between skin and parotid fascia is supported by histologic examination using Masson trichrome stain (Fig. 36.11) [32].

36.3.5 Mandibular Ligament

Furnas reported that the mandibular ligaments originated from bone along a line that was about 1 cm above the mandibular border and that extended along the anterior third of the mandibular body, and that these

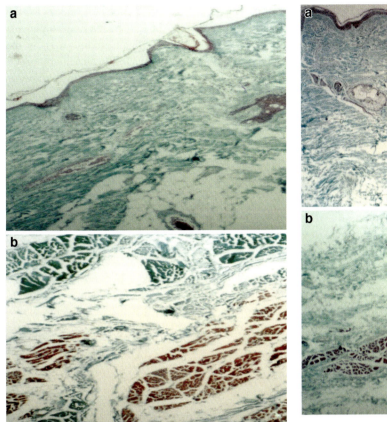

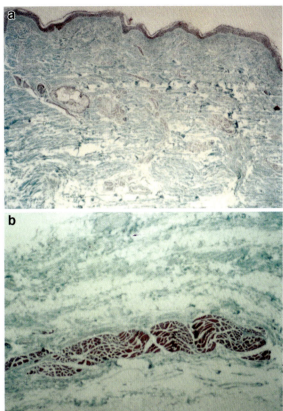

Fig. 36.9 From the dermis (**a**), extending to the parotidomasseteric fascia (**b**), significant collagenized connective tissue formation (Mason trichrome: ×10) [32]

Fig. 36.11 From the dermis (**a**), extending to muscle tissue (**b**), significant collagenized connective tissue formation (Mason trichrome: ×10) [32]

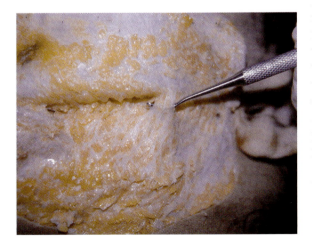

Fig. 36.10 Platysma cutaneous ligament in a cadaver dissection [32]

ligaments usually appeared as a linear series of parallel fibers. It was noted that, typically, a second tier of fibers was aligned 2–3 mm above and parallel to the first tier, and these fibrous bundles interdigitated among the muscle fibers of the platysma and triangularis along their line of attachment. The ligaments were said to be taking a path perpendicular to the skin and were about 4–5 mm long, usually accompanied by a sensory nerve and a cutaneous artery. It was also stated that the posterior limit of the mandibular ligament was usually palpable [29, 31, 33].

Mandibular ligament was observed superiorly along the mandibular body and parasymphysis, between skin and bone, and two distinct fibrous structures were obviously dissected. A cutaneous sensory nerve and an artery in between two fibers were identified. The length is 2.4–3.2 cm in men and 2.2–3.1 cm in women. The width is 2.8–3.4 mm in men and 2.5–3.4 mm in women

(Fig. 36.12). The extension between skin and periosteum of the mandible is supported by histologic examination using Masson trichrome stain (Fig. 36.13) [32].

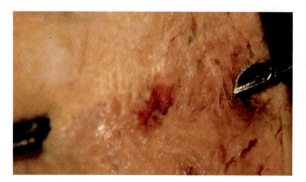

Fig. 36.12 Mandibular cutaneous ligament in a cadaver dissection [32]

Anatomicohistologic studies have revealed that the largest and the thickest one of the retaining ligaments of the face is Mandibular ligament followed by the zygomatic cutaneous ligament, Preauricular parotid cutaneous ligament, Parotidomasseteric cutaneous ligament, and Anterior platysma cutaneous ligament. It is displayed that unlike other ligaments mandibular ligament and zygomatic cutaneous ligament lay between skin and periost, and that parotidomasseteric cutaneous ligament doesn't only consist of masseter fascias but also, parotid fascia (Fig. 36.14). The cutaneous artery and nerve, which are between mandibular ligament and zygomatic cutaneous ligament fibers, are important in terms of the skin flap becoming bloodstained and its sensation. When the SMAS and ligament localizations in the lateral facial region are considered, a more fixed area can be seen compared to the labile, angular area in the middle face region. Studies have determined that these ligaments play a big role in the fixation of the face [32].

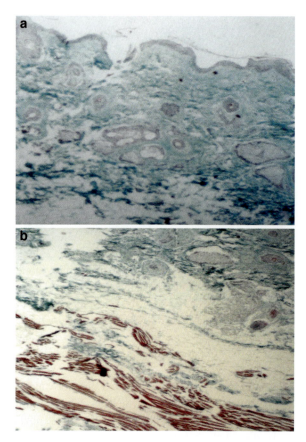

Fig. 36.13 Histologic view of mandibular cutaneous ligament in a cadaver dissection. (**a**) From the dermis (I), extending to the periosteum (II), significant connective tissue formation (Mason trichrome: ×10). (**b**) From the dermis (I), extending to the periosteum (II), significant connective tissue formation (Mason trichrome: ×10) [32]

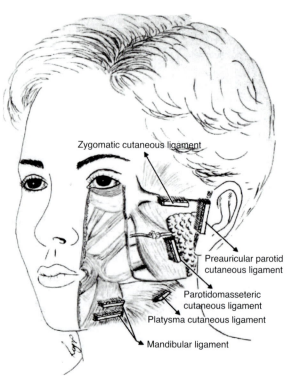

Fig. 36.14 Elongation of retaining ligaments to the skin and dermis [32]

36.4 Aging Changes in the Face

The dermal thickness of the skin decreases progressively and its elasticity begins to disappear. In course of time, telangiectasias, keratosis, and increase of melanosis are to be seen. The aging period differs from one person to the other and the face is especially affected by many factors from smoking habit to climate. Aging doesn't form in a straight line, but in parts and pieces and these parts can vary. Emotional influences can increase the speed of aging. Other exterior impacts that increase the speed of aging process are sunlight, dry air, repeating movements of facial mimetic muscles, progressive loss of the fat tissues of the face, cellular degenerative changes, and attachments of retaining ligaments and muscles to the skin (Fig. 36.15) [1, 2, 4, 5, 10, 11, 16, 22, 31, 35–40].

Aging changes in the face can be histologically arranged as follows: flattening of dermoepidermal intersection, changes in the thickness of epidermis, changes in the cell amount and dimension, atypic changes in nucleus, decrease of melanosis, decrease of langerhans cells. In dermis, the changes are as follows: decrease of dermal volume and atrophy, decrease of fibroblasts, decrease of mast cells, shortening of capillary structures, abnormal nerve outcomes, increase of hydroxyproline, increase of nonfusible collagen, decrease of fusible collagen, increase of collagen resistance, decrease of elasticity, decrease of acid mucopolysaccharide and hexosamin. The changes on the skin are graying of hair, decline in hair amount, increase of vellus in thermal period, abnormal nailfolds, decrease of eccrine sweat glands, increase of apocrine glands, decrease of sebaceous glands [1, 2, 4, 5, 10, 22, 31, 36, 38].

The retaining ligaments of face support facial soft tissue in normal anatomic position, resisting gravitational change. As this ligamentous system attenuates, facial fat descends in the plane between superficial and deep facial fascia and the stigmata of facial age develop. A loss of zygomatic ligament support allows for the inferior descent of the malar pad, influencing nasolabial fold prominence, whereas a loss of masseteric ligament support allows for the inferior descent of facial fat to the mandibular border, leading to the formation of facial jowling. Repositioning of the descended fat pads culminates in a young face.

As a result of aging, the amount of the facial fat as well as its quality decreases. The anatomic location of the facial fat in youth determines the facial shape. Typically, the youthful face is full of well-supported fat, overlying the malar region, and overlying the parotid and masseter in the lateral cheek, secondary to the intact intrinsic support of the retaining ligament system.

The combination of fullness in the malar region and the lateral cheek and concavity overlying the buccal recess accounts for the angular appearance of the youthful face. As the human face ages, facial fat descends and facial shape changes. In the older face, fat situates anteriorly and inferiorly, producing a facial contour that is square in configuration, with little difference between malar highlight and midfacial fat on the frontal view. As facial fat situates inferiorly in the face, the face also appears longer [1–5, 8–12, 22, 26, 31, 33, 34, 36].

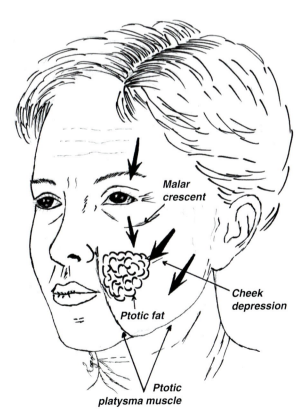

Fig. 36.15 Anatomical changes in the face with aging

36.5 Facelift and Historical Development of Retaining Ligaments of the Face

Midface region has always been the facial part that is aesthetically first noticed. This part of the face has been recognized as a sign of health and beauty. If the exterior view ages while the mind is still youthful, interference is needed. In the last quarter of this century, the operations for repositioning of the face have become very popular.

Repositioning of aging face was first applied by Hollander in 1901 with the subcutaneous face-lift procedure. In 1916 Lexer developed this procedure; in 1921 Joseph also strived to popularize this procedure. In 1920 Bettman used the incision, which is used today as well. In the same year Bettman and in 1927 Bames applied the continuous incision and subcutaneous face-lift procedures. In 1959 McGregor first defined the zygomatic cutaneous ligament. In 1960 Aufricht showed that subcutaneous face-lift border can reach to platysma branches in the submental region. In 1964 Adamson, Horton, and Crawford and in 1972 Pensini and Capozzi defined the submental defatting. In 1969 Baker and Gordon defined the plication of deep tissues in the lateral cheek region and founded the SMAS plication which is being used today. In 1974 Tipton published the postoperative views of 33 patients with deep tissue plications. In 1966, 1973, and 1981 Pitanguy published the anatomical variations of frontal branch and the results of the subcutaneous face-lift which he applied. In 1972 Webster and between 1968 and 1972 Millard defined the submandibular lipectomy. In 1973, 1978, and 1984 Rees described the deep plan plication, SMAS anatomy, and plication and published his clinical series. Between 1974 and 1976, Skoog defined for the first time the deep plane face-lift procedure adding the platysma and SMAS to the skin flap. In 1974 Mitz and Pyronie defined the anatomy of SMAS in the middle and lateral cheek regions. Owsley developed the sub-SMAS platysma face-lift technique in 1977, 1986, and 1993 and he defined the reposition of the malar fat pad. In 1977, 1979, and 1983 Baker studied the surgical anatomy of the face and the facial nerve anatomy with details and strived to obtain the repositioning of the face by applying chemical peeling and deep plane face-lift at the same time. In 1989 and 1995 Furnas studied the retaining ligaments of the face and determined their localizations and dimensions. He also emphasized the extended SMAS surgery and nasolobial fold surgery. In 1989, 1992, and 2000, Stuzin defined the surgical flatting of superficial and deep fascias, buccal fat pad anatomy, extended SMAS dicession, facial nerve frontal branch anatomy, vicryl mesh, increasing of SMAS support, and the fixation of facial forms. In 1990, 1992, 1995, 1998, and 2000 Hamra defined the blepheroplasty and face-lift combination techniques and emphasized the midface plane. He also improved the deep plane composite face-lift technique. Between 1991 and 1996 Ramirez defined the subperiosteal face-lift and endoscopic subperiosteal face-lift techniques. Between 1992 and 1997 Barton published his works on SMAS and nasolabial fold anatomies. Between 1993 and 1996 Gosain studied the nasolabial fold and SMAS anatomies. In 1993, 1994, 1996, and 1998 Yousif studied the nasolabial fold and SMAS anatomy and described the changes in the midface region. In 1995 Hagerty applied and advocated the central suspension technique. In 1996 Robbins did the nasolabial fold restoration by using the SMAS plication technique. In 1996 Har and Shai described the skin and SMAS anatomy with details. In 1997 Whetzel and Mathes published their studies on the topic of face-lift flap becoming bloodstained. In 1997, 1999, and 2001 Mendelson published his study on SMAS plication vectors in retaining ligaments flatting. In 1998 De la Plaza defined the sub-SMAS subperiosteal face-lift technique. In 1999 Camarena defined multiple combined SMAS platysma plication technique [30, 41].

Face-lift surgery has developed progressively until today and a lot of researchers have shared their experiences about rejuvenation.

The development of SMAS surgery revealed the subperiosteal approach, allowing the repositioning of the ligaments of the middle cheek over the periosteum of the zygoma. However retaining ligaments can cause some interior difficulties; first, the mobilization of the vertical limb of the L is not possible because it is bound more to the masseter muscle fascia than the periost. Second, restricted repositioning of the medial cheek and nasolabial fold was encountered because of insufficient tension over the unblocked periosteum of the middle cheek region. While knotting each stur, the probable dimples on the skin are watched; if there is a dimple that probably appeared because the traction is too wide or vertical or the suture is placed too superficial, the suture is changed.

The fundamentals of facelift surgery should include the fixation parallel to the natural anatomic ligaments unrestricting the functional results. The SMAS indicates various properties throughout the regions of face and is strengthened with vertical retaining ligaments including the deep fibrils of the reticula cutis.

The description of the zygomatic and masseteric retaining ligaments of the cheek supports extended SMAS face-lift surgery with the function and the localization of the retaining ligaments taken into consideration in the mobilization of the flaps. For this relief, dissection underlies the expanded SMAS and composite techniques. While identifying the fixation method of mobilized SMAS, the functions and original localizations of these retaining ligaments should be considered. The localizations of retaining ligaments increase more in the middle cheek region rather than in preauricular region for fixation. In medial cheek region and lateral cheek region the attachments of retaining ligaments are more than the neighboring SMAS fixation [10, 11].

Whetzel and Mathes observed that the transverse facial perforating artery provides the major direct blood supply to the lateral cheek and preauricular area following rhytidectomy, if preserved. This perforator was reported to occupy a constant anatomic location 3.1 cm lateral and 3.7 cm inferior to the lateral canthus. The greater variability in localizing the submental perforating artery was depicted. This perforator also contributed significantly to lateral facial blood supply. Both perforator locations were noted to be within the area of standard undermining for rhytidectomy; during this procedure, especially in the clinical setting of a patient with vascular compromise or who is a smoker, the lateral facial perforators were proposed to be preserved [30, 41, 42].

36.6 Retaining Ligament Correction and SMAS Plication in Facelift

The fixation of the face-lift flap rose from the original skin flap technique. A wide area which needs to stick under flap rose through wide decollation. In 1950, Aufricht sutured the subcutaneous layer to the parotidomasseteric fascia [10].

The SMAS or deep plane face-lift surgery described by Skoog included the fixation of the superficial fascial flap to the masseteric muscular fascia. The developments in SMAS surgery provide the attachment of the mobilized SMAS flap to the preauricular region instead of the middle cheek region. Preauricular fixation is attached to the periost of posterior zygomatic arch or to neighboring deep fascia or to undecessed SMAS of that region [43]. Recently the fixation at the middle cheek level has been advocated by Stuzin and Mendelson [8–11].

During the sub-SMAS surgery over the masseteric region, care should be taken to avoid injuring the branches of the facial nerve. The contouring of the facial soft tissue remains a difficult challenge because of the variations in the quality of facial skin and in fascial content of the SMAS from patient to patient. Fixation of the thin superficial layer results in early descent, and the excess SMAS is preferably plicated over instead of being excised [8, 9].

The retaining ligaments of the cheek are stout, firm, and flexible, attaching the facial skin to the facial skeleton and to the deep fascia through subcutaneous tissue. Their efficiency depends on the width of the attachments to the skin and, if small, the ligament stretches in time, but the ripples are not away from the fixation points.

The ptosis of the cheek anterior to the zygomatic ligament and the jowling posterior to the mandibular ligament are evidence.

It provides a more youthful view, to loosen all tissues that prevent the vertical movement of the ptotic facial tissue for the elevation of the nasolobial fold, to lift up the ptotic facial skin with vertical movements, and to fix it so that the ripples disappear and to form a new insertion of the zygomatic ligament. In every four patients facial nerve neuropraxia is reported. The most effective lift can be made if these ligaments separate in the location where the cheek skin severely drapes. Mandibular ligament blocks the skin for a lifting power which has a relation to the cheek flap, which cannot transmit its surgical importance to the submandibular region or cheek region. The surgical release of this ligament provides more effective submental lift and this creates space for lipectomy without doing a submental incision. Platysma auricular ligament is important in terms of making it possible for the surgeon to move to the wrong layer during dicession [31, 33].

The attachments of the facial mimetic muscles, especially the zygomatic muscles, to the SMAS cause difficulties with the sub-SMAS dissection, which ought to be held attentively. These attachments account for the minimal change in the nasolabial crease after a sub-SMAS face-lift dissection [13].

Stuzin et al. mentioned the variability of fat tissue composition from patient to patient and the necessity of the various vectors in lifting. Materials such as Vicryl mesh could be used where the SMAS is weak and in regions where fixation is difficult, such as the inferior SMAS region [8, 9].

Mendelson proposed fixation of the mobilized region to the immobilized region, and claimed that the more suturing was performed to the small area, the better were the results that were encountered.

Sub-SMAS dissection in the middle cheek region and buccal region is difficult. During the dissection and fixation at the middle cheek and buccal region, there's a risk of facial nerve injury. When the laxity and bagginess in the face are lifted up, the resistance of the tissues resumes. The plicated SMAS descends with stress. The lifting vectors should be parallel to the mimetic muscles of the face and should be in at least three vectors, considering the plane in three dimensions, which would not flatten the face, forming the natural view. The plications decrease the tension and also the incision scar [10, 11, 44].

For correction of the aging face, various techniques have evolved and have been used and have both advantages and disadvantages. The understanding of the mechanism of the aging face and the correction depending on this is the basic principle. Anatomic repositioning of the anatomic layers, muscles, fat pads, ligaments, and skin structure seems to be possible [21, 45–47].

36.6.1 Preparations for Surgery and Skin Marking

In the operation room, the face-lift incision plane and probable branch localizations are fixed by drawing after the proper region is cleaned, under general anesthesia, the proper region is diluted 2% lidocaine and half face is diluted HCL+0.025 adrenalin of 6 ml. local anesthetic and 6 ml. saline solution. It starts after the face-lift region is given subcutan. After waiting for 5–10 min, skin incision is planned in oblique posterovertical localization and in preauricular region, and it is planned according to the preauricular skin line from in front of tragus from the line between ear lobe and skin, in postauricular region from postauricular line and in occipital region into the scalp.

36.6.2 Surgical Technique

The skin flap is elevated superior to the superficial temporal fascia and hair follicles in the temporal region according to the supra-SMAS face-lift technique. Under 4x loupe magnification, the zygomatic ligament is dissected in the zygomatic region. If the artery and the nerve are identified, these are preserved to avoid disturbing the nourishment and sensation of the skin, and the attachment of the ligament to the subcutaneous tissue is dissected sharply. The dissection is continued toward the preauricular region, marking the ligament with a suture. In the preauricular region under loupe magnification, the parotid cutaneous ligament is dissected and separated sharply from the skin; meanwhile, the identified cutaneous nerve is preserved and the ligament marked with a suture. The dissection is held anteriorly and inferiorly, reaching the parotidomasseteric and anterior platysma cutaneous ligaments; the attachments are separated and the ligaments are marked. The anterior masseteric border is attained with careful dissection, with the disadvantage of the negative effect on skin flap circulation. A better visualization can be obtained with a headlamp directed toward the mandibular ligament. It is proper to continue with the dissection using a loop coming to the probable part of the ligament which is marked. When the cutaneous nerve and the artery are identified the ligament is separated from the skin and marked with a suture leaving more subcutaneous tissue on the skin flap to avoid dimpling during the anatomic correction of the ligaments (Fig. 36.16). After hemostasis, SMAS plications of

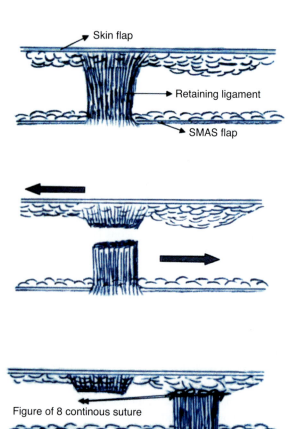

Fig. 36.16 Dissection and suturing design in the anteroinferior portion of the ligament to prevent dimpling [32]

0–1 cm in anterosuperior and anteroposterosuperior vectors with 3–6 cm 5/0 nonabsorbable, colorless propylene sutures are accomplished in the cheek region and with 2–3 cm sutures in the parotid region, the knots localized inferiorly (Fig. 36.17) [32].

The branches of the facial nerve should be cared for, especially in the middle cheek region.

SMAS tension and resistance is increased with SMAS plication. The gravitationally descended facial fat is replaced to the anatomic position. While the skin flap is dispersed over the SMAS, avoiding excessive stretching, the new localizations of the mandibular, parotidomasseteric, zygomatic, anterior platysmal, and preauricular parotid ligaments are pointed out on the skin flap (Fig. 36.18). Suturing of the ligaments to the new localizations is accomplished with colorless 5/0 nonabsorbable propylene using either continuous or figure-of eight sutures every 5–10 mm, depending on the size of the ligament, avoiding stretching and dimpling. With the impact of the edema from postoperative period, dense suturation or tension results in a dimple. After correction of the ligaments, the excess skin flap is excised, preventing the sideburn line displacement and avoiding tension between the incision lines. During excision the ear lobule and the skin flap should be sutured so that the distinct shape of the ear lobule is preserved. An Axiom silicone drain could help to prevent hematoma and control the hemostasis. The incision line is sutured anatomically as two layers of subcutaneous tissue and skin. The operation is finished with a dressing that doesn't cause excessive pressure [32, 48].

Investigation of the cutaneous arterial supply of the face-lift flap is useful during dissection and preservation of sufficient structures, especially in patients with vascular compromise or who are smokers. Although the subperiosteal face-lift, central suspension, deep plane, and multiplane face-lift techniques have been used in face-lift surgery today with the disadvantages determined and explained by the authors, the properties of being physiologic and less traumatic, and having decreased complications and fast healing are

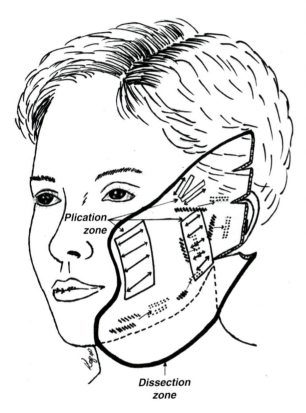

Fig. 36.17 Plication design in the middle and posterior cheek region

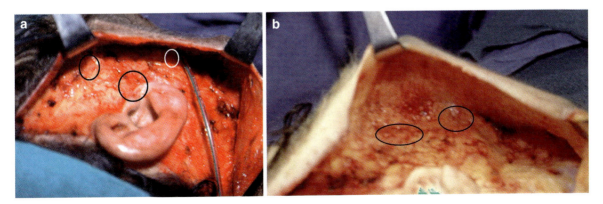

Fig. 36.18 Localization of the facial retaining ligaments in intraoperative period. (**a**) Preauricular parotid cutaneous ligament, Zygomatic cutaneous ligament, platysma cutaneous ligament (**b**) Parotidomasseteric ligament, Mandibular ligament

proposed to be major advantages. However, the lifting of the facial structures superiorly in one vector and the alteration of the anatomic localization of all the structures for repositioning of the facial fat pads correctly is a conflict to be illuminated in the future. Lower eyelid blepharoplasty combined with the same incision is claimed to result in fewer complications, despite the fact that restricted release and fixation of the face-lift flap could have negative effects on the blepharoplasty and face-lift in the long term. The anatomic regions of the face should be considered separately and the surgical procedures should be applied according to the distinct properties of these regions. The author has accomplished these techniques more successfully in selected and exceptional patients recently.

The similar properties of the skin and SMAS are revealed by anatomic studies. The attachments of the mimetic muscles to the skin and subcutaneous tissue in the nasolabial region constitute the nasolabial fold. Because of the redistribution of the cheek fat pad without any alteration in the skin composition and while maintaining the projections of surface landmarks within the cheek mass during smiling, SMAS plication for repositioning of the fat pads, rather than SMAS mobilization, is sufficient. The plication also increases SMAS stability and resistance and, in some instances, Vicryl mesh use is reported. The vectors of plication should be planned perpendicular to the relaxation of the SMAS by the mimetic muscles, so that repositioning of the fat pads is accomplished in addition to the strong stabilization of the SMAS, meanwhile reestablishing the contour of the nasolabial fold. The plication or Vicryl mesh use in the middle cheek region is efficient in accordance with the delicate and loose structure of the SMAS. The rigid and tight property of SMAS in the parotid region prevents excessive relaxation [32].

The dissection in the new localizations of the retaining ligaments of the face should be held deeper, leaving more subcutaneous tissue in the face-lift flap, and the figure-of-eight or continuous suturing techniques with colorless 5–0 propylene could decrease the possible irregularities in the soft tissue and dimpling. The SMAS plication and restabilization of the retaining ligaments of face are necessary for restoration of the normal anatomic structures of the face [32].

The development of SMAS surgery revealed the subperiosteal approach, allowing the repositioning of the ligaments of the middle cheek over the periosteum of the zygoma. However, retaining ligaments may cause some interior difficulties; first of all the mobilization of the vertical limb of the L is not possible, because it is formed by the masseteric fascia rather than the periost. Second, restricted repositioning of the medial cheek and nasolabial fold was encountered because of insufficient tension over the unblocked periosteum of the middle cheek region.

While knotting each suture, the probable dimples on the skin are watched. If there is a dimple that probably appeared because the traction is too wide or vertical or the suture is placed too superficial, the suture is changed. The fundamentals of face-lift surgery should include the fixation parallel to the natural anatomic ligaments unrestricting the functional results. The SMAS indicates various properties throughout the regions of face and is strengthened with vertical retaining ligaments including the deep fibrils of the reticula cutis.

The description of the zygomatic and masseteric retaining ligaments of the cheek supports extended SMAS face-lift surgery with the function and the localization of the retaining ligaments taken into consideration in the mobilization of the flaps.

For this relief, dissection underlies the expanded SMAS and composite techniques. The principle of fixation at the middle cheek region instead of the preauricular region is proposed with the help of the better understanding of the localization of the retaining ligaments and the deep attachments that form a mobile medial cheek and a less mobile part laterally [10, 11].

36.7 Postoperative Care and Complications

To prevent dimples, the dissection should be deep and eight sutures are placed instead of one by one. The dimples caused by postoperative edema disappear in 2–4 weeks and this period decreases by soft massage on this region. The probable tension of the skin flap in preauricular region is reduced by SMAS plication and flatting of retaining ligaments and so the expanded skin can be better contoured. It provides a more reliable dicession plane because the Sub-SMAS dicession is not made. According to observations, blepharoplasty is more useful in terms of midface restoration. Face-lift with blepharoplasty should be kept in mind to be applied for appropriate cases. The risk of hematoma can be prevented by a good hemostasis, an annular 5–8F axiom drain on the face-lift flap region, and a soft dressing that doesn't affect the viability of the skin flap. When no sub-SMAS dicession is applied, the recovery of a pathology in the facial nerve branches will be in 4–6 weeks, specifically in the mandibular branch region, if there is no action.

With this technique, the reposition of the facial fat pad, strengthening of the SMAS, fixation of the retaining ligaments, and tension of the skin flap can be supplied (Figs. 36.19–36.21) [32].

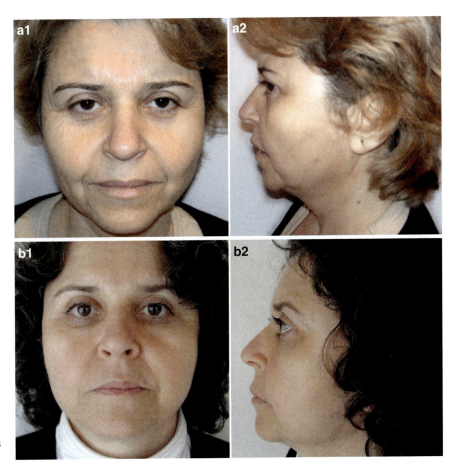

Fig. 36.19 (a) Preoperative patient. (b) Eighteen months after surgery

Fig. 36.20 (**a**) Preoperative patient. (**b**) Thirteen months after surgery

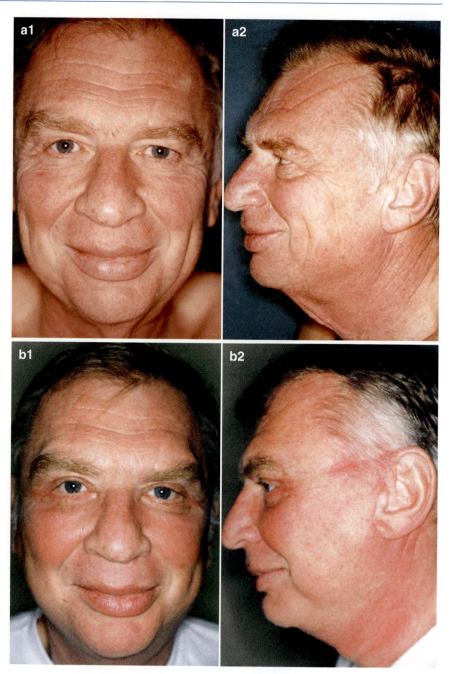

Fig. 36.21 (a) Preoperative patient. (b) Six months after surgery

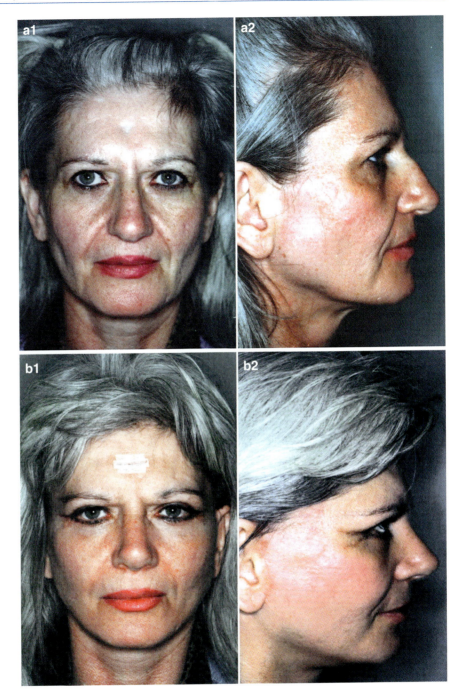

References

1. Rees TD, Aston SJ, Thorne CH. Blepharoplasty and facialplasty. In: McCarthy JG, editor. McCarthy plastic surgery. Philadelphia: W.B. Saunders; 1990. p. 2358–414.
2. Connell BF, Marten TJ. Facial rejuvenation: face lift. In: Cohen M, editor. Mastery of plastic and reconstructive surgery. Boston: Little, Brown & Company; 1994. p. 1873–902.
3. Owsley JQ, Alpert BS. Facial rejuvenation in men. In: Cohen M, editor. Mastery of plastic and reconstructive surgery. Boston: Little, Brown & Company; 1994. p. 1902–10.
4. Thorne CH, Aston SJ. Aesthetic surgery of the aging face. In: Aston SJ, Beasley RW, Thorne CH, editors. Grabb and Smith's plastic surgery. 5th ed. Philadelphia: Lippincott-Raven; 1997. p. 633–49.

5. Aston SJ, Thorne CH, Rees TD. Anatomy and pathogenesis of the aging face. In: Rees TD, LaTrenta GS, editors. Aesthetic plastic surgery. Philadelphia: W.B. Saunders; 1994. p. 662–72.
6. Aston SJ, Thorne CH. Contemporary rhytidectomy. In: Rees TD, LaTrenta GS, editors. Aesthetic plastic surgery. Philadelphia: W.B. Saunders; 1994. p. 722–31.
7. Hamra ST. Composite rhytidectomy. In: Rees TD, LaTrenta GS, editors. Aesthetic plastic surgery. Philadelphia: W.B. Saunders; 1994. p. 722–31.
8. Stuzin JM, Baker TJ, Baker TM. Refinements in face lifting: enhanced facial contour using vicryl mesh incorporated into SMAS fixation. Plast Reconstr Surg. 2000;105(1):290–301.
9. Stuzin JM, Baker TJ, Gordon HL. The relationship of the superficial and deep facial fascias relevance to rhytidectomy and aging. Plast Reconstr Surg. 1992;89(3):441–9.
10. Mendelson BC. SMAS fixation to the facial skeleton: rationale and results. Plast Reconstr Surg. 1997;100(7):1834–42.
11. Mendelson BC. Surgery of the superficial musculoaponeurotic system: principles of release, vectors, and fixation. Plast Reconstr Surg. 2001;107(6):1545–52.
12. Owsley JQ. Superficial musculoaponeurotic system platysma face lift. In: Dudley H, Carter D, Russell RC, editors. Operative surgery. London: Butterworth; 1986.
13. Barton FE. The SMAS and the nasolabial fold. Plast Reconstr Surg. 1992;89(6):1054–7.
14. Keller GS, Cray J. Suprafibromuscular facelifting with periosteal suspension of the superficial musculoaponeurotic system and fat pad of Bichat rotation. Arch Otolaryngol Head Neck Surg. 1996;122(4):377–84.
15. Cardenas Camarena L, Gonzalez LE. Multiple, combined plications of the SMAS- platysma complex: breaking down the face-aging vectors. Plast Reconstr Surg. 1999;104(4):1093–100.
16. Gosain AK, Yousif NJ, Madiedo G, Larson DL, Matloub HS, Sanger JR. Surgical anatomy of the SMAS: a reinvestigation. Plast Reconstr Surg. 1993;92(7):1254–63.
17. Rees TD. The classic operation. In: Rees TD, LaTrenta GS, editors. Aesthetic plastic surgery. Philadelphia: W.B. Saunders; 1994. p. 683–707.
18. Byrd HS, Andochick SE. The deep temporal lift: a multiplanar, lateral brow, temporal, and upper face lift. Plast Reconstr Surg. 1996;97(5):928–37.
19. Williams LP et al. Head and neck. In: Gray's anatomy. 37th ed. New York: Churchill Livingstone; 1992.
20. Gosling JA, Harris PF, Humpherson JR, Whitmore I, Willan PLT. Head and neck. Human Anatomy Coloring Book. Churchill Livingstone; 1996.
21. Har-Shai Y, Bodner SR, Egozy-Golan D, Lindenbaum ES, Ben Izhak O, Mitz V, et al. Mechanical properties and microstructure of the superficial musculoaponeurotic system. Plast Reconstr Surg. 1996;98(1):59–70.
22. Noone RB. Suture suspension malarplasty with SMAS plication and modified SMASectomy: a simplified approach to midface lifting. Plast Reconstr Surg. 2006;117(3):792–803.
23. de Vasconcellos JJ Accioli, Britto JA, Henin D, Vacher C. The fascial planes of the temple and face: an enbloc anatomical study and a plea for consistency. Br J Plast Surg. 2003;56(7):623–9.
24. Gassner HG, Rafii A, Young A, Murakami C, Moe KS, Larrabee WF. Surgical anatomy of the face. implication for modern face-lift techniques. Arch Facial Plast Surg. 2008;10(1):9–19.
25. Hamra ST. The zygorbicular dissection in composite rhytidectomy: an ideal midface plane. Plast Reconstr Surg. 1998;102(5):1646–57.
26. Parry IR, SW BCL, Almand J. The great auricular nerve revisited: pertinent anatomy for SMAS-platysma rhytidectomy. Ann Plast Surg. 1991;27(1):44–8.
27. Hagerty RC. Central suspension technique of the midface. Plast Reconstr Surg. 1995;96(3):728–30.
28. Byrd HS. The extended browlift. Clin Plast Surg. 1997;24(2):233–46.
29. Mendelson BC, Freeman ME, Wu W, Huggins RJ. Surgical anatomy of the lower face: the premasseter space, the jowl, and the labiomandibular fold. Aesthetic Plast Surg. 2008;32(2):185–95.
30. Stuzin JM, Baker TJ. Aging face and neck. In: Mathes JS, editor. Mathes plastic surgery. The head and neck, part 1. Philadelphia: Saunders Elsevier; 2006. p. 159–213.
31. Furnas DW. The retaining ligaments of the cheek. Plast Reconstr Surg. 1989;83:11.
32. Ozdemir R, Kilinç H, Unlü RE, Uysal AC, Sensöz O, Baran CN. Anatomicohistologic study of the retaining ligaments of the face and use in face lift: retaining ligament correction and SMAS plication. Plast Reconstr Surg. 2002;110(4):1134–47; discussion 1148–49.
33. Furnas DW. Strategies for nasolabial levitation. Clin Plast Surg. 1995;22(2):265–78.
34. McGregor M. Face lift techniques. Presented to the annual meeting of the California Society of Plastic Surgeons, Yosemite, 1959.
35. Baker TJ, Stuzin JM. Personal technique of face lifting. Plast Reconstr Surg. 1997;100(2):502–8.
36. Gamboa GM, de La Torre JI, Vasconez LO. Surgical anatomy of the midface as applied to facial rejuvenation. Ann Plast Surg. 2004;52(3):240–5.
37. Barton FE, Gyimesi IM. Anatomy of the nasolabial fold. Plast Reconstr Surg. 1997;100(5):1276–80.
38. Fulton JE. Simultaneous face lifting and skin resurfacing. Plast Reconstr Surg. 1998;102(7):2480–9.
39. Marinetti CJ. The lower muscular balance of the face used to lift labial commissures. Plast Reconstr Surg. 1999;104(4):1153–62.
40. Little JW. Hiding the posterior scar in rhytidectomy: the omega incision. Plast Reconstr Surg. 1999;104(1):259–72.
41. Paul MD, Calvert JW, Evans GR. The evolution of the midface lift in aesthetic plastic surgery. Plast Reconstr Surg. 2006;117(6):1809–27.
42. Whetzel TP, Mathes SJ. The arterial supply of the face lift flap. Plast Reconstr Surg. 1997;100(2):480–6.
43. Skoog T. Plastic surgery: new methods and refinements. Philadelphia: Saunders; 1974.

44. Huggins RJ, Freeman ME, Kerr JB, Mendelson BC. Histologic and ultrastructural evaluation of sutures used for surgical fixation of the SMAS. Aesthetic Plast Surg. 2007;31(6):719–24.
45. Aston SJ, Thorne CH, Rees TD. History. In: Rees TD, LaTrenta GS, editors. Aesthetic plastic surgery. Philadelphia: W.B. Saunders; 1994. p. 658–61.
46. Aston SJ, Thorne CH, Rees TD. Preoperative preparation and evaluation. In: Rees TD, LaTrenta GS, editors. Aesthetic plastic surgery. Philadelphia: W.B. Saunders; 1994. p. 673–7.
47. Herbert JT. Anesthesia for cosmetic surgery. In: Rees TD, LaTrenta GS, editors. Aesthetic plastic surgery. Philadelphia: W.B. Saunders; 1994. p. 678–81.
48. Rees TD, Aston SJ, Thorne CH. Postoperative considerations and complications. In: Rees TD, LaTrenta GS, editors. Aesthetic plastic surgery. Philadelphia: W.B. Saunders; 1994. p. 740–56.

37 Vertical Temporal Lifting: A Short Preauricular–Pretrichal Scar

John Camblin

37.1 Introduction

The cosmetic surgery patient is interested in beautification with minimal scarring and minimal time away from work and social schedule (Figs. 37.1–37.6). Most cosmetic face-lift surgeries have large or visible scars that patients do no want. Recovery from surgery takes days to weeks. Patients wish to return to work or socialize as soon as possible. The technique of a short preauricular–pretrichal scar that is preceded by liposuction of the face and neck gives satisfactory results in a simple manner and with a rapid surgical time.

The simple procedure is done under local anesthesia with or without intravenous sedation. Liposuction of the facial areas is first performed. An incision is made along the superior preauricular area and extended into the pretrichal part of the temporal region. The skin is dissected to the corner of the mouth and the excess that is obtained by strict vertical traction is resected. Three dermoaponeurotic sutures of a nonabsorbable thread involving the malar, jugal, and temporal areas are placed and tied, giving a more lasting result. A fine cross-stitch suture is used to close the skin. This suture is removed in 3 weeks.

37.2 Technique

The patients have the facial aging stigmas that usually necessitate a conventional face-lift (Figs. 37.7–37.18). However, the vertical temporal lifting with a short temporal scar gives the same result and perhaps a more natural look than a classical lifting described by Rees [1] or a sophisticated, but dangerous face-lift, described by Hamra [2].

37.3 Conclusions

This technique is a great asset compared to aesthetic medicine. On the first postoperative day there is cosmetic result of a classical face-lift with minimal surgical care (Figs. 37.19 and 37.20), while aesthetic medicine necessitates several injections to be given to the patient, resulting in an artificial appearance that does not last.

J. Camblin
10 Avenue de L'Opera, 75001, Paris, France
e-mail: john_camblin@yahoo.fr

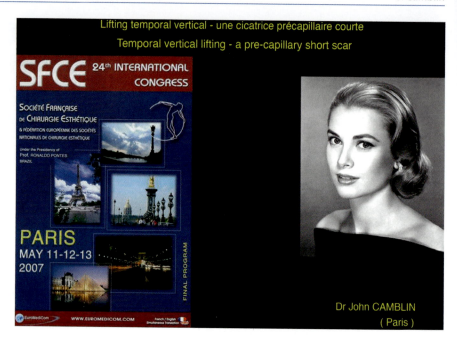

Fig. 37.1 The vertical lifting with a precapillary scar (Presented at the French Aesthetic Surgery Society (SFCE), Paris, May 2007)

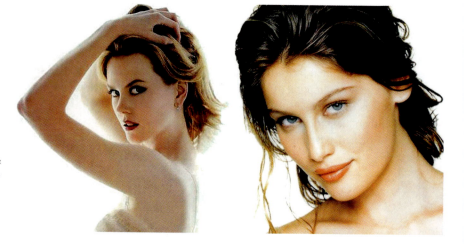

Fig. 37.2 Criterion of facial beauty. The three keys: (1) The external corner of the eye is oblique. (2) The cheekbone and the corner of the mouth are smoothly tilted. (3) The angle of the mandible looks like a capital J

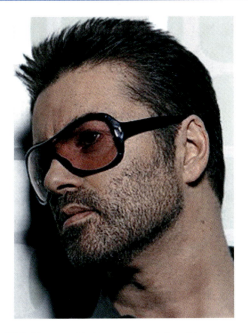

Fig. 37.3 The way this famous singer's beard is cut, gives the typical aspect of a J

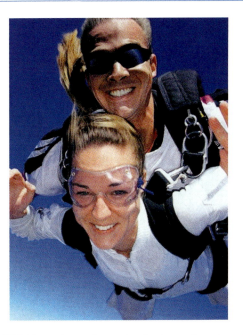

Fig. 37.4 Stupendous rejuvenation is observed on these two parachutists fighting against the air resistance. Vertical traction of the skin results as a vertical face-lift will lift

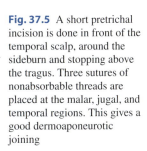

Fig. 37.5 A short pretrichal incision is done in front of the temporal scalp, around the sideburn and stopping above the tragus. Three sutures of nonabsorbable threads are placed at the malar, jugal, and temporal regions. This gives a good dermoaponeurotic joining

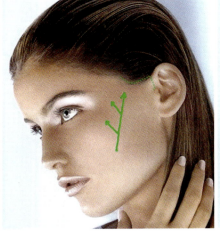
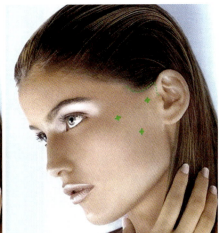

Fig. 37.6 Illusion effect results of the action on the corners of the mouth by a vertical traction. Notice that the same eyes look more attractive and shining when the child is smiling

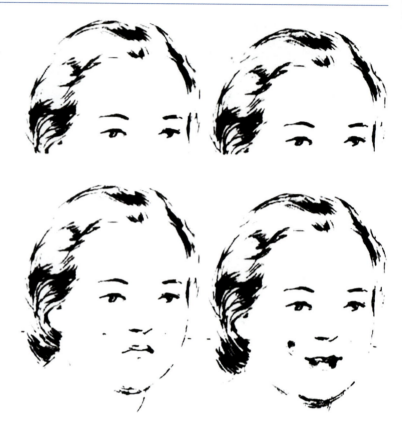

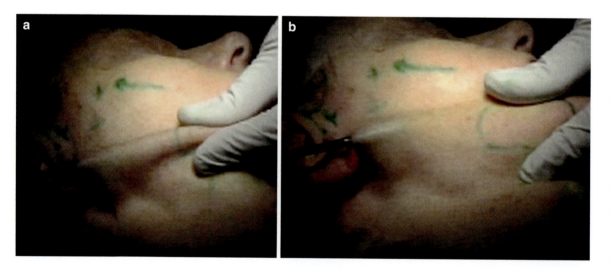

Fig. 37.7 (**a**) Liposuction of the jowls. The fingers are very important to appreciate what is going on. (**b**) When you pull back the cannula, you turn it 180° so that the two holes look superficially and irritate the dermis, facilitating the retraction of the skin

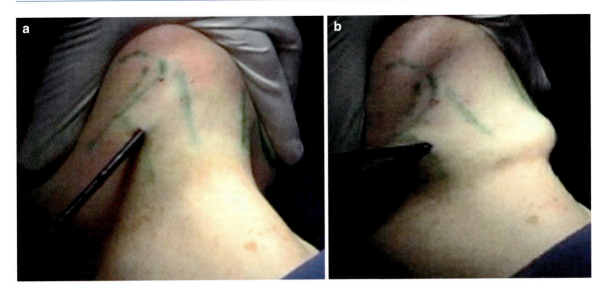

Fig. 37.8 Liposuction of the neck

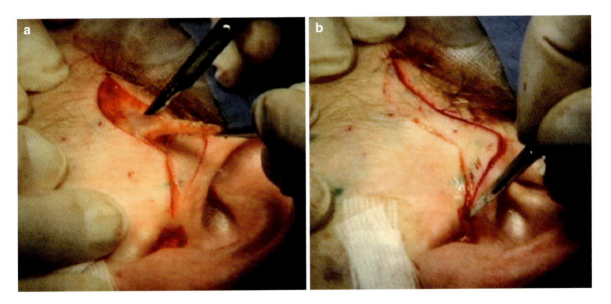

Fig. 37.9 (**a**) The incision of the vertical-lift is short. (**b**) First, a piece of skin is taken off that facilitates the next excision

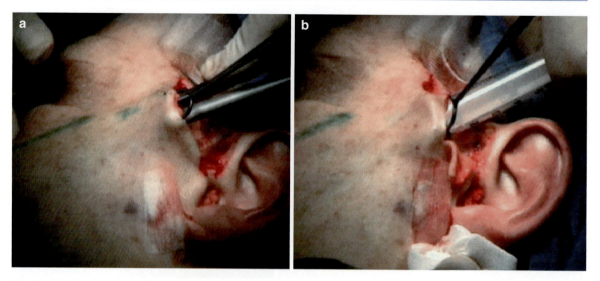

Fig. 37.10 (**a**) Subcutaneous dissection with heavy and thick scissors. (**b**) Vaporization of a hemostatic solution with a syringe

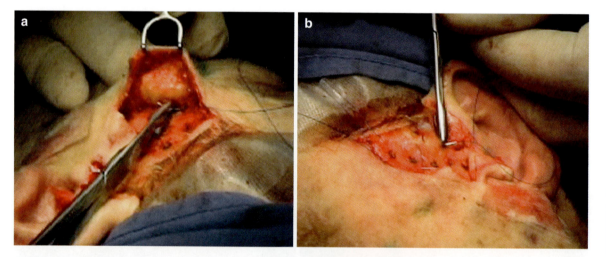

Fig. 37.11 Joining the dermoaponeurosis. (**a**) First, the needle goes across the deep dermis. (**b**) Next the aponeurosis

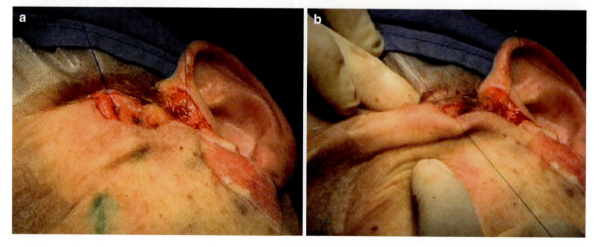

Fig. 37.12 The knots are tied

37 Vertical Temporal Lifting: A Short Preauricular–Pretrichal Scar

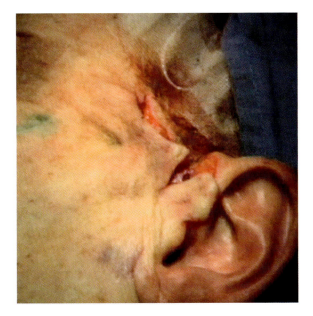

Fig. 37.13 Both flaps resulting from the vertical traction

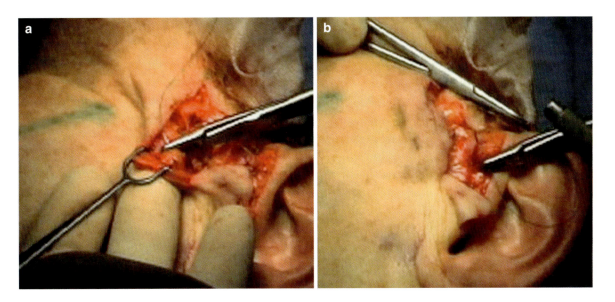

Fig. 37.14 The temporal joining gives better stability to the vertical-lift

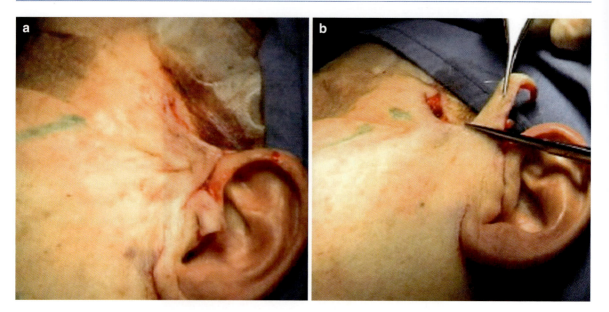

Fig. 37.15 The temporal flap is excised

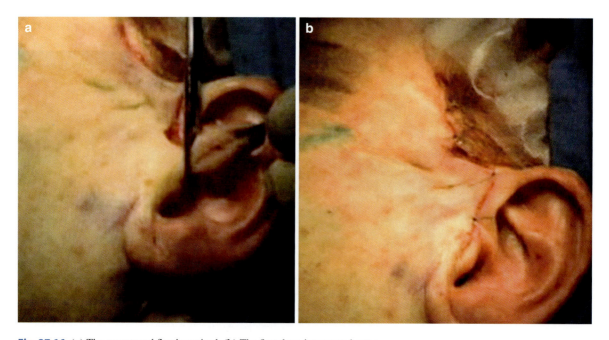

Fig. 37.16 (**a**) The supratragal flap is excised. (**b**) The first three interrupted sutures

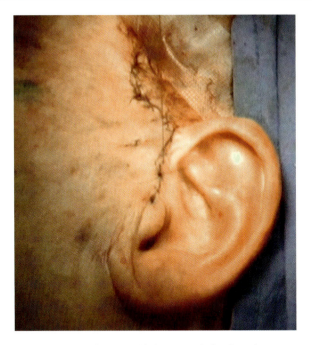

Fig. 37.17 A continuous suture, cross-stitch, is performed. This is removed after 3 weeks

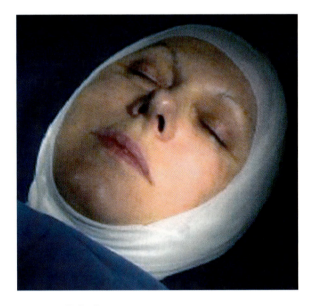

Fig. 37.18 The corners of the mouth are well tilted

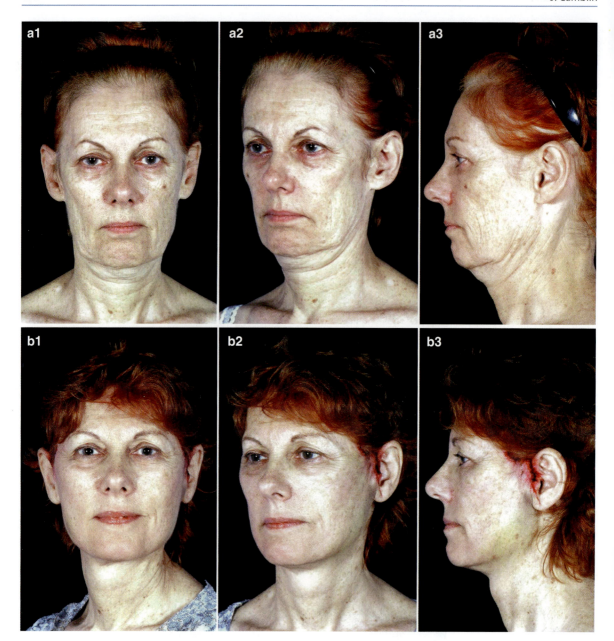

Fig. 37.19 (**a**) Preoperative. (**b**) Postoperative

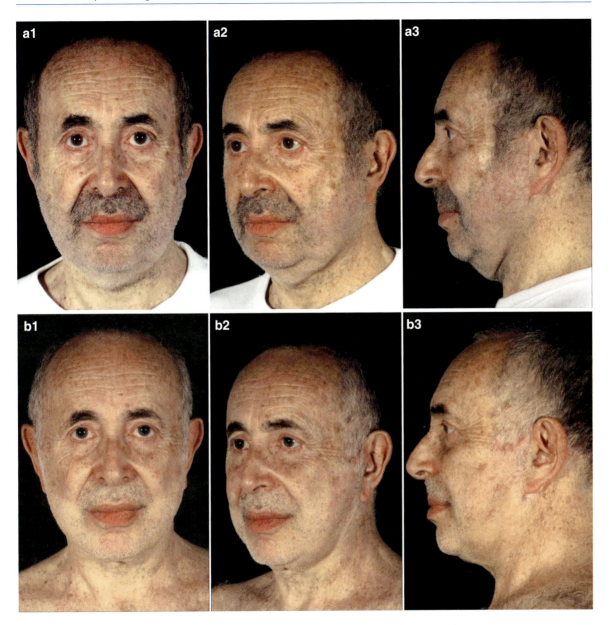

Fig. 37.20 (**a**) Preoperative patient who had undergone previous classical face-lifts. (**b**) Postoperative

References

1. Rees TD, Woodsmith D. Cosmetic facial surgery.: W.B. Saunders; 1973.
2. Hamra ST. Composite rhytidectomy. Philadelphia: Quality Medical Publishing; 1993.

Deep Plane Face-lift: Integrating Safety and Reliability with Results

38

W. Gregory Chernoff

38.1 Introduction

The ongoing improvement in Health Care has yielded an increasingly aged population. As people live longer, healthier lives, they begin to realize that they do not feel as old as they sometimes look. The concurrent improvement in cosmetic surgical techniques has mirrored increased longevity. Worldwide, there has been increased awareness regarding the benefits of cosmetic procedures. Increased awareness has brought about greater acceptance of the concepts of maintenance overruling the stereotypical judgments of vanity. We have therefore seen a younger population of patients in their 30s and 40s seeking aesthetic improvement. This has led to a myriad of modifications to time-tested techniques seeking to decrease invasiveness and healing time. Many trendy techniques have not stood the test of time, especially when longevity of results are objectively studied. Conversely, the ongoing improvement in traditional face-lifting has dramatically improved results.

The acceptance of rhytidectomy in modern times has been slow in the making. A historical perspective on the evolution of this tremendous procedure is found in another chapter of this book. As the procedure has evolved over the years, there has become a greater understanding of facial anatomy, particularly the facial nerve. This enhanced knowledge has led to several modifications, and the subsequent adoption of what are known to be, "deep plane" techniques. There are now many studies from different aesthetic academies highlighting the safety, efficacy, reliability, reproducibility, and the longevity of the results of the procedure.

From a patient's perspective, there are many misconceptions as to what the term "face-lift" means. Many are still intimidated by the term, thinking that everyone who undergoes the operation will end up with a "done" or "over-pulled" look. It is prudent to identify what the patients' preconceived ideas entail. Helping the patient to be realistic as to what to expect, goes a long way to ensuring their satisfaction. Time should be spent in front of a mirror, showing the patient the natural results that can be achieved. They are shown that the entire face is improved with this technique, including the temporal region, the lateral face, the midface, the jaw line, the submental region, platysmal banding, the lateral neck, and the postauricular region. The difference between an overdone look and a natural result can be easily demonstrated to alleviate fears, and educate as to what is realistic to expect. With a successful lift, the scars should be barely noticeable. The hairlines should remain unchanged. Healing time should be no more than a week, with subtle edema resolving over 6 months. Postoperative discomfort should be minimal. Expectations of results should be realistic. Longevity varies from patient to patient. Consistent, long lasting results are the norm to be attained. The patient can expect to always look better having done the procedure than if they had not.

The decision to perform a deep plane lift versus a previously traditional SMAS elevation is based upon the patients' anatomy. This procedure is geared toward the middle-aged patient who is concerned about the relative flattening of the midface, due to decent of the malar fat pad and facial musculature, deepening of the nasolabial folds, decent of the jowl below the oral commissure, and presence of submalar fat in conjunction with loose submalar skin and obvious platysmal banding.

W.G. Chernoff
Chernoff Cosmetic Surgery,
Indianapolis, IN, USA
e-mail: greg@drchernoff.com

An appreciation of the patients' motivation is important. The patient should exhibit a healthy sense of self-esteem. They should be seeking improvement in appearance for themselves, not in an effort to please anyone else in their life. The physician should have an understanding of the condition, Body Dysmorphic Disorder. Questions relating to this underdiagnosed condition should be posed to the patient to ensure they do not suffer from it. No cosmetic procedure should be performed on an individual with BDD. Refer the patient to a psychologist if in question.

38.2 Preoperative Evaluation

A thorough history and pertinent physical examination are important. Any prior surgery should be discussed, with attention to healing patterns. Any preponderance to irregular wound healing, and scarring should be noted. Smokers should not be operated on. A period of 6 months smoke free is preferred. The consequences of poor healing, poor scars, and possible skin necrosis are made clear. A list of medications which should be avoided due to blood thinning should be provided to the patient.

Any medical or surgical issue that would preclude any elective surgical procedure is a contraindication for a face-lift. Medical evaluation and clearance should be sought for any patient that possesses any condition that may adversely affect their health should they undergo the surgery. Say "No" when your gut tells you to. It is seldom wrong.

Preoperative blood work should include a CBC, electrolytes, and bleeding profile. The surgeon should review and sign off on all blood work. Appropriate preoperative photographs should accompany the surgeon into the operating room to act as a road map during the surgery.

38.3 Preoperative Markings

As each patient is different, the marking varies proportionate to the intricacies of each case (Fig. 38.1). The basics are the same and these will be highlighted. Remember what the patient sees and talks about… visible, unsightly, scars, and their hair, especially if there is loss or change in the hair line.

The most controversial portion of the deep plane face-lift is the temporal extension of the incision above the root of the helix. Most authors extend the incision

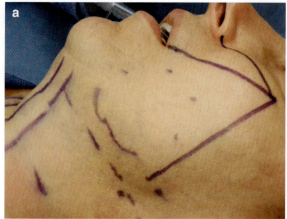

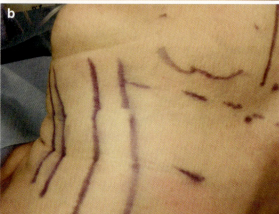

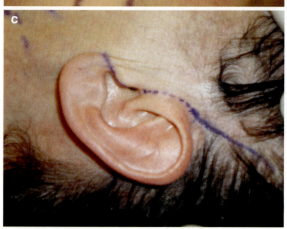

Fig. 38.1 (**a**) External landmarks defined in preoperative patient. The malar eminence is marked. *Lines* are drawn along the course of the zygomatic muscles. The angle of the mandible to the eminence is drawn. The course of the body of the mandible is identified. (**b**) Extent of submental and submandibular dissection. (**c**) Posttragal marking

superiorly from the helical attachment for 5–6 cm. They make this to facilitate the placement of a suture between the elevated scalp and the underlying deep temporal fascia, and to mobilize the temporal scalp to the temporal line. This author does not routinely make this superior extension, unless a composite procedure is necessary to sling the orbicularis muscle laterally. This can cause skin redundancy in the temporal region which necessitates this superior extension. It is not felt by the author that the amount of posterior pull in the temporal region justifies the visible temporal scar that most of these patients complain about several years down the road once they start to lose hair in this region.

The incision is carried inferiorly, behind the tragus in women and men. Most men do not mind shaving up to the tragus if it lessens the visibility of the preauricular component of the incision. This is especially true in patients who do not have a deep natural preauricular fold to hide the incision. The marking then extends inferiorly, around the lobule of the ear, and continues posterosuperiorly on the conchal bowl and then into the hairline where the helix meets the hair. The origin of the zygomatic major and minor muscles is marked at the anterior inferior malar eminence. A line is drawn from this point to the oral commissure. This marks the path of the zygomaticus major. Another line is drawn from this point to the nasal ala, marking the path of the zygomaticus minor muscle. The nasolabial fold occurs between the skin insertions of these two muscles. A line is also drawn from the zygomatic origin to the angle of the mandible. Another line is drawn from the angle of the mandible, along the body of the mandible, toward the chin. The anterior limits of the platysmal bands are also marked.

A submental incision is planned a few millimeters anterior to the natural crease. This allows for the advancement of submental tissues during the imbrications of the platysmal muscle. This allows for the reduction or softening of any "witches' chin" crease that may exist. If a concurrent blepharoplasty or endoscopic brow-lift is performed, these markings are also made with the patient in the sitting position prior to entering the operating room.

38.4 Anesthesia

Improvements in anesthesia techniques have mirrored improvements in operative procedures. Shorter half-lives of medications, a broader scope of induction and maintenance techniques have improved the efficacy and safety of these procedures. The choice of monitored intravenous sedation versus general anesthesia is based upon the comfort of the surgeon and patient with these different techniques. Care should be exercised when offering monitored intravenous sedation. The patient with a short attention span, the easily agitated patient, or the continuous talker, should be advised toward a general anesthetic. MAC versus general is also an anesthesiologist-dependent choice based upon their expertise.

The last thing the operating surgeon needs is to have his attention diverted away from the rejuvenation task at hand to worry about a substandard anesthetic. The choice of anesthesiologist is as important as the patient selection. Experience with cosmetic procedures, and a confidence of the same is required. This is especially true relating to intraoperative induced hypotension, intraoperative steady state, smooth reversal with no coughing or bucking, no nausea, and meticulous postop pain and comfort control. A bad anesthetic will overshadow a great face-lift in the eyes of a patient, and their friends are sure to hear about it.

Once intravenous (IV) sedation or general anesthesia is initiated, subcutaneous infiltration is commenced. The author prefers 0.5% Lidocaine with epinephrine 1:100,000. Initially the neck and left side of the face are infiltrated. At the point of skin suturing on the left face, the right face is infiltrated. This timing provides for optimal vasoconstriction and divides the total amount of infiltrative anesthesia over a greater amount of time. A 25 gauge 1.5 in. needle in a 10 ml syringe is used to infiltrate for a gentle delivery. The first incision is made 10 min after the infiltration process was initiated.

38.5 Deep Plane Technique

The procedure is started in the submental region. A #15 blade is used to make the skin incision anterior to the natural submental crease. Usually, a 2 cm incision is made. This allows for liposuction and adequate visualization and instrumentation for platysmal imbrications. A modified Freeman Rhytidectomy Scissor is used to elevate the submental and submandibular subcutaneous tissue from the platysmal muscle. A single hook is used for retraction during scissor elevation. A flat 4 mm cannula is used to remove excess fat from the region and off the surface of the platysmal. Care is taken to leave 2–3 mm of fat on the dermis so as to avoid any surface irregularities. The extent of dissection inferiorly is to the level of the thyroid cartilage, laterally to the anterior border of the sternocleidomastoid muscles. A determination is then made as whether to imbricate or simply plicate the platysmal bands. This is a crucial decision point as the anterior neck is what the patient looks at in the mirror all the time.

Failure to provide the sharpest defined neck versus not skeletonizing the platysmal muscle is the tightrope the surgeon walks. Preoperative lateral views with the patient respecting the Frankfurt Plane will reveal the answer to the surgeon.

The majority of patients will benefit from subplatysmal dissection of excess fat. A right angle retractor is held by the surgical assistant. The surgeon grasps the most anterior portion of the platysmal bands with a forceps and progressively pinches inferiorly to determine the safe amount of muscle edge to excise. Less is better. At the conclusion, there can be no tension on the sutured muscle bands so as to avoid dehiscence of the suture repair and subsequent unsightly skeletonization of the anterior neck. Once the redundant muscle has been excised, the subplatysmal fat is grasped sequentially, superior to inferior, again to determine the safe amount for excision. This is a vascular area, and a bipolar forceps is used to sequentially cauterize the fat prior to each scissor cut. The excess fat is removed to the level of the thyroid cartilage. The bipolar is then used to sculpt any residual fatty contour anomalies. Clean platysmal edges are desired prior to suturing. Beginning just superior to the thyroid notch, sequential 3–0 Proline buried sutures are used to approximate the freshly cut platysmal edges. During this process, the patients' neck is hyperextended. This allows for smooth approximation and an element of anterior advancement of the muscle which allows for filling in of ant submental depression which may have accentuated a "witches chin" appearance preoperatively. Additional subcutaneous undermining at the lateral edges of the incision is frequently required as a medial indrawing occurs with the platysmal suturing which impedes skin draping and the final contour. Once happy with the neck contour and the proper skin redraping setup, the lateral face can be addressed. The submental incision is left open, covered with moist gauze until the end of the procedure so as to ensure meticulous hemostasis.

Attention is then directed to the lateral face. A #15 blade is again used to make the skin incision. The tissue is grasped with a hook superior to the tragus, and the tissue first dissected off the tragus with the assistant providing medial counter-traction. There must be no damage to the tragus during this stage so as to not create any unnatural contour deficits postoperatively. The skin is elevated from the zygoma in a deep subcutaneous plane, moving in an anterior direction to the skin marked by the line between the malar eminence and the angle of the mandible (Fig. 38.2). This elevation is completed by the outward observance of the progressing scissor tip without internal direct view.

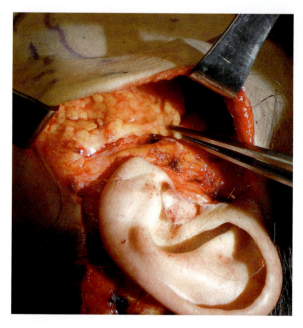

Fig. 38.2 The extent of sharp dissection in the midcheek. The anterior line of sharp dissection between the malar eminence and the angle of the mandible is the posterior margin of the deep plane dissection

If the temporal extension is utilized, the rhytidectomy scissor is used to dissect down to the deep temporalis fascia. Blunt finger dissection is used to separate the superficial temporalis fascia above from the deep temporalis fascia below. These tissues are separated to the temporal line. At this point there is a deep plane of dissection over the deep temporalis fascia and a superficial plane of dissection over the lateral face. The superficial dissection should not go below the line marked along the body of the mandible. The tissue between the superficial and deep dissection contains the superficial temporal artery and vein. The frontal branch of the seventh nerve lies just anterior to the superficial temporal artery. The artery and vein are transected and carefully cauterized so as to lend to adequate posterior mobility of the flap.

After the superior deep dissection is completed, attention is directed to the postauricular dissection. The scalpel is used to complete the skin incision. The rhytidectomy scissor is then used to elevate the flap anteriorly to the angle of the mandible. The cervical dissection separates the platysmal muscle from the neck skin in the subcutaneous plane from the angle of the mandible to the level of the thyroid notch, thus communicating the central submental dissection with the lateral neck dissection. This will ensure smooth redraping of the skin envelope upon completion of the deep muscle lifting. This will ensure longevity of results.

The final portion of the procedure is the anterior face, where the deep plane-lift is performed. A long-blade lighted retractor is recommended for this maneuver. The deep plane dissection divides the face into thirds. The dissection over the masseter muscle is the lower third. Care must be taken here, not to extend the lower dissection deep to the zygomatic muscles. These muscles are innervated on their deep surface, and dissection deep to them carries risk of nerve damage. With the scissor over the masseter muscle, a firm downward motion with the blade on the belly of the muscle is made while opening and closing the scissor. The muscle is easily identified with its deep red color and thin white vertical striations. At this point the surgeon is deep to platysmal inferiorly. Continued dissection is easy by opening the scissor at right angle to masseter. This plane is carried inferior and anterior below the area of jowl fat. Next, dissection is taken over the superior surface of the zygomatic muscles. The tissue is more adherent here than over the masseter. The deep subcutaneous plane is separated until the insertion of the zygomatic major is observed anterior and inferior to the malar eminence. Continuing anteriorly, the zygomatic minor will be encountered lying more toward the nasal ala. Once at this point, notice that the scissor is in a triangle formed by the oral commissure, nasal ala, and the malar eminence. With the upper and lower thirds of the anterior face completed, the middle third is completed by opening the scissor again at right angles to the skin. The buccal nerve will be encountered here. As spreading with the scissor parallel to the nerve is the method used, there is little chance for nerve damage here. If there is excessive cheek fullness, the buccal fat pad can be sculpted at this point. This is a vascular fatty pedicle, so care and caution must be exercised when teasing out the fat.

Upon completion of the dissection, the entire composite flap of midface skin and malar fat pad becomes mobilized. The vector of pull is parallel to the body of the mandible. This repositions the malar fat pad superiorly and brings back the youthful bulk of the midface. Fixation and closure are very important. Care must

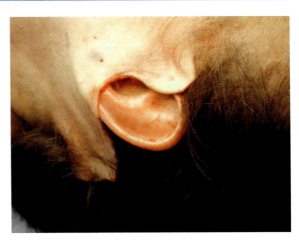

Fig. 38.3 Excess skin is redraped

be taken to adequately reposition the tissue so as to achieve the desired pull. There is a fine line between enough pull and too much, yielding an overdone or "too tight" look. There can be no tension on the skin closure or unsightly scars will follow.

The posterior margin of the platysmal is first addressed. If traction reveals posterior mobility, several 3–0 Proline sutures are used to anchor the platysmal to the capsule of the sternocleidomastoid muscle beneath the earlobe where it is secured. This further tightens the jaw line in addition to the imbrications that was performed in the submental region. In some patients, a bridge of soft tissue is left attached to the body of the mandible to allow a tight closure at this point. Additional 3–0 imbrication sutures are placed, securing the lateral superficial musculoaponeurotic system (SMAS) to the tissue anterior to the tragus and inferior to the zygoma. The composite flap is anchored to the deep temporalis fascia, just above the ear. This suture stabilizes the malar fat pad on the malar eminence. Number 10 Jackson-Pratt drains are inserted and secured with 2–0 silk.

The skin is then redraped (Fig. 38.3). No tension should be placed on the skin. The posterior skin flap is set so as not to change the hairline. A 3–0 Vicryl suture is used here. Excess skin is trimmed and a layered closure obtained with 3–0 chromic and 5–0 Proline interrupted sutures to facilitate meticulous tailoring of tissue. Surgical clips (staples) are not used. The lobule of the ear is set ensuring no tethering, one of the worst signs of a poorly executed face-lift closure. Similarly, the anterior skin is excised. A tragal fixation suture of

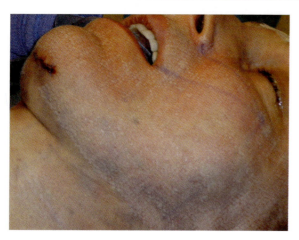

Fig. 38.4 Submental incision closed

3–0 chromic is placed to avoid blunting, one of the surgical telltale signs of a sloppy face-lift. Layered closure anteriorly is performed using 4-0 chromic followed by a 6–0 Proline followed by a 5–0 fast absorbing cat gut. The opposite side is performed in an exact manner to the first side. The submental incision is closed lastly, in a layered fashion using 4–0 chromic followed by 6–0 Proline (Fig. 38.4).

Most patients also undergo CO_2 laser skin exfoliation at the same time. This allows for simultaneous qualitative improvement of the skin at the same time that the gravitational issues are addressed with the face-lift. A light feathering is performed over the elevated skin, while a therapeutic level of exfoliation is performed over the skin of the central zone of the face which was subjected to the deep plane dissection. This does not prolong healing time, and dramatically improves the final aesthetic result. At the conclusion of the procedure, a rhytidectomy dressing is applied, and left on overnight.

38.6 Postoperative Care

The author keeps all rhytidectomy patients overnight. This provides a stress-free course for the patient and family members alike. Reversal of anesthesia is gradual. Postoperative nausea is guarded against religiously. The patient is kept calm, relaxed, and encouraged throughout. The nursing staff suctions the drains every hour for the first 8 h, then every 2 h until discharge. The dressing is removed the following morning. The drains are removed if drainage is minimal. The laser-resurfaced tissue is cleaned. The patients' family members are educated on postoperative care and psychological positive reinforcement. Any edema, bruising is reviewed. The patient is given a glimpse of the result but encouraged to not "microevaluate." The patient is encouraged to ambulate, shower, and resume a normal diet on day 1. One week off work is typical.

The patient is seen daily for the first week, weekly for the next month, then monthly for 6 months. Preauricular sutures are removed on day 7, postauricular sutures removed on day 10. Final postoperative photographs are taken at 6 months.

38.7 Complications

The patient who undergoes a deep plane face-lift is at risk for the usual problems and complications following any face-lift. Generally, the incidence should be 1% or less. These would include infection, bleeding, hematoma, and fifth nerve and seventh nerve weakness. Meticulous surgical technique, coupled with unwavering anatomical knowledge keeps the latter two complications minimal at best. Pencil-thin scars are achieved with tension-free, layered, nonstapled closures, using only finesse hand-sewing. Hair lines are preserved and tragus and lobule irregularities are avoided. Never is there a "pulled" appearance. At all times, from consultation onward, a realistic expectation by the patient is fostered.

38.8 Discussion

There has traditionally been an aura of uncertainty regarding the deep plane face-lift. This historically was propagated by those who felt the procedure subjected the patient to riskier anatomic dissection with subsequent prolonged healing. The same group felt the long-term results did not warrant the perceived additional risks.

The past decade has shown an acceptance of the procedure, particularly for the patient with the heavier neck, flatter midface, deeper nasolabial fold, and fuller jowl. It is especially beneficial with the patient who also has malar festoons. These patients benefit from the additional elevation of the lateral inferior orbicularis over the bony rim, which complements elevation of the malar fat pad. As with other lifting procedures, the deep plane-lift is routinely combined with brow-lift, blepharoplasty, and laser exfoliation. Most authors' experience with the operation has been positive. Initial concerns of a prolonged recovery time are unfounded.

Perhaps the greatest advantage has been the added longevity, particularly in the patient populations identified. These were the patients who, with a traditional SMAS-lift, were seeing a higher revision rate when looseness earlier than expected arose. The use of the composite flap, deep plane rhytidectomy is a valuable addition to the armamentarium of the cosmetic surgeon seeking safe, reliable, and reproducible results.

Recommended Reading

Baker SR. Tri-plane rhytidectomy. Combining the best of all worlds. Arch Otolaryngol Head Neck Surg. 1997;123(11): 1167–72.

Godin MS, Johnson Jr CM. Deep plane composite rhytidectomy. Facial Plast Surg. 1996;12(3):231–9.

Hamra ST. The deep-plane rhytidectomy. Plast Reconstr Surg. 1990;86(1):53–61.

Hamra ST. Composite rhytidectomy. Plast Reconstr Surg. 1992;90(1):1–13.

Hamra ST. The composite rhytidectomy. St. Louis: Quality Medical Publishing; 1993.

Kamer FM. One hundred consecutive deep plane face-lifts. Arch Otolaryngol Head Neck Surg. 1996;122(1):17–22.

Subperiosteal Face-Lift

Lucas G. Patrocinio, Marcell M. Naves, Tomas G. Patrocinio, and Jose A. Patrocinio

39.1 Introduction

Fullness of the cheek represents youthfulness. Aging process initiates during the third decade and in response to gravitational forces, the fat and soft tissue of the cheek drift downward in relation to the underlying bony skeleton. In this process of aging, a constant hollowness of the midface develops. As a result, a patient may display an appearance that is tired, old, or sad [1].

Weakening of the malar and orbital ligaments is a major component of the aging process. The result is a downward and medial displacement of the malar fat pad and other soft tissues over the fixed ligaments of the nasolabial fold. The fat over the malar eminence is left standing, accentuating the malar bag. Another anatomical change that occurs is the weakening of the orbital ligaments that contributes to hollowness under the orbit. The malar fat pad, which in youth was at the level of the orbital rim, falls downward and medially, producing this hollowness. This concavity that is below the convexity of the ocular globe and orbital fat, accentuates and no longer covers the bulge of herniated orbital fat. This produces the "double contour" deformity characteristic of the aging orbital/midface complex. A volume loss of the midface also contributes to the aging process. Finally, the collapse of the zygomaticus major and minor muscles, which suspend the ligamentous and muscular connections of the midface, results in a droop of the corner of the mouth and deepens the labiomental fold (Fig. 39.1) [2].

The purpose of the face-lift procedure is to reverse the aging process that has occurred. This can be achieved through various techniques that have been developed to date. The evolution of face rejuvenation consists in deciding which facial plane is going to be accessed [3].

At the beginning of the nineteenth century, the prior technique consisted of interrupted incisions placed both in front of and behind the ears in natural wrinkles and were combined with limited strips of excised skin. Then in the beginning of the twentieth century, there were the first descriptions of extensive skin undermining and lipectomy. More recently, the discovery of the SMAS (subcutaneous muscle-aponeurotic system) improved the technique (plication, suture, partial sectioning, etc.) aiming for long-lasting results. Trying to address the nasolabial fold, which so far has not been modified by other techniques, the deep plane and composite face-lift were described. They consisted of a deep SMAS dissection, accessing the nasolabial fold; however, their use has been increasingly questioned because of the risk of facial nerve injury [4].

Recent studies emphasize the central third of the face, often referred as midface, the most difficult region of the face to effectively address. In 1979, with the subperiosteal approach, Tessier [5] has revolutionized the treatment of the aging face reducing signs of aging

L.G. Patrocinio (✉)
Division of Facial Plastic, Department of Otolaryngology, Medical School, Federal University of Uberlandia, Uberlandia, Minas Gerais, Brazil and
Rua Arthur Bernardes, 555 – 1o. andar, Uberlândia, Minas Gerais 38400-368, Brazil
e-mail: lucaspatrocinio@clinicaotoface.com.br

M.M. Naves and T.G. Patrocinio
Division of Facial Plastic, Department of Otolaryngology, Medical School, Federal University of Uberlandia, Uberlandia, Minas Gerais, Brazil
e-mail: marcellnaves@yahoo.com.br;
tomaspatrocinio@hotmail.com

J.A. Patrocinio
Department of Otolaryngology, Medical School, Federal University of Uberlandia, Uberlandia, Minas Gerais, Brazil
e-mail: patrocinio@clinicaotoface.com.br

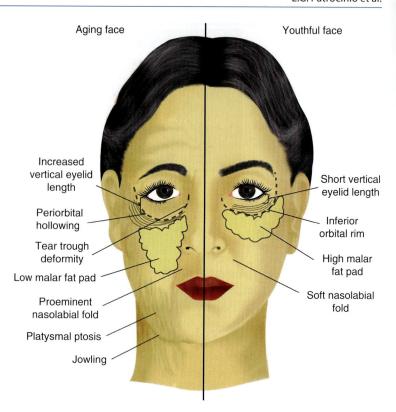

Fig. 39.1 Aged anatomical findings shown on the *right* and youthful contours shown on the *left*

in young and middle-aged patients. Following the studies of Tessier, Psillakis [6, 7], Santana [8], and others have improved the application of subperiosteal dissection in face rejuvenation. Ramirez [9, 10] led to the popularization of this technique in United States with the introduction of the endoscope.

The authors describe their preferred technique for subperiosteal face-lift and discuss its indications, complications, advantages, and limitations.

39.2 Technique

39.2.1 Preoperative Evaluation

A complete medical history has to be obtained before any aesthetic surgery of the face, including allergies, medications, medical problems, previous surgery, and drinking and smoking habits. Smoking cessation is advocated before and after surgery; however, patient disagreement may not affect final results due to the thickness of the flap created during the subperiosteal face-lift. As well, emotional and psychological evaluation is important for elective aesthetic surgery. Preoperative photographs are essential, helping on preoperative planning, intraoperative decisions, patient communication, and medicolegal documentation. At the time of the preoperative consultation the patients are oriented about the planned procedure with written and verbal information provided. Written informed consent is also requested [3].

Subperiosteal face-lift is especially advantageous to patients who had undergone other face-lift procedures, need skin resurfacing, soft tissue augmentation, skeletal disproportion, and patients who need alloplastic implants. The association to forehead-lift is common and produces excellent results [11, 12]. Ramirez [9, 10] and Psillakis [6, 7] demonstrated that subperiosteal face-lift could be applied across the full spectrum of facial aging.

39.2.2 Surgical Technique

The surgery is usually performed with the patient under sedation and local anesthesia (2% lidocaine with

1:100,000 epinephrine) is infiltrated in all areas of planned surgery for anesthesia and vasoconstriction.

Important anatomic structures to consider are the frontal branch of the seventh nerve and the infraorbital neurovascular bundle. The important dissection planes include the dissection deep to the temporoparietal fascia along the deep layer of the deep temporalis fascia and the subperiosteal midface dissection. The surgical technique is divided into three major steps: (1) the endoscopic creation of a temporal pocket, (2) mobilization of the midface by subperiosteal dissection, and (3) elevation and suspension of the mobilized midface to the deep temporalis fascia.

In the temporal region, a 5 cm incision, perpendicular to the temporal line, is placed 3 cm behind the hairline. The dissection is performed to identify the deep layer of the deep temporalis fascia (Fig. 39.2). As the pocket is enlarged, the endoscope is introduced for visualization. The frontal branch of the seventh nerve is contained in the overlying temporoparietal fascia that is analogous to the SMAS found in the lower face, facilitating the mobilization of the entire zygomatic arch periosteum and protecting the frontal branch of the facial nerve from injury. Identification of the superficial temporal fat pad is an important landmark that assures the surgeon that the frontal branch of the facial nerve is lateral to the endoscope.

The dissection continues medially and inferiorly exposing the medial third of the zygomatic arch and orbital rim. An incision is made on the zygoma periosteum and lower subperiosteal elevation is performed to malar imminence, gingival buccal sulcus, and nasolabial fold. It is important to respect the arcus marginalis, the confluence of the periosteum of the orbital rim and the periorbital, in order to minimize the risk of edema and lid eversion in the final result. Care is taken to avoid damage to the infraorbital nerve.

The dissection is extended to the pyriform aperture medially, the oral vestibular mucosa inferiorly, and the superior/anterior border of the masseter muscle laterally. All the dissection detach the eyelids, external canthi and Lockwood ligaments, parotid fascia inferiorly and temporalis fascia superiorly, zygomatic muscles and levator labii superioris, and other muscles from their superior origins (Fig. 39.3). The periosteum is very thin medially and a careful dissection avoids muscle injury.

The final step involves suspension of the mobilized midface to the deep temporal fascia by using three 2–0 polyester sutures (Ethibond, Ethicon, Inc., Somerville, NJ) to secure the cheek. The sutures are crossed and secured to the deep temporalis fascia, creating appropriate superior and lateral vectors of force. Systematization of the midface lifting is made by three main points: Bichat's fat pad, malar fat pad, and suborbicularis oculi fat (SOOF) (Fig. 39.4). The first point is the "B point" (Bichat's fat pad). It is located at a point of intersection of a vertical line from the lateral canthus and a horizontal line from the nasal base. Suspension of this point promotes volumetric augmentation of the midface, elevation of the corner of the

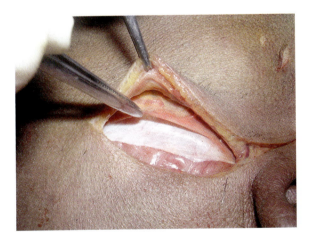

Fig. 39.2 Cadaver dissection showing the temporoparietal fascia (forceps) and the underlying deep temporalis fascia

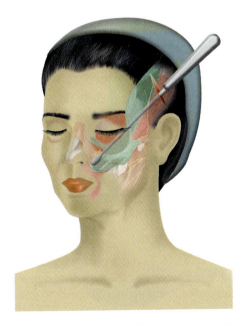

Fig. 39.3 Extent of undermining for the transtemporal subperiosteal face-lift

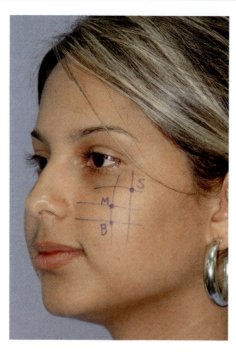 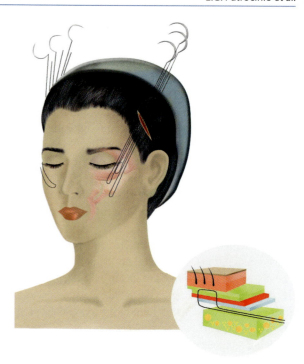

Fig. 39.4 Systematization of the three main points for midface lifting: Bichat's fat pad ("B point"), malar fat pad ("M point"), and sub-orbicularis oculi fat ("S point")

Fig. 39.5 Midface suspension by sutures anchored to the deep temporalis fascia

mouth, and restoration of a triangular face. The second point is the "M point" (malar fat pad) and it is located in a point of intersection of the same previous vertical line and a horizontal line from the superior margin of the nasal ala. The third point is the "S point" (SOOF). This point is located in a point of intersection of a vertical line form the most lateral portion of the brow and a horizontal line from the inferior orbital rim.

These three previously marked points are lifted using Casagrande needle (similar to Reverdin needle) for passing the 2–0 polyester suture (Fig. 39.4). The needle is introduced transcutaneous through the "B point" and, with endoscopic view, is driven through the temporal incision. Then, the polyester suture is passed through the needle's guide-hole and is returned to the Bichat's fat pad area. Keeping the needle inside the soft tissues, a change of direction is performed to grasp more tissue, and the needle is driven to the temporal incision again. There, the suture is removed from the needle and sutured to the deep temporalis fascia. The same procedure is performed at the "M point" and the "S point," bilaterally (Fig. 39.5).

At the deep temporalis fascia, the Bichat's fat pad is suspended and sutured medially, the malar fat pad centrally, and the SOOF laterally. Such fixation lengthens the zygomatic muscles and the soft tissue of the cheeks, correcting tear-trough deformity, softening the nasolabial fold. The zygomatic area is also well modeled because the zygomatic muscle insertions are reinserted in a higher position (Fig. 39.6).

The temporal scalp incision is closed by securing the temporoparietal fascia from the anterior edge of the incision to the deep temporalis fascia posteriorly. The skin is sutured with uninterrupted 4–0 nylon (Ethilon, Ethicon, Inc., Somerville, NJ). A compressive bandage is kept on during the first 6–10 h postoperatively. Supportive taping is placed for 7 days, when the skin sutures are removed. Antibiotics are started prior to surgery and continued for 7 days after surgery.

39.3 Complications

In spite of all care during the surgery, complications can occur. Well-recognized complications of face-lift surgery include hematoma, hair loss, skin slough, hypertrophic scarring, infection, and motor nerve or sensory nerve injury. Major complications including cardiopulmonary emergency, anesthetic disaster, or death are fortunately extremely rare [13, 14].

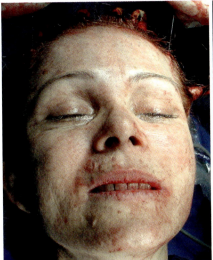 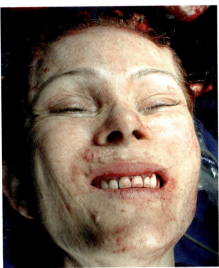

Fig. 39.6 Preoperative (*left*) and immediate (*right*) postoperative outcome of the midface-lift when the surgeon pulls the sutures

Hematoma and seroma are the commonest complication after face-lift. Major hematomas occur in the first 10–12 h postoperatively, due to hypertension, medication use, bleeding abnormality, intraoperative technique, cough, retching, and agitation. Expanding hematoma is a feared complication requiring prompt return to operative room for inspection, hemostasis, supportive taping, and compressive dressing. Due to the bloodless plane of dissection, hematomas are extremely rare. Small hematomas and seromas can be either observed, needle aspirated, or rolled through openings in the incision within the postauricular hairline.

Long-lasting edema, sometimes more than 1 month, may occur and is due to the extensive undermining, especially at the zygomatic arch. It is advocated to avoid dissection over the whole zygomatic arch. Massage is recommended after 7 days of surgery.

Nerve injury is one of the frightening complications for patients. Nerve damage is frequently transient as a result of anesthetic infiltration, direct injection into the nerve, blunt dissection injury, edema of the nerve sheath, traction, or cautery trauma. Injury of branches of the facial nerve can be prevented with a careful dissection under the superficial layer of the deep temporal fascia, as the temporal branch of the facial nerve is located superficially within the temporoparietal fascia. Temporary numbness is caused by interruption of small sensory branches. Sensibility always recovers although it may take months to do so.

Hypertrophic scarring is frequently attributable to excessive tension on the incision closure. Nevertheless, some patients develop hypertrophic scars despite the best efforts of the surgeon. Diluted triamcinolone can be injected into the scars, and usually improves the appearance of the scar considerably.

Asymmetries are rare. They are usually due to the learning curve of the procedure. Careful bilateral suture of the three points of suspension, using the lateral canthus as a parameter is an important rule to follow. An augmentation of the face width may be noted, due to fat pads repositioning in a superior and lateral position.

Patient satisfaction is imperative for face-lift surgery. Although physicians try to help patients understand why complications occur, patients do not fully expect that complications will happen to them. Indeed, any complication detracts from the quality of the outcome. As such, it is difficult for both surgeons and patients to accept complications.

39.4 Discussion

The earliest recorded contributions to the field of facial plastic surgery came from ancient Egypt and India over 2,500 years ago. In 1901, surgeons in Germany performed the first modern face-lift [15]. In these procedures, they excised ellipses of facial skin without any tissue undermining. In 1920 and 1921, Bettman [16] and Bourguet [17] were independently credited with the first subcutaneous rhytidectomy. Unlike previous procedures, this one consisted of extensive undermining and lipectomy. This subcutaneous face-lift was the face-lift most commonly performed prior to the 1970s. Subcutaneous dissection of a variably sized skin flap in the face and neck is performed, followed by redraping of the skin flap, excising the excess skin, and closing the incisions, mostly indicated on young, thin individuals with minimal ptosis of deep structures and no submental fullness. Advantages of this technique include ease of operation, limited postoperative edema due to limited dissection, no risk of facial nerve injury, and a smooth contour of the face immediately following the procedure. The major disadvantage of the subcutaneous lift is the fact that the deeper tissues of the neck have not been lifted.

More recently, technique modifications have occurred to address the dissatisfaction with the lack of long-term correction that occurred with the "classic" skin undermining from the procedures described in the early 1900s. In 1974, Skoog [18] described a technique in which the fascia and platysma muscle were undermined to the level of the nasolabial fold and jowl in an attempt to address the lower third of the face. In 1976, the discovery of the superficial musculoaponeurotic system (SMAS) by Mitz and Peyronie [19] confirmed the existence of a fascial layer investing the facial mimetic musculature. It is also important to note that this was the first approach that advocated the effectiveness of imbrication as a rhytidectomy technique. The SMAS may be incorporated into the face-lift operation in several ways. Making an effort for a longer-lasting procedure, the SMAS dissection and plication, or partial sectioning, can be done; however, this procedure has a longer learning period.

During the past 30 years, various modifications and changes to these traditional face-lift techniques have been developed. These have varied in scope, incisions, and level of tissue dissection. In the 1980s, the emphasis turned to improving the midface, traditionally the most difficult region of the face to effectively address. This was accomplished through the introduction of the deep plane and composite rhytidectomy, which was pioneered by Hamra [20]. He realized that by undermining the orbicularis oculi muscle through a lower blepharoplasty approach and joining this with the face-lift dissection, he could create a composite flap that was composed of the orbicularis oculi, cheek fat, and platysma muscle. Repositioning the composite flap corrected these three ptotic areas while maintaining their relationship with each other and the skin. The SMAS and skin are dissected together as a single flap, rather than independently. The advantage of this procedure is that theoretically the flap is better vascularized and less likely to slough. The disadvantage of the technique is the magnitude of the procedure and the prolonged recovery period and a higher risk of nerve damage.

Psillakis et al. [6, 7] were the first to describe the subperiosteal midface-lift as an open, nonendoscopic procedure. Their technique involved subperiosteal dissection of the midface through a coronal incision in combination with an eyebrow-lift. They thought that since the SMAS was firmly attached to the periosteum through the facial muscles subperiosteal undermining was necessary for adequate mobilization of the cheek.

Ramirez [9, 10] was one of the pioneers in developing the endoscopic approach to the midface. He noted that the midface dissection had several components, which required careful elevation of the suborbicularis oculi fat pad with the underlying periosteum along the inferior orbital rim and malar areas. By starting his dissection in the temporal area and creating a tunnel between the malar-zygomatic arch and the temporal pocket, he was able to suspend the midface suborbicularis oculi fat pad to the temporal fascia. He approached the zygoma from the superior direction along the deep temporalis fascia as Psillakis did. However, at 2–3 cm above the arch, he incised both the superficial and deep layers of the deep temporalis fascia to gain access to the zygomatic arch to separate the periosteum and overlying soft tissue, as the frontal branch of the seventh nerve remained superficial to their dissection. He suspended the midface by placing sutures through the periosteum and the SOOF and the periosteum just superior to the zygomaticus major origin. Each suture was then secured to the deep temporalis fascia.

Several authors have advocated the nonendoscopic elevation of the midface though lower eyelid blepharoplasty incisions. Moelleken [21] described a superficial subciliary cheek-lift with the use of a single subciliary incision with suborbicularis dissection of the malar fat pad (superficial to the zygomaticus major and minor muscles) and fixation to the "intermediate" temporalis fascia located just lateral to the lateral orbital rim. Gunter and Hackney [22] presented a technique in which the cheek is undermined in the subperiosteal plane with fixation of the ptotic malar fat pad to the thick periosteum over the lateral orbital rim. Hester et al. [23] advocate subperiosteal elevation of the midface through an infraciliary incision with suspension of the midface to the lateral orbital rim and deep temporalis fascia.

Subperiosteal face-lift fascinated many authors, since it raises the eyebrows, eyelid lateral corner, forehead, glabella, cheeks, and nasolabial fold, reaching the middle third of the face. This technique includes less incision, use of endoscope, better fixation (especially of the cheeks), and allows for more ancillary procedures, repositioning of the Bichat's fat pad, and jowl treatment.

Subperiosteal face-lift is indicated for patients with significant aging and ptosis of the oval center of the face, tear-trough deformity, sclera-show in severe malar pockets, cases of past facial fractures, when there is the need for simultaneous resurfacing, in cases of facial implants that need to be changed, when there is a need for soft tissue augmentation with fat transfer and even in smokers.

As a result of the procedure the cheek advances upward and backward and a tremendous amount of vertical lift is produced. The fat pad is repositioned, reducing the orbital hollow and the "double contour deformity." A volume augmentation is enhanced by meloplication that fills in both the "orbital hollow" and the "cheek hollow." The nasolabial fold is diminished. The "oral frown" is diminished, to a degree. Malar bags are diminished, to a degree.

The advantages of the subperiosteal face-lift include: easier correction of prominent midface wrinkles, lateral orbital bulging caused by brow ptosis, and ptosis of deep soft tissue and orbital festoons; not compromising the blood supply to overlying tissue, especially for cigarette smokers and those who have thinner tissue; and reduced possibility of facial nerve injury when compared with any other intermediate plane.

The subperiosteal face-lift technique, as originally described by Tessier [5], has benefited from significant technologic advances in medicine. The endoscope now allows extensive subperiosteal undermining of facial soft tissue through minimal access incisions. Improved understanding of facial anatomy and the facial aging process now allows surgeons to reposition and remodel the soft-tissue envelope with excellent aesthetic results. Restoration of facial volume can be achieved with the subperiosteal techniques described and can be applied to the full spectrum of patients with long-lasting results.

Correct diagnosis of the aging changes in the midface, therefore, dictates the most appropriate choice of surgical approach. If the findings are confined predominantly to the periorbital area, with only mild descent of the cheek structures evident, blepharoplasty utilizing a variety of techniques may be all that is required to restore a youthful appearance to the midface. Classical transconjunctival or skin–muscle blepharoplasty is effective when the problem is confined to fat pseudoherniation and skin excess, without deepening of the nasolabial fold. When mild cheek descent is present with resultant thinning of the soft tissues over the infraorbital rim and/or deep nasolabial folds are present, blepharoplasty with fat repositioning is more appropriate (Fig. 39.7). Fat repositioning is especially

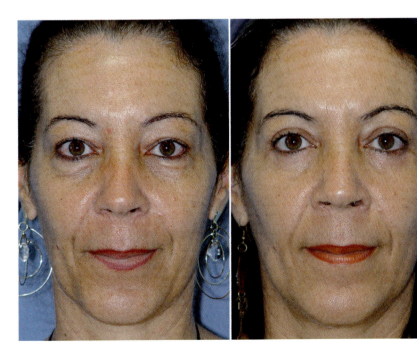

Fig. 39.7 Preoperative (*left*) and 10-month postoperative (*right*) female patient who underwent blepharoplasty with fat repositioning

Fig 39.7 (continued)

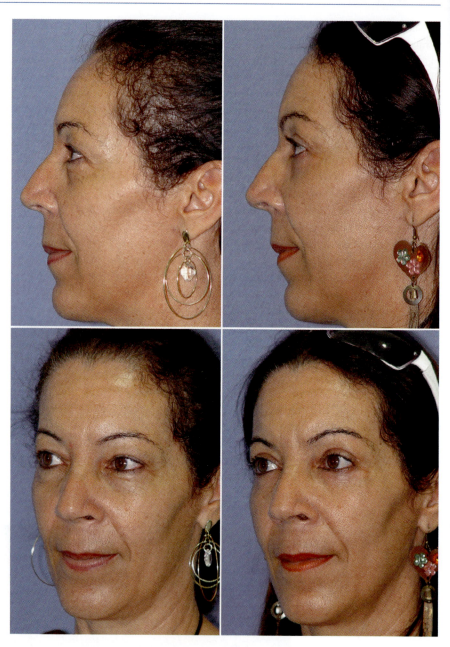

indicated when a negative vector is present, and the bony orbital rim lies posterior to the plane of the cornea. These patients often have scleral show preoperatively, which will often be exacerbated with fat removal as in the traditional blepharoplasty.

As the distance from the infraorbital rim to the malar fat pad increases, the nasolabial folds deepen, and the aging perioral changes are evident, midface lifting should be considered along with blepharoplasty. The subperiosteal face-lift is ideal because all areas of midface aging, from the lower eyelid to the perioral area, can be addressed with a single exposure, and the effects of gravity can be directly opposed by a 180° vertical vector. The transblepharoplasty approach should be restricted to those patients in whom a lesser degree of these aging changes are evident. On the other hand, the transtemporal approach offers the best possible reversion of the aging effects on the midface (Figs. 39.8–39.10).

Fig. 39.8 Preoperative (*left*) and 18-month postoperative (*right*) male patient who underwent subperiosteal midface-lift

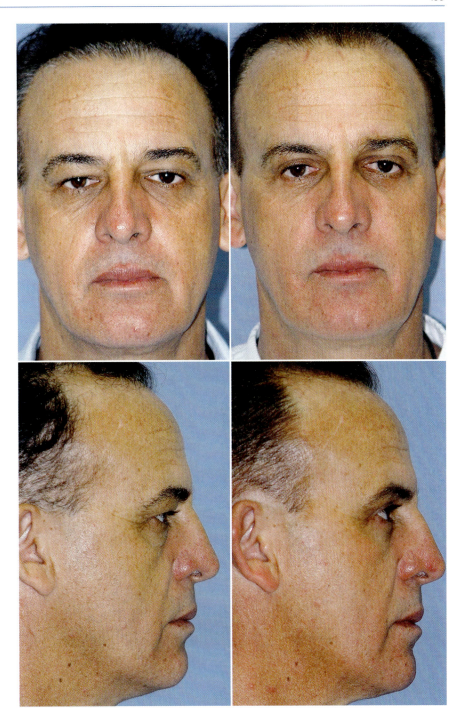

Subperiosteal midface-lift can be enhanced with injection of fat graft (lipotransfer) [24]. The graft helps to restore the youthful appearance in more cases with more severe loss of midface volume (Fig. 39.11).

The demand for face-lift surgery has increased dramatically in recent years as people from all socioeconomic levels become interested in facial rejuvenation. The evolution through surgical correction of the aging midface began with peripheral approaches and, as we

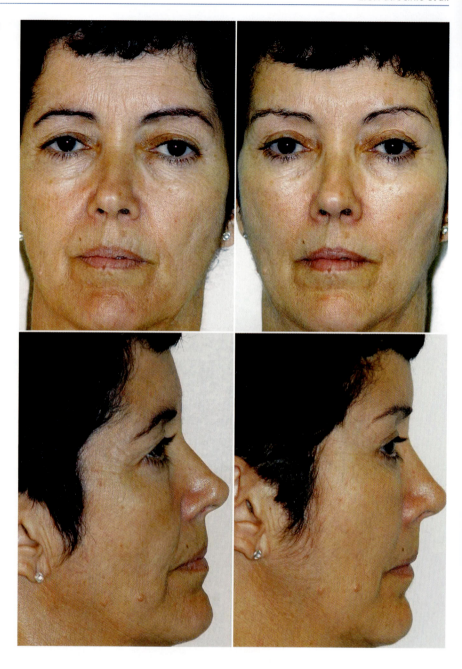

Fig. 39.9 Preoperative (*left*) and 2-year postoperative (*right*) female patient who underwent subperiosteal midface-lift

began to understand the dynamics of midface aging, moved to a vector-based attempt to reposition ptotic soft tissues. Only later did the volumetric component of midface aging become a recognized essential clinical finding. The pathways developed to correct this component were repositioning of soft tissues when the displaced volume was adequate and additive when more volume was required to recapture the soft-tissue fullness of youth.

Anatomic knowledge combined with a thorough understanding of the variety of techniques available will permit to continue serving patients with the best care possible. An important point to understand is that all techniques are simple to those familiar with it, and regardless of the procedure, the results will be better for those who adhere to the fine details and the art of the objective.

Fig. 39.10 Preoperative (*left*) and 1-year postoperative (*right*) female patient who underwent subperiosteal midface-lift and endoscopic forehead-lift

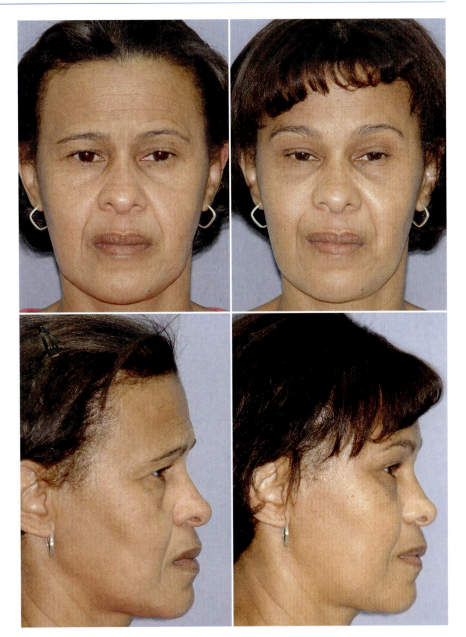

Fig. 39.10 (continued)

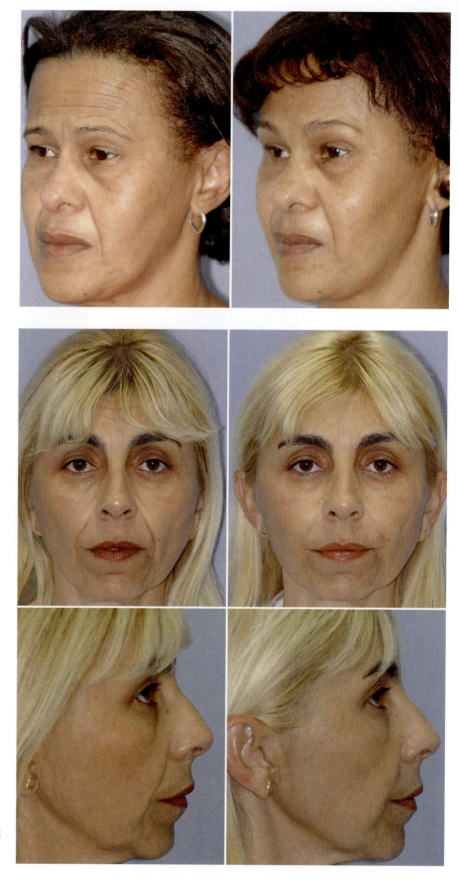

Fig. 39.11 Preoperative (*left*) and 18-month postoperative (*right*) female patient who underwent subperiosteal midface-lift and injection of fat graft to the nasolabial folds

39.5 Conclusions

The subperiosteal face-lift by temporal approach is a procedure designed to rejuvenate the upper and middle thirds of the face. After subperiosteal detachment, the soft tissues of the cheek, forehead, jowls, lateral canthus, and eyebrows can be lifted to reestablish their youthful relationship with the underlying skeleton. It is a technique that produces satisfactory cosmetic results in most of the cases, causing malar augmentation, nasolabial fold improvement, and mild jowl improvement.

References

1. Rees TD, Aston SJ, Thorne CH. Blepharoplasty and facialplasty. In: McCarthy J, editor. Plastic surgery. Philadelphia: W.B. Saunders; 1990. p. 2320–414.
2. Patrocínio LG, Patrocínio JA, Couto HG, de Muniz Souza H, Carvalho PM. Subperiosteal facelift: a 5-year experience. Braz J Otorhinolaryngol. 2006;72(5):592–7.
3. DeFatta RJ, Williams III EF. Evolution of midface rejuvenation. Arch Facial Plast Surg. 2009;11(1):6–12.
4. Adamson P, Litner J. Evolution of rhytidectomy techniques. Facial Plast Surg Clin North Am. 2005;13(3):383–91.
5. Tessier P. Face lifting and frontal rhytidectomy. In: Ely JF, editor. Transactions of the seventh international congress of plastic and reconstructive surgery, Rio de Janeiro, Sep 1979.
6. Psillakis JM. Ritidoplastia: nova técnica cirúrgica. Jornada de Carioca de Cirurgia Estética, Rio de Janeiro, 1982.
7. Psillakis JM, Rumley TO, Camargos A. Subperiosteal approach as an improved concept for correction of the aging face. Plast Reconstr Surg. 1988;82(3):383–94.
8. Santana PM. Craniofacial methods in rhytidoplasty. Cir Plast Ibero-Latinamer. 1984;10:32.
9. Ramirez OM, Maillard GF, Musolas A. The extended subperiosteal facelift: a definitive soft tissue remodeling for facial rejuvenation. Plast Reconstr Surg. 1991;88(2):227–36.
10. Ramirez OM. Endoscopic full facelift. Aesthetic Plast Surg. 1994;18(4):363–71.
11. Patrocínio LG, Reinhart RJ, Patrocínio TG, Patrocínio JA. Endoscopic frontoplasty: 3-year experience. Braz J Otorhinolaryngol. 2006;72(5):624–30.
12. Patrocinio LG, Patrocinio JA. Forehead-lift: a 10-year review. Arch Facial Plast Surg. 2008;10(6):391–4.
13. Patrocínio JA, Patrocínio LG, Aguiar AS. Complicações de ritidoplastia em um serviço de residência médica em otorrinolaringologia. Rev Bras Otorrinolaringol. 2002;68(3):338–42.
14. Sullivan CA, Masin J, Maniglia AJ, Stepnick DW. Complications of rhytidectomy in an otolaryngology training program. Laryngoscope. 1999;109(2 Pt 1):198–203.
15. Paul MD, Calvert JW, Evans GR. The evolution of the midface lift in aesthetic plastic surgery. Plast Reconstr Surg. 2006;117(6):1809–27.
16. Bettman A. Plastic and cosmetic surgery of the face. Northwest Med J. 1920;19:205.
17. Bourguet J. La chirurgie esthetique de la face. Concours Med. 1921;1657–70.
18. Skoog T. Plastic surgery: new methods and refinements. Philadelphia: W.B. Saunders; 1974.
19. Mitz V, Peyronie M. The superficial musculoaponeurotic system (SMAS) in the parotid and cheek area. Plast Reconstr Surg. 1976;58(1):80–8.
20. Hamra ST. Composite rhytidectomy. Plast Reconstr Surg. 1992;90(1):1–13.
21. Moelleken B. The superficial subciliary cheek lift, a technique for rejuvenating the infraorbital region and nasojugal groove: clinical series of 71 patients. Plast Reconstr Surg. 1999;104(6):1863–74.
22. Gunter JP, Hackney FL. A simplified transblepharoplasty subperiosteal cheek lift. Plast Reconstr Surg. 1999;103(7):2029–35.
23. Hester TR, Codner MA, McCord CD. The "centrofacial" approach for correction of facial aging using the transblepharoplasty subperiosteal cheek lift. Aesthetic Surg Q. 1996;16:51.
24. Coleman SR. Structural fat grafts: the ideal filler? Clin Plast Surg. 2001;28(1):111–19.

Progression of Facelift Techniques Over the Years

W. Gregory Chernoff

40.1 Introduction

When compared to non-cosmetic surgical procedures, rhytidectomy is a relatively young procedure, approaching its 100th birthday. Considering this, it is interesting that it has undergone such a high degree of modification, refinement, scrutiny, and in some cases mimicry. As knowledge of facial and neck anatomy grew, the safety, efficacy, and longevity of the procedure have also been maximized. Through the decades, as more "non-mainstream" cosmetic physicians began performing facial procedures, there arose a trend of what has come to be known as "minimally invasive" operations which were portrayed as reasonable facsimiles to the more traditional operation. As with any procedure, patient selection is paramount to success. As younger patients presented for improvement of facial features, these less-invasive procedures gained some popularity, especially with the false stigmata of the term "facelift." Time is showing that when the chief complaint of facial aging includes flattening of the midface, deepening of the nasolabial and mesolabial folds, jowling, and platysmal banding, the "time-tested" traditional rhytidectomy which deals with repositioning of facial musculature, and removal of excess skin and fat, provides the highest intersection of safety, efficacy, and longevity.

The early twentieth century saw the procedure performed primarily by "beauty doctors" in private offices and clinics. Surgical traditionalists felt that the procedure was not worthy of publication. This negativity was at a peak in the early 1920s as evidenced by publications that called for a ban on cosmetic procedures [1]. The majority of the original papers reporting the procedure were in fact retrospective. Texts claiming original contributions arose from America and Europe. These have been attributed to Miller [2], Lexer [3], Hollander [4], Passot [5], Joseph [6], and Noel [7].

The first-described techniques consisted of incisions placed behind and in front of the ears, coupled with minimal excisions of skin strips. Bourguet [8] and Bettman (1920) [9] have both been credited with the first cases involving extensive subcutaneous undermining and lipectomy. Interestingly, the incisions used were similar to those of today, beginning temporally, extending pre-auricular, and posteriorly to the lobule. Joseph, in 1928 [10], introduced the post-tragal refinement.

The subsequent evolution of the technique has occurred primarily in North America [11]. The organization of surgical specialty boards helped foster technique-specific research and the spirited jousting of which techniques were superior. An ongoing evolution of acceptance of the procedure has mirrored the progression of the educated consumer to accepting a theory of maintenance over long propagated misconceptions of vanity. Concurrent improvements in anesthesia and postoperative care have helped the education process accentuating safety and reliability. Ongoing refinements have sought to improve both feature correction and longevity. It has been the latter that has looked down upon some of the supposed "less-invasive" techniques, especially when patients who have undergone them began complaining openly of what was perceived to be "minimal results" with early recurrence of the features which led them to seek the operation in the first place.

Surgical refinement continued to be reported. In 1960, Aufricht [12] proposed improving longevity by suturing deep to fat. Skoog, in 1974 [13], coined the

W.G. Chernoff
Chernoff Cosmetic Surgery, Indianapolis, IN, USA
e-mail: greg@drchernoff.com

term "buccal fascia," which incorporated the platysmal muscle and the superficial fascia of the lower third of the face. This fascia was undermined to the level of the jowl and melolabial fold and then sutured to the mastoid fascia and parotidomasseteric fascia, respectively. In 1976, Mitz and Peyronie [14] described the superficial musculoaponeurotic system (SMAS). This finding confirmed a fascial layer distinct from the underlying parotidomasseteric fascia, which invests the facial musculature. They found that the SMAS was in a tissue plane continuous with the platysma in the neck, and the temporoparietal fascia in the scalp. Fibrous adhesions to the overlying subcutaneous tissue and skin allowed for SMAS manipulations to effect desired skin improvements. This benefit can be lost if the relationship between SMAS and overlying skin is not maintained due to extensive undermining. This "SMAS rhytidectomy" has remained a popular technique, which combines a subcutaneous dissection with a separate SMAS elevation via plication (pulling back, folding over, and suturing), as described by Webster in 1982 [15] or imbrication, (advancement, shortening, and suturing), as described by Lemmon and Hamra [16]. Throughout these papers, maintaining a natural look while minimizing complications was repeatedly advocated.

The 1990s and the first decade of this century showed research into improving the midface, the most difficult region of the face to obtain consistent long-term results. Deep-plane and composite rhytidectomy, as pioneered by Hamra [17, 18], were the next steps in the evolution of facelift. Versions of this technique then evolved as the bi- and tri-plane dissections by Baker [19] and modifications by Kamer [20]. Ramirez [21] took the deep-plane to its full extent by reporting a subperiosteal approach.

The most important aspect of providing meticulous results is the ability of modifying one's technique proportional to what the patient would benefit from, based upon the chief complaint at the time of the initial consultation. Applying all that has been learned over time from skin excision to composite dissections must be weighed with the potential for complication and delivering the result that has been assured. Assessing the degree of midfacial aging, nasolabial and melolabial folds, jowling, platysmal banding, subplatysmal fat, and skin quality play into the surgeons' decision of choosing the appropriate rhytidectomy for the patient. What is paramount is that the surgeons have available in their armamentarium all potential techniques and know when to offer each one.

40.2 Limited Flap Rhytidectomy Procedures

Various limited techniques have been popularized under different names. These include the short flap technique, the S-lift, the mini-lift, the "lunchtime lift," the "weekend lift," and the most recent moniker – the "lifestyle lift." This essentially comprises a limited pre-auricular incision terminating at the lobule, a short amount of skin undermining, limited SMAS imbrication or plication, coupled with platysmal plication and cervical liposuction.

Indications include younger patients with limited midfacial ptosis and jowling and mild skin laxity. Professed advantages include shorter operative and recovery periods, increased safety, and the ability to be more aggressive with concomitant skin exfoliative procedures with chemicals or lasers. As one might expect, detractors profess limited and transitory benefits yielding patient dissatisfaction and the need for reoperation. It does seem appropriate for the patient who seeks a subtle, safe procedure with a shorter recovery time than the procedures discussed hereafter.

40.3 Extended Flap Rhytidectomy Procedures

This group encompasses several techniques, which involve extensive tissue undermining on the lateral face, and may extend across the midline in the submental region. Indications include those patients with more advanced signs of aging, such as flattening of the midface, moderately deep nasolabial and melolabial folds, significant platysmal banding, and significant elastosis. Multiple procedures can be performed simultaneously without adding to recovery time or compounding postoperative discomfort. The procedure has increased potential for complications, given the extensive undermining. Surgical skills with uncompromising anatomical knowledge are prerequisites to the successful completion of this rewarding procedure.

The classic long flap technique is safe and easy to learn. It is coupled with SMAS imbrication proportionate to what the patient would benefit from as determined in consultation. It offers significant improvement to the neck and lower third of the face. Its shortcoming would be the limited correction of the ptotic midfacial tissues. Extensive skin undermining can lead to vascular compromise and flap necrosis. Excessive closure tension and hematoma can exacerbate these unfortunate sequelae.

The developments of more extensive SMAS procedures were the result of efforts to minimize the aforementioned problems. The "sub-SMAS rhytidectomy" expands on simple imbrication by extending the dissection anterior to the parotid gland. The "extended sub-SMAS" approach takes the dissection to the lateral edge of the zygomaticus muscle. This technique redistributes some tension forces from the skin to the SMAS, but does not totally negate the flap risk associated with the wide undermining. The fact that the SMAS is attenuated at the level of the melolabial fold reflects this procedure's inability to enhance the midface as reliably as it does the neck and jawline.

Subsequently, efforts continued to attempt to improve the malar complex. In 1988, Faivre [22] described the deep temporal lift. Temporal soft tissues were elevated in the submusculoaponeurotic plane and fixed to the temporalis muscle. This produced correction of temporal, lateral brow, and jugal ptosis. Similarly, Psillakis et al. [23] reported a subperiosteal approach to the midface. The ptotic malar skin, fat, and muscle were mobilized and suspended by anchoring the periosteum overlying the lateral orbit, malar arch, and zygoma. This procedure was ideally suited for midfacial ptosis without lower face rejuvenation requirements. Disadvantages included prolonged midfacial swelling, lateral canthal elevation, widening of the midface, and the necessity of performing a standard rhytidectomy to correct lower third aging features.

The 1990s saw debate surrounding appropriate vectors of midfacial elevation, and proper plane of dissection. The infraorbital approach was added to the temporal lift as a viable technique [24]. Proponents favored the vertical vector of this approach as compared to the superolateral pull observed with the temporal lift. This dissection was either performed in the subperiosteal plane or in the plane deep to the suborbicularis oculi fat pad (SOOF) via a blepharoplasty incision. Elevated tissue is suspended to the infraorbital rim.

40.4 Deep-Plane Rhytidectomy

The latest frontier of facial rejuvenation has been the deep-plane rhytidectomy as described by Hamra [17]. This procedure modifies Skoog's technique by including superolateral elevation of the malar fat pad in addition to the lower facial tissues. Hamra previously described a tri-plane rhytidectomy in which he combined midfacial subcutaneous elevation with subplatysmal elevation of the lower face and a pre-platysmal neck dissection.

In the deep-plane technique, the amount of skin undermining is limited to the amount suitable for redraping, once the SMAS has been elevated and repositioned. The dissection is performed deep to platysmal SMAS, also cheek fat. It is carried medially over the zygomaticus major and minor muscles, to a point lateral to the melolabial fold. The mobilized fat pad is suspended to the body of the zygoma in a superolateral vector. Hamra's work has been instrumental in the understanding and refinement that have dramatically improved the results in selected patients.

Hamra [18] continued to adapt this process through the description of the "composite rhytidectomy." This modification includes superolateral advancement of the orbicularis oculi muscle to improve the inferolateral descent of the malar crescent or malar festoon. This denotes the most inferior extent of the orbicularis oculi muscle in the midface. This procedure creates a musculocutaneous flap pedicled on the facial artery perforators inferiorly and the angular and infraorbital vessels superiorly. The orbicularis mobilization is performed through a subciliary approach. This approach may cause orbicularis weakness, abnormal alteration of lower lid position if not performed correctly.

The deep-plane technique provides a robust cervicofacial flap that restores youthful contours. It is technically challenging and poses an increased risk of nerve injury, especially to those facial nerve branches which course deep to the SMAS to enter the mimetic muscles from their undersurfaces. Their remains a lack of long-term follow-up studies that conclusively demonstrate a definitive long-term improvement when the deep-plane technique is employed. Short-term reduction in tension of the undermined flap is established.

Many expert facelift surgeons have reported the evolution of their technique to include the deep-plane lift. Kamer [25] reported substantial improvement upon moving to the deep-plane lift, with fewer tuck-ups required for loss of correction. It appears that the technique achieves a more natural, long-lasting improvement in the midface, jawline, and neck.

40.5 Adjuvant Procedures

There has been a trend to performing total facial rejuvenation in a single session. The ability to deal with the upper, middle, lower thirds of the face, as well as the neck in a single operation has been afforded primarily due to the improvements in anesthesia technique. Combining brow lift, blepharoplasty, deep-plane rhytidectomy, platysmaplasty, and some form of skin exfoliation provides a consistent, reproducible, safe method of facial rejuvenation which affords a long-lasting natural result for which the patient will have a high level of satisfaction. Surgeon skill is the main factor that dictates the ability of completing this combination in less than 6–8 h. Many surgeons will keep their full facial rejuvenation patients overnight to ensure patient comfort and safety.

The addition of fillers and neurotoxins at the time of surgery is also an acceptable adjuvant as patients seek to maximize their experience. These are typically performed at the start of the procedure to enhance the surgeon's aesthetic advantage. On an individual basis, concurrent procedures should be performed only if benefits outweigh any added risk and patient safety is not compromised. Patient satisfaction will reflect the highest intersecting points of safety and efficacy. The surgeon's comfort level will dictate which procedure will best accomplish this goal.

References

1. Ryan RF. A 1927 view of cosmetic surgery. Plast Reconstr Surg. 2000;106(5):1211.
2. Miller CC. The correction of featural imperfections. Chicago: Oak Printing; 1907.
3. Lexer E. Zur gesichtsplastik. Arch Klin Chir. 1910;92:749.
4. Hollander E. Cosmetic surgery. In: Joseph M, editor. Handbuch von Kosmetik. Leipzig: Vering von Velt; 1912. p. 688.
5. Passot R. La chirurgie esthetique des rides du visage. Presse Méd. 1919;27:258.
6. Joseph J. Plastic operation on protruding cheek. Dtsch Med Wochenschr. 1921;47:287.
7. Noël A. La chirurgie esthétiqaue son rôle sociale. Paris: Masson et Cie; 1926. p. 62–6.
8. Bourguet J. La chirurgie esthétique de la face. Le Concours Med 1921;1657–1670.
9. Bettman AG. Plastic and cosmetic surgery of the face. Northwest Med. 1920;19:205.
10. Joseph J. Nasenplastic and sonstige Gesichtsplastik nebst einem Anhan uber Mamaplastik. Leipzig: Verlag von Curt Kabitzsch; 1928. p. 31.
11. Haiken E. The making of the modern face: cosmetic surgery. Soc Res. 2000;67:82–99.
12. Aufricht G. Surgery for excess skin of the face and neck. In: Wallace AB, editor. Transactions of the second congress of the international society of plastic surgeons. Baltimore: Williams & Wilkin; 1960. p. 495–502.
13. Skoog K. Plastic surgery: new methods and refinements. Philadelphia: W.B. Saunders; 1974.
14. Mitz V, Peyronie M. The superficial musculoaponeurotic system (SMAS) in the parotid and cheek area. Plast Reconstr Surg. 1976;58(1):80–6.
15. Webster RC, Smith RC, Papsidero MJ, Karolow WW, Smith KF. Comparison of SMAS plication with SMAS imbrication in face lifting. Laryngoscope. 1982;92(8 Pt 1):901–12.
16. Lemmon ML, Hamra ST. Skoog rhytidectomy: a five year experience with 577 patients. Plast Reconstr Surg. 1980;65: 283–97.
17. Hamra ST. The deep-plane rhytidectomy. Plast Reconstr Surg. 1990;86(1):53–61.
18. Hamra ST. Composite rhytidectomy. Plast Reconstr Surg. 1992;90(1):1–13.
19. Baker SR. Triplane rhytidectomy. Combining best all worlds. Arch Otolaryngol Head Neck Surg. 1997;123(11):1167–72.
20. Kamer FM. One hundred consecutive deep plane face-lifts. Arch Otolaryngol Head Neck Surg. 1996;122(1):17–22.
21. Ramirez OM. The subperiosteal rhytidectomy: the third-generation face-lift. Ann Plast Surg. 1992;28(3):218–32.
22. Faivre J. Deep temporal facelift: techniques and indications. Fr Rev Cosmet Surg. 1988;14:53.
23. Psillakis JM, Rumley TO, Camargos A. Subperiosteal approach as an improved concept for correction of the aging face. Plast Reconstr Surg. 1988;82(3):383–94.
24. Freeman MS. Transconjunctival sub-orbicularis oculi fat (SOOF) pad lift blepharoplasty: a new technique for the effacement of nasojugal deformity. Arch Facial Plast Surg. 2000;2(1):16–21.
25. Kamer FM, Frankel AS. SMAS rhytidectomy vs. deep-plane rhytidectomy: an objective comparison. Plast Reconstr Surg. 1998;102:878–81.

Facial Contouring in the Postbariatric Surgery Patient

Anthony P. Sclafani and Vikas Mehta

41.1 Introduction

Morbid obesity is a worldwide problem, with 1.7 billion people considered overweight [1]. Approximately two-thirds of adults in the USA are overweight, and half are obese [2]. In 1991, the National Institute of Health established indications for bariatric surgery, BMIs >40 or >35 with significant comorbidities, and these guidelines may be further liberalized. According to Buchwald et al., patients who undergo bariatric surgery lose 61.6% of their actual excess body weight and a majority of patients with diabetes, hyperlipidemia, hypertension, and obstructive sleep apnea experience complete resolution or improvement of these comorbidities [3]. Overall 5–10 weight loss retention rates vary from 30% to 80%. Despite the drastic improvement in health, two-thirds of massive weight loss patients are unhappy with their appearance secondary to copious sagging skin [4] and may experience dysphoria, depression, and discrimination. According to the American Society of Plastic Surgeons, 47% of these (roughly 150,000) patients underwent body contouring procedures in 2007 after significant postsurgery weight loss [5].

Bariatric surgery leads to significant (mostly trunkal) weight loss, with relatively less weight loss in the face and neck. However, this small but disproportionate fat reduction can cause secondary facial and cervical aesthetic deformities. The loss of cervicofacial fat often leaves the patient with noticeable soft tissue volume deficiencies and skin laxity. These post-bariatric changes result in a "hollowed," prematurely aged appearance (Fig. 41.1a). Specifically, patients will often present with prominent nasolabial and nasojugal grooves, lip atrophy, and a turkey-neck deformity. Although the truncal skin excess can be significantly more dramatic, many patients report that the facial changes are of greater concern as they cannot easily be hidden with clothing. Similar to HIV-associated antiretroviral therapy (HAART) patients, this weight loss is often (ironically) perceived as an indication of chronic illness. Often, these patients pursue cosmetic facial surgery prior to addressing other body contour issues. As more Americans undergo weight loss surgery, it is useful to identify and address the operative and perioperative challenges that affect this unique and growing population. The mechanics, physiology and demographics of these patients differ significantly from the typical patient with an aging face. Understanding these variations is the key to successful and safe cervicofacial rejuvenation in the massive weight loss patient.

41.2 Pathomechanics

Fundamentally, postbariatric contouring surgeries focus on skin laxity and fat loss. An analysis of the biomechanical properties of skin following weight loss showed decreased stiffness, increased laxity, greater

A.P. Sclafani (✉)
Division of Facial Plastic Surgery, The New York Eye & Ear Infirmary, 310 East 14th Street, New York,
NY 10003, USA and
Department of Otolaryngology, New York Medical College, Valhalla, NY, USA
e-mail: asclafani@nyee.edu

V. Mehta
Department of Otolaryngology, The New York Eye & Ear Infirmary, 310 East 14th Street, New York, NY 10003, USA
e-mail: vmehta@nyee.edu

Reprinted with permission of Springer

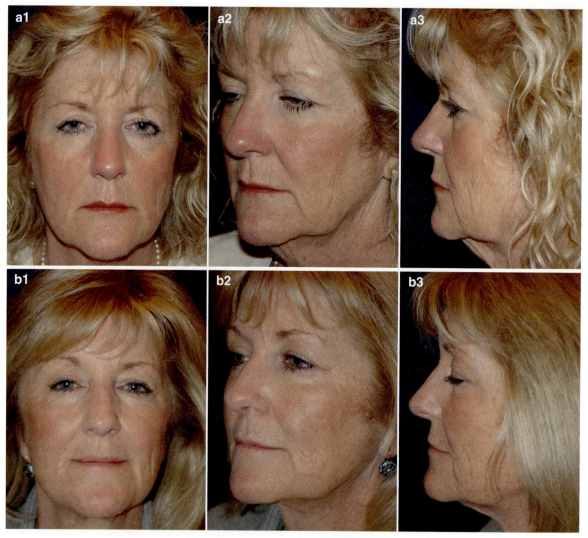

Fig. 41.1 Postbariatric surgery patient. (**a**) This patient appears prematurely aged, with significant malar flattening and midfacial volume loss, as well as lateral cheek and cervical skin redundancy. (**b**) Six months after endoscopic brow-lift, submental liposuction and SMAS face-lift with volume enhancement of the midface. The natural structural features of the midface are highlighted postoperatively. A minor revision procedure was performed subsequently to further improve the lax cervical skin

skin compliance, and increased elastic deformation [6]. In addition to these cellular abnormalities, there are location-specific trends in fat loss that contribute to aesthetic concerns in the cervicofacial area. In the submental region, the expanded, stretched, and redundant skin is the principal cosmetic deformity. In contrast, deformities in the perioral and midface region are primarily due to loss of fat volume.

Within the midface, areas that are most notably affected by volume loss are the nasojugal groove, the malar eminence, the submalar region, and the nasolabial crease. Traditionally, age-related changes in the midface were attributed to a decrease in the suspension properties of the fibrous tissue. Therefore, aesthetic surgery in this region was primarily focused on techniques to lift and redistribute the fat compartments. Motivated by desire for less invasive and more conservative techniques, recent trends place a greater emphasis on volume augmentation. Using various imaging techniques, connective tissue laxity, bone remodeling, and facial lipoatrophy have all been shown to play an important role in pathomechanics of the aging midface [7, 8]. This is an important point of difference between the aging and massive weight loss patients.

Overall, postbariatric surgery (PBS) patients are relatively young. Similar to patients with HIV-associated lipoatrophy, the suspension properties of the midfacial skin have not been altered drastically. Instead, it is the massive weight loss that creates a hollowed appearance in otherwise convex areas of the face [9]. Therefore, more traditional midface lifting techniques are usually not indicated, and a variety of temporary and permanent volume restoration options have been developed and applied to the midface, perioral complex, and lip of the PBS patient.

In contrast to the midface, deformities in the jaw and neckline are caused primarily by skin excess and laxity and, therefore, are addressed solely by rhytidectomy techniques. Prior to bariatric surgery, pre and subplatysmal fat accumulation leads to stretching of the skin and platysma muscle. As in the rest of the body, postsurgical fat loss reveals stretched, inelastic, and redundant skin. In the neck, the anatomic area of interest is typically the anterior compartment between the sternocleidomastoid muscles. Again, however, a key difference between the aging patient and massive weight loss patient must be highlighted. The primary distinction lies in the pathomechanics, and subsequently the treatment, of the platysma muscle. In the aging neck, the platysmal muscle undergoes a decrease in tone as well as an increase in diastasis. However, in the PBS patient, there is less muscle diastasis and greater skin excess that is the principal issue. More conservative treatment of the midline platysma by plication is performed in these patients.

41.3 Preoperative Evaluation

As with all patients seeking cosmetic surgery, a thorough preoperative consultation will include not only the patient's particular aesthetic defect, but also their exact expectations, a complete history, and physical and a quick assessment of their psychological and emotional well-being. In each of these areas, there are issues specific to the massive weight loss patient that must be addressed. First, timing of cosmetic surgery should be carefully planned. As mentioned previously, many PBS patients seek to correct their facial deformity prior to addressing other body contouring surgery. A recent meta-analysis has shown that the patient's weight is likely to fluctuate within the first year and long-term weight loss is poorly described in the literature [10]. Additionally, it is well known that skin will undergo some degree of contraction after 60% of the body fat is lost. Therefore, it is prudent to wait for 6–12 months to allow the skin to reach its final position and the patient's weight to stabilize to avoid overcorrection.

Correction of midface deformities focuses on volume restoration. Areas of the midface that require particular attention are the tear trough/infraorbital rim, the malar eminence, the submalar region, and the nasolabial crease. These areas typically undergo the greatest volume loss. Additional areas of concern are the temporal fossa, jawline, and perioral region, and less commonly, the glabella and lateral brow. It is important to decide preoperatively (1) which areas to address, (2) the specific type of filler to be used and lastly, (3) the amount needed for effective volume replacement. There are scales described for both autologous fat transfer [11] and hyaluronic acid derivatives [12], but a universally accepted, standardized grading scale has yet to be established. If the surgeon is considering autologous fat, it is imperative to anticipate the amount of volume needed so that an appropriate amount can be harvested.

In the preoperative evaluation, there are unique anatomic considerations in each area of the face. Symmetry is of particular importance in the midface, as it is frequently variable and easily correctable. In the perioral region, restoration of the normal curves and convexities of the lip is essential to both redefine the shape of the lips as well as to reestablish the lip volume. With fat volume loss, the vermilion margin will flatten, and volume augmentation will allow the patient to regain the healthy, "pouty" look.

Evaluation of the lower face focuses not only on the skin, muscle, and fat of the submental region, but also the bony substructure, including the strength of the anterior jaw projection and position of the hyoid bone. Anterior mandibular deficiency, unless corrected, will allow cervical skin to hang in unaesthetic positions in the PBS patient. Failure to treat weak anterior bony projection seriously compromises the final results of rejuvenative surgery in these patients.

Even in the PBS patient, a significant amount of submental fat may still be present, and cervical liposuction is generally necessary to adequately define the cervicomental angle and lower jawline. Fat removal should be thorough, and also should be feathered peripherally. Excessive liposuction should be avoided, but "cobra neck" deformity [13] is uncommon because of the relatively lower incidence of midline platysma diastasis. Finally, the overall degree of skin laxity must be assessed in order to counsel the patient set appropriate postoperative expectations. In cases of severe skin laxity, a truly youthful appearing neck and jawline may be impossible or require several revisions to fully redrape the skin.

Other preoperative considerations specific to the PBS patient include those related to their extensive comorbidities. While weight loss surgery can have a positive impact on related diseases, such as diabetes, the literature is controversial. Several authors have reported large cohorts of weight loss patients with significant reductions in comorbidities [14, 15] and mortality over time [16, 17] (up to 89% reduction at 5 years). However, a meta-analysis [10] which included only studies with greater than 3 years postoperative follow-up noted several flaws in the above-mentioned studies' claims, as well as a statistically significant regain in weight for all of the series included at 10 years. For the cosmetic surgeon, the key to this controversy lies in the possibility that despite the initial weight reduction, many patients may return to obesity and retain their comorbidities, especially diabetes. It is important, therefore, that any contouring surgery be deferred for at least a year and extensive preoperative medical screening is performed on every PBS patient.

Other well-documented issues in treating the PBS patient include cardiac arrhythmias and nutritional deficiencies. Up to 10% of patients will develop new cardiac arrhythmias after bariatric surgery, and if any anomalies are identified on a preoperative electrocardiogram, a complete cardiac evaluation is warranted. PBS patients may develop hypokalemia and hypomagnesemia, and appropriate electrolyte evaluation should be performed preoperatively. Massive weight loss patients are at significant risk for caloric and nutritional deficiencies in vitamin A, vitamin B12, folate, vitamin C, iron, selenium, zinc, and protein [18]. For the facial plastic surgeon, important considerations are anemia, problems with wound healing, and poor immune response optimization. In an outcomes analysis of 139 patients undergoing contouring procedures after massive weight loss, 14.4% had wound complications [19]. To avoid these and other potential complications, preoperative screening and supplementation is recommended. Also common among these patients is gastroesophageal reflux, especially if any alteration has been made to the GE junction. Some pre- or perioperative reflux medication may be indicated when operating on these patients. Lastly, these patients should be assessed for obstructive sleep apnea and potential difficulties with intubation, both of which are extremely common in all obese individuals.

As with any patient seeking plastic surgery, it is imperative to assess the patient's psychological well-being. This is especially true in the massive weight loss patient. Studies have found a high rate of psychological abnormality among persons with extreme obesity who pursue bariatric surgery. Between 20% and 60% of patients have been diagnosed with axis I psychiatric disorders, the most common of which are mood and anxiety disorders [20, 21]. Additionally, binge eating is common among this population and can return at any time despite the massive weight loss. Patients should undergo preoperative psychological screening, such as a questionnaire to assess potential psychological pathology, especially eating disorders, body dysmorphic disorder, and emotional instability. Positive screening or suspicions should be referred to a mental health professional prior to any cosmetic surgical procedure. Finally, patients may have unrealistic expectations of their final results based on popular figures who have undergone bariatric surgery with contouring. These should be identified and realistic expectations should be discussed explicitly with the patient preoperatively.

41.3.1 Rhytidectomy in the Postbariatric Patient

In tailoring a procedure for the postbariatric surgery patient, it should be kept in mind that the laxity, excess, and ptosis of the skin generally exceed those of the superficial musculoaponeurotic system (SMAS). Rhytidectomy in these patients is still a standard procedure with appropriate modifications. Rather than detail the complete procedure, described here are the important considerations and modifications to a standard SMAS rhytidectomy necessary in postbariatric surgery patients. The skin incision can enter the temporal hairline above the helical root only if the vector of planned facial elevation is predominantly postero-superiorly, not superiorly, oriented; if the vector of flap movement is mostly superior in direction, the incision should course around the sideburn pretrichially to avoid elevation of the temporal hair tuft. It should be remembered that post-bariatric rhytidectomy patients are generally younger than the traditional patient with an aging face, and are undergoing facial surgery to match their facial appearance with their rejuvenated body; these patients are often reluctant to commit to a specific hairstyle to camouflage an occipital scar. The vector of elevation in the neck can be mostly superior in direction, and with care the incision across the mastoid skin and into the hairline can be avoided. Patients appreciate the absence of this obvious portion of the scar, especially when seeking to resume a more active and athletic lifestyle. In patients with severe skin laxity, it may not be possible to contour the postauricular area smoothly without the occipital portion of the skin incision. The skin may "bunch" along the postauricular scar, but this can be redraped if the incision is extended into the hairline, or the scar can be revised 6–8 weeks after surgery as a planned, second stage. These options should be discussed preoperatively with the patient and a plan of action determined before surgery.

Suction-assisted or direct lipectomy, or both, in the submental triangle and jowl areas can be judiciously performed to assist in creating a smooth, contoured, sculpted neckline. In the midline, paramedian platysmal bands are identified and the edges undermined from the submental crease inferiorly to a point 1 cm above the thyroid cartilage. If the bands are particularly thick or prominent, a vertical strip of muscle is excised from the medial edge of each platysmal band. The platysmal edges are then sutured from superior to inferior with a running 3–0 polydiaxone suture, which then returns superiorly with wider tissue bites to be tied in the submental region. This creates a sturdy sling for support of the submentum. Correction of the deformity requires significantly more skin undermining than the typical rhytidectomy to redrape the elevated skin smoothly. Particularly in the patient with massive weight loss, the inelasticity of the skin increases the chance of a "lateral sweep," and it is important that the skin flap be elevated and redraped in a smooth, tension-free fashion. If poor chin projection is present, a chin implant should be placed to assist in defining the cervicomental angle. Occasionally, modest transverse skin excision from the posterior border of the submental incision may be necessary. SMAS elevation and imbrication are performed in the standard fashion, although, as stated earlier, relatively less elevation of this layer is necessary than in the typical rhytidoplasty. The skin is then redraped and trimmed appropriately. The authors now treat all flaps with platelet-rich fibrin matrix (Fibrinet, Cascade Medical Enterprises, Inc, Englewood, NJ) to aid in hemostasis and wound healing. No drains are used, all incisions are closed, and a compressive dressing applied.

Postoperatively, early ambulation of the PBS patient is essential, as Aly et al. [22] noted a 9% incidence of pulmonary embolism in PBS patient undergoing abdominoplasty. Later, the patient should be assessed for residual skin redundancy. A "tuck-up" procedure may be necessary as early as 2–3 months postoperatively to address this additional skin excess; it is preferable to address this severe skin excess at a later date rather than overtighten the skin during the primary procedure, so as to minimize a "lateral sweep deformity." At the same time, contour irregularities in the postauricular sulcus (not uncommon if the occipital portion of the incision is not used) can be treated with conservative resection.

41.3.2 Volume Restoration of the Lower Two-Thirds of the Face

Volume loss out of proportion to skin redundancy is the primary element of acute midfacial aging after bariatric surgery. As such, aggressive skin redraping can easily lead to a "pulled" or "windswept" look, especially in the midface. Appropriate volume augmentation, especially in the submalar area can rejuvenate the face and reduce the chance of a "lateral sweep deformity" [23]. A measured approach to midfacial rejuvenation is essential to maximize results. Moreover, perioral volume loss, particularly in the lips, also ages the PBS patient's appearance, and a comprehensive treatment plan is critical to success in this area as well.

Midfacial fat atrophy after PBS will lead to signs of aging out of proportion to the patient's chronological age. Infraorbital hollowing and nasojugal troughs will lead to a "tired" and "sad" periorbital expression, and may also "unmask" lower eyelid fat pseudoherniation. Fat transposition blepharoplasty can be considered, but the volume of fat available is generally inadequate to correct the severe degree of volume loss present. Midface lifting provides inadequate volume, as the midface has atrophied, not descended. Volume augmentation with extrinsic material is generally necessary to allow the skin envelope to properly drape over the midface skeleton. True bony deficiencies should be corrected with skeletal augmentation. Alloplasts (such as tear trough or malar/submalar implants) can be considered for additional midface volume, but should be used with caution, as a thinned soft tissue envelope will fail to camouflage the implant's edges.

Perioral volumizing is performed in the nasolabial crease, marionette folds, and lips. Relatively speaking, nasolabial crease treatment is less critical in the PBS patient than in the typical aging patient. The nasolabial fold is highlighted by the lateral depression caused by malar soft tissue atrophy. Once malar volume is restored, conservative filling of the nasolabial crease is generally sufficient. However, volume restoration of the labiomandibular groove can further smooth the natural convexities of the lower face. Finally, restoring the volume of the lips not only effaces lip rhytids but reestablishes proper balance of the lower face.

Given the younger age of PBS patients, long-term correction is desirable. Additionally, larger volumes are generally required, which will also have significant financial implications. In light of this volume/persistence need, autologous fat transfer, long-lasting hyaluronic acid derivatives (HA), calcium hydroxylapatite, and poly-L-lactic acid should be considered. A complete description of each filler is beyond the scope of this chapter; however, a brief review of the materials and their uses is reasonable.

Hyaluronic acid products are glycosaminoglycans (GAGs) that are found extensively in the native extracellular matrix of connective tissues. The hydrophilic composition of GAGs attracts water into the extracellular matrix conferring a degree of turgor to the tissue, which acts as a hydrating agent and increases its effect as a volumizing agent. Hyaluronic acid has the unique property of being identical in all species; therefore, its derivatives should not be antigenic across species. Lowe et al. [24] published a series of 709 patients who underwent injections of Hylaform or Restylane without preoperative skin testing. In three patients (0.4%), a delayed inflammatory reaction was observed at the site of injection. After transplantation, the hyaluronic acid derivatives undergo local degradation by hydrolysis and eventual metabolism by the liver. Commercially available injectables consist of hyaluronic acid derivatives that have been cross-linked to form a gel matrix which prolongs their degradation in vivo. Several large series have confirmed the duration of the augmentation achieved with these compounds to be approximately 6–9 months [25–29].

These fillers are approved for mid-deep dermal injection; however, they may be used in an "off-label" fashion to provide large volume augmentation with both deep dermal and subcutaneous placement. Two to six cubic centimeters per side may be necessary, and care should be taken to blend the edges of the treated areas, especially in the nasojugal grooves, where these fillers need to be deposited in a supraperiosteal plane.

Similar in action to hyaluronic acid derivatives that rely solely on their own volume to augment soft tissues, a cross-linked porcine collagen has recently been introduced to use in the United States which can be similarly used and may persist longer [30].

Two other fillers are available that rely in part or fully on the body's response to the injected material. Injectable calcium hydroxylapatite beads are suspended in a mixture of glycerin, water, and cellulose (Radiesse, Bioform Medical, Inc., San Mateo, CA). Once injected subdermally, collagen deposition around the beads provides additional volume correction which can last 12–18 months [31]. Even and smooth subdermal distribution is important; placement in the suborbital grooves should in general be avoided, as the thin overlying skin and soft tissues provide little camouflage or blending to the injected material, which may then be visible as a distinct mass.

Similarly, injectable poly-L-lactic acid (PLLA, Sculptra, Dermik Laboratories, Inc., Berwyn, PA) is a suspension of PLLA beads that are injected subdermally. A progressive fibrosis around the individual beads ultimately generates a thickening of the dermis and volume augmentation, but multiple treatments are generally needed [32]. At the time of this writing, PLLA is approved for HIV antiretroviral therapy-associated lipoatrophy, and FDA approval for cosmetic uses is still pending. However, the longevity of effect of 2 years or more makes PLLA a reasonable option for volume augmentation in PBS patients.

Autologous fat transfer remains the large volume facial filler of choice when a permanent solution is desired. In 1893, Neuber [33] first used autologous fat for soft tissue augmentation. Over the years, the use of adipose grafts in soft tissue augmentation has wavered due to the high rate of graft resorption, as well as the unpredictable degree of volume loss. With the advent of liposuction in the 1970s, autologous fat grafting increased in popularity due to increased ease of harvest. Various other techniques for obtaining adipose tissue have been proposed, including syringe extraction and open harvest. Once extracted, the fat must be pretreated to remove inflammatory mediators and isolate the components necessary for implantation. Many authors have described techniques of fat washing, centrifugation, and filtration; however, no methodology is widely accepted as superior. Harvested and prepared adipose grafts generally are injected with a large-bore (14- to 18-gauge) needle or cannula just below the dermis. Unlike the hyaluronic acid derivatives, a substantial overcorrection is required due to the large degree of resorption with time. Authors report that anywhere between 30% and 60% of the injected fat will be resorbed [34, 35]. However, mixing the adipocytes with an appropriate platelet-rich plasma [36] has been shown to enhance graft survival.

41.4 Postoperative Care and Complications

Postoperative care of the massive weight loss patient following cosmetic surgery is relatively straightforward with a few exceptions. The postrhytidectomy patient is typically observed overnight and discharged in the morning after dressing change. The incidence of minor hematoma following rhytidectomy is relatively low (approximately 0.4–3%) and has recently been shown to improve with the use of fibrin glue prior to closure [37], and this is expected to be similar with the use of a platelet-rich fibrin matrix. Due to severity of the skin laxity, the skin may have a tendency to bunch along the incision lines. The patient must be instructed to massage these areas and the surgeon must note these on early postoperative visits to observe for possible revision. The patient may experience inflammation and ecchymosis for up to 2 months, but typically feel comfortable going out in public after 2 weeks [13]. There is a strong possibility of the need for minor revision procedures, which should be discussed with the patient postoperatively.

The patients injected with volume fillers must be continually assessed for significant absorption of the injected material and an irregular contour once the edema has subsided. Injection site swelling and minor bruising is common, but typically last no more than 4–7 days [38]. If a subcutaneous nodule is prominent (particularly with the use of particulate fillers like calcium hydroxylapatite or PLLA), it may require excision if conservative measures (such as massage or corticosteroid injection) fail. This is especially common in the thin skin of the nasojugal groove if the injection accidentally infiltrates the orbicularis muscle. If hyaluronic acid products have been used, enzymatic degradation with hyaluronidase may be employed. Additionally, if a temporary filler is used, the patient will require periodic follow-up to assess for repeat augmentation; additional injections may be necessary as early as 4 months after the initial treatment, depending on the location, with highly mobile areas such as the lips typically requiring earlier retreatment.

Nutritional deficiencies are common in this patient population and should be suspected if poor wound healing is encountered. In these cases, diet modification, nutritional consultation, and even addition of a daily multivitamin may improve a patient's result.

41.5 Conclusions

Massive weight loss results in an overall improvement in quality of life, but can cause significant facial cosmetic deformity. The loss of volume in the midface and severe skin laxity of the cervicofacial junction often leads PBS patients to seek facial contouring procedures. It is important for the cosmetic surgeon to understand the pathomechanics behind these aesthetic defects in order to appropriately address them. The midfacial and perioral volume loss is easily correctable with injectable fillers. The excess skin laxity can be fixed using the modified rhytidectomy technique (Fig. 41.1). To achieve an optimal result in a safe manner, a good understanding of the special pre- and postoperative needs of the PBS patient is imperative.

References

1. Deitel M. Overweight and obesity worldwide now estimated to involve 1.7 billion people. Obes Surg. 2003;13(3):329–30.
2. National Center for Health Statistics NHANES IV report. Available at: http://www.cdc.gov/nchs/product/pubs/pubd/hestats/obes/obese99.htm 2002.

3. Buchwald H, Avidor Y, Braunwald E, Jensen MD, Pories W, Fahrbach K, et al. Bariatric surgery: a systematic review and meta-analysis. J Am Med Assoc. 2004;292(14):1724–37.
4. Kinzl JF, Traweger C, Trefalt E, Biebl W. Psychosocial consequences of weight loss following gastric banding for morbid obesity. Obes Surg. 2003;13(1):105–10.
5. American Society of Plastic Surgeons. 2007 National plastic surgery statistics. Arlington Heights: American Society of Plastic Surgeons; 2008.
6. Smalls LK, Hicks M, Passeretti D, Gersin K, Kitzmiller WJ, Bakhsh A, et al. Effect of weight loss on cellulite: gynoid lipodystrophy. Plast Reconstr Surg. 2006;118(2):510–16.
7. Gosain AK, Klein MH, Sudhakar PV, Prost RW. A volumetric analysis of soft-tissue changes in the aging midface using high-resolution MRI: implications for facial rejuvenation. Plast Reconstr Surg. 2005;115(4):1143–52.
8. Ascher B, Katz P. Facial lipoatrophy and the place of ultrasound. Dermatol Surg. 2006;32(5):698–708.
9. Ascher BA, Coleman S, Alster T, Bauer U, Burgess C, Butterwick K, et al. Full scope of effect of facial lipoatrophy: a framework of disease understanding. Dermatol Surg. 2006;32(8):1058–69.
10. Shah M, Simha V, Garg A. Review: long-term impact of bariatric surgery on body weight, comorbidities, and nutritional status. J Clin Endocrinol Metab. 2006;91(11):4223–31.
11. Le Louarn C, Buthiau D, Buis J. The face recurve concept: medical and surgical applications. Aesthetic Plast Surg. 2007;31(3):219–31.
12. Raspaldo H. Volumizing effect of a new hyaluronic acid subdermal facial filler: a retrospective analysis based on 102 cases. J Cosmet Laser Ther. 2008;10(3):134–42.
13. Adamson PA, Litner JA. Surgical management of the aging neck. Facial Plast Surg. 2005;21(1):11–20.
14. Sugerman HJ, Wolfe LG, Sica DA, Clore JN. Diabetes and hypertension in severe obesity and effects of gastric bypass-induced weight loss. Ann Surg. 2003;237(6):751–6.
15. Puzziferri N, Austrheim-Smith IT, Wolfe BM, Wilson SE, Nguyen NT. Three-year follow-up of a prospective randomized trial comparing laparoscopic versus open gastric bypass. Ann Surg. 2006;243(2):181–8.
16. Christou NV, Sampalis JS, Liberman M, Look D, Auger S, McLean AP, et al. Surgery decreases long-term mortality, morbidity, and health care use in morbidly obese patients. Ann Surg. 2004;240(3):416–23.
17. Flum DR, Dellinger EP. Impact of gastric bypass operation on survival: a population-based analysis. J Am Coll Surg. 2004;99(4):543–51.
18. Agha-Mohammadi S, Chir SB, Hurwitz DJ. Nutritional deficiency of post-bariatric surgery body contouring patients: what every plastic surgeon should know. Plast Reconstr Surg. 2008;122(2):604–13.
19. Shermak MA, Chang D, Magnuson TH, Schweitzer MA. An outcomes analysis of patients undergoing body contouring surgery after massive weight loss. Plast Reconstr Surg. 2006;118(4):1026–31.
20. Sarwer DB, Cohn NI, Gibbons LM, Magee L, Crerand CE, Raper SE, et al. Psychiatric diagnoses and psychiatric treatment among bariatric surgery candidates. Obes Surg. 2004;14(9):1148–56.
21. Rosenberger PH, Henderson KE, Grilo CM. Psychiatric disorder comorbidity and association with eating disorders in bariatric surgery patients: a cross-sectional study using structured interview-based diagnosis. J Clin Psychiatry. 2006; 67(7):1080–5.
22. Aly AS, Cram AE, Chao M, Pang J, Mckeon M. Belt lipectomy for circumferential trunkal excess; the University of Iowa experience. Plast Reconstr Surg. 2003;111(1):398–413.
23. Lambros V, Stuzin JM. The cross-cheek depression: surgical cause and effect in the development of the "joker line" and its treatment. Plast Reconstr Surg. 2008;122(5):1543–52.
24. Lowe NJ, Maxwell CA, Lowe P, Duick MG, Shah K. Hyaluronic acid skin fillers: adverse reactions and skin testing. J Am Acad Dermatol. 2001;45(6):930–3.
25. Rohrich RJ, Ghavami A, Crosby MA. The role of hyaluronic acid fillers (Restylane) in facial cosmetic surgery: review and technical considerations. Plast Reconstr Surg. 2007;120 Suppl 6:41S–54S.
26. Bousquet MT, Agerup B. Restylane lip implantation: European experience. Operat Tech Oculoplast Orbital Reconstr Surg. 1999;2:172–6.
27. Cantisano-Zilkha M, Bosniak S. Hyaluronic acid gel injections for facial rejuvenation: a 3-year clinical experience. Operat Tech Oculoplast Orbital Reconstr Surg. 1999;2: 177–81.
28. Carruthers A, Carey W, De Lorenzi C, Remington K, Schachter D, Sapra S. Randomized, double-blind comparison of the efficacy of two hyaluronic acid derivatives, restylane, perlane and hylaform, in the treatment of nasolabial folds. Dermatol Surg. 2005;31(11 Pt 2):1591–8.
29. Lupo MP, Smith SR, Thomas JA, Murphy DK, Beddingfield III FC. Effectiveness of Juvéderm Ultra Plus dermal filler in the treatment of severe nasolabial folds. Plast Reconstr Surg. 2008;121(1):289–97.
30. Narins RS, Brandt FS, Lorenc ZP, Maas CS, Monheit GD, Smith SR. Twelve-month persistency of a novel ribose-cross-linked collagen dermal filler. Dermatol Surg. 2008;34 Suppl 1:S31–9.
31. Graivier MH, Bass LS, Busso M, Jasin ME, Narins RS, Tzikas TL. Calcium hydroxylapatite (Radiesse) for correction of the mid- and lower face: consensus recommendations. Plast Reconstr Surg. 2007;120 Suppl 6:55S–66S.
32. Salles AG, Lotierzo PH, Gimenez R, Camargo CP, Ferreira MC. Evaluation of the poly-L-lactic acid implant for treatment of the nasolabial fold: 3-year follow-up evaluation. Aesthetic Plast Surg. 2008;32(5):753–6.
33. Neuber F. Fettransplantation. Kongressbd Dtsch Ges Chir Kongr. 1893;22:66.
34. Chajchir A, Benzaquen I. Fat-grafting injection for soft tissue augmentation. Plast Reconstr Surg. 1989;84(6):921–34.
35. Bucky LP, Kanchwala SK. The role of autologous fat and alternative filler in the aging face. Plast Reconstr Surg. 2007;120 Suppl 6:89S–97S.
36. Azzena B, Mazzoleni F, Abatangelo G, Zavan B, Vindigni V. Autologous platelet-rich plasma as an adipocyte in vivo delivery system: case report. Aesthetic Plast Surg. 2008; 32(1):155–8.
37. Zoumalan R, Rizk SS. Hematoma rates in drainless deep-plane face-lift surgery with and without the use of fibrin glue. Arch Facial Plast Surg. 2008;10(2):103–7.
38. Cohen JL. Understanding, avoiding, and managing dermal filler complications. Dermatol Surg. 2008;34 Suppl 1: S92–9.

Complications of Facelift Surgery

Melvin A. Shiffman

42.1 Introduction

There are a variety of possible complications of facelift surgery. The surgeon should be well aware of all the possible risks and know how to prevent them or make an early diagnosis in order to treat the complication in time. This may reduce tissue damage compared to a late diagnosis.

42.2 Complications

42.2.1 Asymmetry

Asymmetry usually results from excess excision of skin from one side of the face or from unequal pull on the flaps, not in the same direction, on each side. Distortion of the earlobe is common if the closure is performed under any tension around the bottom of the ear. Revision surgery may have to be performed.

42.2.2 Bleeding

Postoperative bleeding may occur if the vessels are not completely ligated or electrocoagulated.

M.A. Shiffman
17501 Chatham Drive, Tustin,
California 92780-2302, USA
e-mail: shiffmanmdjd@yahoo.com

Other causes of bleeding include:

1. Surgical technique
2. Aspirin or nonsteroidal anti-inflammatory drugs (NSAIDS)
3. Hypertension
4. Anticoagulation drugs (coumadin)
5. Blood dyscrasia
6. History of easy bruising

42.2.3 Dehiscence

Tight wound closure with tension may result in wound dehiscence. This may require resuturing but if the tissues are friable, the wound may have to be allowed to heal with secondary intention.

42.2.4 Dog Ear

A dog ear may occur in the temporal region or the posterior neck or scalp. Most will tend to resolve over a few months. It is easier to repair the dog ear at the end of the surgical procedure but revision may be performed at a secondary surgery.

42.2.5 Ear Deformities

Excessive tension is the usual cause of ear deformity. Excision of skin around the ear should be performed after tension sutures have been inserted above the ear and behind the ear. Secondary surgery may be necessary to correct a deformity.

42.2.6 Edema

Edema usually subsides within the first few weeks. Chronic edema should be investigated for causes other than the surgery. Diuretics are not usually recommended.

42.2.7 Hair Loss

Hair loss can occur as the result of a tight closure and tension on the hair-bearing tissues. Most of the time the hair will regrow over time. Repair of the area of chronic hair loss may require excision (after 6 months) of the bare region or hair transplantation can be performed.

42.2.8 Hematoma

An expanding hematoma (pain and swelling of the side of the face) is a surgical emergency and requires early wound exploration with evacuation of the hematoma, ligation of bleeder, and probably needs to be drained at the time of closure [1].

42.2.9 Infection

Infection is rare (11 in 6,166 cases or 0.18% [2]). Inflammation may be treated with topical steroids and any infection should be treated with appropriate antibiotics. Heat applied locally is helpful.

42.2.10 Irregularities

Irregularities may be the result of coming too close to the skin in developing the facial flap. Indentations of the skin following face-lift surgery can be treated with a filler, preferably autologous fat. In one case indentation occurred from a very tight S suture in a modified face-lift (S-lift) (Fig. 42.1). This resolved over a couple of months without treatment except massage of the area.

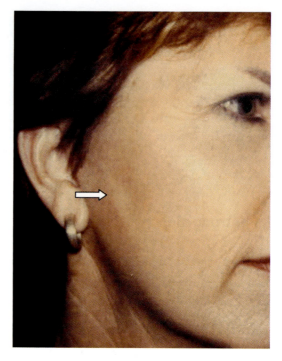

Fig. 42.1 This patient had an S-lift and 1 week after surgery began to develop a swelling of the right cheek. On examination there was a soft swelling that became an indentation when compressed by the finger. Simple observation with mild massage of the area allowed the problem to resolve that originated from too tight a closure of the purse string S suture in the parotid fascia

42.2.11 Necrosis

Necrosis can be the result of the flaps being too thin or the closure being too tight. Smokers are very susceptible to flap necrosis if the smoking is not completely stopped prior to and after surgery [3]. Especially dangerous is electrocoagulation of bleeders on the skin flap. The oozing of blood on the skin flap should be treated with compression only.

42.2.12 Neurological

Any of the facial sensory or motor nerves in the area of the face-lift may be injured. Especially susceptible are the branches of the facial nerve and the anterior and posterior auricular nerves. Prevention is a necessity. The surgeon should understand facial anatomy and the three-dimensional relationship of the nerves.

Temporary paresis can occur with injection of local anesthesia into the area of the nerve or from traction on the nerve. This type of paralysis can be observed until it clears. If there is any question of motor nerve transection then studies should be performed to establish nerve conduction. Early repair of a transected nerve will aid in more complete and earlier return of function.

42.2.13 Pain

Persistent facial pain is rare. If acute following surgery this may suggest an expanding hematoma. If chronic branches of the sensory cervical nerves may have been injured. The pain will usually subside within 6 months. Nerve blocks may give temporary relief.

42.2.14 Pigmentation Changes

Hyperpigmentation may follow facial ecchymoses even with full resolution of the bruising. Sunlight exposure may increase the possibility of hyperpigmentation.

Patients with telangiectasias may develop more after rhytidectomy.

42.2.15 Salivary Fistula

Sutures placed deep in the parotid fascia (part of the SMAS) can result in a salivary fistula (rare) (Fig. 42.2). Treatment would require removal of the offending suture, bland diet, and Donnatol four times daily to reduce the salivary flow. The fistula usually heals very readily with this treatment.

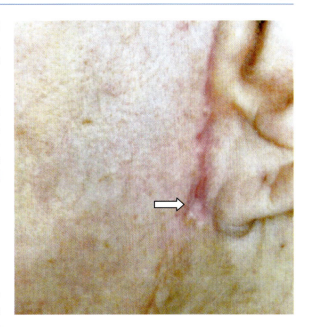

Fig. 42.2 Scar at the anterior inferior portion of the ear following S-lift. Surgical revision was necessary

42.2.16 Scar

Scars are usually a physiologic response to injury and may be hypertrophic or keloid. Keloid scars can be hereditary. Tight closure can contribute to a widened scar (Fig. 42.3).

There are a variety of treatments for keloids and hypertrophic scars including steroid injection, surgery, 5-fluorouracil injection, silicone gel sheeting, bleomycin injection, or a combination of these.

42.2.17 Seroma

Seroma may occur following an unrecognized hematoma under the skin flap. Syringe with needle drainage followed by compression may resolve the problem. Open drainage with suction catheter can be used for persistent seroma.

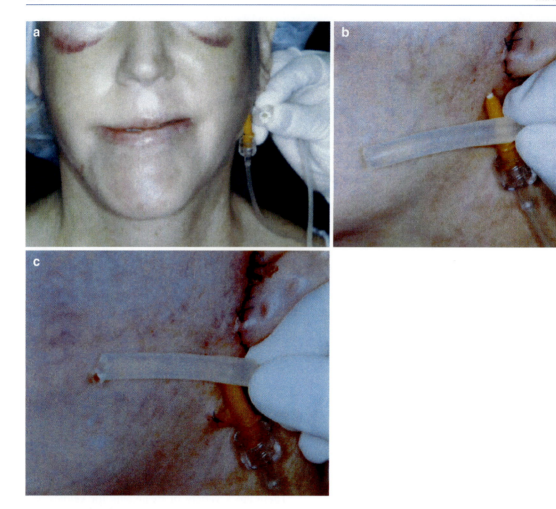

Fig. 42.3 (**a**) Patient developed a soft swelling a few days after modified face-lift. This was drained with a suction catheter. The wound drained 120 ml clear fluid daily. (**b**) Following removal of the vacuum reservoir there was no drainage after 1 min. (**c**) Following biting of a wedge of lime, there was drainage starting at the end of the catheter within 5 s. The diagnosis of salivary fistula was confirmed

References

1. Niamtu III J. Expanding hematoma in face-lift surgery: literature review, case presentations, and caveats. Dermatol Surg. 2005;31(9 Part 1):1134–44.
2. LeRoy JL, Rees TD, Nolan III WB. Infections requiring hospital readmission following face lift surgery: incidence, treatment, and sequelae. Plast Reconstr Surg. 1994;93(3): 533–6.
3. Rees TD, Liverett MD, Guy CL. The effect of cigarette smoking on skin-flap survival in face lift patient. Plast Reconstr Surg. 1984;73(6):911–5.

Forehead Lifting Approach and Techniques

43

Jaime Ramirez, Yhon Steve Amado, and Adriana Carolina Navarro

43.1 Introduction

The procedures of forehead lifting are those that tend to change the apparent descent or the other effects of the soft tissue aging located over the skeletal supraorbital ring, fixing the eyebrow descent and the appearance of wrinkles or furrows and in some cases removing the leftover frontal skin. When speaking of techniques of forehead lifting it is necessary to talk about the diverse ways to deal with the rejuvenation of a specific face area, as it is the superior third. Sometimes the completed procedure, even if is open or with minimum system invasion, does not obtain the expected results, which has generated multiple variations of the surgical approach applied and the suspension techniques.

There is a necessity to treat the superior face segment where the aging process is marked. As a consequence it brings the surgical approach and techniques applied for its adjustment that have been improved trying to diminish the poor result and the appearance of the undesired effects like alopecia, scars, or paresthesia [1, 2].

The object of this chapter is to expose how and when to use a procedure and the advantages and disadvantages of each of the different approaches and techniques used for forehead lifting and also to discuss these based on the experience of the senior author who uses them according to the indications required for each particular case. The selection of the ideal surgical techniques for the patient, that is occasionally a reason of controversy, must be the result of the joint search between the doctor in charge and his patients.

It is understood that the endoscopic forehead lifting is nowadays the most used technique because of its versatility and benefits and this is widely recognized by the majority of authors in facial rejuvenation [3, 4].

The ideal approach for the forehead-lift must allow an efficient loosening and elimination of the adhesions that prevent the free displacement upward of the inelastic structures of the forehead and obtaining reversion of the frontal orbital ptosis generated by aging. This situation is more relevant when the forehead-lift takes part, along with blepharoplasty, as an integral treatment for the facial superior third.

In this chapter the coronal approach is excluded, in spite of being for several years the standard method for superior face rejuvenation. At the moment it has been in disuse for being an invasive technique that requires an ample and notorious incision generating problems of sensitivity and healing as well as greater morbidity.

43.2 Historical Review

The first literary mention referring to the elevation of the facial third superior was by Passot [5], who used elliptic excision in the forehead skin. Hunt in 1926 [6] described

J. Ramirez (✉)
Calle 105 A No. 14-92 Consultorio 107, Bogotá, Colombia
e-mail: info@jaimeramirez.com

Y.S. Amado
Hospital Central de la Policia Ncional,
Cra 11 90-07 cs 208, Bogotá, Colombia
e-mail: steveamadog@hotmail.com

A.C. Navarro
Universidad Nacional de Colombia,
Cll 131 A No 55A – 26 Apto 504, Bogotá, Colombia
e-mail: acnavarrona@unal.edu.co

his technique using incisions by the edge of the hairline in the implantation and in the forehead skin, this being the beginning of the pretrichial approach. In 1930, Passot [7] suggested using a direct incision by the superior edge of the eyebrow end and removing the superfluous skin, which constitutes the first description of the direct eyebrow-lift, as it is actually known. Fomon, in 1939 [8], was the first to indicate that anatomically, the frontal skin continue with the epicranium, and the importance of the muscular fascia implantation, which is important to understand the necessity to dry out the superfluous skin and the possibility to realize a frontal anchorage from the epicranium [9].

Motivated by the short duration of the results of the first forehead lifting the necessity to include the management of the frontal muscle was described; initially with chemical denervation using alcohol, no satisfactory results were obtained, which generate the necessity to evolve in the handling of the corresponding muscles of the frontal region. In 1962, Gonzalez Ulloa [10] described the utility of the frontal myotomies and in 1964 Marino and Gandolfo [11] reported on myotomies of the corrugators, which are still being used [12]. Vinas was the first to enumerate the repair points in the forehead-lift and in order to obtain elevation of the end of the eyebrow it is necessary to perform lateral traction that are elements still in force [1]. The repair points described by Vinas are the inelastic aponeurotic layer on the frontal muscle, which has importance in the vertical traction, necessary for the correction of eyebrow ptosis and the ledge of the orbital bony with its adhesions to the soft tissue that must be dried out to allow mobilization of the glabellar area. In addition Vinas was the first to classify wrinkles into two types: Transitory and persistent according to its relation with the movements of the facial expression [13]. These findings were integrated by Kaye in 1977 [14] who used a coronal approach for the frontal repairs and complementary rhytidectomy.

During the following decades few modifications to the repair points were made until the 1990s when revolutionary change was made to the approach of forehead lifting; Vasconez and Isse [15, 16] presented initial experiences using endoscopy in the correction of the eyebrow ptosis as did Chajchir [17, 18]. Chajchir postulated the bases for the use of surgical endoscopy in the accomplishment of forehead lifting, emphasizing that it is a functional dynamic process.

43.3 Anatomic Guidelines

In order to estimate the anatomy of the facial third superior, it is necessary to specify the anatomic limits of forehead: the superior edge is defined by the hairline implantation, the inferior edge in its medial portion by the frontonasal or glabella suture and laterally to the superior orbital margin. The bony structures are constituted by the frontal bone and its joints with the nasal bones and with the frontal process of the jawbone; laterally, with the frontal zygomatic bone union, and in the temporal cavity with the main wing of the sphenoid [19]. Hairline implantation can be influenced by several factors in its conformation such as age, sex, individual, familial or cultural characteristics, and conditioning of the handling of scars and attenuation of the same [19–22]. The eyebrow thickness, as well, can present similar individual variations too, and in addition to external alteration like shaved and the tattoo, the position and the contour of the same are important in the facial expression and aesthetic, defining gender characteristics, as well as, in men are thicker and more straight than women which are thinner and curved, given the lower implantation through the orbital rim, in man higher than women [22, 23].

The superior orbital margin is a palpable bony prominence or visible in individuals, especially in Latin people; besides, it can be even more notorious creating a fall in the skin over the eyebrow [22–24]. The lateral limit of the forehead corresponds to another bony repair point which is the temporal line that is easily palpable with the mastication movements. It is an important point to locate the temporal artery. To the lateral one, the frontomalar suture is found, located 10 mm from the external canthus. The frontal nerve is usually found at 5 mm previous to the tragus up to 15 mm to the end of the eyebrow, over the zygomatic arc, leading to the external canthal and area of 2.5 cm^2 approximately as a secure area [24–26]. The supraorbital hole described, habitually in literature, in the superior edge of the ciliary arc corresponds properly to 49% foramen, 26% foramina, and present in just one side in 25% of the patients [27]; anatomical dissections realized by the senior author have shown that in some patients a proper orifice does not exist and the supraorbital nerve traverses a channel to the level of the orbital ceiling, to ascend by the frontal region after passing through a notch (Fig. 43.1).

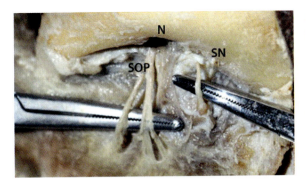

Fig. 43.1 Corpse dissection with the supraorbital package (*SOP*) in relation to the notch (*N*), and the right supratrochlear nerve (*SN*). The frontal soft tissues have been rejected forward and downward (Photo courtesy Dr. Jaime Ramirez)

Anatomically, the frontal muscle has two ways of consideration: the first one, as an individual previous muscular unit and the second one, as a continuation of the digastric muscle that starts from an initial posterior belly, the occipital muscle. This is the primary elevator of the eyebrow; it has multiple insertions, the vertical fibers end up anchoring at the depressor muscle and the longitudinal ones have fibrous digitations along their run to a skin level giving as a result, the vector of contraction of the same going upward and vertically, producing the ascent of all the structures of the forehead and the formation of transverse lines on the skin to the contraction, as a consequence of their fibrous anchorages. This muscle is innervated by the frontal branch of the face [19, 21, 22, 28] (Fig. 43.2).

The corrugator muscle, measuring 2.5 cm/1 cm is thin, with fibers oriented in an oblique direction; it is located in the lateral region glabella, over the nasofrontal suture. Two types of fibers are inserted in the medial portion of the superciliary arc: The short fibers are directed upward up to the deep layer of the skin where the eyebrow begins, to be inserted. The long fibers, in oblique direction are inserted in the middle part and the end of the eyebrow, throughout the frontal muscle and the orbicular muscle. It is a forehead depressor; the simultaneous contraction of both types of fibers produce elevation of the beginning and the middle part of the eyebrow, acting in conjunction with the frontal muscle at the same time; with the orbicular of the eyelids, it produces a depression at the end of the eyebrow, which produces horizontal lines in the glabellar area. With the superciliary depressor it produces vertical lines in the skin. Its innervations take place through the temporal ramification of the facial nerve [19, 21, 22, 24, 28] (Fig. 43.2).

The procerus or pyramidal muscles have their origin in the nasal back; they are two vertical muscular beams, which are inserted in the frontal muscle, from glabella to the lower middle part of the forehead. They are frontal depressors, and create interciliary horizontal lines due to their contraction of the inferior skin of the forehead descend. [19–22, 26, 28] (Fig. 43.2).

The superciliary depressor muscle is the most superficial one of the glabellar area; for some authors, it makes part of the orbicular muscle. It is located in the middle arc of the eyebrow and it is inserted in the nasal in the frontal bone, extending itself to get mixed with the procerus and frontal muscles. Its action elevates the beginning of the eyebrow and descends the middle portion and the skin of it and generates the vertical furrows of the beginning of the region and the middle portion of the eyebrow [22, 26, 28]. It is innervated by the ramification of the facial nerve (Fig. 43.2).

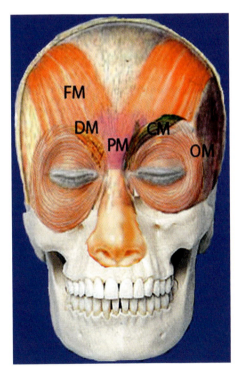

Fig. 43.2 The existing relation in the muscles of the frontal region is observed. Frontal muscle (*FM*), corrugator muscle (*CM*), procerus muscle (*PM*), orbicular muscle (*OM*) and its intimate relation with the superciliary depressing muscle (*DM*)

The orbicular muscle has a concentric disposition over the orbit and circumferential vectors; it is wide, flat, inserted in the nasal portion of the frontal bone and in the frontal process of the jawbone, previous to the middle canthal ligament. It presents two portions: the orbital and palpebral. The palpebral portion has two fibrous insertions in the eyelid; the orbital portion has bony insertions. Its function is to approximate the loosened edge of the eyelid and provoke the occlusion of the palpebral cleavage. Its joint action produces descent of the eyebrow position. It is innervated by the ramification of facial nerve [19, 21, 22, 25, 28] (Fig. 43.2).

The areolar lax tissue is the continuation of the subgaleal tissue. The supraorbital insertion of the orbicular muscle is a strong ligament, formed, as well, by lateral and middle orbital ligaments [19, 20, 29].

The supraorbital and supratrochlear nerves give the sensitive innervations of the skin and the innervation's mechanism comes from the facial nerve [22, 24–27].

The Sentinel vein is an important repair point in the endoscopic surgery; to avoid injuring it, it must be identified. It is located at the superior and lateral tail of the eyebrow and in some cases can be duplicated; it is a structure of transition that perforates the band and it is deepened in company of the frontal facial nerve, toward the lateral superior zone [30] (Fig. 43.3).

The frontal skin is the continuity of the scalp. It presents five well-defined layers: skin, subcutaneous

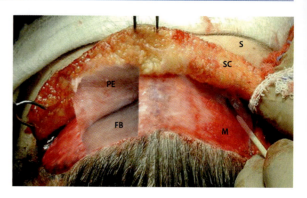

Fig. 43.4 The layers in the dissection of the frontal region are observed. Skin (*S*), subcutaneous cell tissue (*SC*), muscle (*M*), periosteum (*PE*), frontal bone (*FB*)

cell tissue, galea aponeurotic, areolar lax tissue, and periosteum. The skin is thin, rich in sebaceous glands, and sudoriparous; it is anchored in a homogeneous layer of compact adipose tissue and dense fibrous tissue separate it from the muscles label, which generates major quantity of lines of expression. The muscular aponeurosis is the continuation, in double layer of the facial SMAS, [12] keeping the different forehead muscle and the periocular area that possess two types of action: passive by traction and active by contraction. By its passive action it maintains the muscular anchorage and the others structures, while, in contraction puts close together the insertion ends [28, 31] (Fig. 43.4).

43.4 The Eyebrow and Forehead as an Aesthetic Unit

In the surgery of the facial third superior; the forehead, eyebrow, and eyelid must be dynamically analyzed. The patients consult by the apparent excess of palpebral skin, without noticing that in occasions the drop of the eyebrow is one that generates an over dimensioning of redundancy of the eyelid's skin. In the last one is located one of the main keys to establish in the ptotic forehead, when it really corresponds to the drop of the eyebrow, below the orbital bony ledge, whether it is due to looseness or excess in the

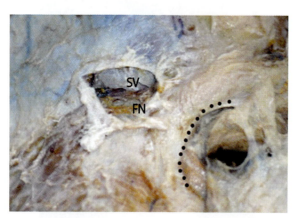

Fig. 43.3 Sentinel vein (*SV*) and frontal branch of the facial nerve (*FN*). The *shaded area* shows the orbital rim (Photo courtesy Dr. Jaime Ramirez)

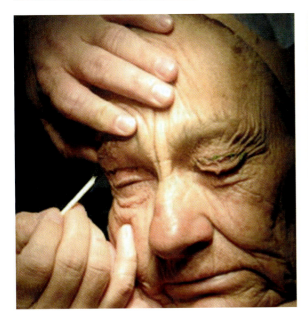

Fig. 43.5 Simulation of the final desired position of the eyebrow and marking in the superior eyelid for the resection of the redundant skin (Photo courtesy Dr. Jaime Ramirez)

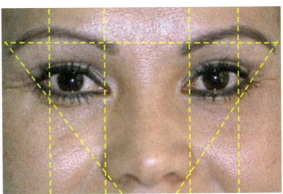

Fig. 43.6 The ideal position of the eyebrow in women is observed (Photo courtesy Dr. Jaime Ramirez)

skin of the eyelid. Bellow regarding, before carrying out a cosmetic blepharoplasty, to make the simulation of the ideal position of the eyebrow, having the patients sitting down or standing up, move the eyebrow with the finger to the new wanted position and visualize the amount of the skin of the eyelid that still looks redundant preventing the definition of superior palpebral furrow. This is done at this moment and not before (Fig. 43.5). It is expected that the doctor realize this presurgical maneuver of measurement and demarcation commenting to the patient his findings. Then the patient will agree with greater facility to the approval of the integral treatment of the suspension forehead lifting with blepharoplasty.

It is also important to do a previous analysis of the factors that influence the eyebrows and forehead aesthetic unit, which must be postsurgically controlled to extend the obtained results, which are: intrinsic factors such as lost elasticity of the tissue and the marked activity of the depressor muscle and the extrinsic factors such as the gravity, the photo exposure, and the tobacco addiction.

43.5 Position of the Eyebrows

The beauty concept must consider the cultural differences and also manage a parameter for each one of the sexes. Aesthetically, the ideal position of the eyebrow in women is defined as a smooth arch, located above the orbital rim, with its higher point coinciding with an imaginary line traced between the lateral limbo and the lateral canthus. The eyebrow descends to the point where the imaginary line ends, drawn up between the facial alar furrow and the lateral canthus [32] (Fig. 43.6).

In men, the eyebrow takes a horizontal line shape to level the orbital rim. With this reference it is understood that the major efforts put in the repositioning of the feminine eyebrow must be directed toward the elevation of the lateral portion; in men the final elevation of the eyebrow must leave the middle portion and the lateral one approximately to the same height preventing in the patient feminine features.

43.6 General Indications

Traditionally, the main indications for forehead-lift include:

1. To elevate the ptotic eyebrows
2. To correct asymmetry of the eyebrows

3. To reduce
   (a) The palpebral redundant skin
   (b) The frontal furrows
   (c) The glabella furrows
   (d) The lines of the lateral canthus expression
4. To elevate the aesthetic unit of the forehead
5. To modify, when desired, the implantation line of the hair
6. To diminish the extension of the frontal skin, when it tends to be redundant

These indications can be presented singly or in conjunction, doing necessary to consider in each case, the best way of possible approach. Intervening a young patient with an asymmetry of the eyebrow without any mark of the glabellar furrows, and a male patient, an adult with scarce hair and frontal marked furrows is not the same.

In literature, the technique and approach terms are frequently distorted, which generates confusion. For the authors, the approach is used to indicate the place where the incision is realized and the used plane for the dissection, whereas the technique refers to the intervention of the repair points and the suspension mechanism that is used for the correction of the eyebrow ptosis and the reduction of the frontal furrows.

43.7 How to Choose the Approach and the Technique?

The technique must be individualized for each patient. Sex, age, physical features, and expectation should be considered. In order to define the way to approach and the technique of frontal suspension the following must be analyzed: degree of ptosis, depth level of the furrows of the skin, eyebrows asymmetry, amount of redundant skin, and the implantation pattern of hair.

43.7.1 Frontal Ptosis Degree

The higher the ptosis degree, the more aggressive the suspension techniques must be, whether this is done through opened or closed approach.

43.7.2 Depth of the Skin Furrows

In patients, especially old men with tendency to baldness and with pronounced frontal furrow, the incisions can be camouflaged in the furrow, allowing a direct approach of the frontal region to suspend.

43.7.3 Asymmetries

The direct approach allows a more precise correction of the asymmetric position of the eyebrow. It would not be an option in patients that do not require a treatment in other areas of forehead and accept a possible visible scar.

43.7.4 Frontal Redundant Skin

This implies the necessity of exeresis for which the open approach of pretrichal type or trichial allows edge to edge suspension.

43.7.5 Implantation Pattern of the Hairline

This can also condition the selection of the approach for the eyebrow and forehead suspension. Once the objectives of the procedure are defined, which can be directed to attenuate the strong expression of the glabella muscle spasms or revert and to correct the asymmetry of the eyebrow position, the approach must be selected considering the line of the hair implantation that can commonly be influenced in men by genetic factors like the alopecia. On the other hand, the line of high implantation in women causes that the approach selected do not elevate the hairline even more and can even facilitate the manipulation to diminish the length of the frontal skin, standing out in this situation the pretrichial–trichial approach (Fig. 43.7).

Fig. 43.7 The implantation lines of the hair and the corresponding approach options are observed

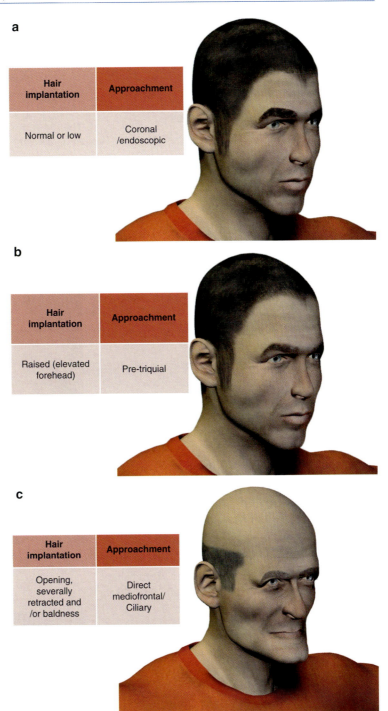

An approach can be chosen, according to Lazor and Cheney [33], considering the implantation line of the hair as it is observed in Fig. 43.7.

43.8 What Fixing Approaches and Techniques Do We Use?

(a) Coronal
(b) Pretrichial/Trichial
(c) Medio-Frontal
(d) Direct Eyebrow Lift
(e) Endoscopic

43.8.1 Coronal

Nowadays a facial approach is rarely used.
Dissection plan: Subgaleal
Advantages: An excellent exposure and direct access to the frontal myotomy.
Disadvantages: It is an invasive surgical approach; there is a risk of hematoma, elevation of the implantation line of the hair and alopecic scar. This can produce vertical enlargement of the forehead. It is not used for the scar and has limited uses in men.

43.8.2 Pretrichial/Trichial

Preparation: The definition of the incision is realized, immediately in front of the hairline, in a zigzag shape reaching to exceed each end of the scalp (Fig. 43.8).

A template designed by the surgeon to demarcate the incision form is used and in the cases where resection of skin is required, in the new edge the same template is used to make the ends coincide when joining (Fig. 43.9). Laterally, the incision can continue in linear shape to 1 cm. behind the hairline, this zone corresponding to the superior part on the temporal region (Fig. 43.10).

The dissection plane in the previous region is subgaleal that allows the loosening of the muscular cutaneous plane above the supraorbital rim, facilitating the exposure of the corrugator muscle and the superior portion of the procerus muscle, as well as the neurovascular supraorbital packages of each side, that must

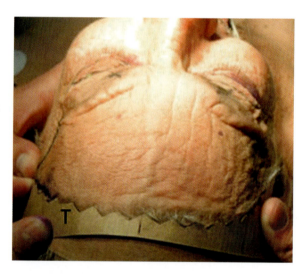

Fig. 43.9 Pretriquial–triquial approach. The template for the demarcation of incision is observed. In case incision of the skin is required, the template is used again in the new incision to allow the edges to coincide (Photo courtesy Dr. Jaime Ramirez)

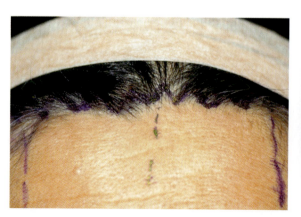

Fig. 43.8 Demarcation of the incision for the pretrichial–trichial approach (Photo courtesy Dr. Jaime Ramirez)

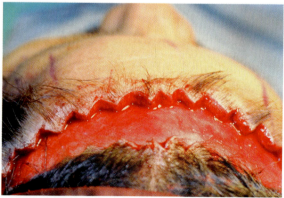

Fig. 43.10 Incision in a zigzag shape, reaching up to exceed in each end of the scalp for the Pretriquial–triquial approach (Photo courtesy Dr. Jaime Ramirez)

be respected (Fig. 43.11). Laterally the dissection is performed in the interfascial plane. In this procedure, fragments of the corrugator (Fig. 43.12) and procerus (Fig. 43.13) muscles and rectangular segments of the superior portion of the orbicular muscle of each side are sectioned and dried out. In addition, when needed, the skin is dried out. The suspension technique uses Ethibond 3–0 to suspend, in the previous region, from galea to galea and in the lateral portion, from superficial fascia to deep fascia (Fig. 43.14).

The advantages are: Excellent visualization of the operating field. It does not change the implantation line of the hair. It allows realizing exeresis of the skin, reducing the length of the forehead and the lax tissue or leftover. By diminishing the depth of furrows when tightening the skin, the scar can be camouflaged (Fig. 43.15).

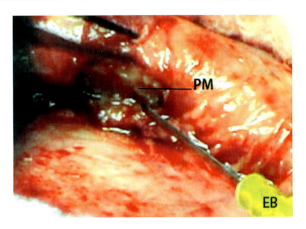

Fig. 43.13 Transverse cut of the procerus muscle (*MP*) with electric scalpel (*EB*) (Photo courtesy Dr. Jaime Ramirez)

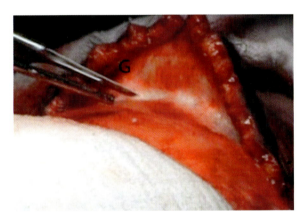

Fig. 43.11 Plane of subgaleal dissection in the pretrichial approach. The Galena is marked with a *G* (Photo courtesy Dr. Jaime Ramirez)

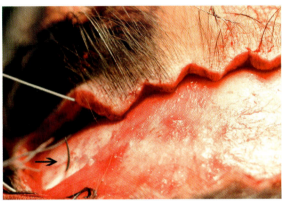

Fig. 43.14 Suspension technique. Anchorage point of the superficial to the deep fascia is observed. The *arrow* indicates the needle of the suture used for the anchorage (Photo courtesy Dr. Jaime Ramirez)

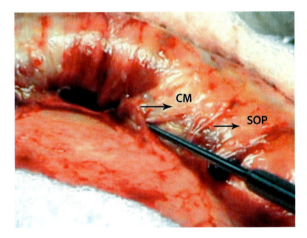

Fig. 43.12 Image of the right corrugator muscle (*CM*) and supraorbital package (*SOP*) (Photo courtesy Dr. Jaime Ramirez)

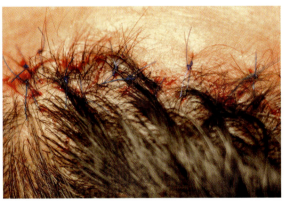

Fig. 43.15 Closing of the incision, without closing the implantation line of the hair and allowing camouflage of the scar (Photo courtesy Dr. Jaime Ramirez)

Disadvantages: It can generate temporal hypoesthesia of the scar and the frontal skin.

The scar can be occasionally visible.

The surgical time is greater.

Ideal for patients with higher hairline, although with restriction in men.

43.8.3 "Half Frontal"

Preparation: the frontal furrows to be intervened must be selected on each side of the forehead, through which the approach will be realized. Later on, it is demarcated and an incision is made in the ellipse in the lateral or middle base according to the case, which increases the inferior flap when the surgical wound is sutured (Fig. 43.16). The incision point can be chosen: throughout the furrow line, centrally, throughout the forehead, or two fusiform excisions to each side (Fig. 43.17).

The initial dissection plane is subcutaneous, to preserve the sensorial innervation; once it is taken to the supraorbital level it affects the galea and the subgaleal plane is introduced (Fig. 43.18) that allows to the superciliary corrugator (Fig. 43.19) and procerus muscles (Fig. 43.20), which can be partially dried out.

The Suspension Techniques: anchorage is realized from the superior portion of the orbicular muscle to the superolateral frontal periosteum with Ethibond 3–0.

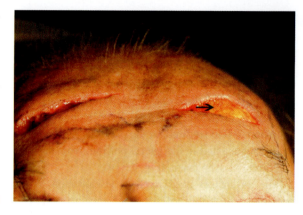

Fig. 43.17 Patient with middle frontal approach. The incisions of the skin in an ellipse and the subcutaneous plane are observed (Photo courtesy Dr. Jaime Ramirez)

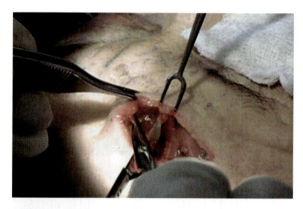

Fig. 43.18 Dissection and direct access to the supraorbital musculature in a half frontal approach (Photo courtesy Dr. Jaime Ramirez)

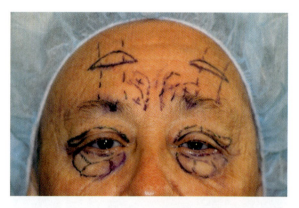

Fig. 43.16 Marking of the incisions in ellipse for the middle frontal approach and the orientation lines of orbicular muscle suspension are observed (Photo courtesy Dr. Jaime Ramirez)

Each side, depending on the necessity to suspend different portions of the eyebrow, needs two or three sutures. One of the key factors in the final results of the scars camouflage is the meticulous closing by planes of the incisions (Figs. 43.21 and 43.22).

Advantages: It is possible to preserve the sensorial innervation.

Good camouflage of the scar in the deep furrows.

A more precise reposition of the eyebrow.

Direct division of the corrugator muscle and the procerus muscle.

Disadvantage: Resultant scar line. It is ideal in male patients, adults with deep horizontal furrows with frontal baldness, with glabellar furrows, and ptosis of the eyebrows.

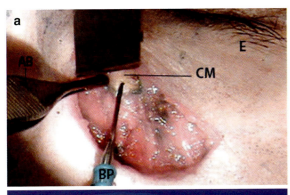
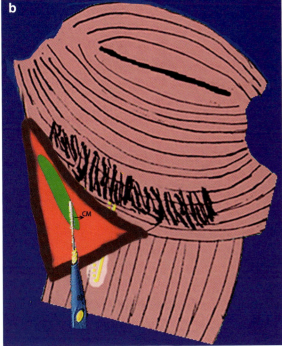

Fig. 43.19 Access to the corrugator muscle (*CM*), through the half frontal incision. Eyebrow (*E*), Adson Brown (*AB*), Bipolar (*BP*) (Photo courtesy Dr. Jaime Ramirez)

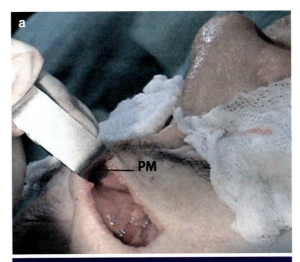
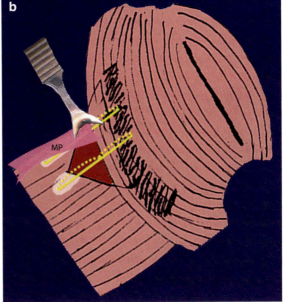

Fig. 43.20 Access to the procerus muscle (*PM*), through the half frontal incision (Photo courtesy Dr. Jaime Ramirez)

43.8.4 Direct Eyebrow Lift

Its name makes reference to the simple way that allows fixing the position of the eyebrow, without including another forehead region.

Preparation: With the patient seated or standing up a marking of the incision is made, preferably more over the lateral region of the eyebrow (Fig. 43.23). The incision of the skin is made in the superior edge of the eyebrow, following the same direction of the hair, to prevent any injury of the follicles. Once the position of the eyebrow is set, the superior line of the ellipse, which is the one that defines the amount of the skin to dry out, the marking of the incision is made (Fig. 43.5).

In some cases when the planned incision is extended to the middle extreme of the eyebrow, there can be limited access to the glabellar musculature. The dissection plane is subcutaneous and is realized downward with scissors up to the frontal muscle. The technique allows to select molding of the eyebrow for modifications of the middle, central, or lateral components of the excision [34].

The Suspension Technique: Although the cutaneous excision can elevate the inferior flap, making the suspension dispensable, this one can be placed from orbicular muscle to the periosteum immediately above the eyebrow (Fig. 43.24). The option to anchor the orbicular to the lateral periosteum of the eyebrow can put in risk the frontal branch of the facial nerve (Figs. 43.25 and

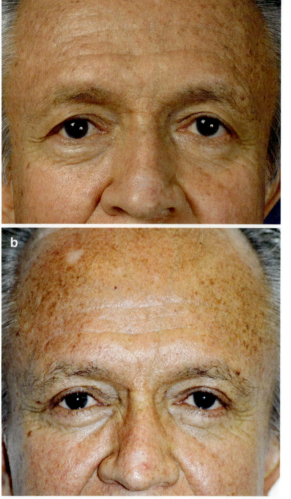

Fig. 43.21 (**a**) Preoperative. (**b**) Two years postoperative following the forehead lifting half-frontal approach and blepharoplasty (Photo courtesy Dr. Jaime Ramirez)

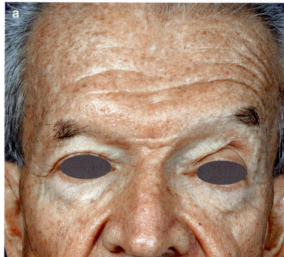

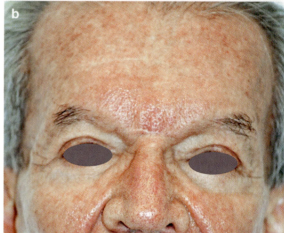

Fig. 43.22 (**a**) Preoperative. (**b**) One year postoperative following the forehead lifting half-frontal approach and blepharoplasty (Photo courtesy Dr. Jaime Ramirez)

43.26). In the case of a preexisting scar, associated to asymmetry of the eyebrow the place of the scar for the approach can be used (Figs. 43.27 and 43.28).

Advantages: Excellent approach for the treatment of asymmetric ptotic eyebrow.
 Less invasive surgical dissection.
 Low cost, security, effectiveness, and simplicity [35].
 Quick recovery.
 Disadvantages: Scar sometimes visible.
 Limited access to the glabellar musculature.
 Not recommended in young patients.
 Ideal in adult patients with thick eyebrows, average ptosis, and/or unilateral ptosis.

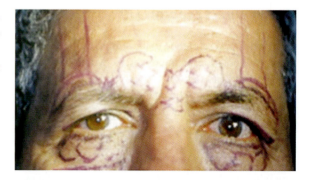

Fig. 43.23 Marking of the incisions in the lateral edge of the eyebrows for the direct approach of the eyebrow lifting (Photo courtesy Dr. Jaime Ramirez)

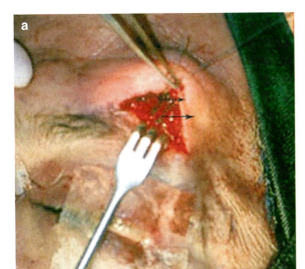

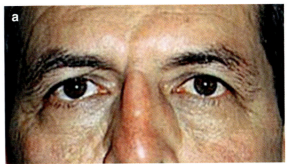

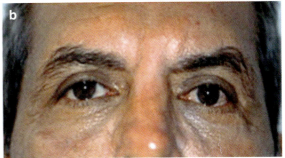

Fig. 43.25 (a) Preoperative. (b) Three years postoperative after direct eyebrow lift, blepharoplasty, and rhinoplasty (Photo courtesy Dr. Jaime Ramirez)

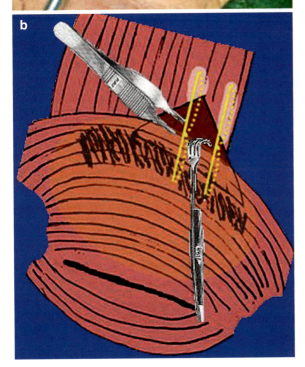

Fig. 43.24 Suspension point of the orbicular muscle to periosteum, immediately above the eyebrow. The *arrows* indicate the ends of the suture (Photo courtesy Dr. Jaime Ramirez)

43.8.5 Endoscopic

At the moment, it is the technique more used, in spite of requiring a curve of learning in the manipulation and exploitation of the specific instrumentation. It is a favorable technique as much for the patient because it diminishes the sequels of the opened approach as for the surgeon, when magnifying the structures allowing a more precise and conservative work of them. The applied anatomy of the area, referred in general to the beginning of this chapter, has repairs in the endoscopic approach that are important as much for the novel surgeon as for the more experienced surgeon:

Dissection Planes: (a) In the previous frontal region: subperiosteum plane (Fig. 43.29). (b) In the temporary region: interfascial plane (between fascia temporoparietal, superiorly and temporary deep fascia in the inferior part) (Fig. 43.30). (c) In the parietoccipital fissure the subgaleal plane.

Repair Points:

- Temporal Line: Zone that delimits the interphase between the previous subperiosteal plane and the interfacial plane laterally, constituted by fiber connective tissue or joint sinew (Fig. 43.31)

Orbital Ligament: It extends from the external part of the orbital rim to the orbicular muscle of the eyelids and the dermis.

Sentinel Vein (v. zigomaticotemporal): Located 1 cm approximately to the superior and lateral part of the lateral orbital rim (Fig. 43.32).

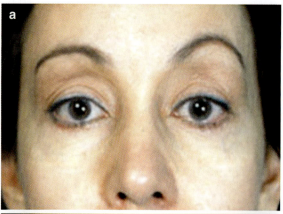

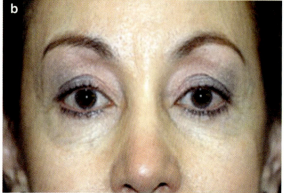

Fig. 43.26 (**a**) Preoperative for eyebrow lift. (**b**) Two years postoperative after eyebrow lift with correction of the asymmetry of the left eyebrow without any notorious scar (Photo courtesy Dr. Jaime Ramirez)

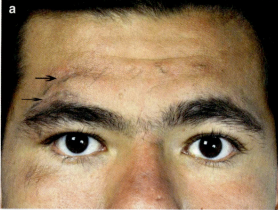

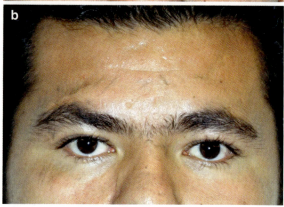

Fig. 43.27 Presurgical and postsurgical image of direct eyebrow lift using as a way of approach a preexisting scar in the superior edge of the right eyebrow. Two years postoperative. The old scars are indicated with *arrows* (Photo courtesy Dr. Jaime Ramirez)

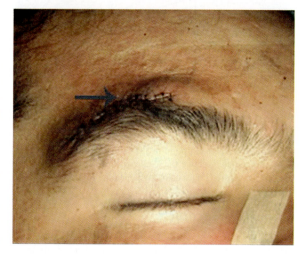

Fig. 43.28 Immediately postoperative showing suspension with direct eyebrow lift used as a way of approach with a preexisting scar (Photo courtesy Dr. Jaime Ramirez)

- Facial Nerve. Frontal branch. Attending closely near the superior portion of the sentinel vein, throughout the temporoparietal fascia. It ascends from the posterior to the anterior to 1.5 cm of the eyebrow tail approximately.
- Supraorbital Package: Artery, vein, and fascia emerging from the orbit throughout the same notch that is easily palpable in the middle portion of the superior orbital rim for its identification and protection.

Preparation: The marking is performed in the skin of the forehead of the temporal, midforehead, and paramedian lines, these last ones coinciding with an imaginary line between the extern canthus and the lateral limb (Fig. 43.33). Later on and limited by portions of hair previously isolated, they are demarcated in the scalp using five incisions of approximately 2 cm in length and 1.5 cm behind the hairline. Three out of these incisions become sagittal, corresponding in the scalp thus: one

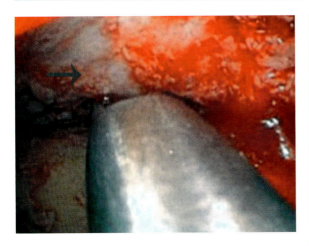

Fig. 43.29 Endoscopic view of subperiosteum plane. The *arrow* indicates the dissected periosteum (Photo courtesy Dr. Jaime Ramirez)

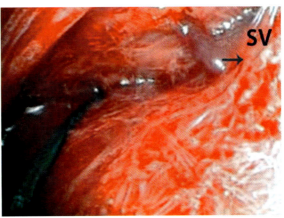

Fig. 43.32 Endoscopic view of sentinel vein (*SV*) (Photo courtesy Dr. Jaime Ramirez)

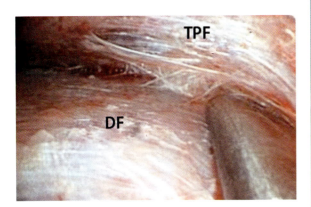

Fig. 43.30 Endoscopic view of interfacial dissection in the temporary region. The temporary deep fascia (*DF*) and the temporoparietal fascia. (*TPF*) are observed (Photo courtesy Dr. Jaime Ramirez)

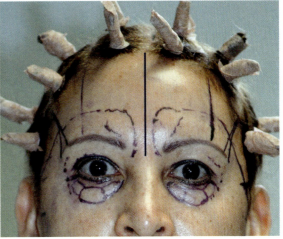

Fig. 43.33 Frontal lines for the preparation of the endoscopic approach (Photo courtesy Dr. Jaime Ramirez)

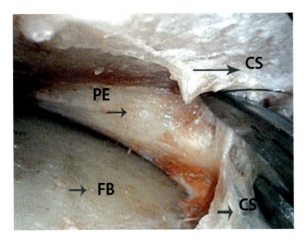

Fig. 43.31 Corpse dissection. Endoscopic image, the *arrows* indicate the frontal bone (*FB*), the periosteum (*PE*), and the conjoin sinew (*CS*) (Photo courtesy Dr. Jaime Ramirez)

with the midforehead line and the other two with paramedian lines. The lateral incisions, in the scalp, become parallel with an imaginary line that goes along the prolongation of the line of the external orbital rim to the implantation line of the sideboards (Fig. 43.34). The zone of the glabellar musculature is also marked making the patient to pucker the frown. If the presurgical analysis shows the necessity of complementary eyelid lift (blepharoplasty), in the same operating act, it is carried out before the forehead lifting, to avoid a consecutive edema in the eyelids.

After infiltrating the marks with 1% lidocaine with 1:100,000epinephrine the described incisions are realized. The sagittal ones extend to the bone to previously make a subperíosteal plane that can be dissected up to 1.5 cm over the orbital rim and toward the

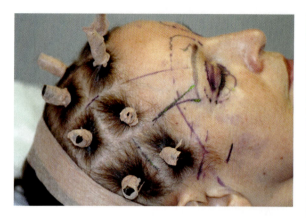

Fig. 43.34 Lateral lines for the preparation of the endoscopic approach (Photo courtesy Dr. Jaime Ramirez)

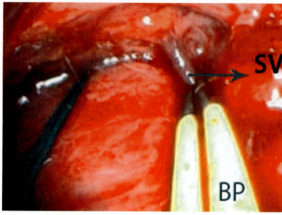

Fig. 43.37 Endoscopic bipolar (*BP*) cauterization of the sentinel vein (*SV*) at its base (Photo courtesy Dr. Jaime Ramirez)

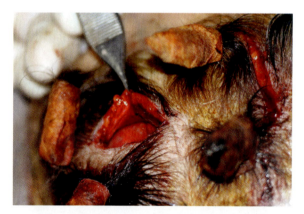

Fig. 43.35 Transverse and sagittal incisions for the endoscopic approach (Photo courtesy Dr. Jaime Ramirez)

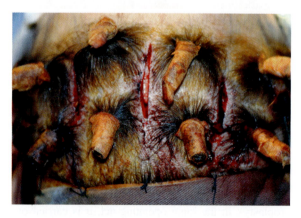

Fig. 43.36 Sagittal incisions for the endoscopic approach (Photo courtesy Dr. Jaime Ramirez)

parietoccipital region a subglaleal plane rises. The transverse incisions are deepened to the temporary fascia to identify and to raise endosmotically the temporoparietal fascia (Figs. 43.35 and 43.36). Once there, from lateral to medial, to prevent any injury of the frontal branch of the facial nerve, a cut of the joint fascia is done communicating the interfacial and subperiosteal planes. In the inferior part of this incision the orbital ligament is released and the sentry vein laterally must be repaired and if not possible, can be inferiorly dissected and cauterized with bipolar in its base, not in the superior part, because of the risk of injuring the frontal branch of the facial nerve (Fig. 43.37). After repairing and cutting the vein, the subperiosteal dissection of the lateral orbital rim and the anterior zygoma is continued, until finishing in the superior orbital edge, which can be identified, guiding externally with a nondominant finger of the surgeon or the assistant. Next, the periosteum is cut with microscissors from lateral to medial, until getting at the repairs of the supraorbital package. In this area, the periosteum is weaker and usually it is necessary to carefully incise with a curved, thin, and blunt dissector. The cut of periosteum is then completed toward the middle line, where the glabellar musculature is found (Fig. 43.38). The cut of periosteum is realized in the same way in the contralateral side. The superior flap of the periosteum is discreetly elevated to expose the musculature.

The superciliary corrugator muscle and procerus muscle are incised and partially dried out making use of microforceps, respecting the supratrochlear innervations. Besides the myotomies of the procerus and corrugator, a resection of a small rectangular segment of the superior portion of the orbicular muscle, lateral to the supraorbital package, can be realized to complete the lysis of the depressant function.

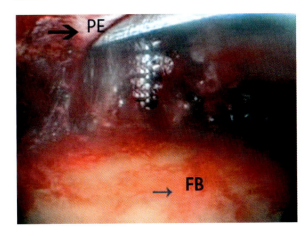

Fig. 43.38 Endoscopic periosteum dissection (*PE*), being careful with the supraorbital package, frontal bone (*FB*) (Photo courtesy Dr. Jaime Ramirez)

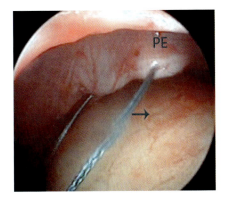

Fig. 43.39 Endoscopic suspension point (*arrow*) of the bottom edge of periosteum (*PE*) to the galea point (Photo courtesy Dr. James Ramirez)

Suspension technique: It is realized beginning with the more lateral suspension, corresponding with the correction vectors of each patient. The points of suspension are placed with Ethibond 3–0, generally three in the temporal area from temporoparietal fascia to deep fascia; two paramedium from periosteum to galea (Fig. 43.39), and a central one from periosteum to galea.

The point of central suspension is indicated if there is medial ptosis of the eyebrow. The suspension points in the temporary region must avoid getting close to the temporoparietal fascia, to prevent injury of the frontal branch of the facial nerve. It is more important that the dissection completely liberates the supraorbital periosteum than the suspension with sutures. Hemovac type drains are left, throughout the more lateral portion but lateral of the fixed transverse incisions to the scalp and the incisions with instruments holding the wound.

Advantages: Well-hidden scars, less invasive approach, amplification of the operative field. Selective manipulation of the glabellar muscles and less bleeding (Figs. 43.40 and 43.41).

Disadvantages: Elevation of the hair line, variable results, requires learning and familiarization with special instrumentation.

Contraindications to this technique include severe ptosis of the brow, thick sebaceous skin, and high frontal hairline [36].

Ideal in young and middle-aged patients, with a normal or low hair line.

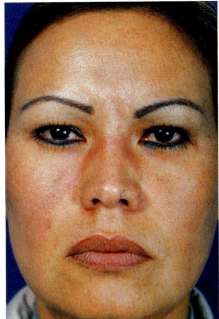
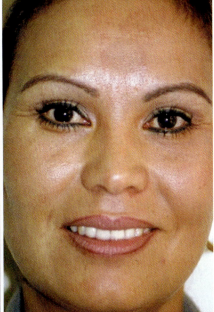

Fig. 43.40 (**a**) Preoperative. (**b**) One year following endoscopic forehead lift (Photo courtesy Dr. James Ramirez)

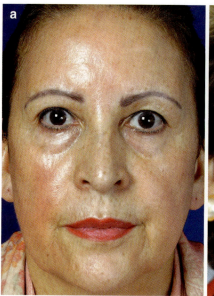
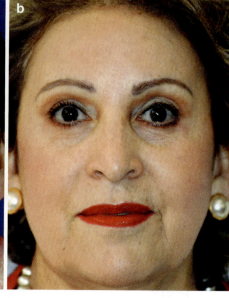

Fig. 43.41 (a) Preoperative. (b) Eight months postoperatively after endoscopic forehead lifting and blepharoplasty (Photo courtesy Dr. James Ramirez)

43.9 Complications

The possible complications depend on the technique and the choice of approach, also on the patient's condition.

1. Based on the area of the incision, visible scarring or alopecia may occur.
2. The extension of the dissection may produce a neurological alteration with hypoesthesia or vascular damage caused by the occurrence of hematomas.
3. Other possible complications include:

Asymmetry or deformation of the brow with a surprised expression.
    Excess or undercorrection of the frontal skin
    Injury to the facial nerve
    Necrotic tissue
    Infection

43.10 Discussion

As a surgeon, it is important to acquire the experience in recognizing the most suitable approach or surgical technique that offers advantages and complies with the needs and expectations of each patient and to know that there is not a single approach that is useful for all cases.

Currently endoscopic surgery is an excellent option for the forehead-lift procedure, given its versatility, advantages, and safety profile that allow optimum results in most patients. In cases when only the elevation of the brow tails and diminishing of the lateral furrows is required, it is possible to limit the dissection to a trough to single bilateral incisions that allows the suspension of this specific area.

Neither the effectiveness of the diverse suspension methods has been studied comparatively nor has its cost effectiveness has been analyzed. Currently there are different methods for anchorage such as nails, bone perforations to allow sutures, endothelial sutures [37], and multiple suture materials. The authors have only used Ethibond 3–0 for suspension, with favorable results.

43.11 Conclusions

Facial aging is a multifactor process, especially in the superior third of the face. Manipulation of this area must be integral in the process of rejuvenation. The chosen technique must be individualized for each patient, and gender, age, physical features, and expectations should be taken into consideration. The plastic facial surgeon who has diverse techniques in his operational resources can provide the best results depending on each patient. The technique to minimize incisions and reduce scarring has led to the development of advanced procedures.

References

1. Paul MD. The evolution of the brow lifting aesthetic plastic surgery. Plast Reconstr Surg. 2001;108(5):1409–24.
2. Pedroza F, dos Anjos GC, Bedoya M, Rivera M. Update on brow and forehead lifting. Curr Opin Otolaryngol Head Neck Surg. 2006;14(4):283–8.
3. Daniel R, Tirkanits B. Endoscopic forehead lift: an operative technique. Plast Reconstr Surg. 1996;98(7):1148–57.
4. Ramirez O. Why I prefer endoscopic forehead lift. Plast Reconstr Surg. 1997;100(4 Suppl):1033–9.
5. Passot R. La chirurgie esthetique des rides du visage. Presse Med. 1919;27:258.
6. Hunt HL. Plastic surgery of the head, face, and neck. Philadelphia: Lea & Febige; 1926.
7. Passot R. Chirurgie estheetique pure: techniques et results. Paris: Gaston Doin & Cie; 1930.
8. Fomon S. The Surgery of injuries and plastic repair. Baltimore: Williams & Wilkins; 1939. p. 1409.
9. Patrocinio Lucas G, Patrocinio Jose A. Forehead-lift. A 10 year review. Arch Facial Plast Surg. 2008;10(6):391–4.
10. Gonzales-Ulloa M. Facial wrinkles: integral elimination. Plast Reconstr Surg. 1962;29:658–73.
11. Marino H, Gandolfo E. Treatment of wrinkles of the forehead. Prensa Méd Argent. 1964;51:1368–71.
12. Isse NG. Endoscopic facial rejuvenation: endoforehead, the functional lift, case reports. Aesthetic Plast Surg. 1994;18(1):21–9.
13. Vinas JC, Caviglia C, Cortinas JL. Forehead rhytidoplasty and brow lifting. Plast Reconstr Surg. 1976;57(4):445–54.
14. Kaye BL. The forehead lift: a useful adjunct to face left and blepharoplasty. Plast Reconstr Surg. 1977;69(2):161–71.
15. Vasconez LO, Core GB, Oslin B. Endoscopy in plastic surgery: an overview. Clin Plast Surg. 1995;22(4):585–9.
16. Isse NG. Endoscopic facial rejuvenation. Clin Plast Surg. 1997;24(2):213–31.
17. Chajchir A. Endoscopic subperiosteal forehead lift. Aesthetic Plast Surg. 1994;18(3):269–74.
18. Chajchir A. Endoscopic facelift: two years experience. Aesthetic Plast Surg. 1997;21(1):1–6.
19. Sullivan PK, Salomon JA, Woo AS, Freeman MB. The importance of the retaining ligamentous attachments of the forehead for selective eyebrow reshaping and forehead rejuvenation. Plast Reconstr Surg. 2006;117(1):95–104.
20. Knize DM. Reassessment of the coronal incision and subgaleal dissection for foreheadplasty. Plast Reconstr Surg. 1998;102(2):478–89; discussion 490–2.
21. Patel BC. Endoscopic brow lifts uber alles. Orbit. 2006;25(4):267–301.
22. Patel BCK. Surgical eyelid and periorbital anatomy. Semin Ophthalmol. 1996;11(2):118–37.
23. Steinsapir KD, Shorr N, Hoenig J, Goldberg RA, Baylis HI, Morrow D. The endoscopic forehead lift. Ophthal Plast Reconstr Surg. 1998;14(2):107–18.
24. Walden JL, Orseck MJ, Aston SJ. Current methods for brow fixation: are they safe? Aesthetic Plast Surg. 2006;30(5):541–8.
25. Schmidt BL, Pogrel MA, Hakim-Faal Z. The course of the temporal branch of the facial nerve in the periorbital region. J Oral Maxillofac Surg. 2001;59(2):178–84.
26. Stuzin JM, Wagstrom L, Kawamoto HK, Wolfe SA. Anatomy of the frontal branch of the facial nerve: the significance of the temporal fat pad. Plast Reconstr Surg. 1989;83(2):265–71.
27. Webster RC, Gaunt JM, Hamdan US, Fuleihan NS, Giandello PR, Smith RC. Supraorbital and supratrochlear notches and foramina: anatomical variations and surgical relevance. Laryngoscope. 1986;96(3):311–5.
28. Isse NG. Orbiculari oculii muscle myotomy, its role in the functional and passive brow lift/forehead lift. Plast Surg Forum. 1994;18:7–9.
29. Fodor PB, Isse NG. Endoscopically assisted aesthetic plastic surgery. Mosby: St. Louis; 1996. p. 39–61.
30. Trinei FA, Januszkiewicz J, Nahai F. The sentinel vein: an important reference point for surgery in the temporal region. Plast Reconstr Surg. 1998;101(1):27–32.
31. Isse NG. Endoforehead plasty. Lipoplasty Newsl. 1995;12:8–15.
32. Lam S, Williams III E. Enfoque integral del rejuvenecimiento facial. Venezuela: Editorial Amolca; 2006. p. 55.
33. Lazor JB, Cheney ML. The forehead lift. In: Cheney ML, editor. Facial surgery: plastic and reconstructive. Baltimore: Williams & Wilkins; 1997. p. 905–11.
34. Chand MS, Perkins SW. Comparison of surgical approaches for upper Facial rejuvenation. Curr Opin Otolaryngol Head Neck Surg. 2000;8:326–31.
35. Dailey R, Saulny S. Current treatments of brow ptosis. Curr Opin Ophthalmol. 2003;14(5):260–6.
36. Henderson JL, Larrabee W. Analysis of the upper face and selection of rejuvenation techniques. Facial Plast Surg Clin North Am. 2006;14(3):153–8.
37. Jacovella P, Tuccillo F, Zimman O, Repetti G. An alternative approach to brow lift fixation: temporoparietalis fascia, galeal, and periosteal imbrication. Plast Reconstr Surg. 2007;119(2):692–702.

Endoscopic Forehead Lift

Jorge Espinosa and José Rafael Reyes

44.1 Forehead Aging Process

The aging process is characterized by a progressive loss of firmness and elasticity of the soft tissues of the face, compounded by the pull of several vectors on the tissues [1]. This process is particularly evident in the upper third of the face, leading to changes in eyebrow and lid position that give the person a tired and aging look. Tissue descent results not only from the effects of the pull of gravity but also from the persistent action of the corrugator (corrugator supercilii), procerus and orbicularis (orbicularis oculi) muscles which act as eyebrow depressor. On the other hand, the frontalis muscle loses its ability to elevate and maintain forehead structures in position (Fig. 44.1).

This muscle group is also responsible for the horizontal lines of the forehead, the vertical glabellar lines, the horizontal radix lines, and the radiated periorbital lines creating the well-known "crow's feet." Lines that appear only during muscle activity are considered "dynamic" and may become "static" or permanent when there is damage to the deep layers of the skin due to repeated muscle contraction (Fig. 44.2).

Although the first reports about modern facial lift date back to the earlier part of the past century with the work of Miller in 1907 [2], the forehead and brow area began to receive similar attention only in the mid twentieth century [2]. It was around 1992 that a new era began with the work by Core [3], Lyand [4], and Isse [5] and with the use of optical instruments for endoscopic procedures. Thus began endoscopic forehead lift as a method for rejuvenating the forehead and the periorbital with the new ability to produce optimal, natural-looking, and lasting results with minimal, well-camouflaged scars.

Despite the need for special instruments and a very well-defined learning curve, endoscopic forehead lift has become a most valuable tool in the rejuvenation of the forehead and periorbital area [6].

44.2 Indications

The earliest signs of aging tend to manifest in the periorbital area, particularly in eyebrow position. A tired, premature-aging look is common as a result of a low-set eyebrow tail. Although brow position and shape vary significantly depending on race, gender, and age, in general, an attractive female eyebrow should be set above the upper orbital rim and the tail should be slightly higher than the head. Starting at the tail, the brow must follow a smooth curve toward the midline and the head, sometimes with a small elevation at the point where the lateral third joins the two medial thirds. In men, eyebrows are usually horizontal in shape and are set at the same level of the upper orbital rim. Endoscopic forehead lift is indicated in young patients with a

J. Espinosa (✉)
ENT Service, Universidad de la Sabana: Campus Universitario del Puente del Común, Km. 7, Autopista Norte de Bogotá, Colombia and
Faculty of the Integrated Otolaryngology Service, Central Military Hospital, San Rafael Hospital Clinic, Universidad Militar Nueva Granada, Calle 123 # 7–60, Consultorio 304, Bogotá, Colombia
e-mail: jorgespinosa@gmail.com

J.R. Reyes
Colombian Society of Facial Plastic Surgery and Rhinology, Av. 7 # 119-14, Consultorio 211, Pontificia, Universidad Javeriana, Av 7 No 40-32, Bogotá, Colombia
e-mail: joserafaelreyes@gmail.com

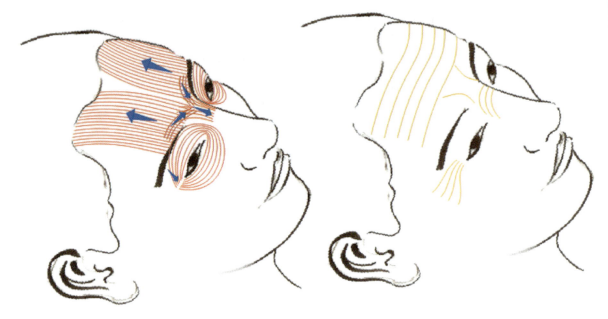

Fig. 44.1 Aging process of the forehead. Facial lines and their relationship with muscle contraction

low-set hairline and few dynamic forehead lines. Usually, this group of patients requests a change in the shape and position of the eyebrows in order to eliminate the tired or sad look in their faces (Fig. 44.3).

Another group of patients that can benefit from the endoscopic technique are men with a frontal baldness pattern in whom the coronal approach will create a notorious unacceptable scar.

Frequently, patients who come for an upper lid blepharoplasty because of the presence of redundant

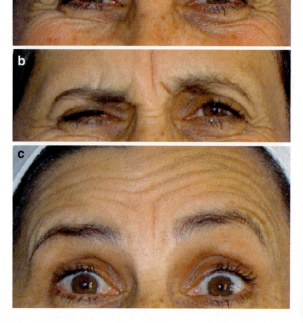

Fig. 44.2 (**a**) Lines produced by the contraction of the forehead muscles, and crow's feet lines. (**b**) Glabellar lines produced by the contraction of the procerus and corrugator supercilii muscles. (**c**) Horizontal lines produced by the contraction of the frontalis muscle

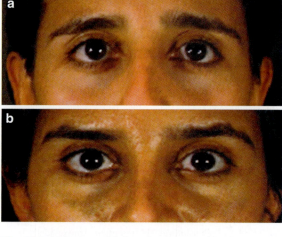

Fig. 44.3 (**a**) Patient with lateral eyebrow ptosis giving him a sad appearance. (**b**) Six months after endoscopic forehead lift

skin in fact only require repositioning of the brow in its original position, thus making blepharoplasty unnecessary, or reducing significantly the amount of skin to be resected [7, 8].

In some patients, brow ptosis becomes more pronounced after upper lid blepharoplasty, usually as a result of aggressive surgical techniques in which an important portion of the orbicularis muscle is removed with an excision that extends laterally. This creates significant scarring of the muscle that pushes the brow down and creates a stigma in the form of a pronounced wrinkle in the crow's feet area associated with brow ptosis, resulting in patient dissatisfaction (Fig. 44.4).

The physical preoperative examination is done with the patient standing in front of a mirror. The distance from the lateral cantus, the pupil, and the medial cantus to the lower edge of the brow is measured, and asymmetries are recorded (Fig. 44.5).

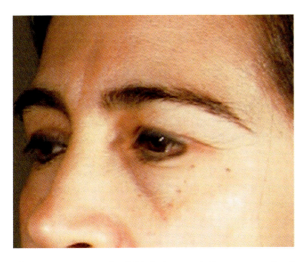

Fig. 44.4 Pronounced wrinkle in the crow's feet area associated with eyebrow ptosis after blepharoplasty with excessive muscle resection

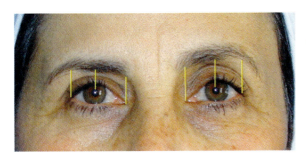

Fig. 44.5 Distance is measured from the lateral canthus, the pupil at the medial canthus to the lower edge of the eyebrow and asymmetries are recorded

44.3 Alternative Methods

Facial plastic surgeons must have access to other alternatives in order to address specific problems such as asymmetries resulting from facial paralysis or lateral descent of the eyebrow, and in order to offer solutions to those patients who cannot, or will not, undergo a surgical intervention.

Direct resection of an ellipse of skin at the tail of the eyebrow allows for a precise correction of asymmetries resulting from facial paralysis, since it not only repositions the brow but also provides an approach for suspension to the periostium of the orbicularis oculi. In lifting the lateral portion of the brow, the skin resection is performed over the temporal area taking an ellipse of scalp skin. The amount of tissue to be resected must be carefully assessed in order to avoid asymmetries and create the smallest possible shortening of the sideburn.

The use of botulinum toxin has become one of the most widely used cosmetic procedures in facial plastic surgery. With a good knowledge of the forces exerted by the muscle groups of the upper third of the face, it is possible to achieve excellent results of brow tail repositioning and "crow's feet" elimination. Occasionally, botulinum toxin can be used before endoscopic forehead lift to weaken the depressor muscles and help the frontalis muscle with brow elevation [9].

Several suspension methods using subcutaneous sutures and anchoring devices have been designed to improve long-term outcomes, although with variable results. Overall, nonabsorbable materials tend to extrude and produce granulomas and, for this reason, they have lost popularity.

44.4 Anatomy

From superficial to deep, the following layers are found in the forehead: skin, subcutaneous cellular tissue, aponeurotic galea (enveloping the frontalis muscle), lax areolar tissue, and periosteum. Periosteum and galea meet approximately 1 cm above the orbital rim.

In the forehead, the frontalis is the only muscle that elevates the eyebrow. This muscle proceeds upward and backward along with the occipital muscle through the attachment of its aponeurotic envelope. With no bone attachments, this muscle inserts into the skin of the brow after crossing the orbicularis oculi. Its multiple insertions on the forehead dermis give rise to the characteristic horizontal lines that develop as time goes by.

The procerus and corrugator supercilii muscles are the eyebrow depressors. They act on the head of the eyebrow, while the orbicularis of the lids acts on the lateral two-thirds of the eyebrow.

The procerus inserts onto the external aspect of the nasal bones and the upper nasal cartilages and on the intercilliary skin. When it contracts, it forms horizontal lines on the radix and pulls the head of the eyebrow down and inward.

The corrugator supercilii is located deep to the orbicularis and inserts onto the most medial portion of the supercilliary arch and the deep aspect of the eyebrows after crossing the orbicularis. When it contracts, this muscle forms the vertical lines of the glabella and pulls the head of the brow medially. It is the deepest muscle and the first we come across in endoscopic forehead lift. The depressor supercili muscle emerges from the dermis and inserts just above the medial cantus. The orbicularis oculi muscle inserts on the orbital rim and then superiorly on the deep layer of the skin. When it contracts, its fibers become intertwined with the frontalis and the corrugator supercilii muscles, closing the palpebral fissure and lowering the eyebrow, creating the crow's feet lines (Fig. 44.6).

Motor innervation is supplied by the frontal branch of the facial nerve arising from the parotid gland, deep to the superficial musculoaponeurotic system (SMAS). This branch crosses the zygoma over an area 2 cm anterior to the helix radix and 2 cm posterior to the lateral cantus and enters into the frontalis muscle divided into several separate branches. The most inferior branch goes to the corrugator supercili and depressor supercili muscles and to the medial region of the orbital portion of the orbicularis oculi.

This facial nerve runs along a plane deep to the superficial temporalis fascia (superficial fascia) inside the superficial temporal fat pad.

Deep to this superficial temporal fat pad is the superficial layer of the deep temporalis fascia (intermediate fascia) that is a continuation of the superficial zygomatic periosteum and of the masseteric fascia.

Deep to the intermediate fascia is the intermediate temporal fat pad and deep to it is the deep layer of the deep temporalis fascia (deep fascia) that extends into the periosteum of the deep aspect of the zygomatic arch.

The deep temporal fat pad lies between the deep fascia and the temporalis muscle.

Endoscopic forehead lift dissection is performed on the deep plane of the superficial termporal fat pad allowing the fat pad to protect the temporal branch of the facial nerve.

From there, the dissection may then proceed toward the middle third of the face, passing through the intermediate fascia toward the intermediate temporal fat pad. At this point, an incision is performed on the periosteum of the zygomatic arch, and the dissection then proceeds inferiorly (Fig. 44.7).

Consequently, the dissection is safe if performed along the subcutaneous plane or immediately superficial to the intermediate fascia. This is the usual plane for endoscopic forehead lift dissection. The deep temporalis fascia merges with the periosteum of the forehead at the level of the upper temporal line. In performing the dissection for endoscopic forehead lift, it is important to elevate the temporal portion and communicate this pocket with the frontal subperiosteal dissection. This is done from lateral to medial, creating a sufficiently large pocket to allow the continuation of the endoscopic procedure.

The sensory innervation to the forehead region is supplied, medially, by the ophthalmic branch of the trigeminal nerve through its supratrochlear and

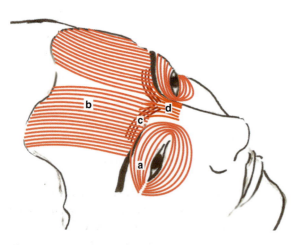

Fig. 44.6 Forehead muscles that depress and elevate the eyebrows. (*a*) Orbicularis oculi. (*b*) Frontalis. (*c*) Corrugator supercili. (*d*) Procerus

44 Endoscopic Forehead Lift

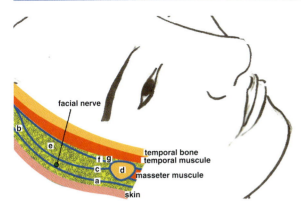

Fig. 44.7 Dissection planes in endoscopic forehead-lift. (*a*) Superficial temporal fascia (superficial fascia). (*b*) Superficial temporal fat pad. (*c*) Superficial layer of the deep temporalis fascia (intermediate fascia). (*d*) Zygomatic arch. (*e*) Intermediate temporal fat pad. (*f*) Deep layer of the deep temporalis fascia (deep fascia). (*g*) Deep temporal fat pad

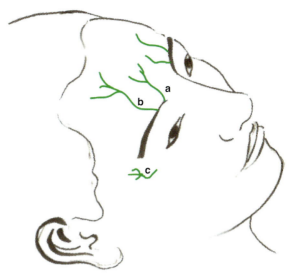

Fig. 44.8 Sensory forehead innervation. (*a*) Supratrochlear branch. (*b*) Supraorbital branch. (*c*) Zygomatic facial branches

supraorbital branches and, laterally, by the facial zygomatic branches. The supratrochlear branch arises from the orbit at the level of the superior oblique muscle pulley and crosses the corrugator supercilii. The supraorbital branch arises at the level of the supraorbital orifice. On occasions, this orifice is replaced by a cleft that does not form a true bony conduit.

These nerves cross the forehead periosteum and muscles after they emerge from the bony conduit before proceeding cephalad. This emergence of the nerve bundles makes dissection difficult and requires the use of endoscopic visualization for correct management and preservation (Fig. 44.8).

44.5 Endoscopic Forehead Lift Surgery: Rationale

Endoscopic forehead lift is a permanent method to elevate the position of the brows. Moreover it provides significant improvement of horizontal forehead lines, glabellar furrows, and crow's feet.

In essence, the surgery consists of detaching and cutting the periosteum through small incisions inside the scalp under the eyebrow implantation in order to weaken the brow depressor muscles. This allows the frontalis muscle to apply upward traction on the periosteum and subsequent fixation of the brow in a higher position. It also reduces lines produced by the action of

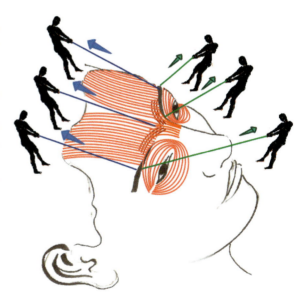

Fig. 44.9 The key in endoscopic forehead-lift is to weaken the action of the muscles that pull the brow down, allowing the frontalis to act without opposition. This will lift eyebrow position

the procerus, corrugator supercilii, and orbicularis oculi muscles. In this technique, the elevation of the entire periosteum and of the arcus marginalis is mandatory [6, 9, 13], in order to obtain consistent long-term results [10–12] (Fig. 44.9).

Potential fixation systems include screws, sutures, bone tunneling, and more recently, periosteal suspension and fixation mechanisms by means of anchoring devices [13, 14]. The technique described below uses suture fixation from the periosteum to the galea.

The endoscopic forehead lift technique performed by the authors is designed to create a harmonious natural-looking result and to give the patient a non surgical look.

For this reason, it does not aim to eliminate mobility of the procerus, corrugator supercilii, and orbicularis oculi muscles. It seeks to diminish the lines created as a result of the action of these muscles, and to elevate the brow naturally.

Glabellar, forehead, and crow's feet lines may reappear after surgery if the patient has a habit of frequent muscle contraction. Consequently, the periodic use of botulinum toxin is required in order to avoid their reappearance in many cases. However, since the eyebrows are set at a higher position, the patient does not feel the need to contract the frontalis muscle frequently and there is a smaller chance of the forehead lines forming again in the short run.

Endoscopic forehead lift may be combined with other facial plastic procedures in order to produce a more harmonious overall result. When performed simultaneously with upper lid blepharoplasty, skin resection must be very accurate if postoperative open-eye complications are to be avoided. This technique can also be combined with an endoscopic middle third face-lift.

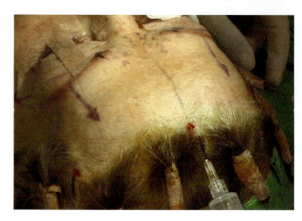

Fig. 44.10 Infiltration of working incisions

emerge. In some instances it is important to have a long cautery tip at hand for hemostasis.

44.6.2 Anesthesia

The procedure may be performed under local anesthesia and mild sedation. The incision areas in the scalp and the areas where sensory nerves (supratrochlear, supraorbital, and temporomalar nerves) emerge in the forehead are infiltrated with lidocaine 1:200,000, with 1% epinephrine (Fig. 44.10).

44.6 Technique

44.6.1 Instruments

Only three dissectors are required in the vast majority of cases: a sharp dissector, a blunt dissector, and a 90° angled dissector used to detach the arcus marginalis at the upper orbital rim. The 30° endoscope with its protective sheath and continuous saline solution irrigation channel allows for constant flushing of the lens and clear visualization of the surgical field. Metzembaum scissors may be used instead of endoscopic scissors, because they enable an accurate sectioning of muscle and periostium and dissection at the sites where the supratrochlear and supraorbital neurovascular bundles

44.6.3 Delimitation of the Working Areas

1. Hair implantation line: serves as a guide for hiding scalp incisions.
2. Middle vertical line: reference for the vertical incision.
3. Vertical line on the lateral corneoscleral limbus: reference for intermediate incisions.
4. Superior temporal line: defines the point of insertion of the temporalis muscle on the frontal and parietal bones and the place where the lateral and medial dissection planes will meet.
5. Zygomatic arch: helps determine the inferior extension of the dissection and the safe dissection area in order to protect the frontal branch of the facial nerve.

6. Site of emergence of bilateral supratrochlear and supraorbital neurovascular bundles: although there is no 100% certainty that these structures will always emerge through the supraorbital cleft, this structure is marked as a landmark for surgery.
7. Site for the periosteum and bilateral orbicularis oculi sectioning.
8. Marking of the horizontal lines of the forehead, crow's feet, and horizontal and vertical glabellar lines.
9. The following working incisions are marked:
   (a) Vertical midline, 5 mm superior to the hairline, approximately 2.5 cm in length.
   (b) Bilateral vertical lines crossing the lateral sclerocorneal limbus, above the hairline, approximately 2.5 cm in length.
   (c) Oblique incisions in the temporal region, 2.5–1 cm from the hairline and parallel to it (Fig. 44.11).

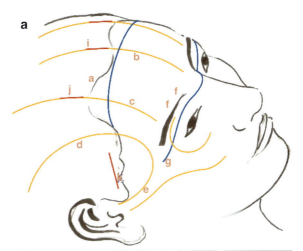

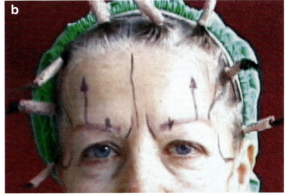

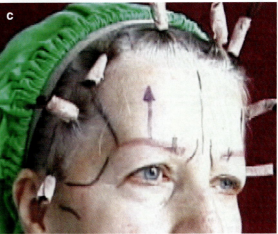

Fig. 44.11 Incision and dissection delimitation. (*a*) Hairline. (*b*) Middle vertical line. (*c*) Vertical line that crosses the lateral sclerocorneal limbus. (*d*) Superior temporal line. (*e*) Zygomatic arch. (*f*) Supratrochlear and supraorbital neurovascular bundles emergence site. (*g*) Site for periosteal and bilateral orbicularis oculi sectioning. (*i*) Midline incision. (*j*) Paramedian vertical line incision. Note the marking of the horizontal forehead lines, crow's feet, vertical and horizontal glabellar lines, and incision in the temporal region

44.6.4 Skin Incisions

A number 15 blade is used for skin and subcutaneous cellular tissue incisions. Scissors are used to find the supraperiosteal subaponeurotic plane in the frontal vertical incisions and the interfascial plane (between the superficial temporalis fascia and the superficial layer of the deep temporalis fascia) in the temporal region. This plane is readily identifiable because the deep temporalis fascia does not move when skin edges are pulled. However, when in doubt, a small incision will reveal the characteristic temporalis muscle (Fig. 44.12).

44.6.5 Subaponeurotic Supraperiosteal Dissection

The subaponeurotic supraperiosteal dissection is performed through the vertical frontal incisions using the blunt dissector over a length of approximately 4 cm toward the vertex. This is an avascular plane that usually has little or no bleeding (Fig. 44.13).

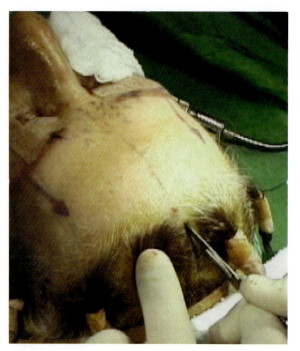

Fig. 44.12 Skin incisions

44.6.6 Subperiosteal Dissection

A frontal periosteal incision is performed using a number 15 blade through the frontal vertical incisions, and the sharp dissector is then used to elevate the periosteum of the frontal region, up to 1 cm above the brow implantation and laterally out to the upper temporal line at the site of implantation of the temporalis fascia (Fig. 44.14).

44.6.7 Interfascial Dissection

Once the plane between the deep and superficial layers of the deep temporalis fascia (interfascial plane) has been identified, the blunt dissector is then used to bring the dissection up to the upper temporal line, 1 cm short of the lateral orbital rim (Fig. 44.15).

44.6.8 Communication Between the Two Pockets

The same dissector is then used to connect both pockets – the interfascial pocket of the temporal region and the subperiosteal pocket of the frontal region. This creates a sufficiently broad flap to allow the use of the endoscope and the surgical instruments (Fig. 44.16).

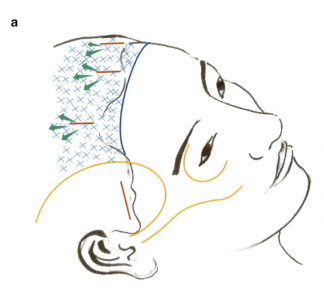
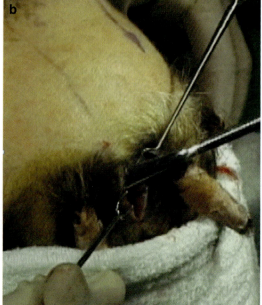

Fig. 44.13 Dissection in the supraperiosteal subgaleal plane

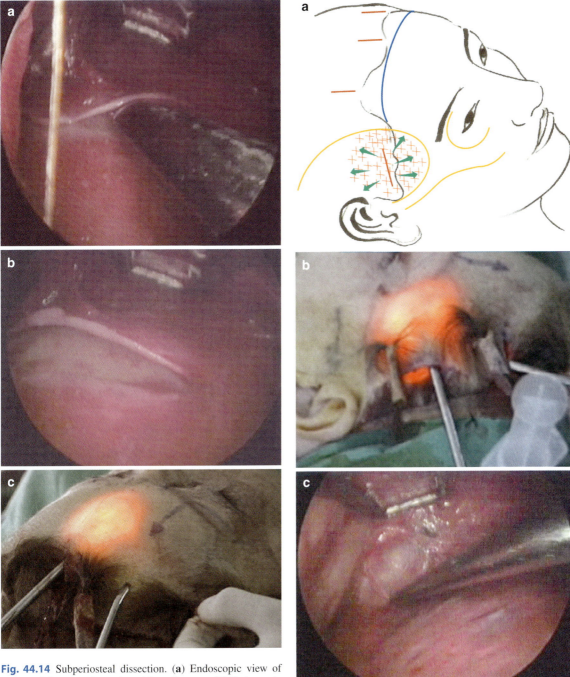

Fig. 44.14 Subperiosteal dissection. (**a**) Endoscopic view of periosteal flap elevation using a blunt dissector. (**b**) Endoscopic view of the raised periosteal flap. (**c**) External view of the placement of the endoscop and the dissector

Fig. 44.15 Dissection along the interfascial plane down to 1 cm off the lateral orbital rim. (**a**) Identification of the dissection plane. (**b**) Blunt dissection. (**c**) Endoscopic view of the interfascial dissection

44.6.9 Endoscope Placement and Use

The endoscope is placed through the lateral vertical incision in the frontal region, and blunt dissection is then performed through the temporal incision. This dissection proceeds up to the lateral orbital rim until the sentinel vein is encountered. This vein is protected as much as possible, working around it in order to

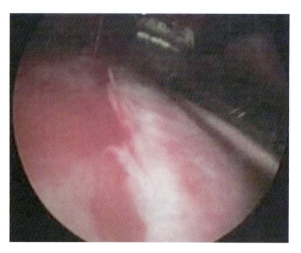

Fig. 44.16 Communication between the subperiosteal and interfascial pockets. Endoscopic view of the communicated pockets: on the left the subperiosteal pocket and on the right the interfascial pocket

avoid injury. In the event there is a need for coagulation, it must be done with extreme care, avoiding cauterization toward the superficial plane where the vein is associated with the path of the frontal branch of the facial nerve [15, 16].

The arcus marginalis (junction between the periosteum and the lateral orbital rim) is released using the angled dissector. This release is critical for long-term results.

44.6.10 Periosteal and Muscular Sectioning

Endoscopic scissors are used to cut the periosteum below the site of eyebrow and palpebral orbicularis muscle implantation. At this point, it is sometimes necessary to cauterize the sentinel vein in its portion closest to the skull. A bipolar cautery is preferable in that instance. Continuing with the dissection medially, once the site of emergence of the supratrochelar and supraorbital nerves is reached, the dissection proceeds carefully, always following a vertical direction, the same followed by the neurovascular bundle as it emerges from its orifice. The procerus and corrugator muscles are then sectioned at the site corresponding with the skin lines marked in advance (Fig. 44.17).

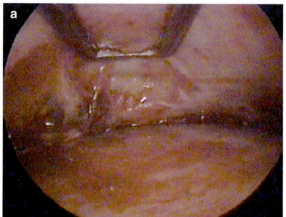
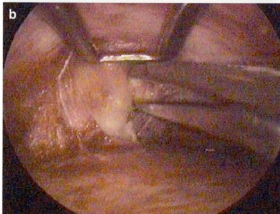
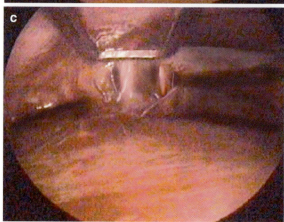

Fig. 44.17 Periosteal elevation. (**a**) Endoscopic view of lateral periosteal sectioning. (**b**) Dissection at the site of emergence of supratrochlear and supraorbital nerve bundles. (**c**) Endoscopic view of the nerve bundles

44.6.11 Fixation Suture Placement

Once the muscle is sectioned, several fixation sutures are placed from the periostium to the galea on the frontal vertical incisions, and from the deep layer of the deep

pressure bandage is placed on the frontal area in order to avoid dead space and hematoma formation.

44.6.13 Postoperative Follow-Up

The patient is discharged on oral paracetamol-type analgesics, 500 mg every 6 h. Next day, on the first follow-up visit, the bandage and Penrose drain are removed, and staples are removed 1 week later.

Photographic follow-up is critically important for final result assessments. Photographs taken at 1, 3, and 6 months will ensure adequate follow-up and control (Fig. 44.19, 44.20, 44.21, 44.22, 44.23, 44.24, 44.25).

44.7 Complications

Complications are infrequent. The most feared complication is frontalis muscle paralysis as a result of injury to the temporal branch of the facial nerve. This is quite improbable if the dissection is performed on the safe planes as described above. There may be cases of transient frontalis paresis, perhaps due to inflammation along the path of the facial nerve. This may take between 15 days and 6 months to recover. When paresis persists for more than 1 month, the use of botulinum

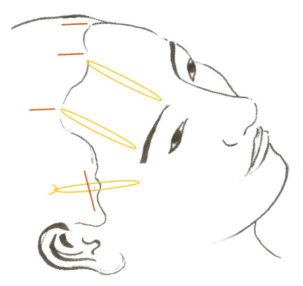

Fig. 44.18 Placement sites for maintenance sutures

temporalis fascia to the superficial layer of the same fascia on the incisions in the temporal area. Braided polyester 3/0 sutures are used for this purpose (Fig. 44.18).

44.6.12 Closure

Incisions are closed with fine metal staples. A Penrose drain is left in the temporal incisions and a mild

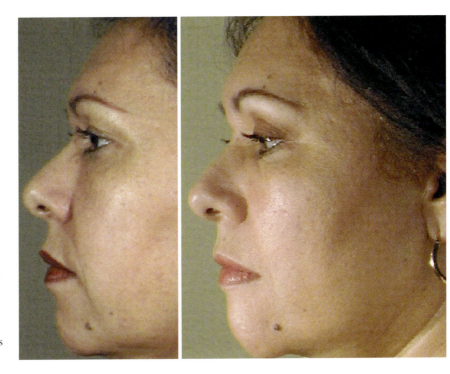

Fig. 44.19 A 50-year-old patient who underwent endoscopic forehead-lift and upper lid blepharoplasty: eyebrow elevation and improved orbital appearance are observed. (*Left*) Before surgery. (*Right*) Eight months after surgery

Fig. 44.20 A 48-year-old patient who underwent endoscopic forehead-lift and upper lid blepharoplasty. (*Left*) Before surgery. (*Right*) Eight months after surgery. The height of the new upper lid sulcus and the persistence of a few expression lines in the glabellar and crow's feet areas are observed

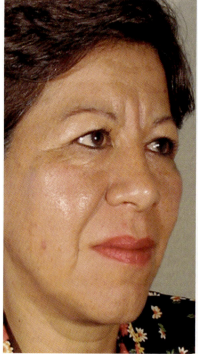
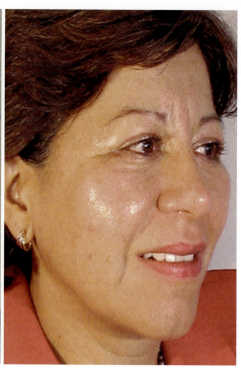

Fig. 44.21 A 54-year-old patient who underwent endoscopic forehead-lift, upper lid blepharoplasty, and facelift. (*Left*) Preoperative patient showing a lateral wrinkle and eyebrow ptosis resulting from prior upper lid blepharoplasty with excessive orbicularis oculi muscle resection. (*Right*) One year after surgery showing a more youthful appearance of the orbit

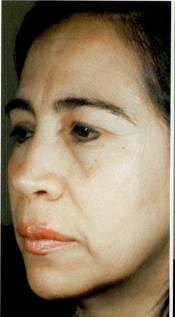
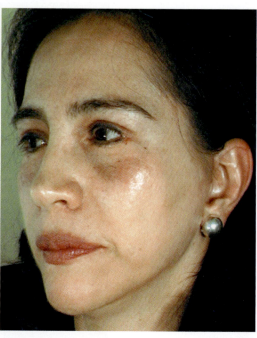

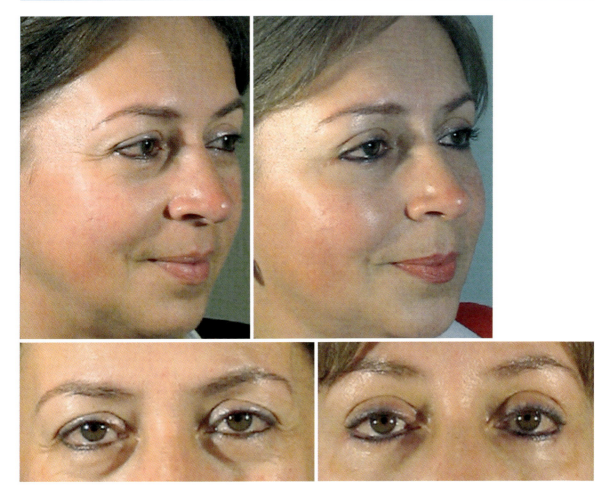

Fig. 44.22 A 54-year-old patient who underwent endoscopic forehead-lift and upper lid blepharoplasty. (*Left*) Before surgery. (*Right*) One year after surgery

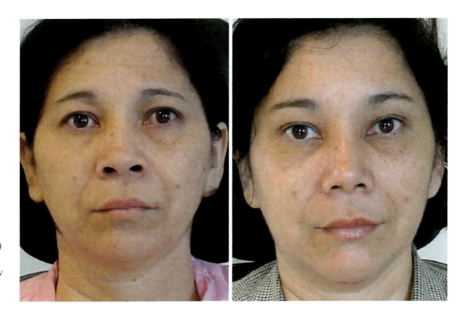

Fig. 44.23 A 45-year-old patient who underwent endoscopic forehead-lift. (*Left*) Before surgery. (*Right*) One year after surgery showing a change in eyebrow direction and a slight lift of the lateral canthi

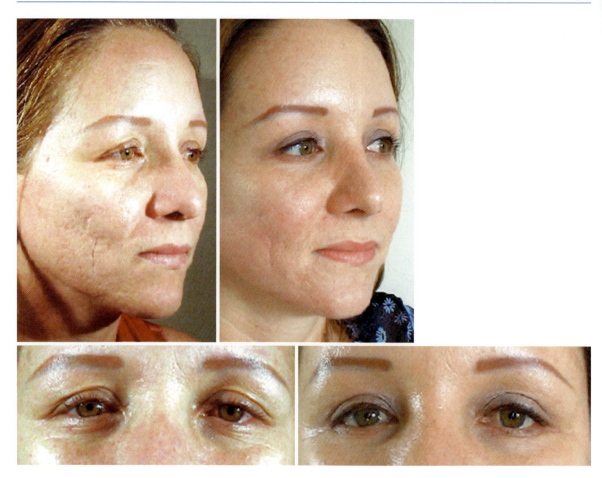

Fig. 44.24 A 32-year-old patient who underwent endoscopic forehead-lift, upper lid blepharoplasty, and dermabrasion. (*Left*) Before surgery. (*Right*) One year after surgery

toxin in the nonaffected side must be considered in order to restore movement symmetry and reduce patient anxiety while mobility is fully restored.

It is common to see paresthesias in the frontal region and in the scalp during the postoperative period. These can last up to 6 months. Careful manipulation of the areas where the supratrochlear and supraorbital nerves emerge may reduce the occurrence of this complication.

Scars are usually imperceptible since they are hidden under the hair. In bald patients or patients with little hair density, incisions that follow facial tension lines, such as Lange's lines, may be used in order to improve the cosmetic results of the scars. In any event, patients must be informed of the possibility that incisions may be visible during the first few months after surgery. Hair loss in the incision areas is rare [17, 18].

44.8 Discussion

Endoscopic forehead lift is one of the least invasive and most effective methods for eyebrow elevation and for controlling glabellar lines. Long-term results are excellent and very well accepted by patients. The degree of eyebrow elevation must be carefully assessed in order to attain natural-looking, "nonsurgical" harmonious results. Although this technique requires a slightly longer learning

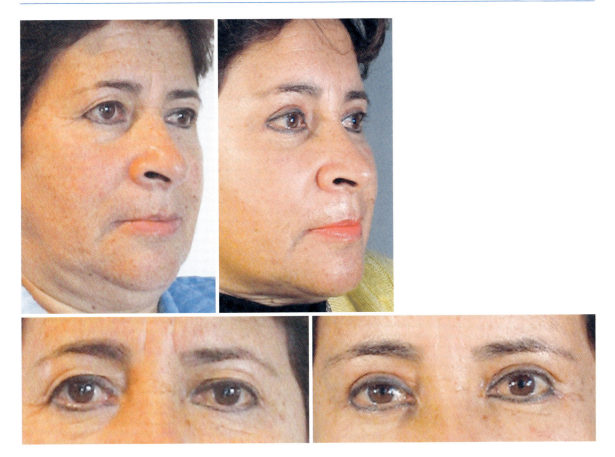

Fig. 44.25 A 49-year-old patient who underwent endoscopic forehead-lift. (*Left*) Before surgery. (*Right*) One year after surgery

curve than other brow-lift procedures, mainly because of the use of endoscopes, cameras, and special instruments, its excellent and lasting results warrant its application.

References

1. Pitanguy I. Indications and treatment of frontal and glabellar wrinkles in an analysis of 404 consecutive cases of rhytidectomy. Plast Reconstr Surg. 1981;67:157–66.
2. Miller CC. Subcutaneous section of the facial muscles to eradicate expression lines. Am J Surg. 1907;21:235.
3. Gonzales-Ulloa M. The history of rhytidectomy. Aesthetic Plast Surg. 1980;4:1.
4. Core GB, Vasconez LO, Askren C, et al. Coronal facelift with endoscopic techniques. Plast Surg Forum. 1992;15:227.
5. Liang M, Narayanan K. Endoscopic ablation of the frontalis and corrugator muscles, a clinical study. Plast Surg Forum. 1992;15:58.
6. Isse N. Endoscopic forehead lift. Paper presented at the annual meeting of Los Angeles County Society of Plastic Surgeons; 1992.
7. Castanares S. Forehead wrinkles, glabellar frown and ptosis of the eyebrows. Plast Reconstr Surg. 1964;34:406.
8. McKinney P, Mossie RD, Zukowski ML. Criteria for the forehead lift. Aesthetic Plast Surg. 1991;15(2):141–7.
9. Zimbler MS, Nassif PS. Adjunctive applications for botulinum toxin in facial aesthetic surgery. Facial Plast Surg Clin North Am. 2003;11(4):477–82.
10. Nassif PS, Kokoska MS, Cooper P, et al. Comparison of subperiosteal vs subgaleal elevation techniques used in forehead lifts. Arch Otolaryngol Head Neck Surg. 1998;124(11): 1209–15.
11. De La Fuente A, Santamaria AB. Facial rejuvenation: a combined conventional and endoscopic assisted lift. Aesthetic Plast Surg. 1996;20:471–9.
12. Oslin B, Core GB, Vasconez LO. The biplanar endoscopically assisted forehead lift. Clin Plast Surg. 1995;22:633–8.
13. Holzapfel AM, Mangat DS. Endoscopic forehead-lift using a bioabsorbable fixation device. Arch Facial Plast Surg. 2004;6(4):389–93.

14. Stevens WG, Apfelberg DB, et al. The endotine: a new biodegradable fixation device for endoscopic forehead lifts. Aesthetic Surg J. 2003;23(4):103–7.
15. Larrabee WF, Makielski KH, Cupp C. Facelift anatomy. Facial Plast Surg Clin North Am. 1993;1:135–52.
16. Pitanguy I, Ramos AS. The frontal branch of the facial nerve: the importance of its variations in face lifting. Plast Reconstr Surg. 1966;38:352–6.
17. Tardy ME, Thomas JR, Brown R. Facial aesthetic surgery. 1st ed. St. Louis: Mosby; 1995.
18. Sclafani AP, Fozo MS, Romo T, et al. Strength and histological characteristics of periosteal fixation to bone after elevation. Arch Facial Plast Surg. 2003;5(1):63–6.

Minimally Invasive Ciliary-Frontoplasty Technique

German Guillermo Rojas Duarte

45.1 Introduction

Since his origin, man has possessed a sense of beauty that is innate and is accompanied by the desire to keep youthfulness and this has led him to look for different methods to get his objective of keeping himself beautiful and young.

The forehead is considered as a very important aesthetic unit in the facial appearance. The eyebrows, as well as the eyelids and the lips are expression signs that reveal the emotions, feelings, and state of mind and they accompany the person's oral language. For being a mobile unit, it is here where the aging signs are most marked. In some occasions, the forehead crosswise wrinkles can be comparable to a scar.

We can see that in children or young patients, the eyebrow tail goes over the orbital flange. In advanced aged patients, this relation is reversed and it can be observed that a lower eyebrow tail than the eyebrow head is a sign of aging.

Aging with subsequent gradual eyebrow decrease and the changes in the forehead is attributed to different causes. Among them is age, the flaccidity occasioned by fat reabsorption, the mass loss, the muscular tone, and the three-dimensional loss of the bony volume. Also involved besides the mobility are the gravity effects on the tissues and the environment effects such as the sun, the wind, etc.

45.2 History

Traditionally, facial rejuvenation surgical treatments were centered in the cheeks and neck. Nowadays, in the handling of the face it has become very important to get a harmonic balance of the facial contour by attempting to obtain a natural state.

The first description on forehead lifting was reported in 1919 by Lexer [1]. It consisted of lifting the skin and the muscles superiorly, cutting the skin excess, and suturing. In 1926, Noel [2] presented his frontal lift technique. In 1931, Joseph [3], considered as the father of the modern plastic surgery, proclaimed his technique of skin elliptic resection immediately above the hair implantation line. In 1926, Hunt [4] published his technique through frontal bone incision. In 1957, Edwars proposed to carry out selective neurotomies of the facial temporary line to produce a facial paralysis of the frontal muscle. In 1951, Fomón [5], through eyebrow incisions, proposed to carry out avulsion of the insertions of the corrugator, procerus, frontal, and orbicular muscles, performing resection of the facial nerve frontal line also.

In 1956, Ichi-Uchida [6] proposed to dry up skin beneath the hairy implantation line and frontal muscle resection. In 1962, González-Ulloa recommended to use a skin elliptic wedge beneath the hairy front implantation line with no skin dissection. In 1973, Marino published his frontal bone incision technique, following the McIndoe postulates, with skin dissection up to the orbital edge and partial resection of the front, procerus, and corrugator muscles. In the 1970s and 1980s, with the boom of the reconstruction surgical techniques of the cranial-facial surgery through frontal bone incisions and mobilization of big facial flaps with satisfactory results, the application of these techniques led to the aesthetic surgeries [7].

G.G.R. Duarte
Plastic and Reconstructive Surgeon, San Martín University,
Cra. 18 No. 80-35, Bogotà D.C., Colombia, CES University,
Calle 10 A No. 22 - 04, Medellín, Antioquia, Colombia and
Cra 18 No. 85-36 Of. 201, Bogota, DC, Colombia
e-mail: contacto@germanrojas.com

In 1969, Viñas [8] presented his technique of frontal facelift, by using a prehairy and intrahairy treatment (front bone); cutting the skin and the galea in both cases and inverting the flap for a better treatment of the frontal and corrugator muscles. In 1981, Coiffman [9] published a technique for treating the forehead and eyelid wrinkles. He recommended, besides other aspects, drying up the eyelid muscles. Then, he stopped this technique since it left an eyelid depression over time. There exist a lot and very important contributions of surgeons such as Regnault Kaye, Pitanguy, Riefkohl, Owsley, Adamson, Papillon, Connell, McKinney, Matarasso, Terino, Psillakis, Hinderer, and many others, who presented innovative techniques always looking for the perfection of the face higher third part [10].

In the last decade of the twentieth century, Isse, Ramírez, Vasconez, and Chajchir disclosed their first experiences of forehead-lift by means of small incisions and use of the endoscope. These techniques revolutionized the surgical practices of the aesthetic surgery, but controversies were presented later on since there were those who defended the traditional surgery with the argument that where there was skin excess, it was necessary to remove it and reposition the loosened tissues, whereas others continued to prefer the endoscopic surgery.

45.3 Forehead Anatomy

Knowledge of the forehead's complex anatomy gives us the basis for choosing a good surgical technique according to each patient's situation.

We can consider the frontal region as an aesthetic subunit limited in the higher and lateral part by the hairline and in the lower part by the eyebrows. When making the incisions, the lines of less skin tension should be kept in mind. In the facial higher third part, the following structures are found: (1) The skin and the subcutaneous cellular tissue. (2) The superficial aponeurotic muscle determined by the eyelid's orbicular muscle, the frontal muscle, and the occipital muscle joint by the epicranial aponeurosis or aponeurotic galea. (3) The deep muscular system including the superciliary depressor muscle, the nose procerus-pyramidal muscle, and the corrugator muscle. (4) The vascular–nervous system formed by the supratrochlear vascular–nerve package, supraorbital vascular–nerve package, and the periosteum. (5) The retaining ligaments where we find the higher septum-temporal, lower septum-temporal, and the periorbital septum. (6) The motor innervation of the frontal region and the scalp depending on the facial nerve [11] (Fig. 45.1).

45.4 Ciliary Ptosis Classification

It is important to evaluate the eyelid position to be able to provide the best treatment since this influences the forehead and eyelids. The eyebrows have a head, body, and tail. We can see the following characteristics in the eyebrows:

Normal (Fig. 45.2): The eyebrows should go on the orbital edge in young people. The ideal eyebrow is limited by taking an imaginary line that passes by the internal border of the eye, extending it up to the nasal base, an oblique line drawn from the nasal base up to the orbital edge, another line that unites the higher points of the lines previously described, a parallel line to the first one that passes through the external edge of the ocular iris and finally, one that joins the intersection of the first one with the third one extending it up to the external border, giving us the ideal eyebrow limits.

Eyebrow Ptosis, Medial Position: The eyebrow is seen fallen in its central part (Fig. 45.3).

Eyebrow Ptosis: The eyebrow is seen fallen. It is lower than the orbital edge and the swollen eyelids, giving an aspect of tired and bored person (Fig. 45.3).

Lateral Ptosis: Observed is a decrease of the eyebrow tail with increase of the crow's-feet wrinkles (Fig. 45.3).

45.5 Nonsurgical Techniques in Forehead Rejuvenation

Botulinum Toxin: It is the capacity of the botulinum toxin type A to produce muscle paralysis for cosmetic purposes that occurs by inhibiting the muscle movement of the corrugator, procerus, and frontal muscles. This has a duration of 3 to 6 months. It is used in patients that do not want surgery [12].

Soft Tissue Filling: There exist in the market a number of products to fill forehead and eyebrow

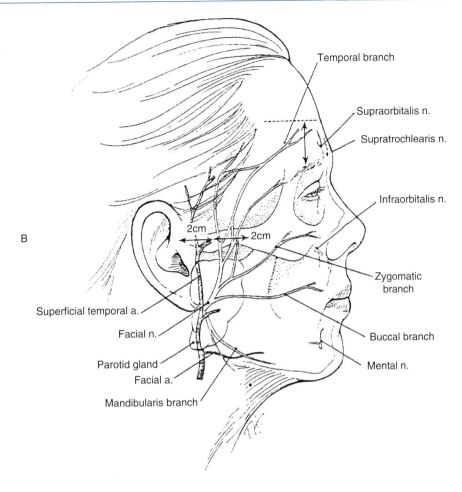

Fig. 45.1 Motor innervation of the frontal region and the scalp depending on the facial nerve

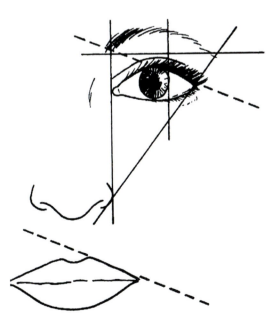

Fig. 45.2 Ideal eyebrow

depressions. Among those most used are collagen and the hyaluronic acid.

45.6 Surgical Techniques in Frontal Rejuvenation

Although there are a great number of techniques, we will only mention the most common ones.

45.6.1 Autogenous Fat Injection

This consists in the transfer of fat from a donor zone to fill the forehead and eyebrow crosswise wrinkles using syringe and needle. Generally, it is done with ambulatory local anesthesia. This technique does not entirely remove the wrinkle depressions but it is useful in young

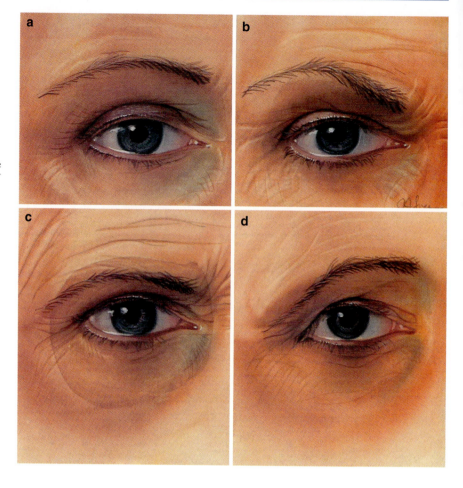

Fig. 45.3 Classification. (**a**) Normal eyebrow. (**b**) Medial eyebrow ptosis: The eyebrow is seen fallen in its central part. (**c**) Eyebrow ptosis: The eyebrow is seen fallen. It is lower than the orbital edge and the swollen eyelids, giving an aspect of tired and bored person. (**d**) Lateral eyebrow ptosis: Observed is a decrease of the eyebrow tail with increase of the crow's-feet wrinkles

patients and those who do not want invading procedures [13].

45.6.2 Moisturizing Graft

This is mainly used to fill the eyebrow wrinkles. Its absorption is less than the autogenous fat. A block of fatty tissue and dermis is obtained and are applied through small incisions [11].

45.6.3 Open Frontal Lift

This surgery is indicated in cases of advanced ptosis where there is need to remove skin. This technique can be intrahairy when the hair implantation line is low and the person has abundant hair, or prehairy when the patient has a very broad forehead or the hair implantation line is much behind.

45.6.4 Periorbital Approach

The ciliary-frontoplasty is made through an incision at the superciliary level. It is used to lift eyebrows and eyelids.

45.6.5 Transpalpebral Resection of the Corrugator Muscle

This is used in patients who present hyperactivity of the corrugator muscles. It can be done by a standard incision when the patient recovers from a blepharoplasty. Otherwise, a medial incision is performed.

45.6.6 Forehead Endoscopic Rejuvenation

This is done through endoscopy and small incisions in the scalp. The aim is to lift the eyebrows, stretch the forehead, and hold the galea up by fixing it to the parietal bone.

45.6.7 Minimally Invasive Ciliary-Frontoplasty

This is done through small incisions in the scalp. When it is the sole procedure, it can be performed with sedation using local anesthesia containing 2% lidocaine with epinephrine. The incisions are those used in endoscopic surgery in the scalp temporal region 1.5–2 cm from the hairline (Fig. 45.4), with No. 15 blade, at a 45° angle in order to avoid injuries of the hairy follicles that will cause alopecia and scars in the zone. When there is need to lift the eyebrow body, the dissection is extended to the eyebrow body and to the hairline level using a 1.5 cm. incision, parallel to the imaginary line previously drawn. Once the incisions are made to the surgical plane that we look for in the temporal region between the superficial and deep temporal fascia, dissection is beneath the orbital edge and the orbicular myotomies in its superior-external part are carried out. The plane is subperiosteal in the frontal medial region.

Later on, both these planes are joined in order to get the zone detachment. The technique principle is to slide two blades one over the other. Then according to the vectors drawn, the suspension points are fixed with Ethibond 3–0 in the temporal region (2–3) of the superficial fascia to the deep fascia and in the periosteum frontal–medial to the galea. The scalp is closed with mechanical suture (staples). Later on, it is splinted with one inch skin colored Micropore tape.

45.7 Complications

With the technique of minimally invasive ciliary-frontoplasty, there has been no type of complications since it was established. In the universal medical literature the following complications are detailed:

- Loss of sensitivity
- Pain, swelling, and hematoma
- Temporal loss of the expressive movements
- Sensation of oppression in the forehead
- High initial position of the eyebrows
- Muscular paralysis of the frontal nerve
- Necrosis
- Infection
- Hematoma and haemorrhage
- Scar
- Eyebrows or eyelids asymmetry
- Chronic pain
- Overcorrection

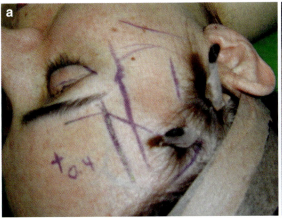
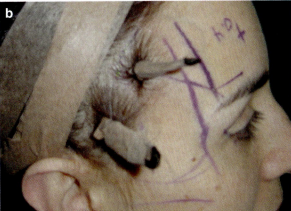

Fig. 45.4 Demarcation surgically repaired

45.8 Conclusions

The minimally invasive ciliary-frontoplasty was used in 290 patients with ptosis of the eyebrow tail and eyebrow ptosis during a 7-year period (2000–2007). The results were very good and improvement between 98% and 100% was noted with minimum or zero complications (Figs. 45.5–45.7).

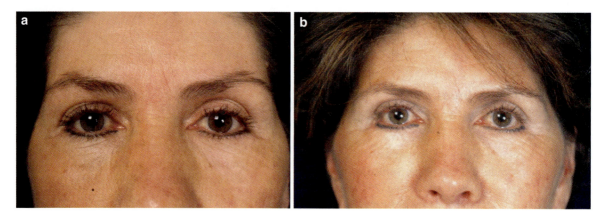

Fig. 45.5 (**a**) Preoperative. (**b**) Postoperative

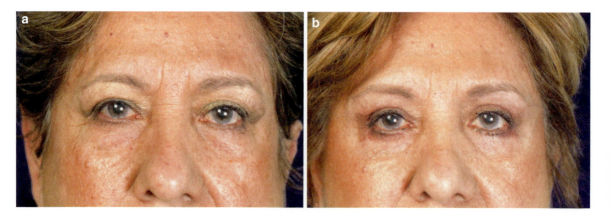

Fig. 45.6 (**a**) Preoperative. (**b**) Postoperative

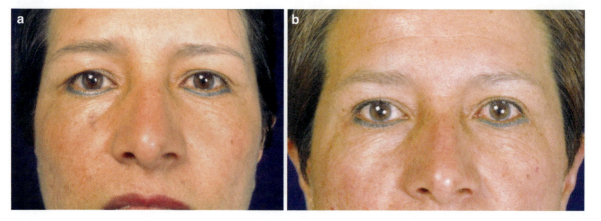

Fig. 45.7 (**a**) Preoperative. (**b**) Postoperative

References

1. Lexer E. Die gesamte Wiederherstellungs-Chirurgie, Vols. 1 and 2. Leipzig: Jahann Ambrosius Barth; 1931.
2. Noel A. La chirurgie esthetique et son role social. Paris: Masson; 1926. p. 62–6.
3. Joseph J. Nasenplastik und sonstige Gesichtplastik nebst einen Anhang uber Mammaplastik. Leipzig: Kabitzch; 1931. p. 507–9.
4. Hunt HL. Plastic surgery of the head, face, and neck. Philadelphia: Lea & Febiger; 1926.
5. Fomon S, Goldman IB, Neivert H, Schattner A. Face-lift operation by rotation flaps. Arch Otolaryngol. 1951;54(5): 478–92.
6. Uchida JI. A method of frontal rhytidectomy. Plast Reconstr Surg. 1965;35:218–22.
7. Marino H, Gandolfo E. Treatment of forehead wrinkles. Prensa Méd Argent. 1964;51:1368–71.
8. Vinas JC. Plan general de la ritidoplastia y zona tabu. In: Transactions of the 4th Brasilian congress on plastic surgery, Porto Alegre, 5–8 Oct 1965; p. 32.
9. Coiffman F. Elevación de cejas y frente por incisiones mínimas y sin endoscopio. Enfoque personal. In: Coiffman F, editor. Cirugía Plástica, Reconstructiva y Estética. Tomo II. Venezuela: Amolca; 2007. p. 1108–15.
10. Paul M. The evolution of the brow lift in aesthetic plastic surgery. Plast Reconstr Surg. 2001;108(5):1409–24.
11. Latarjet M et al. Anatomia humana, Buenos Aires. Médica Panamericana 2005:304–315.
12. Sastoque C et al. Estudio de tres diluciones de toxina botulínica tipo A. Rev Colombiana Cir Plast Reconstr. 2002; 8(2):1.
13. Guerrerosantos J. Autologous fat grafting for body contouring. Clin Plast Surg. 1996;23(4):619–31.

Treatment of Eyebrow Ptosis Through the Modified Technique of Castañares

Giovanni André Pires Viana and Giovanni Pires Viana

46.1 Introduction

Fascination with beauty as well as with the orbits and their surrounding tissues dates back to early human civilization. The lid–eyebrow complex is perhaps the most expressive part of the face; one can express anger, worry, surprise, and other emotions by his or her brows [1, 2]. A high eyebrow positioned above the orbital rim and small eyebrows with the eyebrow arch positioned in the middle were preferred for many decades [1–3].

Gravity and senescence are the main causes of aging of the entire periorbital region and brow; however, numerous etiologies for eyebrow ptosis exist, including those that were congenital, posttraumatic, iatrogenic, facial paralysis related, and functional (usually age related) [4–7]. One of earliest signs of facial aging, starting in the third decade, is descent or flattening of the lateral eyebrow [4, 6, 7]. Eyebrow ptosis gives the eyes a heavy, tired, and sad look, and enhances aesthetic deformities of the upper eyelid. The resultant brow ptosis manifests in lateral hooding of the eyelid and has implications for functional visual field obstruction [4–7].

There is a great diversity among individuals with respect to eyebrow position and shape and, the notion of an "ideal" eyebrow has changed quite significantly over the past several decades [1].

G.A.P. Viana (✉)
Member of Brazilian Plastic Surgery,
Department of Ophthalmology, Vision Institute,
Federal University of São Paulo, São Paulo, SP, Brazil
e-mail: info@cliniplast.com

G.P. Viana
Alameda Jauaperi 732, São Paulo, SP 04523-013, Brazil
e-mail: info@cliniplast.com

Many brow lift surgical procedures have been described over the last 100 years, including direct eyebrow lift, midforehead lift, coronal brow lift, transpalpebral brow lift, and endoscopic brow lift [1, 6, 8–16]. More recently, nonendoscopic, limited-incision approaches to correct the descent of the lateral eyebrow alone have been reported by several authors [4, 7, 9, 17–19]. A nonsurgical option for brow lift using botulinum toxin A injections has been described for temporary paralysis of the depressor muscles of the brow [20].

46.2 Patient Marking

After identification of eyebrow ptosis, one must determine the patient's optimal eyebrow position. The "butterfly wing" incision was proposed initially by Viñas and popularized by Castañares [9, 10].

The amount of skin resection depends on the elevation desired and the amount calculated ahead of time to be excessive. Viñas has suggested a simple but accurate method to determine the amount of skin resection: by pinching the skin with thumb and index finger above the lateral end of the brow with the patient in the erect position and watching for the desired effect. The widest part of the drawing is marked above the tail of the brow, and the lateral extension is then carried out to complete it beyond the tail of the brow in an upward and lateral direction (Fig. 46.1) [10]. It is important to place the lower margin of the incision along the superior border of the brow abutting the hair follicles.

Another way to draw the "butterfly wing" incision would be with the patient in a supine position, doing the same maneuver described by Viñas with forceps, but the disadvantage would be no gravity acting on the tissues (Fig. 46.2).

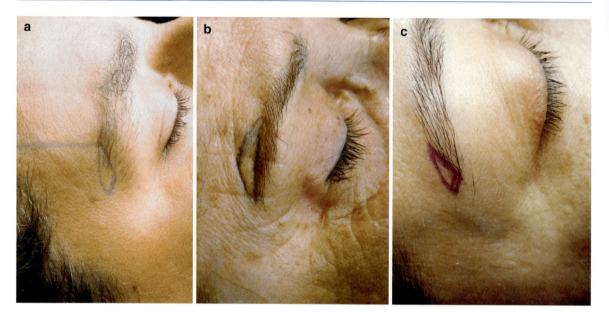

Fig. 46.1 Schematic drawing. (**a**, **b**) and (**c**) show how the "butterfly wing" incision adapts to each patient

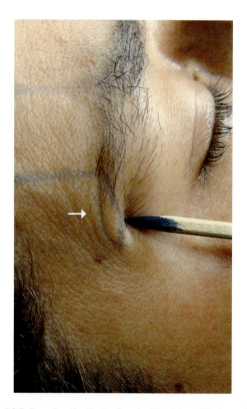

Fig. 46.2 Drawing the "butterfly wing" incision with the patient in a supine position. *Arrow*: The superior limit of surgical scar often fell within or parallel to a preexisting crease of the crow's feet

46.3 Surgical Procedure

The patient is placed in a supine position, the face and brows are cleaned with antiseptic solutions and draped. Under intravenous sedation, local anesthesia along the incision lines and into the "butterfly wing" incision is administered (Fig. 46.3). An incision is made and it is beveled to parallel the hair follicles, preventing damage to the brow hair follicles, then the authors undermine superficially (epidermis dissection), like Schwartzman's maneuver in breast reduction surgery (Fig. 46.4). There is no undermining underneath this level. Thereafter, the epidermis is removed, following meticulous hemostasis of the wound (Fig. 46.5) and, the closure is carried out in the conventional manner (Fig. 46.6). A pressure dressing is applied to the incision for 5 days. The stitches are usually removed between 7 and 10 days postoperatively.

46.4 Complications

The overall rate of complications was low. The most common complication was epidermal cyst (3.3%) and suture dehiscence due to local trauma (2.2%). Reoperation was performed in the unsatisfied patients (2%).

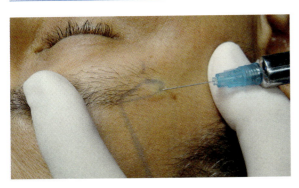

Fig. 46.3 Anesthetic injection into the "butterfly wing" incision

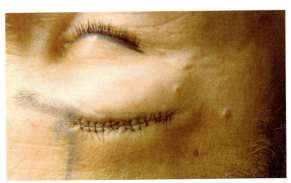

Fig. 46.6 Closure of the wound

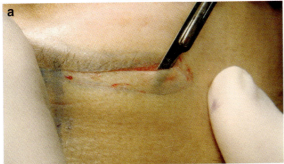

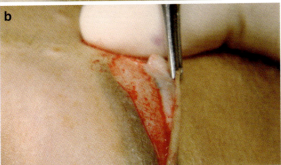

Fig. 46.4 Undermining superficially (**a**, **b**)

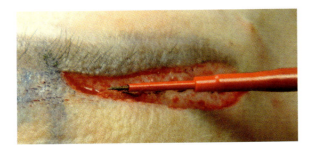

Fig. 46.5 Meticulous hemostasis

The surgical scar became scarcely noticeable over time, and often fell within or parallel to a preexisting crease of the crow's feet. There were no hypertrophic or keloid scars, no infection, no lagophthalmos, and no postoperative hematoma. Neither brow hair loss nor scar widening was noticed.

46.5 Discussion

Since 1996 the authors had done 910 eyebrow elevations in 455 consecutive patients whose ages ranged from 35 to 85 years. Almost 94% of the patients were female. Over 90% of the cases were performed simultaneously with rhytidectomy and blepharoplasty, 16.9% were performed in association with blepharoplasty and eyebrow lift alone represented 4% of the cases. The procedure was completed on average in 30 min (20–45 min). The follow-up in this series was from 10 months to 12 years. Good brow elevation that lasted through the period of follow-up was uniformly demonstrated (Figs. 46.7–46.12).

Brow positioning is considered a "cornerstone" with respect to the appearance of the periorbital region, and ptosis of the eyebrow is considered a characteristic feature of the aging face [4]. Even a minor change in brow position can alter the expression of an individual's face. With the correction of lateral drooping of the brow, the facial expressions of sadness and fatigue caused by brow ptosis can be improved to achieve a more tranquil facial aesthetic [4].

The modern concept of "ideal" brow position was described by Westmore in 1974 [1]. Optimal eyebrow position is both objective and subjective and, ideal

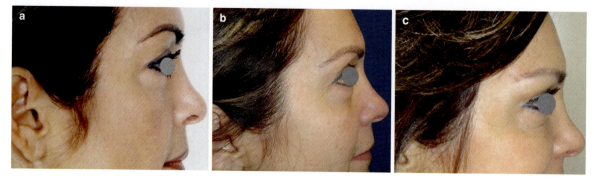

Fig. 46.7 (**a**) Preoperative 50-year-old female. (**b**) Three years postoperative. (**c**) Five years postoperative after a touch-up

Fig. 46.8 (**a**) Preoperative 38-year-old female. (**b**) Ten months postoperative

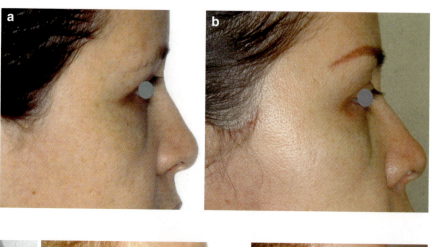

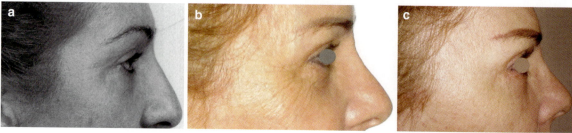

Fig. 46.9 (**a**) Preoperative 61-year-old female. (**b**) Ten years postoperative. (**c**) Two years postoperative after a touch-up

criteria vary from surgeon to surgeon and continue to be debated [1, 5, 21]. According to Feser et al. there is not one single beauty ideal for eyebrows, but at least three, this being determined by the patient's age and trends. For instance, trends are generally introduced by young people and not by older individuals and the young tend to prefer eyebrows in a lower position. This way, it seems plausible to assume that the trend currently appears to be moving away from arched eyebrows toward lower-positioned eyebrows with maximum height in the lateral third [1].

Knize discussed several mechanisms contributing to brow ptosis, including depression of the medial eyebrow from overaction of the brow depressors and descent of the lateral eyebrow from unopposed lateral orbicularis oculi contraction [22].

To recreate the aesthetically pleasing brow, several surgical procedures have been published over the past century [2, 6–13, 15–19]. Many different surgical corrective procedures and types of incisions for raising the eyebrow have been characterized including direct eyebrow lift, midforehead lift,

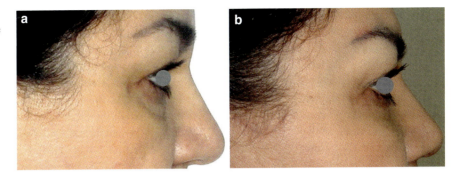

Fig. 46.10 (**a**) Preoperative 60-year-old female. (**b**) Three months postoperative

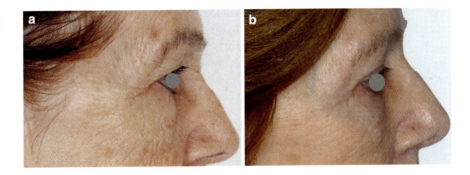

Fig. 46.11 (**a**) Preoperative 69-year-old female. (**b**) One year postoperative

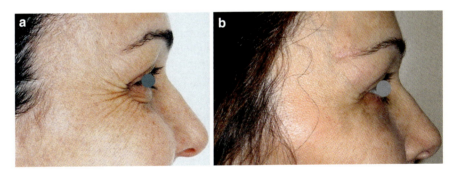

Fig. 46.12 (**a**) Preoperative 51-year-old female. (**b**) One month postoperative

coronal brow lift, transpalpebral brow lift, endoscopic brow lift, and the use of botulinum toxin [1, 6, 8–16]. More recently, nonendoscopic, limited-incision approaches to correct the descent of the lateral eyebrow alone have been reported by several authors [2, 7, 9, 17–19]. Sometimes a combination with brow-lift and blepharoplasty is necessary to achieve the desired results [16, 23]. Performing upper blepharoplasty in conjunction with brow lift is not a problem if care is given to proper preoperative analysis, quantification, and marking [16].

The authors have presented their experience with "butterfly wing" incision based on Viñas' study [10].

Indication for surgery is more dependent on the aging signs than on the patient's chronological age. The authors use this approach to correct the lateral end of the brow (tail), mostly in patients with hairless eyebrow or in patients wearing makeup to disguise the brow ptosis. Nevertheless, this approach would be carried out in all patients because they have been warned ahead of time of the scar extension. It is important to stress to the patient that the scar would be visible for a period of time but it may be concealed temporarily with cosmetics. Another important fact is to identify and discuss any preoperative eyebrow asymmetry with the patient, because he or she will be more likely to notice the asymmetry postoperatively during focused attention on the surgical results.

Viñas [10] and Castañares [9] correct the eyebrow ptosis by resection of a roughly elliptical section of the forehead skin immediately above and lateral to the eyebrow. Through this approach the forehead is undermined to the hairline, severing all epicranial fibers, the corrugator supercilii, and the procerus [9]. Different from Viñas and Castañares, the authors' resection is performed superficially, like Schwartzman's maneuver in breast reduction surgery, without undermining underneath the epidermis level. In this manner, the authors believe that this approach reduces the prevalence of unaesthetic scar formation by avoiding injury to the dermis. Further, the maximal amount of skin is excised laterally, allowing a favorable elevation of the lateral portion of the eyebrow with respect to the medial part.

In this series, the most common complication was epidermal cyst (3.3%), suture dehiscence due to local trauma (2.2%), and reoperation of unsatisfied patients (2%). Reoperation was performed in nine patients with minimal recurrence of brow ptosis due to previous inadequate resection. Viñas et al. [10] revealed an extremely low complication rate (0.4%) of hematoma formation, permanent alopecia, and "nerve damage." They also reported a 2.4% dissatisfaction rate, which is comparable with the numbers presented in this series and other studies in literature [2, 8, 10, 12–14, 16, 18, 19]. According to Viñas, the advantage of this approach is its simplicity, it is well tolerated as an outpatient procedure under local anesthesia and that most patients can resume their activities the following day [10]. The authors agree with Viñas on this advantage; another is that it carries a direct one-to-one correction of brow ptosis. The disadvantage of this procedure is the scars on the forehead, but to quote Viñas: "The scars usually become inconspicuous with time. Also because of their location, they can be easily disguised (if necessary) with a couple of strokes of an eyebrow pencil" [10]. If these factors are properly explained beforehand and with the visible improvement, these patients accept the temporary inconveniences with conformity and understanding.

46.6 Conclusions

The key to correction of eyebrow ptosis in patients undergoing cosmetic surgery is to first recognize it and include this component in each patient's evaluation.

The "butterfly wing" incision provides a useful alternative in situations in which the surgeon may not be familiar with endoscopic techniques, does not have access to endoscopic equipment, or when frontalis modification is not required. Although this operation yields sustained improvements, it does not remove all underlying factors involved in brow aging. The effects of gravitational forces continue and may result in the need for future enhancements. The final results of this operation are consistently very gratifying to the patient and to the plastic surgeon alike.

References

1. Feser DK, Gründl M, Eisenmann-Klein M, Prantl L. Attractiveness of eyebrow position and shape in females depends on the age of the beholder. Aesthetic Plast Surg. 2007;31(2):154–60.
2. Tabatabai N, Spinelli HM. Limited incision nonendoscopic browlift. Plast Reconstr Surg. 2007;119(5):1563–70.
3. Gunter JP, Antrobus SD. Aesthetic analysis of the eyebrows. Plast Reconstr Surg. 1997;99(7):1808–16.
4. Har-Shai Y, Gil T, Metanes I, Scheflan M. Brow lift for the correction of visual field impairment. Aesthetic Surg J. 2008;28(5):512–7.
5. Noel CL. Eyebrow position recognition and correction in reconstructive and cosmetic surgery. Arch Facial Plast Surg. 2009;10:44–9.
6. Karabulut AB, Tümerderm B. Forehead lift: a combined approach using subperiosteal and subgaleal dissection planes. Aesthetic Plast Surg. 2001;25(5):378–81.
7. Strauch B, Baum T. Connection of lateral brow ptosis: a nonendoscopic subgaleal approach. Plast Reconstr Surg. 2002;109(3):1164–7.
8. Paul MD. The evolution of the brow lift in aesthetic plastic surgery. Plast Reconstr Surg. 2001;108(5):1409–24.
9. Castañares S. Forehead wrinkles, glabellar frown and ptosis of the eyebrows. Plast Reconstr Surg. 1964;34:406–13.
10. Viñas JC, Caviglia C, Cortiñas JL. Forehead rhytidoplasty and brow lifting. Plast Reconstr Surg. 1976;57(4):445–54.
11. Herzog Neto G, Sebastiá R, Viana GAP. Brow ptosis: transpalpebral approach. Rev Soc Bras Cir Plast. 2005;20:231–6.
12. Pitanguy I. Indications for and treatment of frontal and glabellar wrinkles in an analysis of 3, 404 consecutive cases of rhytidectomy. Plast Reconstr Surg. 1981;67(2):157–68.
13. Berkowitz RL, Jacobs DI, Gorman PJ. Brow fixation with the endotine forehead device in endoscopic brow lift. Plast Reconstr Surg. 2005;116(6):1761–7.
14. Elkwood A, Matarasso A, Rankin M, Elkowitz M, Godek CP. National plastic surgery survey: brow lifting techniques and complications. Plast Reconstr Surg. 2001;108(7):2143–50.
15. Troilius C. Subperiosteal brow lifts without fixation. Plast Reconstr Surg. 2004;114(6):1595–603.
16. Friedland JA, Jacobsen WM, TerKonda S. Safety and efficacy of combined upper blepharoplasty and open coronal

browlift: a consecutive series of 600 patients. Aesthetic Plast Surg. 1996;20(6):453–62.
17. Lassus C. Elevation of the lateral brow without the help of an endoscope. Aesthetic Plast Surg. 1999;23(1):23–7.
18. Kikkawa DO, Miller SR, Batra MK, Lee AC. Small incision nonendoscopic browlift. Ophthalmic Plast Reconstr Surg. 2000;16(1):28–33.
19. Viana GP, Viana GAP. Approach to eyebrow ptosis through the modified technique of Castañares. Indian J Plast Surg. 2009;42:58–62.
20. Fagien S. Botox for the treatment of dynamic and hyperkinetic facial lines and furrows: adjunctive use in facial aesthetic surgery. Plast Reconstr Surg. 1999;103(2):701–13.
21. Roth JM, Metzinger SE. Quantifying the arch position of the female eyebrow. Arch Facial Plast Surg. 2003;5(3):235–9.
22. Knize DM. An anatomically based study of the mechanism of eyebrow ptosis. Plast Reconstr Surg. 1996;97(7):1321–33.
23. Rohrich RJ, Coberly DM, Fagien S, Stuzin JM. Current concepts in aesthetic upper blepharoplasty. Plast Reconstr Surg. 2004;113(3):32e–42e.

Endobrow Lift

47

Anthony Erian

47.1 Introduction

The eyebrow (Fig. 47.1) deserves special mention within the context of the balance of the upper face and therefore forehead rejuvenation. The author has a simple new technique and concept, that of the endobrow lift, which is the direct elevation of the brow through the upper blepharoplasty incision. There are various other procedures in the context of forehead rejuvenation that are discussed.

The Endobrow Lift is a procedure that restores a more youthful, refreshed look to the area above the eyes by correcting drooping of the brows. The main advantage of this procedure is avoiding an extrascar or hair loss that other procedures might cause.

Most imbalances involve the middle and lower areas of the face. The eyebrows should be located at least 2–2.5 cm above the upper lid margin level when the eyes are closed. The medial aspect of the eye brow is caudal to the lateral extreme, and the highest portion of the eye brow arch is at the junction of the lateral third with the medial two-thirds of the eye brow corresponding to the lateral limits of the limbus in a straight forward gaze [1].

The eyebrow droop can cause significant overhang of upper eyelid skin over the lashes, and these are suitable candidates for the eyebrow lift. The cause of eyebrow ptosis is unknown but simple ptosis and true excess of skin on the upper eyelids (dermatochalasis) can occur due to gravity and aging, which can cause thinning and descent of the tissue of the forehead. Occasionally, eyebrow ptosis is caused by a paralysis of the facial nerve (facial palsy), or the weight of a tumor, or trauma on one side. It can interfere with visual function or appear unsightly. It is usually bilateral but can be asymmetrical, appearing on one side only [2].

First the surgeon must assess the appearance of the forehead, eyebrows, upper eyelids, and the periocular region. The surgeon must assess the lines of the forehead, how active the eyebrows are, whether the

A. Erian
Pear Tree Cottage, Cambridge Road,
Wimpole 43, SG8 5QD Cambridge, United Kingdom
e-mail: plasticsurgeon@anthonyerian.com

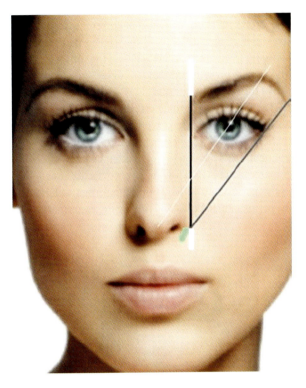

Fig 47.1 (*white*) Ala to inner canthus (*green*) ala to outer corner of eye and brow

eyebrows are used a lot to keep the eyelids open, or whether they are immobile, suggesting a nerve palsy. Measurements will be made and photographs taken. The amount of associated upper eyelid ptosis and excess skin on the eyelids is determined. According to the findings, the surgeon may recommend brow ptosis surgery.

47.2 Anatomy

The brows (Fig. 47.2) come in different shapes and sizes and gender differences exist. The male brow is naturally lower and less arched than that of the female. The female brow is finer, more curved, and is situated above the bony rim [3, 4].

The forehead (Fig. 47.3) is a highly dynamic region of the face, and patients who are more animated use each muscle of the forehead more frequently. This frequent use undoubtedly causes changes to the skin. A major factor stabilizing the eyebrow is its attachment to the periosteum in the supraorbital region. Dividing the periosteum laterally and freeing the arcus marginalis is mandatory to free the lateral brow and thereby enable elevation. Anatomically one muscle elevates the brow which is frontalis, and four muscles depress the brow, namely corrugator, procerus, fibers of the orbicularis, and superficial supercilii (Fig. 47.4).

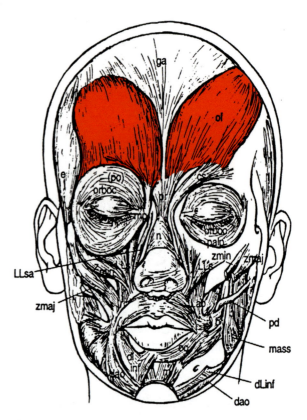

Fig. 47.3 Extent of brow area, anatomically

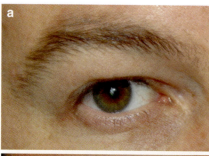

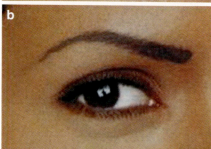

Fig. 47.2 Different shapes of brow in male and female. (**a**) The male brow is naturally lower and less arched than that of the female. (**b**) The female brow is finer, more curved, and is situated above the bony rim

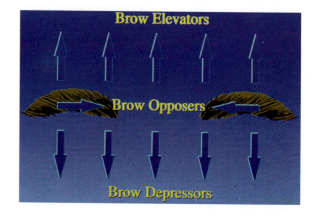

Fig. 47.4 Elevators and depressors of the brow. Anatomically the frontalis muscle elevates the brow and the corrugator, procerus, fibers of the orbicularis, and superficial supercilii depress the brow

47.3 Endobrow Lift

47.3.1 Objectives of a Brow Lift

A forehead lift is most commonly performed to minimize the visible effects of aging. It can help to:

1. Correct a low, heavy or droopy brow, achieving a more alert and refreshed look.
2. Correct furrows and frown lines which have developed around the brow and eye.
3. Achieve a better overall result from facial surgery, for example, when used in conjunction with blepharoplasty (eyelid surgery), where addressing aging of the eyelids alone does not always yield the best results, or in conjunction with a face-lift to rejuvenate the face.

Drooping eyebrows can cause a visual field problem. Fatigue and headaches at the end of the day may be caused by overaction of the forehead muscles which raise the eyebrows. There are also aesthetic/cosmetic reasons [5].

47.3.2 Preoperative Counseling

It is important to spend time with patients and ascertain what exactly is bothering them. The options open to the patients must be discussed in detail, including possible complications, as well as both pre and postoperative instructions (Table 47.1). To avoid problems, it is imperative to make sure that the patient has realistic expectations.

47.3.3 Learning Curve

It is of paramount importance that the cosmetic surgeon achieves a leaning curve to understand the procedure and its effects toward the best results. This reduces

Table 47.1 Pre and postoperative instructions

Forehead (brow) lift
BEFORE SURGERY
1. For your comfort, please bring a headscarf or hat and a pair of sunglasses to wear after surgery
2. No make-up or lotions on your face prior to surgery
3. If you bleach, tint, color, or perm your hair, then please do so no later than 1 week prior to surgery. It will be at least 6 weeks before you can have this done again
4. Do not cut your hair before surgery, in order for incisions to be covered postoperatively
AFTER SURGERY
1. You may experience some swelling of the face and you may also have bruising on the neck and chest. This is normal and should disappear within 2 weeks
2. Ice compresses to the exposed areas of your face for the first 48 h at home will be helpful to reduce any expected swelling
3. Should you have pain not relieved by your prescribed medications or if you are bleeding through your bandages, do contact the surgeon or the hospital immediately
4. When sleeping, lie on your back with you head at approximately a 45° angle for seven nights after surgery to help minimize any swelling. This can be accomplished with two pillows under your head
5. You may wash your hair 3 days after surgery
6. No alcohol should be taken for 1 week after surgery
7. Do not go out into direct sunlight for 6 weeks after surgery and protect your skin daily with a sunblock factor 30
8. Limit activities such as bending, straining, and lifting. Avoid excessive neck turning movements and heavy physical exertion for the first month. Avoid also any movements that will give you the feeling of pulling or tightness along the incision line. We do not want you to stretch your incisions
9. Postoperatively massage your face with moisturising cream where you are able to. Arnica cream works well
10. You may have a facial after 6 weeks

operative time and minimizes postoperative complications. Towards this aim, a solid knowledge of anatomy is vital as well as an understanding of the aesthetic elements of brow rejuvenation.

47.3.4 Patient Satisfaction and Cost-Effectiveness

In order to guarantee success in one's practice, it is important to achieve patient satisfaction and cost-effectiveness. One must be able to understand the needs of the patient and the downtime they will require, in order to suggest the correct treatment. One must also be able to give the patient an idea of the longevity of a particular procedure.

47.3.5 Surgical and Nonsurgical Treatments of Forehead Rejuvenation

There are various approaches used to raise the eyebrows, ranging from a direct incision, just above the eyebrow, to incisions within the scalp, above the hairline using a coronal incision.

47.3.6 Direct Operations to the Brow

This involves removal of a segment of scalp tissue from above the eyebrow. It does not correct the forehead position nor remove forehead wrinkles and lines; it only corrects the eyebrow position. This type of operation is mostly recommended for the older and frailer patient, or the patient with facial palsy, as it can be done under local anaesthesia. It leaves a small scar which is hidden within natural creases and wrinkles of the eyebrow.

47.3.7 Endoscopic Brow Lift

The endoscopic brow lift has revolutionized forehead rejuvenation and has almost certainly made coronal incisions obsolete. It can be performed under intravenous sedation or general anesthesia. It is performed through four incisions, two on each side of the midline. The first is a longitudinal incision 7–10 cm from midline. The second is a transverse incision in the temporal region. The area is infiltrated with a tumescent solution of saline, lignocaine, and epinephrine. The transverse incision is dissected to the deep temporal fascia and the midline incision is dissected subperiosteally. This is important in order to avoid injury to the superficial branch of the temporal nerve as well as other nerves including the supraorbital and supratrochlear nerves. The endoscope will be able to demonstrate these clearly.

The arcus marginalis and the periosteum must be released in order to allow free movement and elevation of the brow and this is accomplished endoscopically. For this, the author uses the Ramirez dissectors. Fixation can be achieved by three methods: (1) by suturing in two different planes, one superficially and one deep to anchor to the temporal fascia, (2) by screw fixation, or (3) by the use of surgical glue. Each has positive and negative aspects, and the surgeon must decide which method is best in their practice.

Both the eyebrows and the forehead are lifted and this removes the horizontal lines. Surgery is done through incisions in the scalp above the hairline. Incisions can be long (coronal incision), or short Y to V shaped, or short and straight. Usually two or three small incisions are made above the hairline, and a further two small incisions placed a small distance above the ears. A tunnel is made underneath the forehead, to free up all the ligaments holding it down and raise the forehead and eyebrows upward. An absorbable embedded fixation plate is used to secure the new brow-height, or tissue may be excised, in which case fixation is not required.

Forehead and brow lifting is usually done under general anaesthesia, with addition of local anaesthesia to the scalp to reduce bleeding during the surgery. Endoscopic forehead and eyebrow lift is very suitable for patients aged 30–60 years, who have furrows between the eyebrows, eyebrow ptosis, and deep horizontal forehead lines. It gives a good brow and forehead lift, but is a longer operation than the direct or transeyelid/blepharoplasty incision approach.

47.3.8 Risks

When complications arise during an endoscopic forehead lift, which occurs in about 1% of cases, a switch to the open forehead lift method must be performed.

Complications are rare when a forehead lift is performed by a surgeon trained in the technique. However, it is possible for the surgical process to damage the nerves that control eyebrow and forehead movements. Hair loss can also occur along the scar edges in the scalp when an incision is made through the hairline. Moreover, infection and bleeding are possible with any surgical procedure.

Patients who have Endotine implants in their foreheads risk moving their newly adjusted tissues with relatively small movements just after the operation and before complete healing takes place. While the implant absorbs into the body, the Endotine generally does not support the very thick forehead skin and heavy brows often seen in some overweight males [6, 7].

47.4 Variations of Forehead and Brow Lift

If the patient requires upper eyelid blepharoplasty and eyebrow and forehead lift, this can be done simply through a combination of the transeyelid and scalp incisions above the hairline (Fig. 47.5). An endoscope and fixation may not always be required.

47.5 Transpalpebral Corrugator Resection

This operation is done while the patient is under intravenous sedation. The area is infiltrated with lignocaine and adrenaline (1/100,000 concentration). The operation is done through the same upper blepharoplasty incision, with dissection to reach the orbital rim (Fig. 47.6) [8, 9].

47.6 Coronal Incision

This operation was the most commonly performed procedure some years ago; however, due to the advent of endoscopic forehead rejuvenation this procedure is less frequently seen now. The author recommends that every plastic or cosmetic surgeon should see this procedure performed to a patient, or to a cadaver, as it is extremely useful in demonstrating the anatomy of

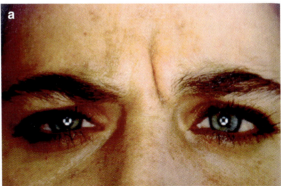
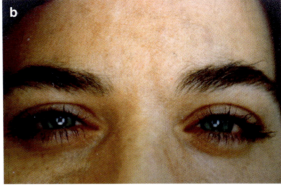

Fig. 47.6 Transpalpebral corrugator resection. (**a**) Before. (**b**) After procedure

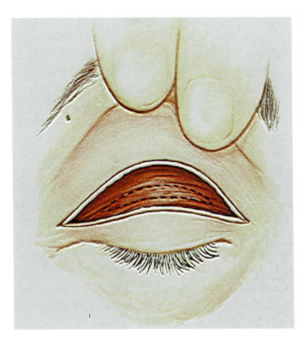

Fig. 47.5 Routine incision for endobrow

the forehead. This procedure is done while the patient is under intravenous sedation; the incision is marked approximately 5 cm behind the hair line extending from one temple to the other, a few centimeters above the ear. Generally it is not necessary to shave the hair; however, techniques like braiding, elastic bands, and hair gel should be used. The area is infiltrated in its entirety with a modified tumescent solution, using lidocaine hydrochloride, 2%, and epinephrine, one in one thousand, as a local anesthetic. The incision is taken down to the subgaleal plane and laterally becomes superficial to the deep temporal fascia to avoid injury to the superficial branch of the facial nerve. The dissection is continued anteriorly and extended supraperiosteally to the superorbital rim. The arcus marginalis and the fibrous bands are released to allow the brow to be elevated. The supraorbital and supratrochlear nerves are carefully dissected and preserved. The corrugator muscle and the procerus are released and resected as extensively as possible to eliminate the frown lines. Fat grafting can be considered to fill the defect caused by surgery. Drains may minimize the postoperative bruising and swelling; however, the author does not tend to use them and results have been excellent. The incision is closed in two layers and normally surgical clips are used after surgery. Antibiotic ointment is placed on the incision. The patient will be allowed to wash their hair 3–4 days after the operation. Slight bruising is expected that can take up to 2–3 weeks to clear and normally instructions for pre and postoperative care are given [10, 11].

47.7 Fat Grafting

Fat grafting has seen renewed interest as research has shown that fat can survive if it is used in small droplets and placed near a good blood supply. In his practice, the author is able to achieve survival between 5 and 7 years. The use of autologous fat graft has been advocated since 1893, when Neuber [12] first published his paper. The success of this technique relies on obtaining the fat using a large bore syringe, thereby not macerating it. The author does not centrifuge the fat. Reinjection is done by using the pearl technique, which has been

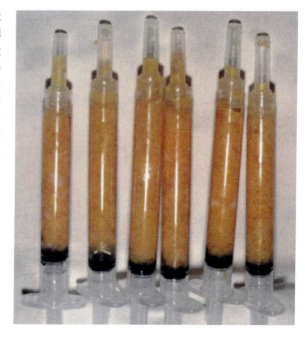

Fig. 47.7 Fat ready for transfer

pioneered by Fischer [13] and yields extremely favorable results. The operation is normally combined with another procedure such as a face-lift, and so it can be done under sedation (Figs 47.7 and 47.8).

The donor site is infiltrated with small volumes of a saline solution that contains one in one thousand adrenaline and 20 units of lignocaine 1%. The fat reinjection site for the brow is usually just underneath the brow and this has an elevating effect and fullness especially in patients who loose fat due to atrophy or aging (Fig. 47.9). Slight absorption is always expected and the patients can have a touch-up on a yearly basis, in which case a fat-bank could be justifiable. In the author's practice in England a fat-bank is not permitted; however, this is a very popular option in Japan, Argentina, and China, among others. It is also possible to inject the frown lines with autologous fat after performing subcision, in order to create a pocket for the insertion of the fat. The major warning is that one or two dramatic cases that resulted in death have been reported due to the fact that the fat was injected by mistake into a vein causing embolization. Patients must be informed about absorption, which can be irregular and which is a rare disadvantage of this operation. In addition, in thin patients it could be difficult to obtain enough graft.

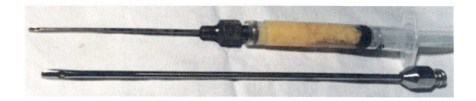

Fig. 47.8 Cannula and syringe for fat extraction by hand

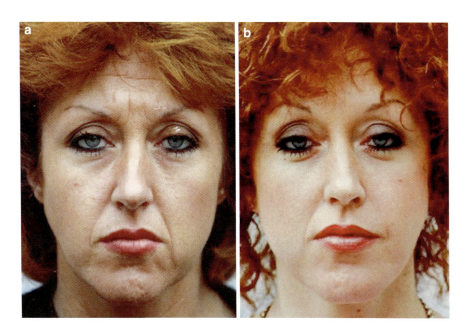

Fig. 47.9 (**a**) Preoperative. (**b**) Postoperative

47.8 Suspension and Suture Techniques

47.8.1 Thread Lift Guide

A thread lift addresses sagging underlying tissues of the cheek and jaw line by threading 4–12 barbed sutures into the skin and deeper soft tissues. The nonabsorbable threads stay within the deep tissues and provide support. A thread lift is often referred to as a minimally invasive surgical procedure. This is a relatively new procedure developed in Russia in 1999 by Sulamanidze [14] who pioneered the technique. The thread lift procedure can use Aptos threads (blue nylon) or clear sutures such as the contour thread lift that contains a series of cogs or microbarbs. Contour lifts may be best for a fair skin tone, since the Aptos threads may appear visible through the skin. In cases of more severe sagging or facial folds and furrows, a traditional face-lift may achieve more dramatic results.

During the procedure local anesthetic is used. A hollow stainless tube with a needle-sharp end is inserted under the skin at specific entry points on the face and through the fat layer under the skin along a designated path (Fig. 47.10). The exit point is then made and the thread is inserted into the tube. The thread is pulled through the other side of the tube, the tube is removed, and the thread stays in place. The threads are positioned, tugged into the desired placement, anchored, cut just at the skin, and then inserted under the surface of the skin. Where the thread ends are inserted into your face, they are taped for a few days to prevent movement. Excessive movement can dislodge the intended placement of the threads, altering the desired thread lift result. For endobrow lifting the thread lift can be adapted to lift the brows using suspension and in this technique the sutures are tied to the temporal fascia.

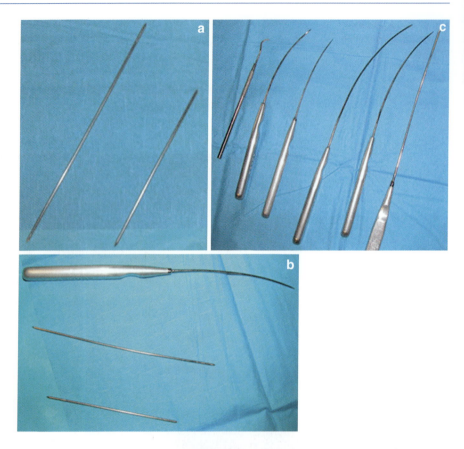

Fig. 47.10 (**a–c**) Mendes needles and serdev needles for threading

47.8.2 Thread Lift Risks

These include bruising, swelling, and tenderness. Additional potential complications of a thread lift are puckering where the barb is pulling, visibility of the blue thread through the skin, and threads poking through the skin. A thread lift, while less invasive than a face-lift, is nonetheless surgery with its inherent risks. The most serious complication is injury to the temporal branch of the facial nerve which can get caught in the treads, and this could be temporary or permanent.

47.9 Botox (Chemodenervation with Botulinum Toxin)

Botulinum toxin, the most lethal poison known to mankind has provided hope and relief to countless victims with certain neurological conditions (Fig. 47.11). More recently, its application for cosmetic use has been established. In particular, it is of prime importance in forehead rejuvenation. It is known to work on

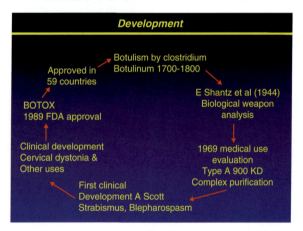

Fig. 47.11 Development of Botox

the neuromuscular junction through a blocking process (Fig. 47.12).

In forehead rejuvenation, the basic applications work well to improve the following areas:

- Horizontal forehead lines (Figs. 47.13 and 47.14)
- Glabellar frown lines (Fig. 47.15)
- The results of lateral and medial brow lifts
- Crow's feet (Fig. 47.16)

Fig. 47.12 Mechanism of action of botulinum toxin. (**a**) Binding. (**b**) Internalization. (**c**) Blockade. (**d**) Reinnervation

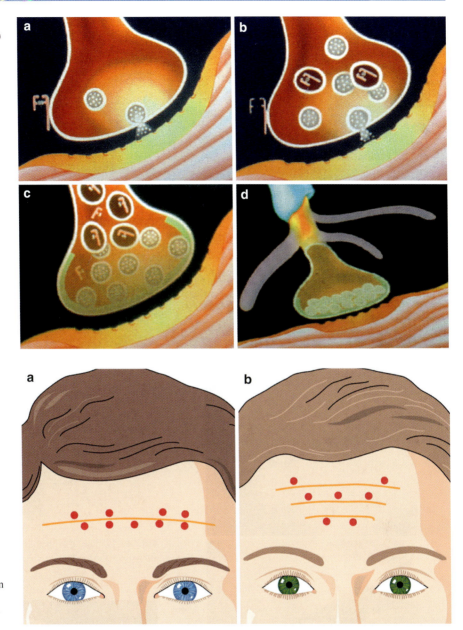

Fig. 47.13 Sites of injection of Botox for (**a**) horizontal and (**b**) multiple frown lines

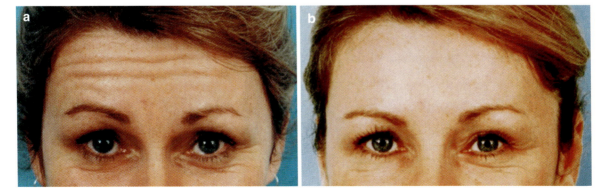

Fig. 47.14 Partial elimination of frontalis muscle by Botox. (**a**) Before treatment. (**b**) After treatment

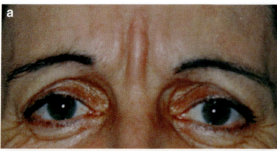
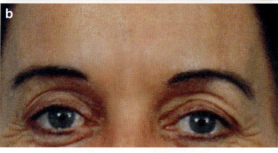

Fig. 47.15 Good result by injecting the corrugator and procerus for glabellar lines. (**a**) Before treatment. (**b**) After treatment

Table 47.2 Botox vial dilutions

BOTOX®: Vial Dilutions		
Saline diluents volume	U/mL	U/0.1 mL
1.0 mL	100.0	10.0
1.5 mL	66.7	6.7
2.0 mL	50.0	5.0
2.5 mL	40.0	4.0
3.0 mL	33.3	3.3

47.10 Endobrow

A relatively new technique to elevate the brow through a blepharoplasty incision using absorbable screws (LactoSorb®) has been described (Figs. 47.17–47.19). The procedure is relatively easy to learn but requires a steep learning curve to perfect.

Through the blepharoplasty incision, one must elevate the brow and dissect to the periosteum. The

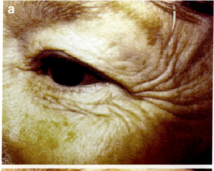
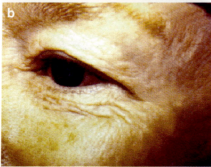

Fig. 47.16 Botox injection for crow's feet. (**a**) Before treatment. (**b**) After treatment

The dilution used by the author is 1 ml of saline to 50 units of Botox. While this works well, dilutions vary and many practitioners prefer different dilutions (Table 47.2).

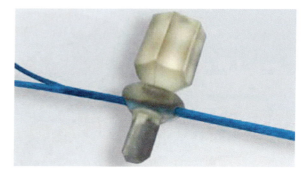

Fig. 47.17 The dissolvable screw and thread (LactoSorb Endobrow Push screw)

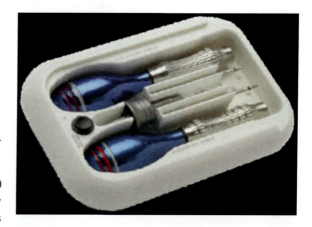

Fig. 47.18 915–3007 LactoSorb® Hex Head Driver

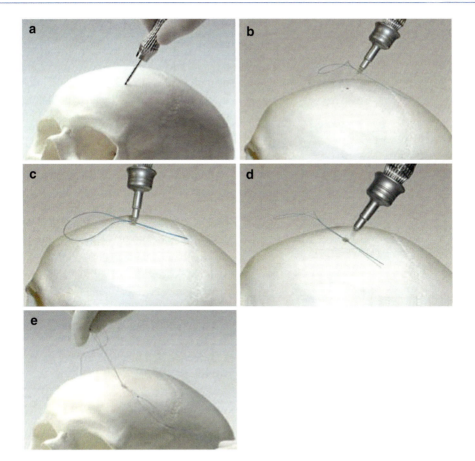

Fig. 47.19 (a) Initial screw placement should be determined by the surgeon. Drill a pilot hole using the 1.8 mm drill bit at the desired location for brow suspension. No tapping is required. (b) Load the Endobrow Push screw with suture passer onto the Hex Head Driver. If desired, the screw may be threaded with the suture at this step. (c) Position the screw into the pilot hole (perpendicular to the bone) and push straight down until the screw is fully seated. No twisting is required during insertion. (d) Disengage the hex head from the screw after insertion by gently turning the Hex Head Driver clockwise. (e) Suture is easily passed through the screw head utilizing the suture passer (if screw is not already threaded with suture) and is fixed to both the periosteal tissue and the LactoSorb®

periosteum must be released from the bone, in addition to the arcus marginalis in a cephald direction, to allow the brow to be elevated. Two to three positions for the screws must be marked and positioned. It is vital to avoid injuring the temporal branch of the facial nerve. It is important to use the drill which has shoulders to prevent deeper penetration.

The screw must be inserted fully loaded with the stitch attached. The stitch must be tied at the chosen level and height. The results will be seen immediately on the operating table. The stitch will be secure in the periosteum and surrounding muscle, but one must be careful not to catch the tissues during closure. A standard closure is used for the blepharoplasty incision.

The LactoSorb® Endobrow screw combines the push screw technology with a proven resorbable material. This allows for predictable resorption, requiring only two instruments for insertion. LactoSorb® Endobrow push screws are low in profile and resorb within 1 year. Designed specifically for the brow lift, the unique screw design features an eyelet in the screw head to allow insertion of the suture. The LactoSorb® Endobrow push screw has in many cases been found to afford quicker and easier brow lifting [15–18]. Results are excellent (Figs. 47.20 and 47.21)

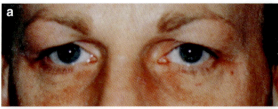
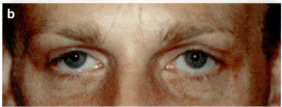

Fig. 47.20 (**a**) Preoperative. (**b**) Postoperative following lateral brow elevation

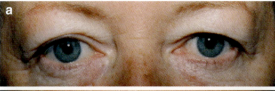
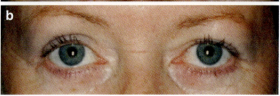

Fig. 47.21 (**a**) Preoperative. (**b**) Postoperative after endobrow lift

47.10.1 Screw Placement

1. Initial screw placement should be determined by the surgeon. Drill a pilot hole using the 1.8 mm drill bit at the desired location for brow suspension. No tapping is required.
2. Load the Endobrow Push screw with suture passer onto the Hex Head Driver. If desired, the screw may be threaded with the suture at this step.
3. Position the screw into the pilot hole (perpendicular to the bone) and push straight down until the screw is fully seated. No twisting is required during insertion.
4. Disengage the hex head from the screw after insertion by gently turning the Hex Head Driver clockwise.
5. Suture is easily passed through the screw head utilizing the suture passer (if screw is not already threaded with suture) and is fixed to both the periosteal tissue and the LactoSorb® (Fig. 47.19).

47.10.2 Possible Complications

All surgery carries some uncertainty and risk. Complications are rare and usually minor when a forehead lift is performed by an experienced cosmetic surgeon. Yet, the possibility of complications must be considered.

1. Numbness of the forehead, just beyond the incision line can occur. It is usually temporary, but on rare occasions, may be permanent in some patients.
2. Asymmetry of the brows may occur which may be due to postoperative swelling or premature dissolving of the sutures involved in the surgery. This is usually amenable to correction by the surgeon.
3. In rare cases, the nerves that control eyebrow movement may be injured on one or both sides, resulting in a loss of ability to raise the eyebrows or wrinkle the forehead. Additional surgery may be required to correct the problem.
4. Infection and bleeding are very rare, but are possibilities [19, 20].

References

1. Knize DM. Anatomic concepts for brow lift procedures. Plast Reconstr Surg. 2009;124(6):2118–26.
2. Codner MA, Kikkawa DO, Korn BS, Pacella SJ. Blepharoplasty and brow lift. Plast Reconstr Surg. 2010; 126(1): 1e–17e.
3. Goldstein Scott M, Katowitz JA. The male eyebrow: a topographic anatomic analysis. Ophthal Plast Reconstr Surg. 2005;21(4):285–91.
4. Freund RM, Nolan III WB. Correlation between brow lift outcomes and aesthetic ideals for eyebrow height and shape in females. Plast Reconstr Surg. 1996;97(7):1343–8.
5. Ramirez OM. Why I prefer the endoscopic forehead lift. Plast Reconstr Surg. 1997;100(4):1033–9.
6. Punthakee X, Mashkevich G, Keller GS. Endoscopic forehead and brow-lift. Facial Plast Surg. 2010;26(3):239–51.
7. Keller GS, Mashkevich G. Endoscopic forehead and brow lift. Facial Plast Surg. 2009;25(4):222–33.
8. Cintra HP, Basile FV. Transpalpebral brow lifting. Clin Plast Surg. 2008;35(3):381–92.
9. Langsdon PR, Metzinger SE, Glickstein JS, Armstrong DL. Transblepharoplasty brow suspension: an expanded role. Ann Plast Surg. 2008;60(1):2–5.
10. Cilento BW, Johnson Jr CM. The case for open forehead rejuvenation: a review of 1004 procedures. Arch Facial Plast Surg. 2009;11(1):13–7.
11. Huijing MA, van der Lei B. Gull wing midforehead lift: when a poor man's forehead lift becomes the treatment of choice for brow ptosis. Ann Plast Surg. 2010;64(6): 713–7.
12. Neuber F. Fettransplantation. Chir Kongr Verhandl Dtsch Gesellsch Chir. 1893;22:66.

13. Fischer G. Fat transfer with rice grain-size fat parcels. In: Shiffman MA, editor. Autologous fat trans-plantation. New York: Marcel Dekker; 2001. p. 55–63.
14. Sulamanidze MA, Shiffman MA, Paikidze TG, Sulamanidze GM, Gavasheli LG. Facial lifting with Aptos threads. Int J Cosmet Surg Aesthetic Dermatol. 2001;3(4):275–81.
15. Hönig JF, Frank MH, Knutti D, de La Fuente A. Video endoscopic-assisted brow lift: comparison of the eyebrow position after Endotine tissue fixation versus suture fixation. J Craniofac Surg. 2008;19(4):1140–7.
16. Byrne PJ. Efficacy and safety of endotine fixation device in endoscopic brow-lift. Arch Facial Plast Surg. 2007;9(3): 212–4.
17. Foustanos A. Suture fixation technique for endoscopic brow lift. Semin Plast Surg. 2008;22(1):43–9.
18. Berkowitz RL, Apfelberg DB. Preliminary evaluation of a fast-absorbing multipoint fixation device. Aesthetic Surg J. 2008;28(5):584–8.
19. Kim BP, Goode RL, Newman JP. Brow elevation ratio: a new method of brow analysis. Arch Facial Plast Surg. 2009;11(1):34–9.
20. del Campo AF. Update on minimally invasive face lift technique. Aesthetic Surg J. 2008;28(1):51–61.

Minimally Invasive Midface Lift

48

Enrique Andrade

48.1 Introduction

Aesthetic facial rejuvenation has gained widespread acceptance among the general public. As more younger patients have requested facial invigoration, surgeons have rushed to find improved techniques amended in the sense of providing longer lasting, natural-appearing results with decreasing perioperative and postoperative sequels.

The youthful midface is described as triangular shape with high cheeks, smoothness toward the midface, and minimal nasolabial folds. The aged midface is represented by a more rectangular shape due to sagging of not only the skin but also the malar fat pad (cheek).

As the malar fat pad descends inward and downward against the nasolabial line, at least four signs of midface aging occur. These include: the full nasolabial fold, hollowness to the midface, tear-trough hollow at the lower lid–cheek interface, and a slight prominence of the cheek profile.

48.2 Surgical Goals

Meloplication goals are to elevate volumetrically the malar fat pad, thereby recreating a more youthful triangular midface shape, lessening the fullness lateral to the nasolabial line, filling the hollow from the midface, and smoothing out the infraorbital areas in a lesser degree. A secondary benefit can be a slightly improved reduction of the fullness contour at the jowl and sagging of the labial–mandibular fold above the mandibular margin. This procedure may be used as a "closed" technique to correct an isolated malar fat pad ptosis in cases without excess of the facial skin. Meloplication may also be incorporated in an "open" rhytidoplasty, as one of the maneuvers to correct the midface ptosis, as in the lower lid blepharoplasty, a transcutaneous approach to performing a vertical fat pad elevation.

48.3 Indications and Contraindications

The ideal candidate for "closed" meloplication is a 35–45 year-old patient with early midface laxity involving primarily ptosis of the malar fat pad. Such a patient has exhibited an incipient facial skin excess, jowls, labial mandibular folds, or platysmal bands.

48.4 Surgical Technique

48.4.1 Preoperative Markings

"Closed" meloplication technique was introduced in 2000 by using two permanent sutures, each fixed by Gore-Tex anchor grafts. The fan-shaped malar fat pad and the anterior ramus of the temporal branch of the facial nerve are marked on the upright patient. The classical course of the anterior ramus of the temporal nerve is drawn to extend from 0.5 cm inferior to the antihelix-tragus landmark toward 1.5 cm superolateral

E. Andrade
Plaza Corporativa Zapopan, Blvd. Puerta de Hierro
5150 suite 404-B, Zapopan, Jalisco CP 45116, Mexico
e-mail: eandrade99@hotmail.com

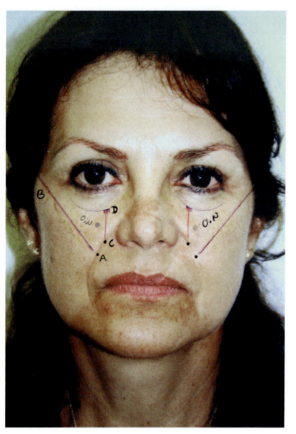

Fig. 48.1 Two point incisions on the nasolabial fold on dots A and C. One 1–1.5 cm incision is done behind B, 1 cm behind the hair line (temporal zone incision). Letter D shows the point of attachment of the vertical suture, in the orbital rim periosteum by an external incision for blepharoplasty

and from C-D – these will be the pathways for suspension sutures of one of the two lifting vectors.

48.4.2 Anesthesia

The "closed" meloplication suspensions may be done under local anesthesia. A 5–10 ml buffered 1% Xylocaine with 1:400,000 epinephrine solution is injected into the subcutaneous layer of the midface, extending from the nasolabial fold to the temporal region and following the line from A-B. Selective nerve blocks from the zygomatic–facial, zygomatic–temporal, and infraorbital nerves with 0.5% Marcaine (1:200,000 epinephrine) complete the anesthetic requirement.

48.4.3 Sutures and Gore-Tex Suspension System

Figure 48.2 shows the sutures and suspension system: 3–0 Ethibond at the main suture and 4–0 Vicryl for the suture guide. Both suture endings are tied together at 10 cm. Keith needles. Two small pieces of Gore-Tex 4×4 mm are used. One is inserted in the 3–0 Ethibond tied in the Keith needle. The other Gore-Tex is used to anchor the sutures up to the temporalis fascia. For vertical vector 6 cm Keith needles are preferred because of a minor distance. The 4–0 Vicryl is used to guide and seesaw the tissue to avoid forming a dimple at the place the Gore-Tex is anchored, in the soft tissues at the nasolabial fold.

Four sets of sutures and needles are used if the two vectors are placed, two sets per side.

48.4.4 Elevation of the Temporalis Vector A-B

The surgical procedure begins first by incising 1–1.5 cm (Fig. 48.3) within the temporal hairline using a #15 blade at an angle through the 1 cm. temporal marking. A small pocket is created with Iris scissors between the temporoparietal fascia and the deep temporal fascia. Then, the dot incisions A-C on the nasolabial fold, are done using the tip of an 11 blade, making it a little deep and wide with the tip of an iris scissors.

to the tail of the eyebrow; however, determination pathway of the anterior branch of the temporal nerve to bony landmarks is variable.

As shown in Fig. 48.1, dot C is marked lateral to the nasal alae, on the nasolabial fold. Dot A is marked 1 cm inferior to dot C. Line B passes 1 cm lateral to the lateral orbital cantus, going behind into the hair line 1 or 2 cm. Incisions A and C are performed using an 11 blade knife tip. Incision B is done and dissected toward the temporalis fascia. Incision D is done as an external blepharoplasty in the traditional way; a mark is drawn over the infraorbital nerve. Infraorbital rim is located and dissected leaving the periosteum intact. Once the midpart between the internal cantus and the infraorbital nerve is set, place dot D here.

Two vectors are marked, A-B and C-D, the Temporal Vector and the Vertical Vector. Draw lines from A-B

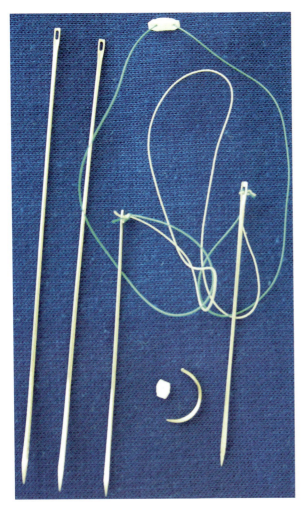

Fig. 48.2 Keith needles 10 and 6 cm, 3–0 Ethibond, 4–0 Vicryl, Gore-Tex 4×4 mm, and eyed ½ circle French needle

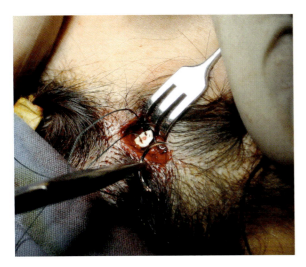

Fig. 48.3 Temporal incision with anchoring the Gore-Tex to deep temporalis fascia

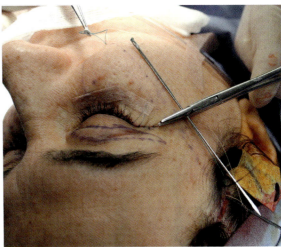

Fig. 48.4 Pathway from nasolabial fold to temporal incision

The first Keith needle is introduced into dot incision A, deeply touching the bone, then lifted a few millimeters, and then oriented laterally following the line toward the temporal incision. The subcutaneous tissue is pinched along the safe pathway upward along the temporal incision B. This maneuver allows the needle to remain safe until is retrieved at the temporalis pocket (Fig. 48.4).

The other Keith needle is passed through the same incision in a similar way but slightly inferior to the previous one and retrieved at the temporal pocket tract.

Working with the 4–0 Vicryl, each limb of the suture is grasped and see-sawed through the soft tissue until the dimpling at the nasolabial fold is eliminated. The Vicryl suture is then removed. The permanent 3–0 Ethibond suture is pulled and the anchor Gore-Tex is passed into the incision, so that the fat malar pad can be elevated; a mosquito clamp secures the suture end.

48.4.5 Anchoring the Suture to the Deep Temporalis Fascia

An eyed ½ circle French needle is used, securing each end of the suture, and passed through the previously pinched Gore-Tex 5×5 mm. A sliding knot elevates the nasolabial fold 3–5 mm and it is fixed with several knots. The anchor Gore-Tex is covered with several square knots with an reabsorbable suture. The closure of the incision is done with 4–0 Prolene, and the dots at the nasolabial fold with 6–0 Prolene (Fig. 48.3).

48.4.6 Elevation of the Vertical Vector C-D

This vector is done through a subciliary incision for a transcutaneous external blepharoplasty. Dissection is performed over the orbital septum to the orbital rim.

The periosteum is located and blunt dissected at the rim region between the medial cantus and the pupillary line, and a 4–5 mm curved cut is done. A small flap is elevated with a small sharp dissector. The Keith needle sutures system is set in place.

Starting in the C dot incision, as in the temporal vector, Keith needles are directed to the D flap in the orbital rim. The dimple is see-sawed using the 4–0 Vicryl suture and removed. The 3–0 Ethibond suture is pulled, also the Gore-Tex anchored in the soft tissues of the malar fold. The Ethibond is secured with eyed ½ circle French needles in each limb, passed through the 4 mm Gore-Tex anchor and secured to the periosteum flap (Fig. 48.5), first with a sliding knot pulling the cheek 3–4 mm, and three more knots. The knots are covered with soft tissue and reabsorbable 5–0 Vicryl.

Close the incisions as in the blepharoplasty technique and the dot incision with 6–0 Prolene.

48.5 Complications

There are almost no complications with these techniques. The pathways are safe and no permanent nerve lesions have been seen. Early transitory asymmetry that resolved by itself was observed in the first

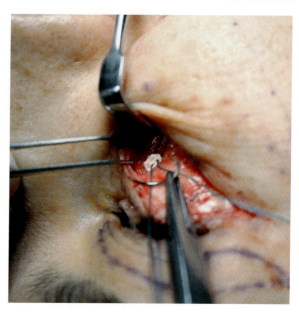

Fig. 48.5 Orbital rim, anchoring Gore-Tex to periosteal flap

4–6 weeks and one spontaneous weakness of the zygomaticus major muscle.

Antibiotics are given to avoid Gore-Tex infection.

48.6 Conclusions

Repositioning of the cheek corrects most of the midface ptosis (Figs. 48.6 and 48.7). The closed procedure is minimally invasive and the temporal vector assures 4–6 mm of elevation by the time the vertical vector resolves or improves the nasojugal groove. Most of these patients combine meloplication with blepharoplasty or other procedures.

The temporal vector is versatile and can be as open technique during the rhytidectomy. Long-lasting results are seen after 3–5 years. More outcome studies are required for further evaluation.

Fig. 48.6 (**a**) Before minimally invasive midface lift and lower blepharoplasty. (**b**) Six months after close temporal vector and vertical vector, note improvement of nasolabial fold and upper position of the cheek

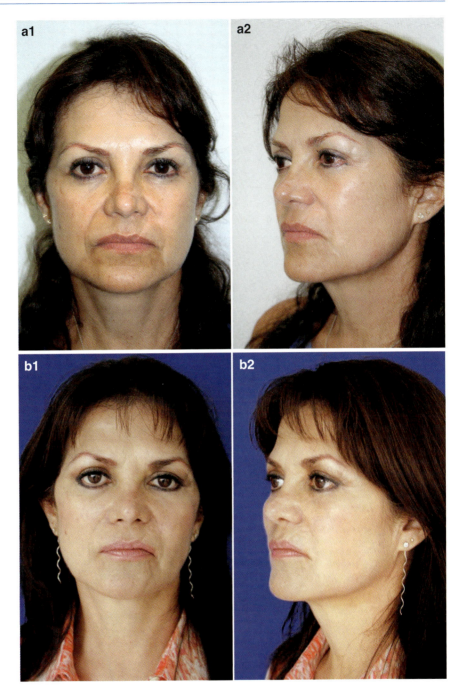

Fig. 48.7 (**a**) Before rhinoplasty, blepharoplasty, and minimally invasive midface lift. (**b**) After 8 months note improvement of the nasolabial folds, cheek elevation, and smoothness of the infraorbital region

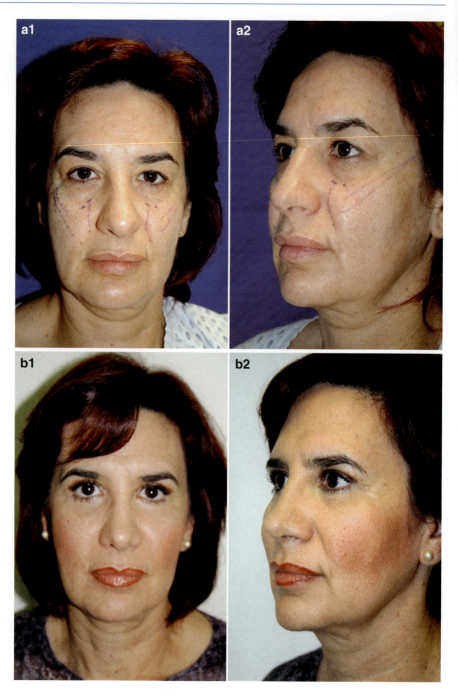

Recommended Reading

Anderson RD, Lo MW. Endoscopic malar/midface suspension procedure. Plast Reconstr Surg. 1998;102(6):2196–208.

Freeman MS. Endoscopic techniques for rejuvenation of the mid face. Facial Plast Surg Clin North Am. 2005;13(1):141–55.

Gordon H. Sasaki MD. TACS meloplication of the malar fat by percutaneous cable sutures technique for midface rejovenation. Presented at new horizons symposium incosmetic surgery, La jolla, California, January 21, 2000.

Gunter JP, Hackney FL. A simplified transblepharoplasty subperiosteal cheek lift. Plast Reconstr Surg. 1999;103(7):2029–35.

Larrabee WF, Makielski KH. Superficial musculoaponeurotic system. In: Larrabee WF, Makielski KH, editors. Surgical anatomy of the face. New York: Raven; 1993.

Owsley JQ. Lifting the malar fat pad for correction of prominent nasolabial folds. Plast Reconstr Surg. 1993;91(3):463–74.

Ramirez OM. Endoscopic full face lift. Aesthetic Plast Surg. 1994;18(4):363–71.

Upper Eyelid Blepharoplasty

49

Amir M. Karam and Samuel M. Lam

49.1 Introduction

Aging of the upper periorbital region is often one of the first signs of aging noted by patients. The pathogenesis of upper lid aging is a process involving both soft tissue excess and volume loss. The goal of any facial rejuvenation procedure is to restore the individual's youthful appearance – not to create morphologic change that is novel. Hence, successful rejuvenation of this region requires a thorough understanding of the aging process as well as how this process has affected the individual patient. Overall, there has been a trend away from aggressive removal of skin, muscle, and fat which had resulted in hollowing and skeletonization of the upper lid complex. Hollowing of the upper eyelid complex was seen in the postoperative period, which often left the patients looking older or simply "different." The modern approach is to perform conservative excisional blepharoplasty targeted primarily at the excess upper eyelid skin coupled with some level of volume augmentation of the lateral eyebrow and infrabrow region. This translates to recreation of the youthful and healthier-appearing upper eyelid region, which can be generally defined by a fullness of the soft-tissues without obvious skin excess. In this chapter, we evaluate the periorbital aging process and how upper eyelid blepharoplasty can be used in addition to other treatments to restore the youthful structure of this area.

49.2 Periorbital Aging

The youthful upper eyelid has a minimal degree of eyelid skin excess [1]. The superior orbital rim and infrabrow region appears soft as a smooth layer of subcutaneous and submuscular fat exists over the contour of the bony orbital rim. The lateral aspect of the eyelid should be free of lateral hooding. The supratarsal crease should be clearly visible with a corresponding degree of lid show inferior to the crease. The degree of eyelid show varies even in youth. It varies most among Asian patients. There is no "norm" to measure the degree of eyelid show. With age, dermatochalasis gives way to skin redundancy which extends down below the supratarsal crease and shortening the preexisting eyelid show. As the volume of the peribrow region diminishes there is a descent of the lateral brow further contributing to lateral hooding. The infrabrow volume loss results in skeletalization of the superior orbital rim. In certain cases, there may be mild prolapse of the medial fat pad; however, this is often unmasked as a result of the regional volume loss.

49.3 Anatomic Considerations

In no other area of facial aesthetic surgery is such a fragile balance struck between form and function as that in eyelid modification. Owing to the delicate

A.M. Karam (✉)
Carmel Valley Facial Plastic Surgery, 4765 Carmel Mountain Road, Suite 201, San Diego, CA 92130, USA
e-mail: md@drkaram.com

S.M. Lam
Willow Bend Wellness Center, Lam Facial Plastic Surgery Center & Hair Restoration Institute, 6101 Chapel Hill Boulevard, Suite 101, Plano, TX 75093, USA
e-mail: drlam@lamfacialplastics.com

nature of eyelid structural composition and the vital role the eyelids serve in protecting the visual system, iatrogenic alterations in eyelid anatomy must be made with care, precision, and thoughtful consideration of existing soft tissue structures. A brief anatomic review is necessary to highlight some of these salient points.

49.4 Musculature

Directly under the thin upper eyelid skin lays the orbicularis oculi muscle [2]. It is grossly defined as a relatively large, flat, elliptical muscle that encircles both the upper and lower eyelid. It covers the orbit but extends into the temple and eyebrow in the superior half and into the upper cheek on the lower half. In the upper eyelid it is comprised of the orbital and palpebral portions. The orbital portion is darker and thicker than the palpebral segments. Many fibers insert into the skin and subcutaneous tissues of the eyebrow, which in the lateral portion forms the depressor supercilii. This segment is partly responsible for pulling down the lateral brow and is often the target of neurotoxin injection. The thin palpebral portion of the muscle lies directly over the upper eyelids and is divided into the preseptal and pretarsal segments [2–4]. The transverse facial, supratrochlear, and supraorbital vessels supply the muscle. The innervation is derived from the temporal, zygomatic, and buccal branches of the facial nerve.

The main function of the orbicularis is to serve as the sphincter of the upper and lower eyelids. The palpebral portion acts involuntarily to close the eyelids or reflexively to blink. The orbital portion is under voluntary control. When the orbital portion of the muscle contracts, it draws the skin of the cheeks and temple together resulting in crow's feet and eyelid wrinkle formation. Neurotoxin is used to relax the contraction of the lateral portion of the orbital orbicularis to minimize crow's feet formation.

49.5 Orbital Septum

Directly under the palpebral portion of orbicularis oculi muscle lays the orbital septum. This is a continuation of the periosteum of the orbit (periorbital) and skull which extends over the eyelid. It is subdivided into an upper and lower portion. In the upper portion (above the tarsus), it divides the muscular compartment from the orbital fat compartment. The inferior portion fuses with the anterior part of the tarsus [3]. The insertion with the levator aponeurosis varies with ethnicity. In Asians, it inserts around 3 mm from the base of the eyelid margin while in westerners, it attaches higher around 8–10 mm, thus accounting for a higher eyelid crease.

49.6 Levator Palpebrae Superioris

Directly beneath the superior portion is the aponeurosis of the levator palpebrae superioris muscle. This is the main muscle responsible for the eyelid opening. It is powered by CN III. In addition, Mueller's muscle which is deep to the tarsus is a smooth muscle responsible for 3–4 mm of eyelid opening. Beneath the orbital septum are the orbital fat compartments. Unlike in the lower eyelids, the upper fat compartments consist of only the medial and central compartments. In occasional cases, the medial fat pad may prolapse requiring surgical extraction. Removal of the central fat pads is rarely required, as it may often create an iatrogenic hollowing years later (A-frame deformity).

Beneath the inferior portion of the septum, lies the tarsal plate. In the upper eyelids, it typically measures 8–12 mm, unlike 4–7 mm in the lower eyelid. Beneath the septum about the tarsus lies the preaponeurotic fat, which when removed or retracted identifies the aponeurosis. The aponeurosis of the levator palpebrae superioris muscle attaches to the anterior portion of the tarsus, forming the superior palpebral fold. Weakening or dehiscence of the attachment results in eyelid ptosis.

49.7 Orbital Fat

Contained behind the orbital septum and within the orbital cavity, the orbital fat has been classically segmented into two discrete pockets (central and medial). Unlike the lower eyelid, a lateral fat pad does not exist [2–4]. Of these, the medial fat pad is more commonly seen to have mild prolapse. Similar to the lower eyelid, the medial pad has characteristic differences from its other counterparts, including a lighter color, a more fibrous and compact lobular pattern, and a frequent association with a sizable blood vessel near its medial aspect. The orbital fat can be considered an adynamic structure because its volume is not related to body habitus, and once removed it is not thought to regenerate.

49.8 Preoperative Evaluation

Patient analysis is directed to understanding the patient's desires and expectation, the etiology of the problem at hand, and development of the optimal treatment plan for the patient's unique needs. The preoperative assessment of the anatomical characteristics must be directed at presence of:

1. Dermatochalasis or blepharochalasis (younger patients)
2. Volume status of the superior orbital rim and infrabrow region
3. Pseudoherniation of medial orbital fat
4. Glabellar lines and wrinkles

The treatment plan needs to include treatment of each of these potential anatomic issues.

In addition, a systematic and thorough preoperative assessment of blepharoplasty candidates is essential to minimize potential postoperative complications. Patients need to be specifically questioned about the history of dry-eye syndrome, hypertension, smoking, visual problems, ocular disorders (i.e., glaucoma), bleeding disorders, recent use of NSAIDS, aspirin, and other anticlotting medications. Appropriate workup is required depending on the patient's history.

49.9 Ocular Assessment

Examination of the eyes should begin with an overall inspection. The eyelid should be assessed for symmetry (by noting palpebral fissure height and length), position of the upper eyelid margin with respect to the superior limbus, presence of eyelid ptosis, and lagophthalmus.

As a minimum, baseline ocular assessment should document visual acuity (i.e., best corrected vision if glasses or contact lenses are worn), extraocular movements, gross visual fields by confrontation, corneal reflexes, the presence of Bell's phenomenon, and lagophthalmus. If there is any question of dry-eye syndrome [5–7], a conservative approach must be taken and postoperative lubricating drops and ointment must be used as directed. In severe cases, the patient should be evaluated with Schirmer testing [8] (to quantify tear output) and tear film break-up times (to assess stability of precorneal tear film). Patients who demonstrate abnormalities in either or both of these tests or who have past or anatomic evidence that would predispose them to dry-eye complications should be thoroughly evaluated by an ophthalmologist preoperatively.

49.10 Operative Procedure

Upper eyelid blepharoplasty is an operation which is commonly performed to rejuvenate the upper eyelid region. Today, conservatism is favored and the surgical target is primarily excess eyelid skin. The underlying orbicularis oculi muscle and orbital fat are preserved in the vast majority of cases.

49.11 Upper Eyelid Blepharoplasty Approach

The ideal candidate is a patient of any age that exibits redunent upper eyelid skin resulting in a reduction of the individuals aesthetic potential. In other words, is there enough skin excess that is negatively affecting the individuals appearance? If so, the patient may be considered a candidate for surgical excision of this skin excess. Younger patients affected by familial blepharochalasis often benefit from upper blepharoplasty in their 30s or 40s. Whereas the typical "aging face" patient may benefit from surgical excision in their 40s and beyond.

49.12 Preparation

While sitting upright, the patient is asked to look forward and to open and close their eyes. This helps to define the superior palpebral fold (or crease) which when present should be marked. This line represents the inferior border of the skin excision. Placing the incision into the natural crease helps ensure that the incision will fall into the natural crease postoperatively minimizing the potential of "looking different" as well as optimizing scar placement. This inferior limb is extended slightly past the lateral canthus depending on the degree of lateral hooding present (Fig. 49.1). The more hooding, the longer the extension, so make certain to include the hooding into the excision. A crow's feet wrinkle is chosen and the line is extended superiorly at an angle toward the lateral brow. The patient is then asked to close their eyes. With a nontoothed forceps the excess skin is pinched and marked (Fig. 49.2). Care is taken to avoid eyelid opening while pinching. This is essential in preventing postoperative lagophthalmus.

One percent lidocaine (Xylocaine) with 1:100,000 epinephrine to which is added a 1:10 dilution of sodium bicarbonate is then injected into the subcutaneous plane using a 30-gauge needle. Experience has demonstrated that this mixture affords analgesic effect while minimizing the sting of initial infiltration through alkalinization of the local agent. Care is taken to avoid injection into the underlying muscle. Typically 1–1.5 ml is sufficient. After waiting a full 10 min for vasoconstriction to occur, the outline of the incision is made using a 15 blade scalpel. Next, the skin is elevated off the underlying muscle using a scalpel. Hemostasis is then obtained using bipolar coagulation.

In cases in which a prominent medial fat pad is present, the skin over the medial aspect of the incision is retracted using a narrow double prong skin hook and the orbicularis is incised using scissors and the septum is penetrated. The medial fat pad which is lighter in color is exposed and expressed through the septal incision (Fig. 49.3). A fine-toothed hemostat is used to clamp the fat pad at its base. Prior to sharply excising the fat, bipolar is used to coagulate the fat above the clamp. Care is taken to remain conservative in order avoid postoperative hollowing. The incision is then carefully reapproximated using a running 6–0 Prolene suture; however, a variety of skin sutures and techniques can also be used. The key to a fine scar outcome is excellent approximation and limited wound tension (Figs. 49.4 and 49.5). Both eyes should then be irrigated with sodium chloride (Ophthalmic Balanced Salt Solution).

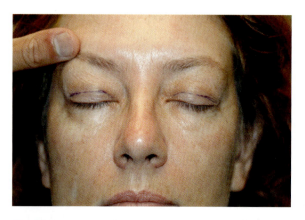

Fig. 49.1 Surgical markings along the supratarsal crease with an extension into a crow's feet wrinkle to include lateral hooding

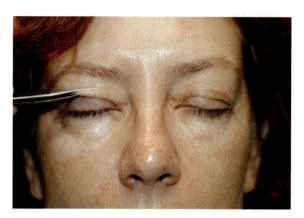

Fig. 49.2 Skin excess following pinching of the skin while the eyes are closed. If too much skin is pinched, then the eyes will open. This is an indication that too much skin excision is marked and the patient may be at risk for postoperative lagophthalmus

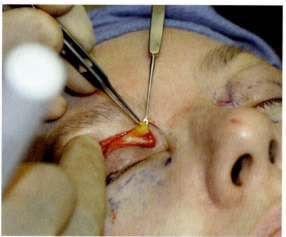

Fig. 49.3 The medial fat pad which is lighter in color is exposed and expressed through the septal incision. A fine-toothed hemostat is used to clamp the fat pad at its base prior to cauterization

Fig. 49.4 (*Left*) Preoperative patient. (*Right*) Five weeks postoperative following upper eyelid blepharoplasty in addition to fat augmentation and lower eyelid blepharoplasty

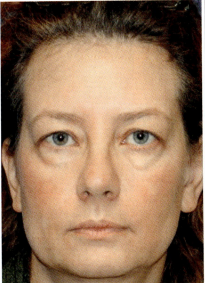
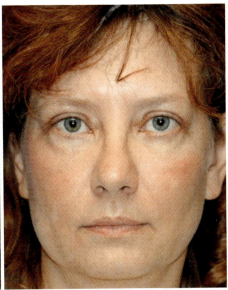

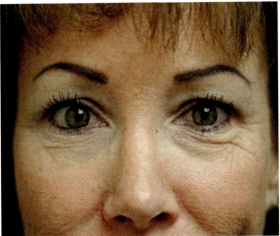
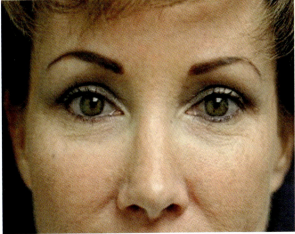

Fig. 49.5 (*Left*) Preoperative patient. (*Right*) Postoperative following upper eyelid blepharoplasty alone

49.13 Postoperative Care

Immediately after surgery, the patient is kept quiet with head elevated at least 45°. Cold compresses are placed on both eyes and changed every 20 min. The patient is observed closely for at least an hour for any signs of bleeding complications. The patient is given strict instructions to limit physical activity for the next week. The patient who is diligent about the cold compresses and head elevation during the first 48 h will experience substantially less swelling.

49.14 Complementary Treatments

49.14.1 Restoration of Infrabrow and Lateral Brow Volume

Restoration of volume in the infrabrow and lateral brow areas must be addressed in the appropriate candidate. Two reliable methods exist. These include injectable hyaluronic acid fillers and autologous microfat grafting.

49.14.2 Injectable Fillers

Recent trends in nonsurgical treatment of facial aging have resulted in the creative application of the widely available injectable fillers in the periorbital area. Specifically, the use of nonanimal, stabilized, hyaluronic acid (NASHA) fillers have enabled the treatment of early signs of aging in the periorbital complex.

Filling infrabrow hollows can be preformed in the office setting with topical and/or local anesthesia. Following infiltration of a small amount of local anesthesia containing 1% lidocaine with 1:100,000, epinephrine can be injected directly into the treatment areas for vasoconstriction. Alternatively, ice packs may be applied before and after injection to decrease bruising. The filler is injected in a retrograde linear threading fashion in the submuscular plane.

The material should be injected only during retraction of the needle to prevent vessel embolization. Layered injections are suggested. These injections should be attempted only after one has gained sufficient experience injecting in more forgiving locations. Gentle massage should be preformed after every few injections to disperse small isolated collections of material that may become palpable or visible as edema subsides. Risks specific to this treatment include bruising, palpable subcutaneous bumps, fluid collection in the injected area, and very remote risk of retinal embolus.

49.14.3 Structural Fat Grafting of the Infrabrow Region

Autologous fat grafting along the superior orbital region is used to restore volume loss along the skeletonized superior bony rim and infrabrow hollows. This helps restore the natural fullness and smooth convexity of the youthful eye. The fat is typically harvested from the abdomen or thighs using a low-pressure liposuction technique. Then the fat is prepared by separating the serum and blood using a centrifuge. Once purified adipose tissue is isolated, it is injected using a microcannula along the superior orbital rim using a microinjection technique (Fig. 49.6). The most common complication of this technique in this region is contour irregularities and palpable nodules. Due to the thin skin and bony nature of the periorbital region, successful treatment requires experience. When successfully performed the results are extremely pleasing (Fig. 49.7).

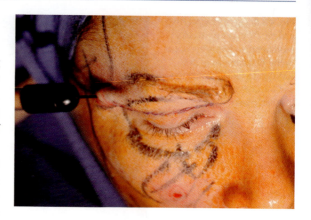

Fig. 49.6 Fat injected using a microcannula along the orbital rim using a microinjection technique

49.15 Complications

Complications after blepharoplasty are usually the result of overzealous skin or fat resection, lack of hemostasis, or an inadequate preoperative assessment [9, 10]. Less commonly, an individual's physiologic response to wound repair may lead to undesirable sequelae despite execution of the proper technique. The goal in minimizing complications consequent to blepharoplasty must therefore focus on prevention by identifying and managing known risk factors.

49.15.1 Hematomas

Collections of blood beneath the skin surface can usually be minimized before surgery by optimizing coagulation profiles and normotensive status during surgery through delicate tissue handling and meticulous hemostasis and after surgery through head elevation, cold compressing, a controlled level of activity, and appropriate analgesic support. Should a hematoma develop, its extent and time of presentation will guide management.

Small, superficial hematomas are relatively common and are typically self-limiting. If organization occurs with the development of an indurated mass and resolution is slow or nonprogressive, conservative steroid injections may be used to hasten the healing process. Moderate or large hematomas recognized after several days are best managed by allowing the clot to liquefy (7–10 days) and then evacuating the hematoma through large-bore needle aspiration or by creating a

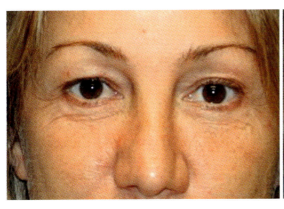
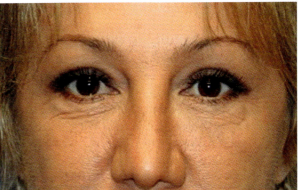

Fig. 49.7 (*Left*) Preoperative patient. (*Right*) Postoperative following upper eyelid blepharoplasty and fat augmentation to the infra-brow region

small stab wound over it with a no. 11 blade. Hematomas that are large and present early, that are expanding, or that represent symptomatic retrobulbar extension (decrease in visual acuity, proptosis, ocular pain, ophthalmoplegia, progressive chemosis) demand immediate exploration and hemostatic control. In the case of the latter, urgent ophthalmologic consultation and orbital decompression are the mainstays of treatment.

Although many methods of management have been described to manage threatened vision resulting from elevated intraocular pressures (reopening the wound, lateral canthotomy, steroids, diuretics, anterior chamber paracentesis), the most effective definitive treatment is immediate orbital decompression, which is usually accomplished through medial wall and orbital floor resections. Certainly, ophthalmologic consultation is advisable.

49.15.2 Blindness

Blindness, though rare, is the most feared potential complication of blepharoplasty. It occurs with an incidence of approximately 0.04%, typically presents itself within the first 24 h after surgery, and is associated with orbital fat removal and the development of a retrobulbar hematoma (medial fat pocket most commonly involved). Commonly implicated causes of retrobulbar hemorrhage include the following: (1) excessive traction on orbital fat resulting in disruption of small arterioles or venules in the posterior orbit; (2) retraction of an open vessel beneath the septum after fat release; (3) failure to recognize an open vessel because of vasospasm or epinephrine effect; (4) direct vessel trauma resulting from injections done blindly beneath the orbital septum; and (5) rebleeding after closure resulting from any maneuver or event that leads to an increased ophthalmic arteriovenous pressure head.

Early recognition of a developing orbital hematoma can be facilitated by delaying intraoperative closure (first side), avoiding occlusive-pressure eye dressings, and extending the postoperative observational period.

49.15.3 Epiphora

Assuming dry-eye syndrome was ruled out before surgery or managed appropriately intraoperatively (conservative and staged resections), a dysfunctional lacrimal collecting system rather than a high glandular output state is typically responsible for postoperative epiphora (although reflex hypersecretion may be a contributing factor because of coexistent lagophthalmus or vertical retraction of the upper lid). This response is common in the early postoperative period and is usually self-limited. Long-term cases can result from excessive skin excision, resulting in lagophthalmus and retraction.

49.15.4 Suture Line Complications

Milia or inclusion cysts are common lesions seen along the incisional line resulting from trapped epithelial debris beneath a healed skin surface or possibly from the occlusion of a glandular duct. They are typically associated with simple or running cuticular stitches. Their formation is minimized by subcuticular closure. If they develop, definitive therapy is aimed at uncapping the cyst (#11 blade or epilation needle) and teasing out the sac. Granulomas may develop as nodular thickenings within or beneath the suture line and are typically treated by steroid injections if small and by direct excision if large. Suture tunnels develop as a result of prolonged suture retention and epithelial surface migration along the suture tract. Preventive treatment includes early suture removal (3–5 days), and definitive treatment involves unroofing the tunnel. Suture marks are also related to prolonged suture retention and their formation can usually be avoided by using a rapidly absorbing suture (fast-absorbing gut or mild chromic), by removing a monofilament suture early, or by employing a subcuticular closure.

49.15.5 Wound Healing Complications

Wound dehiscence may develop as a result of closure under excessive tension, early removal of sutures, extension of an infectious process (unusual), or hematoma (more common). Treatment is directed to supportive taping or resuturing.

49.15.6 Ocular Injury

Corneal abrasions or ulcerations may result from inadvertent rubbing of the corneal surface with a gauze sponge or cotton applicator, instrument or suture mishandling, or desiccation developing as a result of lagophthalmus, ectropion, or preexistent dry-eye syndrome. Symptoms suggestive of corneal injury, which include pain, eye irritation, and blurred vision, should be confirmed by fluorescein staining and slit-lamp examination by an ophthalmologist. Foreign body sensation like a grain of sand scratching the eye during eye opening and closure can signify that a corneal abrasion has occurred. Therapy for mechanical injury typically involves use of an antibiotic ophthalmic drop with lid closure until epithelialization is complete (usually 24–48 h). Treatment for dry-eye syndrome includes the addition of ocular lubricants, such as Liquitears and Lacri-lube.

49.15.7 Contour Irregularities

Contour irregularities are generally caused by technical omissions. Failure to remove enough fat, particularly in a patient with a prominent medial fat pad, can lead to surface irregularities and persistent bulge. Overzealous fat resection, on the other hand, can lead to deep hollows in the medial infrabrow region. Areas of induration or lumpiness below the suture line can usually be attributed to unresolved or organized hematoma, tissue reaction, or fibrosis secondary to electrocauterization or thermal injury, or soft-tissue response to fat necrosis. Treatment in each case is directed at the specific cause. Persistent fat bulges are managed by resection, whereas areas of depressions from excess fat removal can be managed by volume augmentation.

References

1. Volpe CR, Ramirez OM. The beautiful eye. Facial Plast Surg Clin North Am. 2005;13(4):493–504.
2. Zide BM. Anatomy of the eyelids. Clin Plast Surg. 1981;8(4):623–34.
3. Aguilar GL, Nelson C. Eyelid and anterior orbital anatomy. In: Hornblass A, editor. Oculoplastic, orbital and reconstructive surgery. Vol. 1: Eyelids. Baltimore: Williams & Wilkins; 1988.
4. Jones LT. New concepts of orbital anatomy. In: Tessier P, Callahan A, Mustarde JC, Salyer K, editors. Symposium on plastic surgery in the orbital region. St Louis: CV Mosby; 1976.
5. Rees TD, Jelks GW. Blepharoplasty and the dry eye syndrome: guidelines for surgery? Plast Reconstr Surg. 1981;68(2):249–52.
6. Jelks GW, McCord CD. Dry eye syndrome and other tear film abnormalities. Clin Plast Surg. 1981;8(4):803–10.
7. Holt JE, Holt GR. Blepharoplasty: indications and preoperative assessment. Arch Otolaryngol. 1985;111(6):394–7.
8. McKinney P, Zukowski ML. The value of tear film breakup and Schirmer's tests in preoperative blepharoplasty evaluation. Plast Reconstr Surg. 1989;84(4):572–6.
9. Adams BJ, Feurstein SS. Complications of blepharoplasty. Ear Nose Throat J. 1986;65(1):11–28.
10. Castanares S. Complications in blepharoplasty. Clin Plast Surg. 1978;5(1):149–65.

Lower Eyelid Blepharoplasty

50

Amir M. Karam and Samuel M. Lam

50.1 Introduction

Aging of the lower periorbital region is a complex process involving both soft-tissue excess and volume loss. As a result, successful rejuvenation of this region requires a thorough understanding of the aging process and its influence on the complex anatomy. Lower eyelid blepharoplasty is the principle operation performed to rejuvenate the lower eyelid region.

It is considered a technically challenging operation with a myriad of variations and paradigms. The technical challenge of this procedure is due to the fact that a very fine line exists between an enhanced aesthetic outcome and significant functional and aesthetic complications.

Traditional blepharoplasty techniques have been criticized for their failure to truly restore a refreshed and youthful appearance. Often, following aggressive removal of skin, muscle, and fat, the infraorbital region is left looking hollowed, which actually has the opposite effect on the appearance. Modern periorbital rejuvenation paradigms involve a combination of treatment modalities, ranging from conservative blepharoplasty techniques, volume restoration, and skin resurfacing.

An intimate and thorough understanding of the anatomy coupled with an understanding of the natural history of lower eyelid aging is required to achieve a successful surgical outcome. In this chapter, we evaluate the periorbital aging process and how blepharoplasty can be used in addition to other treatments to restore the youthful structure of this area.

50.2 Periorbital Aging

The youthful lower eyelid should have a short lid–cheek junction and a smooth gentle convexity that blends into the upper cheek mound as a single convexity [1]. With age, a combination of fat volume loss overlying the inferior orbital rim, weakening of the orbital septum resulting in fat pseudoherniation, descent of the malar fat pad, sagging of the orbicularis oculi muscle resulting in lengthening of the lid–cheek junction, exposure of the bony outline of the inferior orbital rim occur. These factors combined results in a double-convexity contour deformity. The orbital fat is the superior convexity, directly below this is the relative concavity defined by arcus marginalis along the skeletonized inferior orbital rim, and the second convexity is defined by the cheek mound. This finding is a telltale sign of aging of the central face. Tear-trough deformity or nasojugal fold is described by a depression at the transition of the medial aspect of the lower eyelid and upper cheek. The resultant deformity causes the periorbital region to have fatigued and aged appearance. This finding is caused by a deficiency of tissue, not excess. Therefore, removing skin, muscle, or fat from the lower eyelid will worsen this deformity.

A.M. Karam (✉)
Carmel Valley Facial Plastic Surgery, 4765 Carmel Mountain Road, Suite 201, San Diego, CA 92130, USA
e-mail: md@drkaram.com

S.M. Lam
Willow Bend Wellness Center, Lam Facial Plastic Surgery Center & Hair Restoration Institute, 6101 Chapel Hill Blvd., Suite 101, Plano, TX 75093, USA
e-mail: drlam@lamfacialplastics.com

50.3 Anatomic Considerations

In no other area of facial aesthetic surgery is such a fragile balance struck between form and function as that in eyelid modification. Owing to the delicate nature of eyelid structural composition and the vital role the eyelids serve in protecting the visual system, iatrogenic alterations in eyelid anatomy must be made with care, precision, and thoughtful consideration of existing soft tissue structures. A brief anatomic review is necessary to highlight some of these salient points.

With the eyes in primary position, the lower lid should be well apposed to the globe, with its lid margin roughly tangent to the inferior limbus and the orientation of its respective palpebral fissure slanted slightly obliquely upward from medial to lateral (occidental norm). An inferior palpebral sulcus (lower eyelid crease) is usually identified approximately 5–6 mm from the ciliary margin and roughly delineates the inferior edge of the tarsal plate and the transition zone from pretarsal to preseptal orbicularis oculi [2].

50.3.1 Lamellae

The eyelids have been considered as being composed of two lamellae: [3] an outer lamella, composed of skin and the orbicularis oculi muscle and an inner lamella, which includes tarsus and conjunctiva. The skin of the lower eyelid is thin over the eyelid and as it extends beyond the lateral orbital it becomes gradually thicker. The skin is devoid of a subcutaneous fat layer and is interconnected to the underlying musculus orbicularis oculi by fine connective tissue attachments in the skin's pretarsal and preseptal zones.

50.3.2 Musculature

The orbicularis oculi muscle can be divided into a darker and thicker orbital portion (voluntary) and a thinner and lighter palpebral portion (voluntary and involuntary). The palpebral portion can be further subdivided into preseptal and pretarsal components. The larger superficial heads of the pretarsal orbicularis unite to form the medial canthal tendon, which inserts onto the anterior lacrimal crest, whereas the deep heads unite to insert at the posterior lacrimal crest. Laterally, the fibers condense and become firmly attached at the orbital tubercle of Whitnall, becoming the lateral canthal tendon [4]. Although the preseptal orbicularis has fixed attachments with the medial and lateral canthal tendons, the orbital portion does not and instead inserts subcutaneously in the lateral orbital region (contributing to crow's feet).

Immediately beneath the submuscular fascia, extending along the posterior surface of the preseptal orbicularis, lays the orbital septum. It originates at the arcus marginalis along the orbital rim (continuous with orbital periosteum), and after fusing with the capsulopalpebral fascia posteriorly about 5 mm below the lower tarsal edge, it forms a single fascial layer that inserts near the tarsal base. The orbital septum delineates the boundary between anterior eyelid (outer lamella) and intraorbital contents.

50.3.3 Orbital Fat

Contained behind the orbital septum and within the orbital cavity, the orbital fat has been classically segmented into discrete pockets (lateral, central, and medial), although interconnections truly exist [5]. The lateral fat pad is smaller and more superiorly situated, and the larger nasal pad is divided by the inferior oblique muscle into a larger central fat compartment and an intermediate medial compartment. (During surgery, care must be taken to avoid injury to the inferior oblique.) The medial pad has characteristic differences from its other counterparts, including a lighter color, a more fibrous and compact lobular pattern, and a frequent association with a sizable blood vessel near its medial aspect. The orbital fat can be considered an adynamic structure because its volume is not related to body habitus, and once removed it is not thought to regenerate.

50.3.4 Infraorbital and Midface Anatomy

The infraorbital area consists of skin, subcutaneous soft tissues, and fat overlying the bony orbital rim, arcus marginalis, and malar eminence. Two distinct fat pads in this area have been identified – the malar fat pad, and the suborbicularis oculi fat (SOOF) pad. The SOOF is defined as a collection of fat deep to the orbital portion of the orbicularis oculi muscle, overlying the inferior arcus marginalis [6]. The malar fat pad is inferior to the orbicularis oculi muscle. These tissues mask the visibility of the inferior orbital rim in the youthful face. Volume loss, inferior and medial descent of the malar fat and SOOF result in the aging infraorbital area characterized by volume reduction and exposure of the inferior orbital rim. Descent of these tissues coupled with pseudoherniation results in the tear trough or nasojugal deformity [6].

50.4 Preoperative Evaluation

Patient analysis is directed to understanding the patient's desires and expectation, the etiology of the problem at hand, and development of the optimal treatment plan for the patient's unique needs. The preoperative assessment of the anatomical characteristics must be directed at presence of:

1. Pseudoherniation of orbital fat
2. Volume status of the inferior orbital rim and upper cheek
3. Dermatochalasis
4. Fine lines and wrinkles

The treatment plan needs to include treatment of each of these potential anatomic issues.

In addition, a systematic and thorough preoperative assessment of blepharoplasty candidates is essential to minimize potential postoperative complications. Patients need to be specifically questioned about the history of dry-eye syndrome [7, 8], hypertension, smoking, visual problems, ocular disorders (i.e., glaucoma), bleeding disorders, recent use of NSAIDS, Aspirin, and other anticlotting medications. Appropriate workup is required depending on the patient's history.

50.4.1 Ocular Assessment

Examination of the eyes should begin with an overall inspection. The eyelid should be assessed for symmetry (by noting palpebral fissure height and length), position of the lower eyelid margin with respect to the inferior limbus, scleral show, and the presence of ectropion/entropion or exophthalmos/enophthalmos.

As a minimum, baseline ocular assessment should document visual acuity (i.e., best corrected vision if glasses or contact lenses are worn), extraocular movements, gross visual fields by confrontation, corneal reflexes, the presence of Bell's phenomenon, and lagophthalmus. If there is any question of dry-eye syndrome, the patient should be evaluated with Schirmer testing (to quantify tear output) and tear film break-up times (to assess stability of precorneal tear film) [8, 9]. Patients who demonstrate abnormalities in either or both of these tests or who have past or anatomic evidence that would predispose them to dry-eye complications should be thoroughly evaluated by an ophthalmologist preoperatively.

50.4.2 Assessment of Lid-Supporting Structures

Because the most common cause of lower lid ectropion after blepharoplasty is failure to recognize a lax lower lid before surgery, it is essential to properly assess the lid-supporting structures. Two simple clinical tests aid in this evaluation. A lid distraction test (snap test) is performed by gently grasping the midportion of the lower eyelid between the thumb and index fingers and outwardly displacing the eyelid from the globe. Movement of the lid margin greater than 10 mm indicates an abnormally lax supporting lid structure and suggests the need for a lid-shortening procedure. The lid retraction test [10] is used to assess lid tone as well as medial and lateral canthal tendon stability. By using the index finger to inferiorly displace the lower lid toward the orbital rim, observations are made in terms of punctal or lateral canthal malposition (movement of puncta greater than 3 mm from the medial canthus indicates an abnormally lax canthal tendon and suggests the need for tendoplication). Releasing the eyelid, the pattern and rate of return of the lid to resting position should be observed. A slow return, or one that requires multiple blinks, indicates poor lid tone and eyelid support. Again, a conservative skin–muscle resection and lower lid-shortening procedure would be warranted.

50.4.3 Assessment of Tear Trough or Nasojugal Deformity

The tear trough deformity is frequently one of the first signs of aging in the central face. Often initially noticed in the early 30s, this deformity is defined as a loss of volume in the skin and soft tissues of the infraorbital area resulting in a depression in the medial lower eyelid–cheek junction extending obliquely from the medial canthus (Fig. 50.1). It may also be associated with volume loss in the lateral aspect of the inferior orbital rim compounding the "tired" or "worn out" appearance of which affected patients complain. The tear trough deformity is important to recognize as is not generally addressed by standard lower eyelid procedures. Anatomically, the thinning of this area caused by descent of the infraorbital soft tissues exposes the infraorbital rim. This deformity may be accentuated by pseudoherniation of lower eyelid fat. The restoration of volume over the inferior orbital rim has been shown to improve the results of lower eyelid rejuvenation in affected patients.

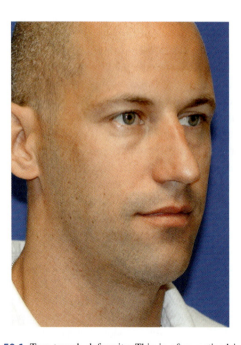

Fig. 50.1 Tear trough deformity. This is often noticed in the early thirties. Note the loss of volume in the skin and soft tissues of the infraorbital area resulting in a depression in the medial lower eyelid–cheek junction extending obliquely from the medial canthus

50.5 Operative Procedure

Lower eyelid blepharoplasty is an operation which is commonly performed to rejuvenate the lower eyelid region. It is considered a technically challenging operation with a myriad of variations and paradigms. The technical challenge of this procedure is due to the fact that a very fine line exists between an enhanced aesthetic outcome and significant functional and aesthetic complications. An intimate and thorough understanding of the anatomy coupled with an understanding of the natural history of lower eyelid aging is required to achieve a successful surgical outcome.

50.5.1 Technique

The two most common surgical approaches described in lower lid blepharoplasty are: (1) transconjunctival and (2) skin–muscle flap blepharoplasty.

50.5.1.1 Transconjunctival Approach

The transconjunctival approach to lower eyelid blepharoplasty was first described in 1924 by Bourguet [11]. Although it is not a new procedure, over the last 10 years there has been a surge of interest and a growth of proponents for this approach. The transconjunctival lower lid blepharoplasty respects the integrity of the orbicularis oculi, an active support structure of the lower eyelid. This minimizes the incidence of ectropion. Also, an external scar can be avoided.

Proper patient selection for the transconjunctival approach is required. Ideal candidates include older patients with pseudoherniation of orbital fat and a limited amount of skin excess, young patients with familial hereditary pseudoherniation of orbital fat and no excess skin, all revision blepharoplasty patients, patients who do not want an external scar, patients with a history of keloids, and dark-skinned individuals who have a small possibility of hypopigmentation of the external scar [12, 13]. Because several authors have reported a significant reduction in short and long-term complications with the transconjunctival approach to lower eyelid blepharoplasty compared with the skin–muscle method, the indications for the technique have been gradually expanding [12, 14]. The presence of excess lower lid skin does not preclude use of the transconjunctival approach. In the authors practice, the most commonly performed lower lid procedure consists of transconjunctival fat excision, pinch excision of skin, and 35% trichloroacetic acid (TCA) peeling (described later) [12–16]. The skin excision is needed to recontour the lower eyelid once the fat has been removed. There is frequently less excess than one initially estimates before the fat excision is performed [17].

Preparation

While sitting upright, the patient is asked to look upward. This helps to refresh the surgeon's memory as to which fat pads are the most prominent, and these are marked. The patient is then placed supine. Two drops of ophthalmic tetracaine hydrochloride 0.5% are then instilled into each inferior fornix. Prior to the local injections, patients typically will receive some intravenous sedation of the surgeon's choice. Ten milligrams of intravenous dexamethasone (Decadron) is also given to help minimize postoperative edema. A local anesthetic consisting of 1% lidocaine (Xylocaine) with 1:100,000 epinephrine to which is added a 1:10 dilution of sodium bicarbonate, is then injected into the lower lid conjunctiva using a 30-gauge needle. The needle is advanced through the conjunctiva until the bony orbital rim is palpated. The local is slowly injected as the needle is withdrawn. This is performed medially, centrally, and laterally.

After waiting a full 10 min for vasoconstriction to occur, the lower lid is gently retracted by an assistant using a double-pronged skin hook. The upper lid is placed over the globe to protect it. Either a guarded needle-tip Bovie on a low setting or a 15-blade is used to make the transconjunctival incision 2 mm below the inferior edge of the inferior tarsal plate. This inferior tarsal edge appears gray through the conjunctiva. The medial aspect of the incision is in line with the inferior punctum. The incision is carried just 4–5 mm shy of the lateral canthus.

Immediately after the transconjunctival incision is made, a single 5–0 nylon suture is placed in the conjunctiva closest to the fornix and used to retract the posterior lamella over the entire cornea (Fig. 50.2). Mosquito hemostats snapped onto the patient's head wrap are used to hold the sutures under tension.

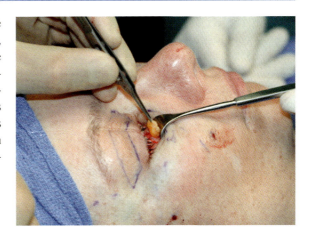

Fig. 50.2 Immediately after the transconjunctival incision is made, a single 5–0 nylon suture is placed in the conjunctiva closest to the fornix and used to retract the posterior lamella over the entire cornea. The orbital septum is then opened to expose the orbital fat

The conjunctiva acts as a natural corneal protector and the superior retraction allows for easier plane dissection. The skin hook is then carefully removed and a Desmarres retractor is now used to evert the free edge of the lower lid.

After the 5–0 suture retraction and Desmarres retractor are in place, the preseptal plane is developed with a combination of blunt dissection with a cotton swab and sharp dissection with scissors. It is mandatory to maintain a dry surgical field. Therefore, a bipolar cautery, "hot loop," or monopolar cautery is used to cauterize any bleeders.

The preseptal plane is an avascular plane between the orbicularis oculi and the orbital septum. Because the orbital septum is still intact while the preseptal plane is being developed, orbital fat does not bulge into one's view. The visualization obtained is closely similar to the orientation one is used to having when performing a skin–muscle flap blepharoplasty. The orbital septum will still have to be opened to access the orbital fat below (Fig. 50.2).

The medial, central, and lateral fat pads are each individually identified through the septum with the help of some gentle digital pressure on the conjunctiva covering the globe. The orbital septum is then opened with scissors. Using forceps and a cotton-tipped applicator, the excess fat is carefully teased above the orbital rim and septum. Care must be taken to remove only the excessive and herniated fat because the eyes may take on a hollowed-out appearance following excessive fat excision. The ultimate goal is to achieve a lower eyelid contour that forms a smooth, gentle concave transition between it and cheek skin.

A 30-gauge needle is then used to inject a small amount of local anesthetic into the excess fat. The bipolar cautery is used to cauterize across the base (Fig. 50.3). When one is sure the entire stalk has been cauterized, scissors are used to cut across the cauterized area. Others, notably Cook [20], reduce fat volume with electrocautery, minimizing surgical excision. Many surgeons feel that the lateral fat pocket should be explored initially because its volume contribution becomes more difficult to assess after removal of its adjacent and interconnected central fat pad. After excess fat has been removed from each compartment, the field is examined to make sure there is no bleeding. The Desmarres retractor should be removed periodically and the lower eyelid redraped over the fat that remains in place to facilitate examination of the contour of the eyelid. The fat that is removed is retained on gauze on the surgical field in order from lateral to medial, allowing for comparison with the fat removed from the opposite side. For example, if preoperatively the surgeon felt that the right lateral fat pad was much larger than all others, then intraoperatively that compartment would have the most fat removed.

The medial and central fat compartments are separated by the inferior oblique muscle. This muscle must be clearly identified prior to the excision of excess fat from these compartments to prevent muscle injury. The medial fat pad is whiter than the central and lateral fat pads. This helps in its identification. The lateral compartment is usually isolated from the central one by a fascial band off the inferior oblique muscle. This fascial band can be cut safely.

After each successive fat compartment is treated, the entire field must again be examined for bleeding. After all of the bleeding has been cauterized with the bipolar, the Desmarres and the retraction sutures are removed. The lower lid is gently elevated upward and outward and then allowed to snap back into its proper position. This allows for proper realignment of the edges of the transconjunctival incision. No suture is required, although some surgeons feel more comfortable closing the incision with one buried 6–0 fast-absorbing gut stitch. Both eyes should then be irrigated with sodium chloride (Ophthalmic Balanced Salt Solution) (Figs. 50.4 and 50.5).

In an older patient with skin excess, a lower lid skin pinch or chemical peel may now be performed. Using fixation forceps or Brown–Adson forceps, a 2–3-mm raised fold of redundant skin is raised just below the ciliary margin. The skin fold is excised with sharp scissors, with care taken not to cut the lower eyelashes. The edges of the skin pinch are then brought together with interrupted 6–0 fast-absorbing gut stitches.

Patients with crepey or fine lower eyelid rhytids are then treated with a 25–35% trichloroacetic acid (TCA) peel. The TCA is applied immediately below the skin pinch incision. A typical "frost" is generated.

Postoperative Care

Immediately after surgery, the patient is kept quiet with head elevated at least 45°. Cold compresses are placed on both eyes and changed every 20 min. The patient is observed closely for at least an hour for any signs of bleeding complications. The patient is given strict instructions to limit physical activity for the next week. The patient who is diligent about the cold compresses and head elevation during the first 48 h will experience substantially less swelling. Some physicians place their patients on sulfacetamide ophthalmic drops during the first 5 postoperative days to help prevent an infection while the transconjunctival incision is healing.

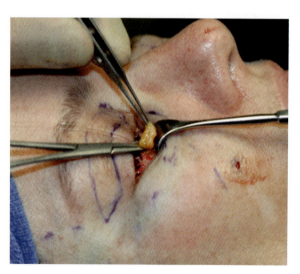

Fig. 50.3 Removal of the excess orbital fat. The bipolar cautery is used to cauterize across the fat stalk followed by sharp excision

Fig. 50.4 (*Left*) Preoperative. (*Right*) Six weeks postoperatively following lower eyelid transconjunctival blepharoplasty and upper eyelid blepharoplasty

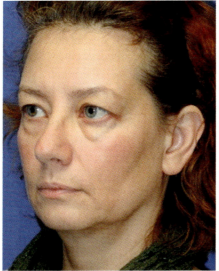
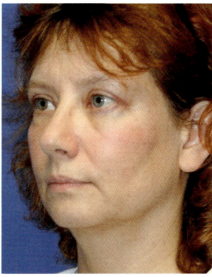

Fig. 50.5 (*Left*) Preoperative. (*Right*) Six months postoperatively following lower eyelid transconjunctival blepharoplasty

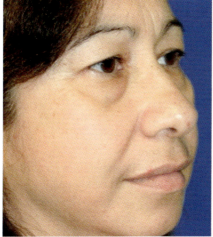
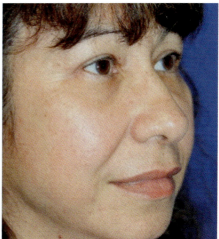

50.5.1.2 Skin–Muscle Flap Approach

The skin–muscle flap approach was perhaps the most commonly used method in the 1970s and early 1980s. In patients with a large amount of excess skin and orbicularis oculi as well as fat pseudoherniation, this is an excellent procedure [19, 20]. The advantages of this approach are related to the safety and facility of dissecting in the relatively avascular submuscular plane and the ability to remove redundant lower eyelid skin. One must realize that even with the skin–muscle flap one is limited by how much skin can safely be removed without risking scleral show and even an ectropion. Persistent rhytids often remain despite attempts to safely resect redundant eyelid skin. Further, the skin–muscle approach also risks the eyelid canthus moving upward and inward which often changes the intrinsic shape of the eyelid and hence chances the individual's appearance.

Preparation

Preparation for this method is similar to that for the transconjunctival approach, except that tetracaine drops are not necessary. A subciliary incision is planned 2–3 mm beneath the eyelid margin and is marked with a marking pen or methylene blue with the patient in the sitting position. Any prominent fat pads are also marked. The importance of marking the patient in the upright position before injection relates to the changes in soft-tissue relationships that occur as a result of dependency and infiltration. The medial extent of the incision is marked 1 mm lateral to the inferior punctum to avoid potential damage to the inferior canaliculus, whereas the subciliary extension is carried to a point approximately 8–10 mm lateral to the lateral canthus (to minimize potential for rounding of the canthal angle and lateral scleral show). At this point, the lateral-most portion of the incision achieves a more horizontal orientation and is planned to lie within a crow's-foot crease line. Care should be exercised in planning the lateral extension of this incision to allow at least 5 mm, and preferably 10 mm, between it and the lateral extension of the upper blepharoplasty incision to obviate prolonged lymphedema.

Patients typically receive intravenous after the preoperative marking has been accomplished and dexamethasone. Before surgical prepping and sterile draping, the incision line (beginning laterally) and entire lower lid down to the infraorbital rim are infiltrated (superficial to orbital septum) with our anesthetic mixture previously described.

Incision

The incision, which is begun medially with a No. 15 scalpel blade, is only through skin to the level of the lateral canthus, but through skin and musculus orbicularis oculi lateral to this point. Using a blunt-tipped, straight-dissection scissors, the incision is undermined in a submuscular plane from lateral to medial and is then cut sharply by orientation of the blades in a caudal direction (optimizing the integrity of the pretarsal muscle sling). A Frost type of retention suture, using 5–0 nylon, is then placed through the tissue edge above the incision to aid in counter retraction. Using blunt dissection (with scissors and cotton-tipped applicators), a skin–muscle flap is developed down to, but not below, the infraorbital rim to avoid disruption of important lymphatic channels. Any bleeding points up to this point should be meticulously controlled with the hand-held cautery or bipolar cautery, with conservatism exercised in the superior margin of the incision to avert potential thermal trauma to the eyelash follicles.

Fat Removal

If preoperative assessment suggests the need for fat-pad management, selective openings are made through the orbital septum over the areas of pseudoherniation and are guided by gentle digital pressure of the closed eyelid against the globe. Although alternatives aimed at electrocauterizing a weakened orbital septum exist [18] that may obviate violation of this important barrier, we are comfortable with the long-term results and predictability of our technique of direct fat-pocket management.

After opening the septum (usually 5–6 mm above the orbital rim), the fat lobules are gently teased above the orbital rim and septum using forceps and a cotton-tipped applicator. The fat resection technique is very much as described in the transconjunctival technique and is not repeated.

Access to the medial compartment may be limited in part by the medial aspect of the subciliary incision. This incision should not be extended; instead, the fat should be gently teased into the incision, taking care to avoid the inferior oblique muscle. The medial fat pad is distinguished from the central pad by its lighter color.

Closure

In preparation for skin excision and closure the patient is asked to open the jaw widely and gaze in a superior direction. This maneuver creates a maximal voluntary separation of the wound edges and assists the surgeon in performing accurate resection of the skin–muscle flap. With the patient maintaining this position, the inferior flap is redraped over the subciliary incision in a superotemporal direction. At the level of the lateral canthus, the extent of skin muscle overlap is marked and incised vertically. A tacking stitch of 5–0 fast-absorbing gut is then placed to maintain the position of the flap. Using straight scissors, the areas of overlap are conservatively resected (medial and lateral to the retention suture) so that edge-to-edge apposition can be maintained without the need for reinforcement. It is important to bevel the blades caudally to allow for a 1–2-mm strip resection of orbicularis oculi on the lower flap edge to avoid a prominent ridge at the time of closure. Some surgeons refrigerate the resected skin (viable for at least 48 h) in sterile saline in case replacement tissue graft is needed after an overzealous resection eventuating in ectropion. It is far better to prevent such complications by performing a conservative resection.

After fat removal from the second eyelid, simple interrupted 6–0 fast-absorbing gut sutures are placed to close the incision on the initial eyelid. Attention can then be redirected back to redraping, trimming, and suturing the second eyelid. Next, sterile strips are placed to aid in temporal support, and an antibiotic ointment is lightly applied to the sutured incision after irrigating the eyes with sodium chloride (Balanced Salt Solution).

Postoperative Care

Postoperative care after the skin–muscle approach is essentially identical to the aftercare used in the transconjunctival approach. Bacitracin ophthalmic ointment is given to the patient for the subciliary incision. Iced saline compresses, head elevation, and limited activity are stressed to all patients.

50.6 Complementary Treatments with Restoration of Infraorbital Volume

Restoration of volume in the infraorbital area must be addressed in the appropriate candidate. Several approaches have been described, including the use of injectable fillers, fat transfer, midface elevation, orbital fat repositioning, and SOOF elevation. Orbital fat repositioning and SOOF elevation may be performed in conjunction with lower eyelid blepharoplasty without the need for additional incisions or approaches.

50.6.1 Injectable Fillers

Recent trends in nonsurgical treatment of facial aging have resulted in the creative application of the widely available injectable fillers in the periorbital area. Specifically, the use of nonanimal, stabilized, hyaluronic acid (NASHA) fillers have enabled the treatment of early signs of aging in the infraorbital complex [21, 22].

Filling of the tear trough deformity and related lateral infraorbital hollows can be preformed in the office setting with topical and/or local anesthesia. Following nerve blocks a small amount of local anesthesia containing 1:100,000 or weaker of epinephrine can be injected directly into the treatment areas for vasoconstriction. Alternatively, ice packs may be applied before and after injection to decrease bruising. The borders of the tear troughs are marked and the filler is injected in a retrograde linear threading fashion in the submuscular plane.

The material should be injected only during retraction of the needle to prevent vessel embolization. Layered injections are suggested, beginning along the infraorbital rim, over the periosteum, and following with gentle layered "feathering" of the injectable material in multiple layers deep to the orbicularis muscle. Injection superficial to the orbicularis muscle can also be preformed, but it is suggested to attempt this only after mastery of the deeper injection technique. Gentle massage should be preformed after every few injections to disperse small isolated collections of material that may become palpable or visible as edema subsides. Risks specific to this treatment include bruising, palpable subcutaneous bumps, fluid collection in the injected area, and very remote risk of retinal embolus (Fig. 50.6).

50.6.2 Orbital Fat Repositioning

Orbital fat repositioning has also been referred to as fat preservation blepharoplasty. This procedure employs the fat of the medial and middle inferior orbital compartments to restore volume over the inferior orbital rim, and efface the tear trough deformity and associated lateral infraorbital hollows [22]. This can be approached through any lower eyelid approach that addresses the postseptal fat compartments. In the increasingly popular transconjunctival approach, the fat of the medial and middle fat compartments are dissected through a septal incision, and left attached as a pedicled flap transposed over the orbital rim and beneath the depression of the tear trough deformity. Fixation can be performed using transcutaneous permanent sutures which are removed in 3–5 days, or absorbable sutures securing the fat to the periosteum of the infraorbital rim. This procedure may also be performed in conjunction with the skin–muscle flap

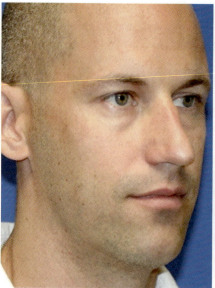 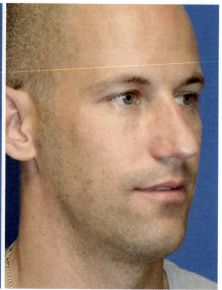

Fig. 50.6 Results of filling the tear trough with Restylane. (*Left*) Preoperative. (*Right*) Postoperative. Note the improvement of the contour along the lid–cheek junction

technique for lower blepharoplasty. In patients with excessive amounts of fat pseudoherniation, a small amount of fat may also be removed according to the techniques detailed above.

50.6.3 Suborbicularis Oculi Fat Lift

SOOF lifting techniques may also be preformed via traditional transconjunctival and skin–muscle flap approaches. The SOOF is exposed by inferior dissection along the deep surface of the orbicularis oculi muscle, and over the periosteum of the inferior orbital rim. This dissection is carried to the inferior aspect of the nasojugal deformity. The SOOF is then encountered inferior to the nasojugal deformity, elevated and secured to the periosteum of the inferior orbital rim with absorbable mattress sutures [7]. Bleeding in this area is controlled with judicious bipolar cautery to prevent infraorbital nerve injury.

50.7 Structural Fat Grafting of the Infraorbital Region

Autologous fat grafting of the inferior periorbital region is used to restore volume loss along the skeletonized inferior bony rim, nasojugal region, and upper cheek in order to create a smooth soft tissue contour from the lower eyelids to the cheek [22, 23]. Specifically, by filling the concavities (orbital rim, nasojugal fold) the double convexity deformity is transformed into a single convexity which is present in youthful eyelids/upper cheek region (Fig. 50.7). The fat is typically harvested from the abdomen or thighs using a low-pressure liposuction technique. Then the fat is prepared by separating the serum and blood using a centrifuge. Once purified adipose tissue is isolated, it is injected using a microcannula along the orbital rim, nasojugal fold, and upper cheeks using a microinjection technique. The most common complication of this technique in this region is contour irregularities and palpable nodules. Due to the thin skin and bony nature of the periorbital region, successful treatment requires experience. When successfully performed the results are extremely pleasing and is synergistic when coupled with a conservative transconjunctival lower eyelid blepharoplasty (Fig. 50.7).

50.8 Complications

Complications after blepharoplasty are usually the result of overzealous skin or fat resection, lack of hemostasis, or an inadequate preoperative assessment [24]. Less commonly, an individual's physiologic response to wound repair may lead to undesirable

Fig. 50.7 (*Left*) Preoperative. (*Right*) Postoperatively after excision of the orbital fat via a transconjunctival lower lid blepharoplasty approach with a skin pinch followed by filling the orbital rim and tear trough with fat. Specifically, by filling the concavities (orbital rim, nasojugal fold) the double convexity deformity is transformed into a single convexity that is present in youthful eyelids/upper cheek regions

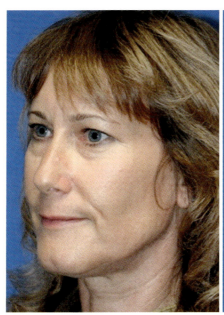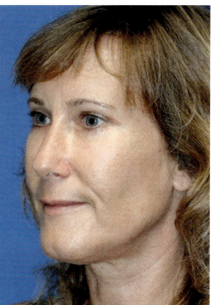

sequelae despite execution of the proper technique. The goal in minimizing complications consequent to blepharoplasty must therefore focus on prevention by identifying and managing known risk factors.

50.8.1 Ectropion

One of the most common complications after lower lid blepharoplasty is eyelid malposition, which may range in presentation from a mild scleral show or rounding of the lateral canthal angle, to a frank ectropion with actual eyelid eversion. In most cases resulting in permanent ectropion, a failure to address excessive lower lid laxity is the etiologic culprit. Other causes include excessive skin or skin–muscle excisions; inferior contracture along the plane of the lower lid retractors and orbital septum (greater in skin flap technique); inflammation of the fat pockets; and, rarely, destabilization of the lower lid retractors (a potential yet uncommon complication of the transconjunctival approach). Temporary ectropion has been associated with lid loading from reactionary edema or hematoma and muscle hypotonicity.

A conservative approach to management may include the following: (1) a short course of perioperative steroids with cold compresses and head elevation to manage edema; (2) warm and cool compresses alternated to hasten resolution of minor established hematomas and improve circulatory status; (3) repeated squinting exercises to improve muscle tonus; (4) gentle massage in an upward direction, and (5) supportive taping of the lower lid (upward and outward) to assist in corneal protection and tear collection.

When skin excisions are recognized to be excessive within the first 48 h, the banked eyelid skin should be used as a replacement graft. If recognition is delayed, conservative measures to protect the eye should be used to allow the scar to mature and a full-thickness graft (preferably upper eyelid skin or, alternatively, postauricular skin, or foreskin in males) used to replace the deficit. In many cases, a lid-shortening procedure is combined with the tissue grafting and is the mainstay of treatment when an atonic lid is present. Management of persistent indurations, resulting from hematoma formation or inflammatory responses of the fat pockets, generally involves direct depot injections of corticosteroid.

50.8.2 Hematomas

Collections of blood beneath the skin surface can usually be minimized before surgery by optimizing coagulation profiles and normotensive status during surgery through delicate tissue handling and meticulous hemostasis and after surgery through head elevation, cold compressing, a controlled level of activity, and appropriate analgesic support. Should a hematoma develop, its extent and time of presentation will guide management.

Small, superficial hematomas are relatively common and are typically self-limiting. If organization occurs with the development of an indurated mass and resolution is slow or nonprogressive, conservative steroid injections may be used to hasten the healing process. Moderate or large hematomas recognized after several days are best managed by allowing the clot to liquefy (7–10 days) and then evacuating the hematoma through large-bore needle aspiration or by creating a small stab wound over it with a No. 11 blade. Hematomas that are large and present early, that are expanding, or that represent symptomatic retrobulbar extension (decrease in visual acuity, proptosis, ocular pain, ophthalmoplegia, progressive chemosis) demand immediate exploration and hemostatic control. In the case of the latter, urgent ophthalmologic consultation and orbital decompression are the mainstays of treatment [24, 25].

50.8.3 Blindness

Blindness, though rare, is the most feared potential complication of blepharoplasty. It occurs with an incidence of approximately 0.04%, typically presents itself within the first 24 h after surgery, and is associated with orbital fat removal and the development of a retrobulbar hematoma (medial fat pocket most commonly involved). Commonly implicated causes of retrobulbar hemorrhage include the following: (1) excessive traction on orbital fat resulting in disruption of small arterioles or venules in the posterior orbit; (2) retraction of an open vessel beneath the septum after fat release; (3) failure to recognize an open vessel because of vasospasm or epinephrine effect; (4) direct vessel trauma resulting from injections done blindly beneath the orbital septum; and (5) rebleeding after closure resulting from any maneuver or event that leads to an increased ophthalmic arteriovenous pressure head.

Early recognition of a developing orbital hematoma can be facilitated by delaying intraoperative closure (first side), avoiding occlusive-pressure eye dressings, and extending the postoperative observational period.

Although many methods of management have been described to manage threatened vision resulting from elevated intraocular pressures (reopening the wound, lateral canthotomy, steroids, diuretics, anterior chamber paracentesis), the most effective definitive treatment is immediate orbital decompression, which is usually accomplished through medial wall and orbital floor resections [26, 27]. Certainly, ophthalmologic consultation is advisable.

50.8.4 Epiphora

Assuming dry-eye syndrome was ruled out before surgery or managed appropriately intraoperatively (conservative and staged resections), a dysfunctional lacrimal collecting system rather than a high glandular output state is typically responsible for postoperative epiphora (although reflex hypersecretion may be a contributing factor because of coexistent lagophthalmus or vertical retraction of the lower lid). This response is common in the early postoperative period and is usually self-limited. Causes include the following: (1) punctal eversion and canalicular distortion secondary to wound retraction and edema; (2) impairment of the lacrimal pump resulting from atony, edema, hematoma, or partial resection of the orbicularis oculi sling; and (3) a temporary ectropion resulting from lid loading. Outflow obstructions, secondary to a lacerated inferior canaliculus, are preventable by keeping the lower lid incision lateral to the punctum. Should laceration injury occur, primary repair over a silastic stent (Crawford tube) is recommended. Persistent punctal eversion can be managed by cauterization or diamond excision of the conjunctival surface below the canaliculus.

50.8.5 Suture Line Complications

Milia or inclusion cysts are common lesions seen along the incisional line resulting from trapped epithelial debris beneath a healed skin surface or possibly from the occlusion of a glandular duct. They are typically associated with simple or running cuticular stitches. Their formation is minimized by subcuticular closure. If they develop, definitive therapy is aimed at uncapping the cyst (No. 11 blade or epilation needle) and teasing out the sac. Granulomas may develop as nodular thickenings within or beneath the suture line and are typically treated by steroid injections if small and by direct excision if large. Suture tunnels develop as a result of prolonged suture retention and epithelial surface migration along the suture tract. Preventive treatment includes early suture removal (3–5 days), and definitive treatment involves unroofing the tunnel. Suture marks are also related to prolonged suture retention and their formation can usually be avoided by using a rapidly absorbing suture (fast-absorbing gut or mild chromic), by removing a monofilament suture early, or by employing a subcuticular closure.

50.8.6 Wound Healing Complications

Albeit rare, hypertrophic or prominent lower eyelid scars may develop because of improper placement of the lower lid incision. If extended too far medially in the epicanthal region, bow-string or web formation may occur (conditions usually amenable to correction by Z-plasty technique). A lateral canthal extension (which normally overlies a bony prominence) that is oriented too obliquely downward or is closed under excessive tension predisposes an incision to hypertrophic scarring, and during healing the vertical contraction vectors act on the lateral lid to favor scleral show or eversion. If the lower lid incision is oriented too far superiorly or too close to the lateral aspect of the upper lid incision, the forces of contraction (now favoring a downward pull) provide conditions that predispose the patient to lateral canthal hooding. Again, proper treatment should be aimed at reorienting the direction of contracting vectors.

Wound dehiscence may develop as a result of closure under excessive tension, early removal of sutures, extension of an infectious process (unusual), or hematoma (more common). Skin separation is seen most often in the lateral aspect of the incision with the skin–muscle and skin techniques, and treatment is directed to supportive taping or resuturing. If tension is too great for conservative management, then a lid suspension technique and lateral grafting should be considered. Skin slough may develop as a result of devascularization of the skin segment. It is almost exclusively seen in the skin-only technique and typically occurs in the lateral portion of the lower eyelid after wide undermining and subsequent hematoma formation. Treatment consists of local wound care, evacuation of any hematomas, establishment of a line of demarcation, and early skin replacement to obviate scar contracture of the lower lid.

50.8.7 Skin Discoloration

Areas of skin undermining frequently evidence hyperpigmentation in the early recovery period secondary to bleeding beneath the skin surface with subsequent hemosiderin formation. This process is usually self-limiting and often takes longer to resolve in darkly pigmented individuals. It is imperative during the healing process, and particularly in this patient population, to avoid direct sunlight because this may lead to permanent pigment changes. Refractory cases (after 6–8 weeks) may be considered for camouflage, periorbital peeling, or depigmentation therapy (e.g., hydroxyquinone, kojic acid). Telangiectasias may develop after skin undermining, particularly in areas beneath or near the incision, and most commonly occur in patients with preexisting telangiectasias. Treatment options may include chemical peeling or dye laser ablation.

50.8.8 Ocular Injury

Corneal abrasions or ulcerations may result from inadvertent rubbing of the corneal surface with a gauze sponge or cotton applicator, instrument or suture mishandling, or desiccation developing as a result of lagophthalmus, ectropion, or preexistent dry-eye syndrome. Symptoms suggestive of corneal injury, which include pain, eye irritation, and blurred vision, should be confirmed by fluorescein staining and slit-lamp examination by an ophthalmologist. Therapy for mechanical injury typically involves use of an antibiotic ophthalmic drop with lid closure until epithelialization is complete (usually 24–48 h). Treatment for dry-eye syndrome includes the addition of ocular lubricants, such as Liquitears and Lacri-lube.

Extraocular muscle imbalance, manifested by gaze diplopia, may be seen and is often transitory, presumably reflecting resolution of an edematous process. However, permanent muscle injury may result from blind clamping, deep penetration of the fat pockets during sectioning of the pedicle, thermal injury resulting from electrocauterization, suture incorporation during closure, or ischemic contracture of the Volkman type. Patients with evidence of refractory and incomplete recovery of muscle function should be referred to an ophthalmologist for evaluation and definitive treatment.

50.8.9 Contour Irregularities

Contour irregularities are generally caused by technical omissions. Overzealous fat resection, particularly in a patient with a prominent infraorbital rim, results in a lower lid concavity and contributes to a sunken-eye appearance. Failure to remove enough fat (common in lateral pocket) leads to surface irregularities and persistent bulges. A ridge that persists beneath the incision line is usually the result of inadequate resection of a strip of orbicularis oculi before redraping. Areas of induration or lumpiness below the suture line can usually be attributed to unresolved or organized hematoma, tissue reaction or fibrosis secondary to electrocauterization or thermal injury, or soft-tissue response to fat necrosis. Treatment in each case is directed at the specific cause. Persistent fat bulges are managed by resection, whereas areas of lid depression can be managed by sliding fat-pad grafts, free-fat, or dermal fat grafts, or orbicularis oculi flap repositioning. Some patients with such bulges or prominences respond to direct injections of triamcinolone (40 mg/cm^3). In selected cases, infraorbital rim reductions distract noticeability from a hollow-eye appearance and may be used as an adjunctive technique. Unresolved hematomas and areas of heightened inflammatory response may be managed with conservative injections of steroids.

References

1. Volpe CR, Ramirez OM. The beautiful eye. Facial Plast Surg Clin North Am. 2005;13(4):493–504.
2. Bashour M, Geist C. Is medial canthal tilt a powerful cue for facial attractiveness? Ophthal Plast Reconstr Surg. 2007;23(1):52–6.
3. Zide BM. Anatomy of the eyelids. Clin Plast Surg. 1981;8(4):623–34.
4. Jones LT. New concepts of orbital anatomy. In: Tessier P, Callahan A, Mustarde JC, Salyer K, editors. Symposium on plastic surgery in the orbital region. St Louis: CV Mosby; 1976.
5. Nesi F, Lisman R, Levine M. Smith's ophthalmic plastic and reconstructive surgery. 2nd ed. St Louis: CV Mosby; 1998. p. 1–78.
6. Freeman MS. Transconjunctival sub-orbicularis oculi fat (SOOF) pad lift blepharoplasty: a new technique for the effacement of nasojugal deformity. Arch Facial Plast Surg. 2000;2(1):16–21.
7. Rees TD, Jelks GW. Blepharoplasty and the dry eye syndrome: guidelines for surgery? Plast Reconstr Surg. 1981;68(2):249–52.
8. Jelks GW, McCord CD. Dry eye syndrome and other tear film abnormalities. Clin Plast Surg. 1981;8(4):803–10.
9. McKinney P, Zukowski ML. The value of tear film breakup and Schirmer's tests in preoperative blepharoplasty evaluation. Plast Reconstr Surg. 1989;84(4):572–6.
10. Holt JE, Holt GR. Blepharoplasty: indications and preoperative assessment. Arch Otolaryngol. 1985;111(6):394–7.
11. Bourguet J. Les hernies grasseuse de l'orbite: notre traitament chirugical. Bull Acad Natl Méd. 1924;3:1270–2.
12. Perkins SW, Dyer II WD, Simo F. Transconjunctival approach to lower eyelid blepharoplasty. Experience, indications, and techniques in 300 patients. Arch Otolaryngol Head Neck Surg. 1994;120(2):172–7.
13. Mahe E. Lower lid blepharoplasty – the transconjunctival approach: extended indications. Aesthetic Plast Surg. 1998;22(1):1–8.
14. Zarem HA, Resnick JI. Minimizing deformity in lower blepharoplasty: the transconjunctival approach. Clin Plast Surg. 1993;20(2):317–21.
15. McKinney P, Zukowski ML, Mossie R. The fourth option: a novel approach to lower lid blepharoplasty. Aesthetic Plast Surg. 1991;15(4):293–6.
16. Baylis HI, Long JA, Groth MJ. Transconjunctival lower eyelid blepharoplasty. Ophthalmology. 1989;96(7):1027–32.
17. Netscher DT, Patrinely JR, Peltier M, Polsen C, Thornby J. Transconjunctival versus transcutaneous lower eyelid blepharoplasty: a prospective study. Plast Reconstr Surg. 1995;96(5):1053–60.
18. Cook TA, Dereberry J, Harrah ER. Reconsideration of fat pad management in lower lid blepharoplasty surgery. Arch Otolaryngol. 1984;110(8):521–4.
19. Klatsky SA, Manson PN. Separate skin and muscle flaps in lower lid blepharoplasty. Plast Reconstr Surg. 1981;67(2):151–6.
20. Wolfley DE. Blepharoplasty: the ophthalmologist's view. Otolaryngol Clin North Am. 1980;13(2):237–63.
21. Goldberg RA, Fiaschetti D. Filling the periorbital hollows with hyaluronic acid gel: initial experience with 244 injections. Ophthalmic Plast Reconstr Surg. 2006;22(5):335–41.

22. Goldberg RA. Transconjunctival orbital fat repositioning: transposition of orbital pedicles into a subperiosteal pocket. Plast Reconstr Surg. 2000;105(2):743–8; discussion 749–51.
23. Trepsat F. Periorbital rejuvenation combining fat grafting and blepharoplasties. Aesthetic Plast Surg. 2003;27(4):243–53.
24. Adams BJ, Feurstein SS. Complications of blepharoplasty. Ear Nose Throat J. 1986;65(1):11–28.
25. Castanares S. Complications in blepharoplasty. Clin Plast Surg. 1978;5(1):149–65.
26. Moser MH, DiPirro E, McCoy FJ. Sudden blindness following blepharoplasty: report of seven cases. Plast Reconstr Surg. 1973;51(4):363–70.
27. Anderson RL, Edwards JJ. Bilateral visual loss after blepharoplasty. Ann Plast Surg. 1980;5(4):288–92.

Upper Blepharoplasty of the Asian Eyelid

Samuel M. Lam and Amir M. Karam

51.1 Introduction

Asian blepharoplasty has a rich and varied history. The primary goal of this procedure is to create a supratarsal crease. The first reported case was performed by the Japanese surgeon Mikamo in the late nineteenth century [1]. Since then, a number of innovative surgeons began to describe their strategies, which can be broadly categorized into suture-based, full-incision, and partial-incision techniques. The other historic trend has been based on Westernization techniques versus methods in which the ethnic identity is preserved. The overlying trend at this point in time appears to be in techniques that maintain the individual's ethnic identity by creating a natural crease. In fact, McCurdy has remarked that over the past 20 years there has been a distinct trend away from Westernization and rather toward enhancement and preservation of ethnicity. It should be noted that the presence of a supratarsal crease is a naturally occurring anatomic finding in the Asian population. The desire to have a "double eyelid" is largely cultural, as this feature is considered attractive. Fascination with epicanthal modulation is also waning given the strong impetus today for an entirely natural look and one that does not appear foreign or westernized.

The method which is advocated in this chapter is the full-incision technique. The rational for this preference can be summarized by the following reasons: (1) relative permanence compared with other methods, (2) no need to rely on any buried permanent sutures to hold the fixation, (3) ease in identifying postseptal tissues through a wider aperture, and (4) ability to modulate excessive skin (dermatochalasis) in the aging eyelid. The major drawback of the full-incision method is the protracted recovery time in which the patient can look grossly abnormal for 1–2 weeks and still not entirely natural for months if not a full year. Scarring has proven to be a nonissue if the delicate tissue near the epicanthus is carefully avoided. Further, the incision line is more difficult to observe in our opinion with the full incision than with the partial-incision method since there is no abrupt ending that is apparent with the more limited incision technique.

S.M. Lam (✉)
Willow Bend Wellness Center, Lam Facial Plastic Surgery Center & Hair Restoration Institute, 6101 Chapel Hill Blvd., Suite 101, Plano, TX 75093, USA
e-mail: drlam@lamfacialplastics.com

A.M. Karam
Clinical Faculty, Department of Surgery, Division of Otolaryngology – Head and Neck Surgery and Facial Plastic and Reconstructive Surgery, University of California, 4765 Carmel Mountain Road, Suite 201, San Diego, CA 92130, USA and
Carmel Valley Facial Plastic Surgery, 4765 Carmel Mountain Road, Suite 201, San Diego, CA 92130, USA
e-mail: md@drkaram.com

51.2 Instrument List

- Fine-tipped gentian violet surgical marking pen
- Castroviejo calipers
- No.15 Bard-Parker blade and knife handle
- Bipolar cautery
- Fine-toothed forceps
- Iris or Tenotomy scissors
- Fine-toothed Mosquito clamp
- Cotton-tipped applicators
- 5–0 Nylon
- 7–0 Nylon

51.3 Operative Technique

The first step is designing the proposed eyelid crease. When counseling a patient regarding which eyelid crease shape would be ideal for him or her, the patient can be encouraged to bring in photographs of Asian models in which they like their crease and to review diligently the surgeon's own previous work to make that decision.

There are several variations ranging from inside fold (the medial incision terminates lateral to the epicanthus) and an outside fold (the medial incision extends medial to the epicanthus by 1–2 mm). There are two variations to the shape of the incision (Fig. 51.1). The first is an oval shape (slight flare of the crease height laterally above the ciliary margin) versus rounded in which the line runs parallel with the ciliary margin. Our preference is the inside fold paired with an oval configuration (Fig. 51.2).

All markings are performed with the patient supine and the upper-eyelid skin held relatively taut to the point that the eyelashes are just beginning to evert. In order to create a natural, low crease design (which constitutes the naturally occurring shape), the degree of skin excision to be performed should err on the side of conservatism with about 3 mm (with the skin under stretch as mentioned above) between the upper and lower limbs and with a distance of about 7 mm from the ciliary margin in most young adults.

After the skin has been marked bilaterally and carefully inspected for symmetry, the patient can undergo infiltration of local anesthesia. Deep sedation should be avoided as patient cooperation is vital to ensure symmetry toward the end of the procedure. A mixture of 0.5 ml of 1% lidocaine with 1:100,000 epinephrine and 0.5 ml of 0.25% bupivicaine with 1:100,000 epinephrine attached to a 30-gauge needle is used to infiltrate the upper eyelid skin by raising two to three subcutaneous wheals which are then manually distributed by pinching the skin along the entire length of the incision (Fig. 51.3). This method that avoids threading the needle limits the chance of a hematoma that can lead to difficulty in gauging symmetry during the procedure. Of note, a total of only

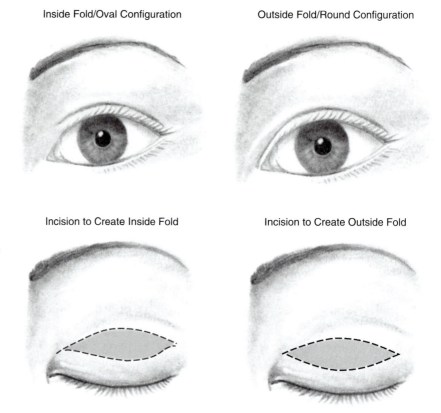

Fig. 51.1 The various eyelid markings and incision configurations. There are several variations ranging from inside fold (the medial incision terminates lateral to the epicanthus) and an outside fold (the medial incision extends medial to the epicanthus by 1–2 mm). There are two variations to the shape of the incision. The first is an oval shape (slight flare of the crease height laterally above the ciliary margin) versus rounded in which the line runs parallel with the ciliary margin. The authors' preference is the inside fold paired with an oval configuration

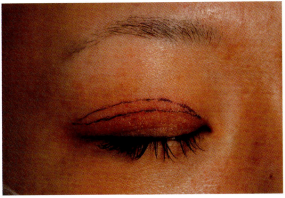

Fig. 51.2 Surgical marking of the inside fold paired with an oval configuration

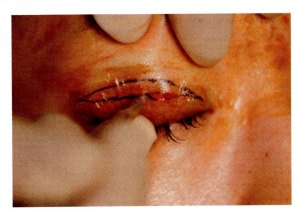

Fig. 51.4 Incision depth. A No.15 blade is used to incise the skin down through orbicularis oculi muscle

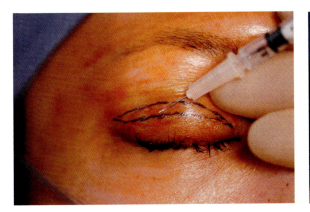

Fig. 51.3 Injection technique. Note that a 30-gauge needle is used to infiltrate the upper eyelid skin by raising two to three subcutaneous wheals which are then manually distributed by pinching the skin along the entire length of the incision

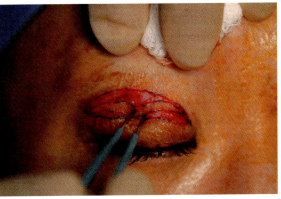

Fig. 51.5 Bipolar cautery used to coagulate the vascular arcades that run perpendicularly across the incision line in order to limit unnecessary bleeding and thereby mitigate swelling and distortion during this delicate procedure

1 ml of the above-stated mixture of local anesthesia is infiltrated along each proposed incision in order to maintain symmetry.

After 5–10 min are allowed to transpire for proper hemostasis and anesthesia, a No.15 blade is used to incise the skin down through orbicularis oculi muscle taking care not to pass the blade much further than that initial depth (Fig. 51.4).

Bipolar cautery is used to coagulate the vascular arcades that run perpendicularly across the incision line in order to limit unnecessary bleeding and thereby mitigate swelling and distortion during this delicate procedure (Fig. 51.5). The depth of the incision can be further deepened with the No.15 blade down toward the orbital septum before removing the skin island with curved Iris scissors. Additional cautery is used as needed. At this point, the exactly same procedure is performed on the contralateral side and continued in this alternating fashion to ensure symmetry.

The same iris scissors are then used to excise an additional 1–2 mm strip of tissue along the inferior edge of the wound so as to remove any remaining orbicularis oculi fibers and some initial fibers of the underlying orbital septum.

With the assistant gently balloting the eyeball above and below the incision line to help herniate the postseptal adipose through, the surgeon makes a small fenestration along the lateral extent of the wound edge just at the point where the strip of orbicularis was previously removed. With the counter traction and balloting of the eyeball mentioned above, the surgeon continues to excise thin films of tissue until the yellow postseptal adipose tissue is encountered. The reason for the small fenestration and the constant attention by the assistant to ballot around the incision to push the fat through the defect is the fact that identifying the postseptal fat is the safety landmark to avoid injury to the deeper levator aponeurosis.

Once the fat is identified, a fine-toothed curved Mosquito clamp is inserted into the fenestration and gently spread medially to lift the remaining orbital septum away from the deeper fat pad and levator aponeurosis. Repeated entry and exit of the tines through the defect can help ensure that the correct tissue plane of dissection is maintained. With the tines open and the orbital septum tented upward, a bipolar cautery with Iris scissors can be used to open the remaining orbital septum to expose fully the deeper postseptal adipose and underlying levator aponeurosis.

A cotton-tipped applicator is used to sweep the preaponeurotic (postseptal) fat pad away from the glistening white levator. At times a thin posterior leaf of the orbital septum can be seen between the levator and the fat pad. Gentle dissection using a fine-toothed Mosquito clamp followed by scissors of this thin orbital septum away from the fat pad can be undertaken to reveal the levator more fully. The same technique is undertaken on the contralateral side to this point.

Many surgeons believe that excessive adipose tissue must be removed to attain a more open eyelid configuration. However, in over 80% of the cases that simple levator-to-skin fixation is all that is necessary to attain the desired eyelid shape configuration and perceived opening of the palpebral aperture. Accordingly, preaponeurotic fat is rarely removed. This bias stems from seeing how much fat loss occurs with aging in the lateral brow and upper eyelid, a condition that is treated with facial fat grafting in the aging eyelid. (If fat is removed, additional 2% plain lidocaine can be infiltrated directly into the fat pad in order to minimize discomfort taking care not to permit any anesthetic to drip onto the levator.) At this point, the first levator-to-skin fixation suture can be placed. With the 5–0 nylon loaded backhanded on the needle driver, the patient is asked to open his/her eyes to determine the position of the midpupil on forward gaze so as to place the suture through the upper skin edge at the midpupil (Fig. 51.6). The suture bite is through the entire epidermis and dermis, as this suture will be removed at 7 days postoperatively.

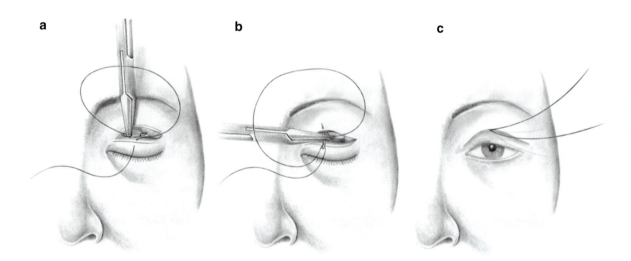

Fig. 51.6 Suture technique used to create the supratarsal eyelid crease. (**a**) A 5–0 nylon loaded backhanded on the needle driver is passed through the lower skin edge at the midpupil. With the 5–0 nylon now loaded normally in a forehand fashion, a horizontal bite is placed through the levator at the approximate lower edge of exposed levator again aligned at the midpupil. (**b**) Next, with the 5–0 nylon loaded in a backhand fashion, the final throw of the needle is placed through the upper skin edge again aligned with the midpupil. The patient is then asked to open his/her eyes after one suture knot to determine proper eyelash position. Slight eversion of the eyelash is desired. (**c**) The crease height will appear grossly too high and should not be used as the desired endpoint

With the 5–0 nylon now loaded normally in a forehand fashion, a horizontal bite is placed through the levator at the approximate lower edge of exposed levator again aligned at the midpupil. Next, with the 5–0 nylon loaded in a backhand fashion, the final throw of the needle is placed through the lower skin edge again aligned with the midpupil. The patient is then asked to open his/her eyes after one suture knot to determine proper eyelash position. The eyelashes should be slightly everted, and that should be the endpoint that is desired. The crease height will appear grossly too high and should not be used as the desired endpoint. If the eyelash position is deemed appropriate, the remaining four square knots are thrown to anchor the suture knot. The same technique is undertaken on the contralateral side and symmetry of the creases is noted and can be adjusted as need be. A higher crease is created by placing the horizontal bite through the levator more superiorly and lowered by placing the suture more inferiorly along the levator.

With the initial fixation suture placed bilaterally and symmetry observed, the two remaining fixation sutures per side can be placed in the same fashion. The second fixation suture is aligned with the medial limbus and the third fixation suture positioned halfway between the lateral limbus and the lateral canthus. Additional fixation sutures can be used as needed to fine-tune any perceived asymmetry.

The skin is then approximated with a running, non-locking 7–0 nylon suture.

51.4 Postoperative Care

Postoperative care is straightforward consisting of icing the eyelid areas for the first 48–72 h and cleansing the incision line twice daily with hydrogen peroxide and dressing it with Bacitracin ointment for the first postoperative week. The patient returns on the seventh postoperative day to have all sutures removed, i.e., the three fixation sutures per side (5–0 nylon) and the running skin closure (7–0 nylon). At times the patient may complain of difficulty opening his or her eyes due to either excessive edema and/or temporary levator dysfunction that can disappear over the first several days but can linger even up to 3–6 weeks following the procedure. The patient is reassured that it often takes a full year to achieve a natural crease configuration owing to persistent pretarsal edema that can linger for many months (Fig. 51.7). Narrow, rectangular-shaped eyeglasses can camouflage some of the exorbitant edema in the immediate postoperative period; and, for female patients, mascara can be used to help hide the abnormal height of the crease during the initial few months following the surgery.

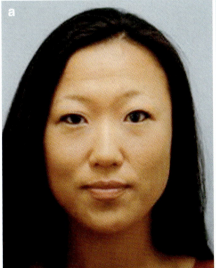
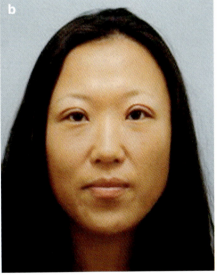

Fig. 51.7 (**a**) Preoperative patient. (**b**) One week postoperative following a full incision procedure. (**c**) Four weeks postoperative. (**d**) Six months postoperative

Fig. 51.7 (continued)

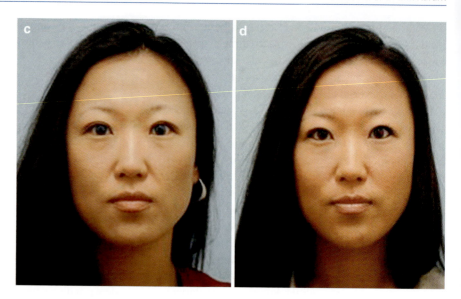

Reference

1. Lam SM. Mikamo's double-eyelid blepharoplasty and the westernization of Japan. Arch Facial Plast Surg. 2002; 4(3):201–2.

Medial and Lateral Epicanthoplasty

Dae Hwan Park

52.1 Introduction

The epicanthoplasty can elongate the length of the eyes, increase the eye size, and improve the aesthetic results of the double-eyelid formation. Epicanthoplasty along with double-eyelid formation is frequently performed on Asians bearing epicanthal folds. Despite the existence of epicanthal fold correction methods frequently practiced on Asians, including the split V-W plasty of Uchida, the V-Y plasty, the modified Mustarde technique, the simple Z plasty, and the complex Z plasty, these correction methods accommodate numerous problems such as the complexity of surgical techniques, the high possibility for generation of scars caused by the tone of the medial canthus flap, and the reoccurrence of the preoperational state. Several techniques have been introduced that remarkably reduce the tension along the skin suture line such as adding plication of the medial epicanthal tendon with medial epicanthoplasty.

52.2 Anatomy and Classification of Epicanthus

The anatomical structure of an Asian's eye is quite different from that of a Westerner's (Fig. 52.1). The eyes of Asians do not have the pretarsal skin attached to the levator palpebrae muscle, so they lack supratarsal folds. While they not only have excessive fat distributed between the orbicularis oculi muscle and the levator muscle, they also have relatively thick palpebral skins and orbicularis oculi muscles. Their orbits are comparatively small so that the orbital margin is more protruded than that of Westerners. Asians also have epicanthic folds that cover up the lacrimal lakes causing the medial canthal area to display fullness. The epicanthal fold indicates the fold initiating from the upper portion of the orbit and covering the medial canthus while being connected to the skin of the nasal bridge. Many muscle and tendon are attached at medial canthal area (Figs. 52.2 and 52.3) and there is fibromuscular tissue below the skin in medial canthal area (Fig. 52.4).

The ideal eyelid for oriental is: The intercanthal distance is 3.0–3.6 cm. The distance ratio between intercanthal distance and horizontal palpebral fissure is 0.90–1.15. The degree of the slant of palpebral fissure is 5–10°. Epicanthus is absent (Fig. 52.5).

There are the epicanthus palpebralis, the epicanthus tarsalis, the epicanthus superciliaris, and the epicanthus inversus [1]. Among these types, the epicanthus tarsalis is displayed most frequently.

52.3 Technique

52.3.1 Medial Epicanthoplasty

The indications of medial epicanthoplasty in Orientals are as follows:

1. Easily visible and severe medial epicanthus.
2. The distance ratio between the intercanthal distance and horizontal fissure of eyelid is larger than 1.3.

D.H. Park
Plastic and Reconstructive Surgery, Catholic University of Daegu, Daegu Catholic Medical Center, 3056-6 Daemyung 4-dong, Namgu, Daegu 705-034, Korea
e-mail: dhpark@cu.ac.kr

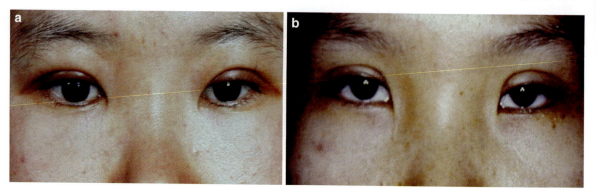

Fig. 52.1 (**a**) Asian's medial epicanthus. (**b**) Blepharoplasty without epicanthoplasty is not good cosmetically

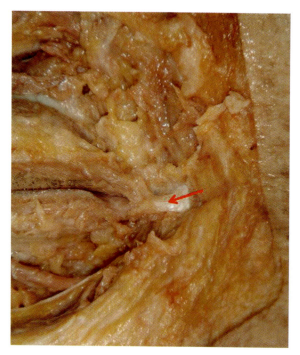

Fig. 52.2 Medial palpebral ligament (*arrow*)

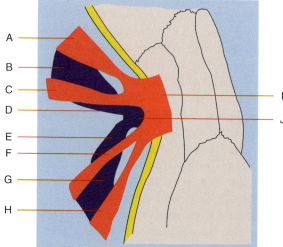

Fig. 52.3 Anatomy of medial canthal area. (*A*) Superficial head of preseptal orbicularis oculi muscle of upper lid. (*B*) Deep head of preseptal orbicularis oculi muscle of upper lid. (*C*) Superficial head of pretarsal orbicularis oculi muscle of upper lid. (*D*) Deep head of pretarsal orbicularis oculi muscle of upper lid. (*E*) Deep head of pretarsal orbicularis oculi muscle of upper lid. (*F*) Superficial head of pretarsal orbicularis oculi muscle of upper lid. (*G*) Deep head of preseptal orbicularis oculi muscle of upper lid. (*H*) Superficial head of preseptal orbicularis oculi muscle of upper lid. (*I*) Medial canthal tendon. (*J*) Lacrimal sac

3. The distance ratio between horizontal fissure and vertical fissure of eyelid is <3.
4. The distance ratio between midpoint of pupil to medial epicanthus and midpoint of pupil to lateral epicanthus is <1.

The classification of epicanthoplasty includes elliptical excision, using Z-plasty, using Y-V advancement, and using W-plasty.

52.3.1.1 Elliptical excision: Von Ammon, Arlt, Hiraga, and Watanabe methods

(a) Von Ammon's method is glabellar resection from radix region [2].
(b) Arlt's method is elliptical resection of skin close to medial epicanthus. But this method makes

Fig. 52.4 Cross section of epicanthus. There is fibromuscular tissue below the skin

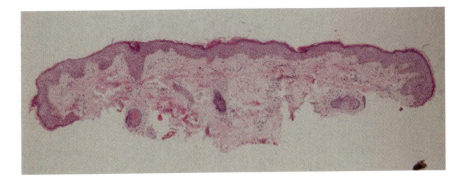

Fig. 52.5 The differences between intercanthal distance and interepicanthal distance

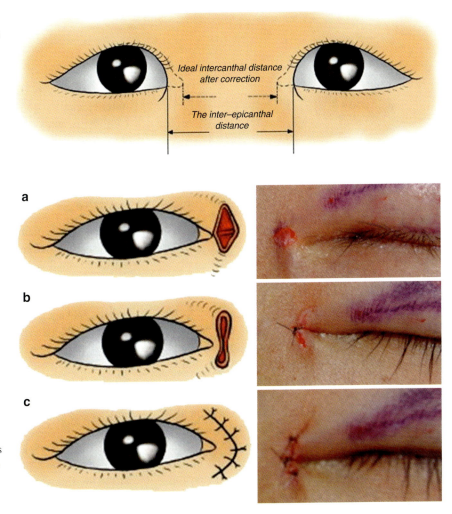

Fig. 52.6 Modified Arlt's method (simple elliptical excision). (**a**) Transverse incision, excision of skin, a small amount of subcutaneous soft tissue and orbicularis muscle of medial epicanthus. (**b**) Suture with Nylon 7–0 and trimming of dog ear. (**c**) Skin suture

remarkable scar. A modified method is used (Figs. 52.6–52.8).

(c) Hiraga's method is transverse incision and trimming of dog-ear.
(d) Watanabe's method is modification of Higara's method to prevent acute angle formation.

52.3.1.2 Z-Plasty Method

Methods using Z-plasty are:

(a) Single Z-plasty:
   Rogman's method: Dictates that the flap, accommodating a pedicle directed toward the superior,

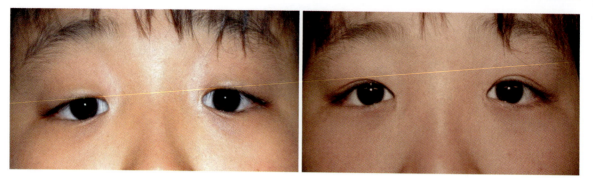

Fig. 52.7 A case of Modified Arlt's epicanthoplasty (simple elliptical excision). (*Left*) Preoperative. (*Right*) One year postoperative

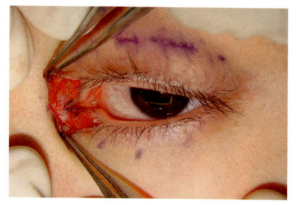

Fig. 52.8 Modified Arlt's method (periciliary approach)

should be positioned not toward the nose but toward the eyes, i.e., toward the lateral direction. The result is a cosmetic surgery method combining Z plasty and VY plasty, while tugging the old toward the medial, i.e., nasal side, with VY plasty. However, the postoperative suture carries the disadvantage of being able to generate a new fold quite easily.

Sheehan's method: Draws a Z on the inferior area of the epicanthic fold and designs the postoperative central angle that is positioned lower than the medial canthus, such that the direction of the suture, postoperatively, would be ideal.

Imre's method: Unlike those of Rogman and Sheehan, has the flap carrying the pedicle on the superior area toward the medial, i.e. nasal side, with the position of Z centered. The resulting disadvantages involve creating unnatural central angles and having difficulty in controlling the supratarsal fold.

Park's Z-plasty method: After marking for Z-epicanthoplasty incisions are made at the outer epicanthus (dotted lines) and the inner epicanthus is marked. After triangular excision, flap elevation is performed. However Park's method although effective makes visible scar. In order to make less scar a modified Park's method (half Z-plasty) is sometimes used (Figs. 52.9 and 52.10).

(b) Methods using double or multiple Z-plasty are various: Blair, Converse (Fig. 52.11) [3], and Mustarde and Spaeth [4].

Blair's method: Consists of two combinations of the Z plasty. Although it is highly effective as it greatly enhances the vertical direction and abolishes the fold better compared to a single Z plasty method, the zigzag-shaped scar on the medial canthal area is quite noticeable and a sutured line is generated horizontally from the medial canthus causing it to lack aesthetics. In addition, huge dog-ears, caused by the rotation of flaps, are sometimes created.

Double opposing Z plasty (Converse): Has two general 60° Z plasty types. When comparing this to the singular Z plasty, its effect on eliminating the fold is great, it is suitable for applying on traumatic epicanthic folds, and the transference of the flap is smoother than in Blair's method. However, even though there is no scar generating horizontally from the medial canthus, the zigzag-shaped scar is frequently and, unfortunately, noticeable. This also has the disadvantage of displaying too much of the medial canthus.

Mustarde's method: Adaptable to severe states of

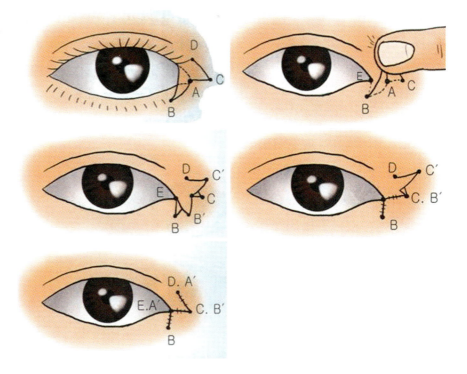

Fig. 52.9 Modified Park's method (half Z-plasty). From *top* to *bottom*: Marking for incision, incision by design, flap elevation, dog-ear removal, postoperative

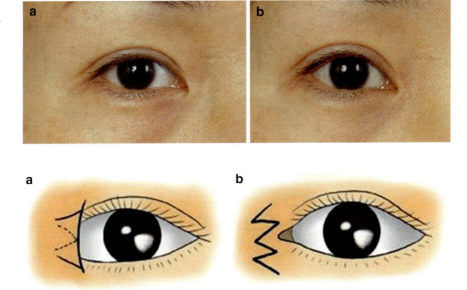

Fig. 52.10 A case of Modified Park's epicanthoplasty (half Z-plasty). (**a**) Preoperative. (**b**) Postoperative

Fig. 52.11 Converse's method. (**a**) Design. (**b**) Postoperative

epicanthus or epicanthic folds with severe scars and is quite efficient in eliminating the folds such that it easily displays the medial canthus into the open, bringing great results. The medial canthal ligament is also shortened and fixed so that there are few cases of reoccurrence after the operation. However, there is the disadvantage of noticeable zigzag scars. In order to improve this, the flap on the superior area of the medial canthal line must be detracted and the epicanthic fold may be corrected by solely using the inferior flap [5]. Mustarde's method can be modified by using a Z-plasty on its lower part [6]. The upper part is trimmed by dog-ear excision (Fig. 52.12).

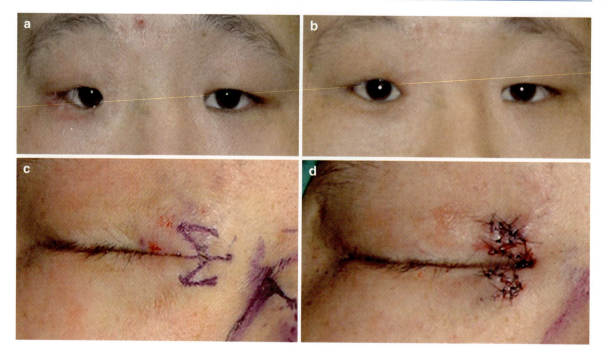

Fig. 52.12 Epicanthoplasty (Mustarde's method) was performed in a 36 year-old man with telecanthus. (**a**) Preoperative. (**b**) Postoperative. (**c**) Design of Mustarde's method. (**d**) Immediately after skin closure

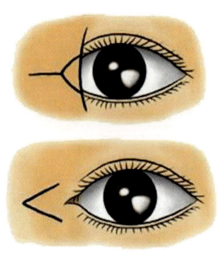

Fig. 52.13 Hughes' simple Y-V advancement flap. (*Above*) Design method. (*Below*) Postoperative

(c) Methods using Y-V advancement flap are Hughes' simple Y-V advancement flap (Figs. 52.13 and 52.14) [7, 8] and del Campo method [9].
(d) Methods using W-plasty are: Mulliken-Hoopes' method [10], Uchida method (Fig. 52.15), and Flowers' method.

Split V-W advancement flap (Flowers' method): Is a modification of Uchida's method [11].

Uchida's method: Is relatively simple in design and obtains geometrical excellence. Although it has the advantage of creating just a relatively short scar, it also has the disadvantage of creating an excessively long bottom side of the central flap when the severity of the epicanthic fold is moderate and an even worse one when the medial canthal area gains an obtuse angle. Further disadvantages include creating a round-shaped eye, having complications such as dog ear, producing hypertrophic scars, etc. But in entropion operation epicanthoplasty by Uchida method is helpful in the cosmetic aspect [12].

52.3.2 Lateral Epicanthoplasty

There are many methods: Von Ammon's method (Figs. 52.16 and 52.17), Fox's method [13], Blaskovics' method, and Uchida's method. Von Ammon's method is performed after transverse incision, V-Y advancement, and lateral cantholysis.

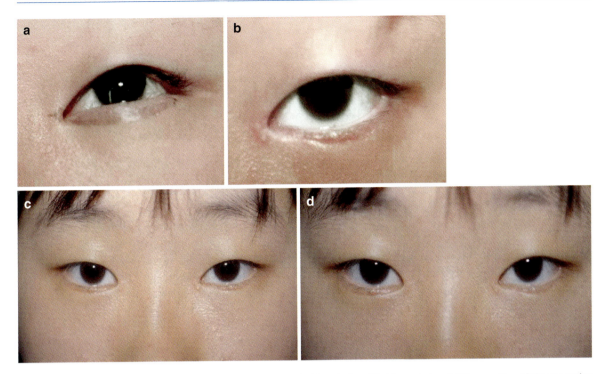

Fig. 52.14 A case of Hughes' simple Y-V advancement flap. (**a**) Incision design. (**b**) After suturing. (**c**) Preoperative. (**d**) Postoperative

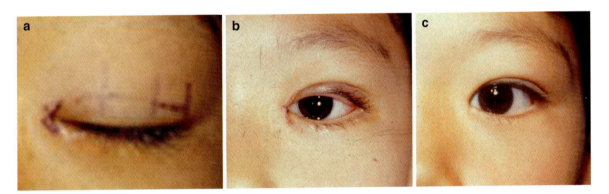

Fig. 52.15 A case of Uchida's method. (**a**) Preoperative design. (**b**) One week postoperative. (**c**) One year postoperative

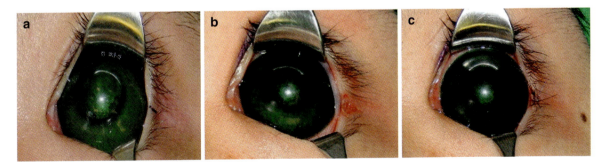

Fig. 52.16 Von Ammon's method. (**a**) Design for incision. (**b**) Skin incision, splitting of conjunctiva, and lateral displacement. (**c**) Sutured incision

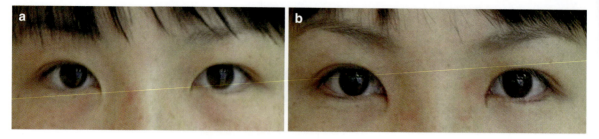

Fig. 52.17 A case of Von Ammon's method lateral epicanthoplasty. (**a**) Preoperative 22-year-old female patient with short length of palpebral fissure. (**b**) Postoperative after lateral epicanthoplasty

52.4 Complications

The most common complication of epicanthoplasty is formation of hypertrophic Scar (Fig. 52.18). Recurrence due to scar Contracture is also common. Other complications are undercorrection and overcorrection. In order to reduce complications, appropriate choice of operative method is important and like loupe or microsurgical operative instruments, the choice of operative instruments is also important (Fig. 52.19).

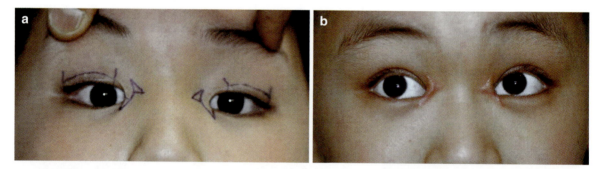

Fig. 52.18 Complication of epicanthoplasty: (**a**) preoperative appearance and design of epicanthoplasty (**b**) hypertrophic scar after epicanthoplasty

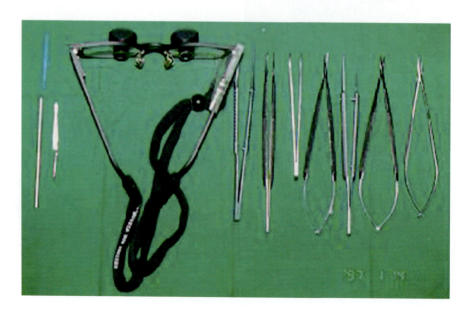

Fig. 52.19 Loupe and microsurgical operative instrument for epicanthoplasty operation

52.5 Conclusions

The normal anatomical structure of an Asian's eye is quite different from that of a Westerner's. The eyes of Asians do not have the pretarsal skin attached to the levator palpebrae muscle, so they lack supratarsal folds. While they not only have excessive fat distributed between the orbicularis oculi muscle and the levator muscle, they also have relatively thick palpebral skins and orbicularis oculi muscles. Their orbits are comparatively small so that the orbital margin is more protruded than that of Westerners. Asians also have epicanthic folds that cover up the lacrimal lakes causing the medial canthal area to display fullness.

The methods of epicanthoplasty are various. Most important point is selection of appropriate operative method.

References

1. Joh SH. Clinical study of epicanthoplasty by Y-V advancement flap. J Korean Soc Plast Reconstr Surg. 1996;23:1495.
2. Park JI. Z-epicanthoplasty in Asian eyelids. Plast Reconstr Surg. 1996;98(4):602–9.
3. Converse JM, Smith B. Naso-orbital fractures and traumatic deformities of the medial canthus. Plast Reconstr Surg. 1966;38(2):147–62.
4. Spaeth EB. Further consideration of the surgical correction of blepharophimosis (epicanthus). Am J Ophthalmol. 1956;41(1):61–71.
5. Mustarde JC. Repair and reconstruction in the orbital region. 2nd ed. New York: Churchill Livingstone; 1980. p. 332–44.
6. Yoon KC. Modification of Mustarde technique for correction of epicanthus in Asian patients. Plast Reconstr Surg. 1993;92(6):1182–6.
7. Hughes WL. Surgical treatment of congenital phimosis: the Y-V operation. AMA Arch Ophthalmol. 1955;54(4):586–90.
8. Iliff WJ. Congenital defects. In: Heilmann K, Paton D, editors. Atlas of ophthalmic surgery. Tokyo: Thieme Maruzen; 1985. p. 1103–25.
9. del Campo AF. Surgical treatment of the epicanthal fold. Plast Reconstr Surg. 1984;73(4):566–71.
10. Mulliken JB, Hoopes JE. W-epicanthoplasty. Plast Reconstr Surg. 1975;55(4):435–8.
11. Flowers RS. Surgical treatment of the epicanthal fold (invited essay). Plast Reconstr Surg. 1983;73:571.
12. Park DH. The correction of entropion using skin-tarsal fixation with epicanthoplasty. Korean Aesthetic Plast Reconstr Surg. 1995;1(1):124.
13. Fox SA. Ophthalmic plastic surgery. 5th ed. New York: Grune & Stratton; 1976. p. 223–5.

Treatment of Tear Trough Deformity with Hyaluronic Acid Gel Filler

53

Giovanni André Pires Viana

53.1 Introduction

Volume loss and muscular hyperactivity are two major components of the aging process that contribute to the formation of the folds and wrinkles [1]. In traditional lower eyelid surgery, the focus is removing tissue. The philosophy coupled with this approach is that facial aging is characterized by excess tissue. The fundamental cosmetic goals are to improve the appearance of the midface while maintaining a natural position of the lower eyelid. The creation of harmonious rejuvenation between the midface and lower lid relies on the preservation of the preoperative shape of eyelids.

The pathogenesis of aging within the lower eyelid is multifactorial and varies among patients. Periorbital age-related changes include crow's feet and lower eyelid rythides, scleral show, infraorbital hollowing, herniated fat pads, excess upper and lower lid skin, festoons, and eyelid hooding. In addition, attenuation of the lateral canthal tendons results in loss of the youthful architecture of the eye secondary to a decrease of the aesthetically pleasing upward tilt [2–6].

However, even with the evolution of these concepts, a problem still affects not only the surgeon, but also the patient himself: the tear trough. The tear trough is a depression centered over the medial inferior orbital rim. It is bounded superiorly by the infraorbital fat protuberance. The inferior border is formed by thick skin of the upper cheek with its abundant subcutaneous fat, suborbicularis oculi fat, and portions of the malar fat pad. In most individuals, the trough is deeper medially, becoming more shallow laterally. Through aging, further loss of soft tissue and, importantly, a loss of osseous support also cause the tear trough to deepen further [7]. Raul Loeb was one of the first surgeons to preserve adipose tissue during the lower eyelid blepharoplasty in an attempt to improve this region [8].

More recently, there has been interest across many disciplines in a philosophy focusing on the volume loss in facial aging. The surgical options for volume replacement have been traditionally more limited; for instance, autogenous fat grafting requires harvesting and can be unpredictable, and the synthetic fillers that were historically available were either permanent or nonpermanent. The arrival of new generation's fillers that are acceptably safe and predictable has provided a practical solution to approach facial volume loss [7, 9–11].

The author began using hyaluronic acid gel filler (Restylane®, Q-MED, Rio de Janeiro RJ, Brazil) for periorbital filling in the beginning of 2007. The purpose of this chapter is to review the results of treatment of tear trough deformity and the lessons learned in 150 patients.

53.2 Hyaluronic Acid Gel Filler

The hyaluronic acid (HA) is a molecule naturally occurring in the extracellular matrix found in many human tissues, including connective tissues, interstitial membranes, dermis, joints, and the vitreous body of the eye. HA is a glycosaminoglycan disaccharide composed of alternately repeating units of D-glucuronic acid and N-acetyl-D-glucosamine (Fig. 53.1) [12–14].

HA is a polyanionic polymer at physiologic pH and is therefore highly charged. The highly charged nature

---

G.A.P. Viana
Member of Brazilian Plastic Surgery, Department of Ophthalmology, Vision Institute, Federal University of São Paulo, São Paulo, Brazil and
Alameda Jauaperi 732, São Paulo, SP 04523-013, Brazil
e-mail: info@cliniplast.com

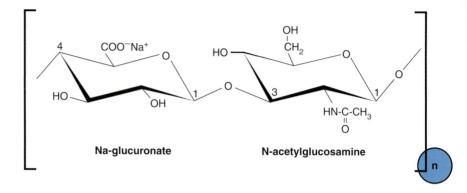

Fig. 53.1 Hyaluronic acid is a glycosaminoglycan disaccharide composed of repeating units of D-glucuronic acid and N-acetyl-D-glucosamine

of hyaluronic acid renders it soluble and allows it to bind water extensively. The average 70 kg man has roughly 15 g of hyaluronic acid in his body, one-third of which is turned over every day [12–14].

Pure hyaluronic acid, even in its longest polymeric form, degrades quickly in tissues. HA derivates have been developed with modified physical and rheological characteristics, making it suitable for tissue augmentation [12–14]. At physiologic pH, hyaluronic acid exists mostly as a sodium salt; this is the most common form of commercially available hyaluronic acid [12–14].

Restylane® is a modified hyaluronic acid. It is nonanimal-derived product obtained by bacterial fermentation of *Streptococcus* strains (*S. equi* or *S. zooepidemicus*) and stabilized by chemical cross-linking process. It has approximately 100,000 particles of gel per millimeter [11–14].

53.3 Patient Marking and Preparation

Before treatment, patients are advised to avoid medications that tend to interfere with platelet function for 2 weeks before treatment. Standard digital photographs are taken with all visits, and informed consent is obtained.

Makeup is removed, the skin is prepped with alcohol, and the morphology of the eyelids is studied. The area to be treated is marked delimiting to the lower and upper borders of the tear trough. When correction of the eyelid–cheek groove is required, the lower and upper limits are marked (Fig. 53.2). As a precaution, the author tends to define the position of the lower bony orbital rim. The lower eyelid area is anesthetized by the topical application of 2.5% lidocaine and 2.5% Prilocaine cream. After 20–30 min the ointment is cleaned off with alcohol.

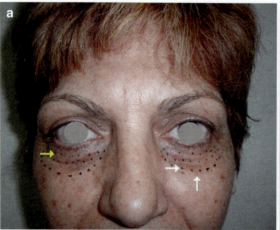
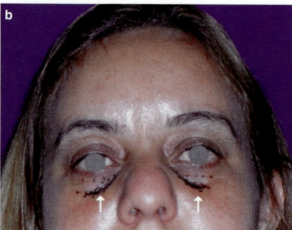

Fig. 53.2 (**a**) *Yellow arrow*: location of the anterior lip of the bony orbital rim. *White arrow*: the area to be treated is marked delimiting to the lower and upper borders of the tear trough and the eyelid–cheek groove. (**b**) *White arrow*: the area to be treated is marked delimiting to the lower and upper borders of the tear trough

53.4 The Injection

Under a bright overhead light and with patient's chair reclined 30° from vertical position, and with the head firmly resting against a solid headrest, the injections begin. The patients are permitted to close their eyes. The goal is to place aliquots of filler in the preperiosteal tissues just inferior to the orbital rim. The filler is introduced by using a serial puncture technique with a 30 gauge needle supplied with the medication (Fig. 53.3). Approximately 0.1 ml is injected at each pass. The needle is withdrawn and the filler is molded to the desired contour. The deepest part of the medial tear trough is treated first and, as the depression becomes less deep, parallel amounts of fillers are injected cephalad and caudal to the first injection until all area is corrected (Fig. 53.4).

If a bruise is noted to be forming, the needle is quickly withdrawn and a gentle pressure is applied to the local area with a cotton tip applicator. If the needle is placed too superficially, visible lumps or wheals of the hyaluronic acid gel will form. It is important to avoid depositing large volumes of the filler in one location. Rather, a gentle continuous pressure is applied to the syringe plunger after the needle touches the periosteal tissue and slowly withdrawn, creating multiple fine vertical stacked deposits, creating smooth three-dimensional contour.

At the conclusion of the procedure, determined by the end points of a successful accomplishment of the goal of artistic filling of the hollow contours, a massage of the treated areas is performed by the surgeon to mold to the desired contour. Afterwards the patient is discharged, and the postoperative instructions consisted of a massage of the treated areas if the patient notices any irregularity in the contour, cold compress on the eyelids for 2 days, makeup to conceal any bruising, and no restrictions on activities is imposed. The patient is scheduled to return to the office in 7 days. When the treated area is reevaluated and if required a touch-up is done.

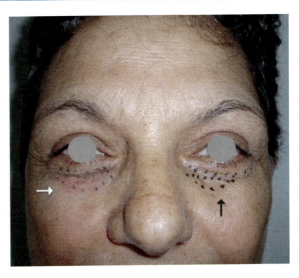

Fig. 53.4 *White arrow* indicates the side treated with HA gel filler. *Black arrow* shows the tear trough before injection

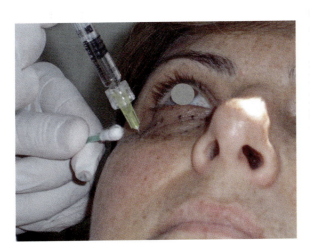

Fig. 53.3 Injection of the hyaluronic acid gel filler below the orbital rim

53.5 Complications

Complications included some degree of bruising, 52% (78/150); erythema, 50% (75/150); local swelling, 8% (12/150); pain at injection site, 4% (6/150); and migraine, 1.3% (2/150). Transient swelling in the lower eyelid is expected for 1 or 2 days. In five cases, persistent swelling was related to bruising and did not resolve until the bruise disappeared. In seven additional cases, swelling subsided after an additional day of observation with no intervention.

53.6 Discussion

The results of this technique are primarily visual (Figs. 53.5–53.8). Approximately 150 subjects have been treated, with the effect of treatment lasting up to

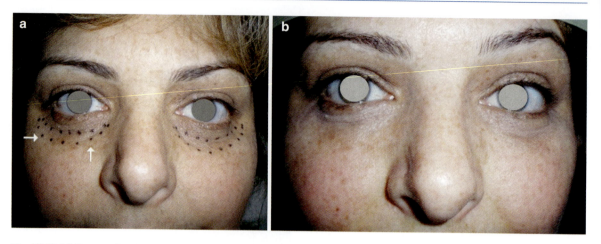

Fig. 53.5 (**a**) Preoperative 45-year-old female with tear trough deformity and the eyelid–cheek groove. (**b**) One and a half years after treatment

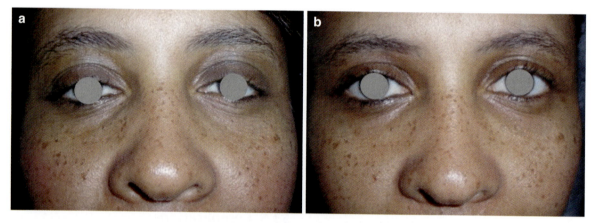

Fig. 53.6 (**a**) Preoperative 38-year-old female with tear trough deformity. (**b**) One year after treatment

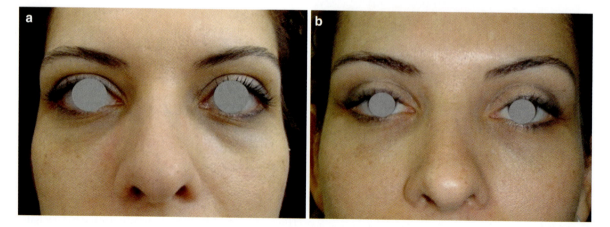

Fig. 53.7 (**a**) Preoperative 25-year-old female with tear trough deformity. (**b**) Eight months after treatment

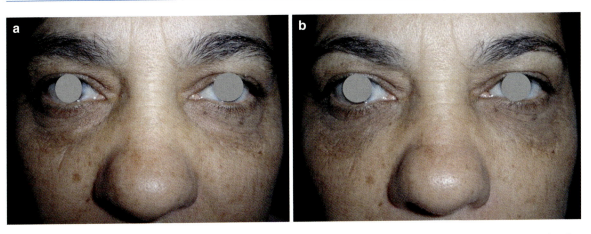

Fig. 53.8 (a) Preoperative 56-year-old female with tear trough deformity and the eyelid–cheek groove. (b) Seven months after treatment

18 months. Patients are told that they will be improved but not perfect. The older and more crepe-like the skin, the less well the treatment works. The mean age was 46.1 (26–62) with 2% male.

The total injection volume per side (baseline + touch-ups) needed to achieve correction of the tear trough was on the right side was 0.63 ml (SD = 0.37) and on the left side 0.6 ml (SD = 0.3). There was a large range in the amount of product used to correct the tear trough, spanning from 0.1 to 2 ml on the right side and on the left side from 0.2 to 1.2 ml. Of the 150 subjects, 15 received a touch-up injection 1 month later. Flowers [15] was the surgeon who described the tear trough saying that, "The deep groove that commonly occurs near the junction of the eyelid and the cheek is the most consistently ignored major deformity of the orbital region. With a characteristic length of about 2 cm, it extends downward and lateral from the inner canthus of the eye…whether limited or extended it gives the face a dissipated, unhealthy, and tired – even haggard-appearance" [15].

The cause of the tear trough deformity is multifactorial, and separating its components exactly may be difficult. The main components of the tear trough are the hollow itself, the fat bulge just superior to it, and the very distinct change of skin quality, color, and thickness between the lid and the cheek [7, 16].

Injectable dermal fillers are rapidly challenging and complementing the market of more invasive cosmetic surgical procedures. Dermal fillers have different tissue-compatibility characteristics that determine their suitability. Thus, no single filler is "ideal" for applications, but certain desirable filler qualities are generally accepted, such as safe and effective; it should be biocompatible, nonimmunogenic, easily obtainable, nonreabsorbable, low in cost, and easily stored. It should be easy to remove if necessary [12–14].

A number of investigators have explored the use of cross-linked stabilized nonanimal hyaluronic acid gel filler to treat the tear trough [7, 9, 16, 17]. Kane described his personal method that places HA gel filler (Restylane®) between the skin and the orbicularis oculi muscle [7]. Goldberg and Fiaschetti demonstrated a method in which they use multiples threads of HA gel filler (Restylane®) injected under the orbicularis oculi muscle [9]. Lambros showed his experience of treating the tear trough with HA gel filler placed in the orbicularis oculi muscle and at the periosteum (1q6) [16]. Steinsapir and Steinsapir reported a 2-year experience of treating the naso-jugal groove (tear trough) with Restylane®, using a deep-fill method [17]. All these methods require considerable experience to achieve acceptable result. The superficial method can easily produce skin irregularities while the deep-fill method places a premium on the skin, maximizing tissue covering and minimizing the risk of intravascular injection. The author prefers to inject HA gel filler in the preperiosteal tissues. With experience, there appear to be some anatomic situations that benefit from a more superficial placement of filler.

One of the concerns of the patient is the durability of the product, usually I explain that the manufacturer states that will be approximately 6–9 months, but what the author has seen in the initial experience is that the effect has persisted for 18 months, and during this time no additional injections were needed. Only few patients needed additional injections, and all were treated 1 month after the first injection. Goldberg and Fiaschetti described that substantial residual effect was noted even at 12 months [9]. Cossío and Oreja noted that HA filler gel (Restylane®) remained basically unchanged 8 months after implantation [12]. Lambros observed that HA gel filler had very long-lasting (1 year or more) effect in the tear trough [16].

Although the goal of HA gel filler products is to enhance one's appearance, there have been some adverse reactions that can occur. The most common reactions described are local edema, erythema, tenderness, bruising, fullness, and contour irregularity [9, 11–14, 17, 18]. The author observed that several patients have had irregularities that were massaged away either at the time of injection or several days later. When irregularities occur, they are usually treatable with massage. The closer one inspects the area, the more effects of the injection that can be seen. Social and casual inspection reveals a smooth contour. If one looks very closely, one can see the sites injected by virtue of very subtle changes in the reflectivity of the skin and its contours. Typically, patients do not notice this degree of imperfection.

Few patients may also present with bluish discoloration in treated areas caused by injections that are placed too superficially. This discoloration can present as a bluish, grayish, or yellowish tint underneath the skin, and it has been known as the Tyndall effect [9–11, 19]. Some surgeons advocate the use of hyaluronidase to solve this problem [9, 19–21]. Others prefer the 1,064 nm Nd:YAG laser to resolve it [22], while Dean & Jacob prefer to extract the superficially placed HA with #11 blade [19].

Much feared is the possibility of an intra-arterial injection, with skin injury or even blindness. The incidence is unknown and at this time there are no reported cases of blindness with HA, although there are a few cases of intra-arterial injection with skin injury [9, 16, 17]. However, the risk of retrograde embolization and consequently visual loss exists with all fillers. Occlusion of the ophthalmic artery with permanent visual loss has been reported with the use of bovine collagen, micronized dermal matrix, injection of autologous fat, silicone oil, and corticosteroids injected into eyelid lesions and nasally [9, 17].

53.7 Conclusions

Periorbital aging often involves soft tissue deflation. Although there is a role for conservatively removing tissue in some patients, almost all patients can benefit from some filling. Even though HA gel filler does not address the root causes of the tear trough, it certainly can improve it without surgery.

The author's opinion is that the use of HA in the tear trough has the following benefits: injection is relatively easy to perform; there is a high degree of patient satisfaction; the material is very long-lasting in the tear trough; most complications are self-limiting and can be easily treated; in the event of an unsatisfactory effect, the material can be dissolved away. Of course there are some disadvantages as follows: it is not permanent and there are no associated improvements in the lower eyelid.

The author was pleased to note an improvement in tear trough deformity in all cases, and all patients were very satisfied with their results. The main indication for leveling the tear trough is the presence of enough deformity to make a visual difference by its improvement.

References

1. Fagien S, Raspaldo H. Facial rejuvenation with botulinum neurotoxin: an anatomical and experiential perspective. J Cosmet Laser Ther. 2007;9 Suppl 1:23–31.
2. Goldberg RA, McCann JD, Fiaschetti D, Simon GJB, Codner MA. What causes eyelid bags? Analysis of 114 consecutive patients. Plast Reconstr Surg. 2005;115(5): 1395–402.
3. Goldberg RA. The three periorbital hollows: a paradigm for periorbital rejuvenation (editorial). Plast Reconstr Surg. 2005;116(6):1796–804.
4. Hirmand H, Codner MA, McCord CD, Hester TR, Nahai F. Prominent eye: operative management in lower lid and midfacial rejuvenation and the morphologic classification system. Plast Reconstr Surg. 2002;110(2):620–8.
5. Pessa JE. An algorithm of facial aging: verification of Lambro's theory by three-dimensional stereolithography, with reference to the pathogenesis of midfacial aging, scleral show, and the lateral suborbital trough deformity. Plast Reconstr Surg. 2000;106(2):479–88.
6. Lambros V. Observations on periorbital and midface aging. Plast Reconstr Surg. 2007;120(5):1367–74.
7. Kane MA. Treatment of tear trough deformity and lower lid bowing with injectable hyaluronic acid. Aesthetic Plast Surg. 2005;29(5):363–7.
8. Loeb R. Fat pad sliding and fat grafting for leveling lid depressions. Clin Plast Surg. 1981;8(4):757–76.

9. Goldberg RA, Fiaschetti D. Filling periorbital hollows with hyaluronic acid gel: initial experience with 244 injections. Ophthal Plast Reconstr Surg. 2006;22(5):335–43.
10. Levy PM, De Boulle K, Raspaldo H. Comparison of injection comfort of a new category of cohesive hyaluronic acid filler with preincorporated lidocaine and a hyaluronic acid filler alone. Dermatol Surg. 2009;35 Suppl 1:332–7.
11. Dover JS, Rubin MG, Bhatia AC. Review of the efficacy, durability, and safety data of two nonanimal stabilized hyaluronic acid fillers from a prospective, randomized, comparative, multicenter study. Dermatol Surg. 2009;35 Suppl 1:322–31.
12. Fernandez-Cossío S, Castana-Oreja MT. Biocompatibility of two novel dermal fillers: histological evaluation of implants of a hyaluronic acid filler and a polyacrylamide filler. Plast Reconstr Surg. 2006;117(6):1789–96.
13. Kablik J, Monheit GD, Yu L, Chang G, Gershkovich J. Comparative physical properties of hyaluronic acid dermal fillers. Dermatol Surg. 2009;35 Suppl 1:302–12.
14. Carruthers J, Cohen SR, Joseph JH, Narins RS, Rubin M. The science and art of dermal fillers for soft-tissue augmentation. J Drugs Dermatol. 2009;8(4):335–50.
15. Flowers RS. Tear trough implants for correction of tear trough deformity. Clin Plast Surg. 1993;20(2):403–15.
16. Lambros VS. Hyaluronic acid injections for correction of the tear trough deformity. Plast Reconstr Surg. 2007;120 (6 Suppl):74S–80S.
17. Steinsapir KD, Steinsapir SMG. Deep-fill hyaluronic acid for the temporary treatment of the naso-jugal groove: a report of 303 consecutive treatments. Ophthal Plast Reconstr Surg. 2006;22(5):344–8.
18. Carruthers JD, Glogau RG, Blitzer A, Facial Aesthetics Consensus Group Faculty. Advances in facial rejuvenation: botulinum toxin type A, hyaluronic acid dermal fillers, and combination therapies – consensus recommendations. Plast Reconstr Surg. 2008;121(5 Suppl):5 S–30S
19. Douse-Dean T, Jacob CI. Fast and easy treatment for reduction of the Tyndal effect secondary to cosmetic use of hyaluronic acid. J Drugs Dermatol. 2008;7(3):281–3.
20. Brody HJ. Use of hyaluronidase in the treatment of granulomatous hyaluronic acid reactions or unwanted hyaluronic acid placement. Dermatol Surg. 2005;31(8 Pt 1):893–7.
21. Soparkar CN, Patrinely JR, Tschen J. Erasing restylane. Ophthal Plast Reconstr Surg. 2004;20(4):317–8.
22. Hirsch RJ, Narurkar V, Carruthers J. Management of injected hyaluronic acid induced Tyndall effects. Lasers Surg Med. 2006;38(3):202–4.

Combined Technique in Otoplasty

Marzia Salgarello

54.1 Introduction

Protruding or prominent ears are a common congenital deformity of the external ear with an incidence rate of 5% which is inherited as an autosomal dominant trait [1, 2]. Interestingly, Matsuo [3] observed that the percentage of protruding ears is 0.4% at birth and increases up to 5.5% at 1 year of age, relating the rate increase to the position of the baby head in the first days of life. He presumes that, when the baby turns its head to one side, the weight of the head keeps the ear folded thus increasing the prominent ear rate.

The normal ear develops in utero between the fifth and the ninth week: the auricular anomalies developing by the tenth week are caused by embryologic maldevelopment and are categorized as malformational auricular anomalies. Those developed in utero after the tenth week (i.e., when the ear is fully developed) or even after the birth result from deformational forces and are considered deformational auricular anomalies [4].

The first group of ear anomalies consists of true malformations with deficient and/or supernumerary auricular components, and comprises from anotia and microtia to auricular sinuses and tags.

Deformational auricular anomalies are caused by abnormal physical forces (from imbalance of the auricular muscles to abnormal positioning) that act on an embryologically normal ear structure. The deforming forces act on a malleable auricular framework, altering its shape. They include the less severe anomalies, which form the majority of the congenital auricular anomalies, such as prominent ears, Stahl deformity, and lop and cup ears.

From an anatomical point of view, the intrinsic and extrinsic auricular muscles stabilize the auricular cartilage. The intrinsic muscles of the anterior auricular surface are the tragicus, the antitragus, and the helicis major and minor muscles. The intrinsic muscles of the posterior auricular surface are the intrinsic transverse and oblique muscles. An interesting theory about the etiology of prominent ears postulates that the prevailing of one among the intrinsic muscles, the antitragus muscle, could exert an anterior pull on the tail of the helicis that contributes to the flattening of the antihelix [5]. These authors, examining the presence and quality of the antitragus muscle when correcting prominent ears, found an inverse correlation with the degree of antihelical folding. When the antitragus muscle was well-developed it was associated with a less-formed antihelical fold. Other Authors also believe that aberrant insertion of the auricular muscles into the auricular cartilage may lead to abnormal muscle vectors which drive to the deformation of the cartilage [3, 6].

As prominent ears have fully developed chondrocutaneous components, they can be manipulated to reach a normal shape. Auricular molding with splinting and taping is an effective way of treating this deformity if started within 3 days of birth [3] and continued for up to 6 months [7, 8]. The pliability of the auricular cartilage in this early period is probably due to the high level of maternal estrogens in the baby [9]. The nonsurgical correction usually requires 1 week in order to obtain the normal shape then it takes months to stabilize it.

Prominent ears show a combination of underdevelopment of the antihelix and overdevelopment of the concha of different degree. Moreover, prominent ears

M. Salgarello
Department of Plastic Surgery, General Surgery Institute, Catholic University of the Sacred Heart, Largo Gemelli 8, 00168 Rome, Italy
e-mail: m.salgarello@mclink.it

show an increased conchoscaphal angle (over 90°) and an increased cephaloauricular distances (superior, medial, inferior). The deformity is usually bilateral, sometimes showing different degrees of the anomaly in the two sides, rarely monolateral.

During plastic surgery consultation, the surgeon has to assess the defect of each ear including the thickness of the auricular cartilage, pointing out the differences between the two sides. The discussion should involve options of correction and the fundamental element of personal motivation. As the patient perception of the deformity is usually very high, each characteristic of the anomaly has to be analyzed in detail with the patient explaining the possibility of the surgery.

At preschool age children do not note this deformity so much, thus they do not suffer from the psychological trauma yet. Moreover, 85% of the auricular growth is completed by 3 years of age, and 90–95% of adult size is achieved by 5 years of age [10, 11] making this time the ideal age for surgery.

The situation changes when the children start social or school activities and the prominent ears become a source of teasing from the other children. At this age the anatomic deformity of the ear can cause such a psychological alteration (personality vulnerability, emotional instability, and very low self-esteem) to recommend the prompt surgical correction [12]. In the adolescence, during which psychological instability can be worsened by an aesthetic deformity such as the prominent ear, and in the adults, where the protruding ears could represent the trauma of an uncomfortable adolescence or even childhood, the psychological perception of the deformity makes the motivation and expectation of surgery very high. It may leave a patient dissatisfied even in case of successful operation from a surgical point of view. Therefore, the surgical correction is now encouraged before school-age without fear of interfering with the growth of the operated ear [13, 14]. Instead, in the majority of cases, they are treated surgically during childhood or even adolescence.

Otoplasty is the surgical correction of the prominent ears, with the aim to restore the normal anatomic features. It has to produce:

1. A smooth, rounded, and well-defined antihelix fold, with the helical rim slightly protruding beyond the antihelix (i.e., being slightly visible from the front view)
2. A concho-scaphal angle of 90°
3. Reduction of conchal excess and reduction of the angle between concha and mastoid
4. Reduction of the cephaloauricular distances
5. Correction of abnormal position of the lobule (if the lobule projection is beyond the helical rim)

Table 54.1 McDowell and Wright's goals of otoplasty (McDowell, Richards)

- All trace of protrusion in the upper one-third of the ear must be corrected. (Some remaining protrusion in the middle third or lower portions may be acceptable, provided the superior aspect is thoroughly corrected; however the reverse does not hold true)
- From the front view, the helix of both ears should be seen beyond the antihelix (at least down the midear and preferably all the way)
- The helix should have a smooth and regular line throughout
- The postauricular sulcus should not be markedly decreased or distorted
- Protrusion should measure between 15 and 20 mm from the helix to the head
- Position of the two ears (i.e. distance from the lateral border to the head should be within 3 mm at any given point)

The analysis of the outcome after the surgical correction of the prominent ears can follow one or more of the following criteria:

- Objective assessment such as McDowell and Wright's goals of otoplasty [15, 16] (Table 54.1)
- Subjective assessment by the surgical team, the patients, their parents

Innumerable surgical techniques have been proposed for the treatment of prominent ears. The multitude of surgical approaches indicates that there is not one definitive technique able to correct all the degrees of the deformities of prominent ears. The ideal technique should be simple, effective, adaptable for the correction of every deformity, successful and with a low complication rate. The technique presented here follows these parameters: it combines elements of various techniques in a graduated approach that is based on anatomical demand [17].

54.2 Technique

The preoperative assessment of the characteristics of the malformation, especially in terms of shape and consistency of the ear cartilage on both sides, is important because it allows the technique to be individually adjusted for each ear.

According to what is needed, surgery can be performed on one ear alone or on both ears, and the surgical techniques can be different on the two sides. In case of severe deformity on one side with minimal anomaly on the other side, we prefer to operate on both sides to achieve a more symmetrical result.

Prophylactic antimicrobacterial agents are used at the beginning of the operation. The surgery is usually done under local anesthesia with sedation. In young children a general anesthetic may be required. In each case infiltration with Xylocaine 1% and adrenaline 1:100,000 is performed on the posterior surface of the ear and on the anterior surface over the antihelix and the concha. This is for a bloodless field and makes undermining of the skin easier.

The helical rim is folded back against the head to visualize the area of the new antihelix which is marked with methylene blue (Fig. 54.1). A linear surgical incision is done on the posterior surface of the ear on the posterior projection of the new antihelical fold, 1–1.5 cm above the retroauricular fold, without removing any skin (Fig. 54.2). In fact, it is not necessary to excise the skin to affect the correction of the auricular cartilage. Cutaneous undermining of the posterior surface of the ear is performed up to the tail of the antihelix inferiorly and laterally toward the helical rim to widely expose the auricular cartilage. The wide exposure helps in positioning of the sutures in order to bend the cartilage of the antihelix.

Accurate hemostasis is performed. Now, a mosquito is inserted at the level of the antitragus–helical fissure (i.e. the fissure located between antitragus and tail of the helix) (Fig. 54.3) to bluntly elevate a tunnel

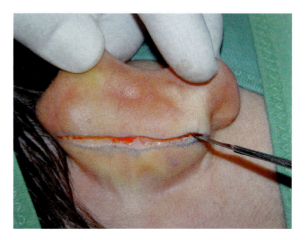

Fig. 54.2 A linear surgical incision is done on the posterior surface of the ear, about 1 cm above the retroauricular fold, without removing any skin

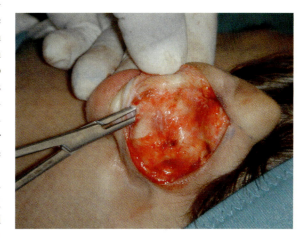

Fig. 54.3 A mosquito is inserted in the antitragus–helical fissure (i.e. the fissure located between the antitragus and the tail of the helix)

from the posterior aspect of the ear toward the anterior surface of the ear. The Stenström otoabrader (Fig. 54.4) is inserted in this tunnel (Fig. 54.5) and is directed toward the anterior surface of the ear in the subcutaneous plane, where the corresponding antihelix is to be formed (Fig. 54.6). Here the perichondrium and cartilage of the antihelix and scapha are rasped making the cartilage more pliable to achieve the correct curve. A careful scoring of the tail of the antihelix and medially scoring toward the concha weakens the cartilage at this level, which is thicker than in the upper third of the ear. This maneuver allows to medialize the tail of the antihelix and to turn the ear lobe toward the mastoid.

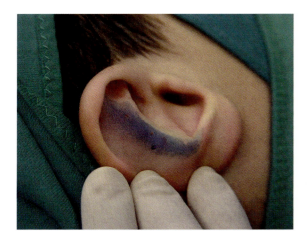

Fig. 54.1 The helical rim is folded back against the head to shape the new antihelix that is marked with methylene blue

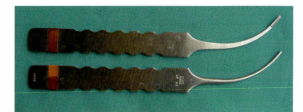

Fig. 54.4 Right and left Stenström otoabraders

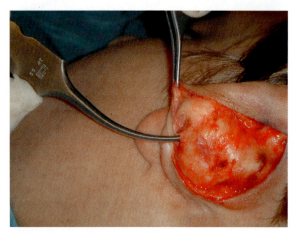

Fig. 54.5 The Stenström otoabrader is inserted at the level of the antitragus–helical fissure to be directed toward the anterior surface of the ear

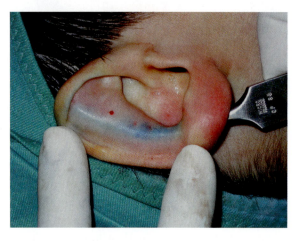

Fig. 54.6 The Stenström otoabrader has been inserted in the subcutaneous plane of the anterior surface of the ear, where the corresponding antihelix is to be formed

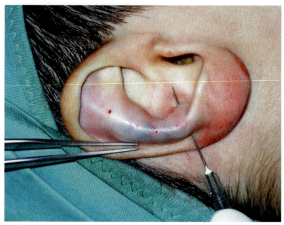

Fig. 54.7 A straight needle dipped in methylene blue is passed through and through the cartilage to mark the inferior pair of points at the tail of the antihelix

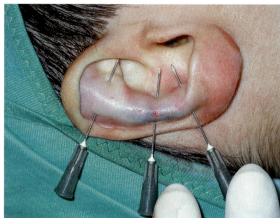

Fig. 54.8 Three straight needles dipped in methylene blue are passed to mark three pairs of points on the skin of the anterior surface of the ear

The helix of the ear is now pressed toward the mastoid to create the correct fold of the antihelix.

Straight needles dipped in methylene blue are passed through and through to mark the cartilage posteriorly with three pairs of points starting inferiorly (Fig. 54.7): the inferior pair of points are set through the tail of antihelix, on the scaphal and on the conchal side, the intermediate points are put down the bifurcation of the antihelix, on the scaphal and on the conchal side, the upper pair of points are placed between the triangular pit and the scapha to delineate the crus lateralis of the antihelix (Figs. 54.8 and 54.9). These pairs of points indicate the position of the mattress sutures that will be tied on the posterior surface of the antihelix to form the antihelix itself.

Three 3–0 Vicryl sutures are now passed through the posterior surface of the cartilage with partial thickness bites (Fig. 54.10) and tied, determining the bending of the antihelix (Fig. 54.11).

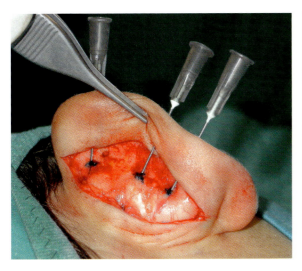

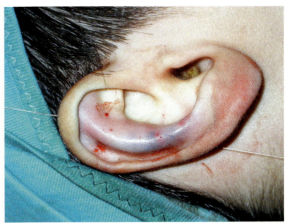

Fig. 54.11 The three sutures have been tied to determine the curve of the antihelix

Fig. 54.9 The three pairs of points already tattooed are visible on the posterior surface of the ear

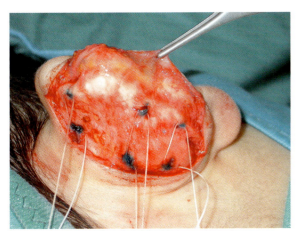

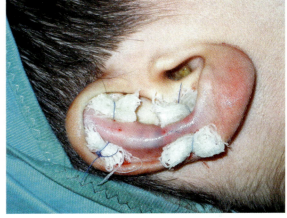

Fig. 54.10 Three sutures are passed through the posterior surface of the cartilage with partial thickness bites

Fig. 54.12 Three transfixion sutures over gauze pads are placed on the anterior surface of the ear to stabilize the curve of the antihelix

It is important to overcorrect the tail of the antihelix moving it medially toward the concha, thus decreasing the conchoscaphal angle and reducing the medial and inferior cephaloauricular distances. It helps in shaping the antihelix and is mainly important to control the positioning of the lobule thus preventing its possible protrusion. The correct positioning of these mattress sutures represents the key point of the operation, because if properly positioned they allow the reorientation of the ear.

If it is necessary to correct a very deep concha, this is done by excising a small crescent of full thickness cartilage (width between 2 and 6 mm) at the junction of the floor and posterior wall of the concha. The edges of this crescent are widely undermined to move them closer. No sutures are needed.

The incision on the posterior surface of the ear is closed with interrupted sutures allowing blood drainage in case of small bleeding.

The curve of the antihelix is then stabilized with transfixion sutures over gauze pads on the anterior surface of the ear (Fig. 54.12). These help in further molding of the cartilage and in maintaining the cartilage in its new position for 10 days before they are removed. An elastic band is worn for about 2 weeks, for compression and prevention of hematomas, so that the patient does not make unintentional movements during sleep that can jeopardize the surgical result [18, 19].

The extent of the dissection implies the amount of postoperative edema: to reduce it the patient has to rest with the head on two pillows, and Arnica medication is used for 2 weeks postoperative.

54.3 Complications

Complications of otoplasty can be divided into early and late groups; each of them may be categorized as major or minor ones. Overall complication rates of otoplasty are low, and when they occur tend to be minor.

Early complications (from hours to days) include major complications such as hematomas, skin necrosis, wound infection, and infection of cartilage. All of these are dreaded ones and require prompt intervention. Minor complications such as a bleeding from the wound a few hours after surgery often require reoperation for exploration. Pain has to be prevented by the use of routine prophylactic analgesics, but excessive pain is a warning symptom as it may indicate a significant auricular hematoma, mandating immediate wound inspection. Pressure wound along the newly formed antihelix and especially at the tail of it may be caused by a too firm bandage and has to be avoided.

Late complications reveal themselves after weeks to months; they include recurrence or residual deformity often due to undercorrection, malposition of the superior crus of the antihelix due to overcorrection, keloids (Fig. 54.13) or hypertrophic scars, and suture extrusion. A peculiar surgical deformity is the telephone ear, due to failure to correct a prominent ear lobule while hypercorrecting the concha (Fig. 54.14) or to removing excessive skin from the middle third of the ear [20].

The most common late complication in the adult patient is patient dissatisfaction [21]. In case the surgery has been properly performed, it may be related to excessive expectation from surgery due to a peculiar psychological status. The preoperative discussion should have emphasized the possibility of slight asymmetries on side-to-side comparison that are considered acceptable.

In case we face a true recurrence of the deformity, it has to be reminded that the cartilage elasticity decreases with advancing age, which may give a higher risk of prominent ear recurrence at this age, thus demanding a more aggressive treatment of the cartilage in patients undergoing otoplasty as adults.

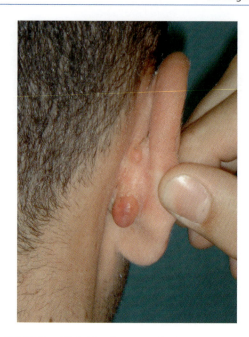

Fig. 54.13 Small keloid at the retroauricular scar

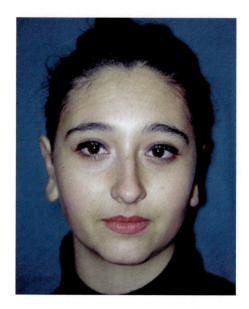

Fig. 54.14 Telephone ear deformity, possibly due to excessive excision of conchal cartilage

Many complications tend to be technically dependent ones. Acute crests and irregular contours along the fold of the antihelix with a tendency to overcorrection are typical deformities seen with the techniques that interrupt the continuity of the cartilage [2, 20] (Figs. 54.15 and 54.16). These residual deformities

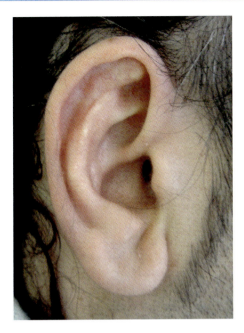

Fig. 54.15 Sharp cartilage edge on the upper part of the antihelical fold after correction of prominent ears with a cartilage cutting technique

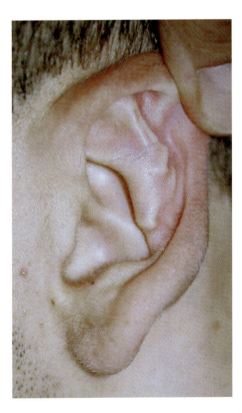

Fig. 54.16 Many acute crests and irregular contour are visible along the antihelix fold after correction of prominent ear with a technique that interrupts the continuity of the cartilage

require secondary correction surgery. They occurred in the past in up to 24% of cases [22], and are rarer today as the interruption of the cartilage is rarely performed.

Suture-related techniques were reported to have suture extrusion in 12.5% of cases [16], and a higher recurrence rate [2, 23]. As suture extrusion is related to the use of permanent sutures, the author's combined technique is recommended since scoring the cartilage helps to weaken it, thus allowing the use of not-permanent stitches for molding the cartilage and extrusion is rare. At present, many Authors agree that the combined techniques show a high success rate with a low complication rate [24].

54.4 Discussion

Over 200 otoplasty techniques have been described since the first otoplasty which is credited to Dieffenbach who used postauricular skin excision to correct prominent ear [25].

Surgical techniques can be grouped into procedures to create the antihelical fold, to correct the concha defect, and to control the position of the lobule. Those addressing the correction of the antihelix keep the fundamental step to correct the prominent ear. They can be grouped into cartilage-cutting techniques and cartilage-sparing techniques. With the cartilage-cutting techniques the cartilage may be incised either full thickness or partial thickness in the anterior or posterior side. They include the ancient methods of full-thickness incisions: a single incision in the posterior surface of the ear at the location of the proposed antihelical fold [26]; two parallel incisions on the posterior surface of the ear behind the antihelix to tube the island of cartilage in between that is secured with sutures to create the antihelical fold [27]; a scaphal incision on the posterior face of the ear to undermine the anterior surface of the cartilage in order to expose it for direct scoring of the antihelical cartilage, then folding the cartilage back and fixing it with buried sutures [28]; two parallel incisions on the posterior surface of the ear behind the antihelix to create a crescent of cartilage, the edges of the adjoining remaining cartilage are undermined and sutured together just under the cartilage crescent to create the antihelix [29, 30]. These methods retain the risk of creating visible contour irregularities and/or sharp edges.

The scoring techniques are partial-thickness methods based on the original observation of Gibson and Davies that cartilage bends away from the side of injury [31]. Following them Stenstrom [32] scored cadaveric auricular cartilage on one side and observed the cartilage curving away from the direction of the scoring. Thus he described scoring the anterior surface of the ear cartilage to create the antihelical fold. He also showed that deeper furrowing resulted in more profound bending.

Many instruments were then used for anterior scoring including rasp, abraders, Adson-Brown forceps, and hypodermic needle [33]. Posterior scoring has been described too by dermabrasion to weaken the cartilage, combined with mattress sutures [34]. The validity of this approach was confirmed by the Weinzweig's studies [35] on rabbits that showed that anterior perichondrium rasping initiated a cartilage regeneration process over the convex surface of the newly created fold.

The cartilage-sparing techniques were developed to avoid the contour irregularities of the cartilage-cutting ones. They basically imply the use of sutures and the cartilage is not incised. Mustarde horizontal mattress sutures for antihelical folding date back to 1963 [36] and Furnas chonchal-mastoid suture for the concha set back and for derotating the ear was introduced in 1968 [37]. It consists of the use of a full-thickness mattress suture placed in the conchal cartilage sutured to the mastoid fascia.

Conchal hypertrophy may be corrected by Furnas suture, by repositioning the posterior auricular muscle [38], through an excision of a crescent of cartilage of the lateral wall, through scoring its anterior surface [2], or by a combination of techniques.

The lobule is the lower noncartilaginous portion of the auricle, the position of which is related to the position of the caudal helix to the conchal bowl. Lobule set back is a difficult objective [2, 23] and may be addressed through a fishtail skin excision [39], wedge-excision, and a deep dermis to scalp periosteum suture [40]. The author's approach to correct the lobule protrusion is through a medial repositioning of the caudal helix toward the concha by scoring the tail of the helix and then fixing it to the adjacent concha with the lower mattress Mustarde suture. This maneuver serves to retropose the lower third of the ear and to medialize the ear lobule as well.

From an historical point of view, after the description of the basic techniques, the combination of techniques to address the deformity started. In 1959, Farrier combined anterior scoring through two cartilaginous incision perpendicular to the antihelix with horizontal mattress sutures and conchal-mastoid suture after weakening the concha through the shaving of an elliptical disk of cartilage [41]. In 1967, Kaye combined cartilage anterior scoring with placement of mattress sutures through three longitudinal stab incisions in the anterior skin [42]. In 1982, Francesconi otoplasty combined anterior scoring with Mustarde sutures and extended the superficial scratching and mattress suture to the helical tail for the repositioning of the ear lobe [43].

Nowadays, otoplasty techniques are continuously modified and refined, and the more recent trend today is the use of a graduated approach that combines elements of various techniques to address the ear deformity [24]. Moreover, as in each person the two ears are neither equal nor symmetric, the surgical technique needs to be individualized.

With the technique presented here the author has attempted to overcome many drawbacks. It is a combined procedure, using the closed anterior scoring technique along with mattress sutures to the posterior cartilage, as it has already been described by some other authors such as Francesconi [43], and Bulstrode [33]. The abrasion of the anterior cartilage represents the best way to obtain a natural and harmonious profile of the ear. Then, the internal mattress sutures combined with external transfixed stitches are used for molding the antihelical fold, for long lasting stabilization and to avoid overcorrection or malposition.

As the author's approach is a graduated one which can be tailored to prominent ear of any grade, it also allows the correction of cup ears of mild degree. In case of cup ear, the feasibility of the technique is tested by bending the antihelix with digital pressure to create the new antihelical fold. If this maneuver corrects the deformity, it is possible to apply the technique for achieving the correction of the defect (Fig. 54.17).

Some technical points render the author's approach peculiar. The avoidance of postauricular skin excision helps in reducing the possibility of cheloids as the skin suture is tension-free. Skin preservation has also been advocated by Kelley et al. [23] to compensate the excessive skin retraction that can obliterate the postauricular sulcus or draw the midhelix into a hidden position on the front view. The use of the Stenstrom

Fig. 54.17 (**a1, a2**) Preoperative 9-year-old girl with right prominent ear and left cup ear of mild degree. (**b1, b2**) Six months postoperative showing the correction of the deformity

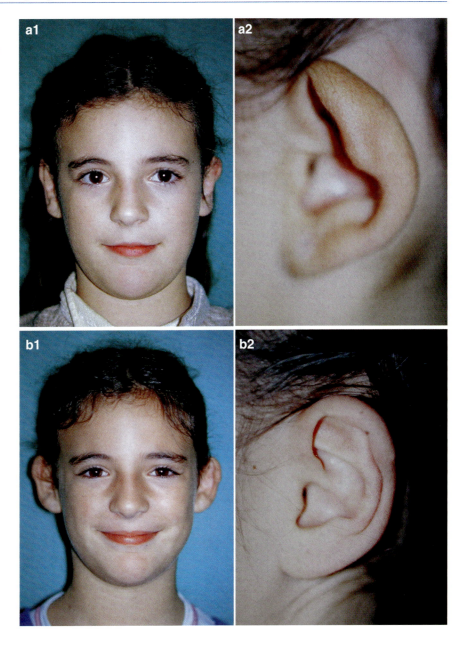

otoabrader that is a standard surgical instrument, makes the anterior scoring safer and more predictable than the modified needle used by Bulstrode and Martin or the Adson Brown forceps used for scoring of the Farrior technique. The use of methylene blue to accurately mark and tattoo the position of the mattress sutures is a useful addition that Francesconi did not describe. It also helps to standardize the method and makes the result more predictable.

Another important point of note is the anterior scoring of the tail of the antihelix and the anterior concha and the inferior mattress suture to derotate the inferior ear. It also turns the ear lobe toward the mastoid allowing a certain degree of repositioning of the ear lobe (Fig. 54.18). This technique allows us to obtain a harmonious antihelical contour with a smooth and well-rounded fold, avoiding cartilage irregularities or sharp edges (Figs. 54.19 and 54.20). It usually leaves the patients very satisfied.

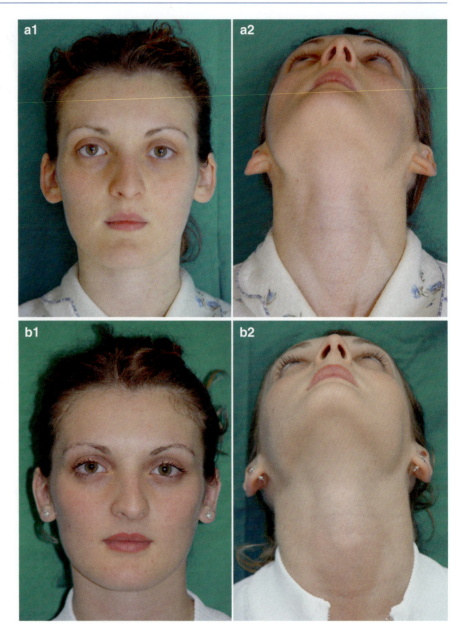

Fig. 54.18 (**a1, a2**) Preoperative 21-year-old woman showing lobule protrusion. (**b1, b2**) Eight months postoperative after lobule set-back by scoring of the tail of the antihelix and the anterior concha and positioning of the inferior mattress suture to derotate the inferior ear

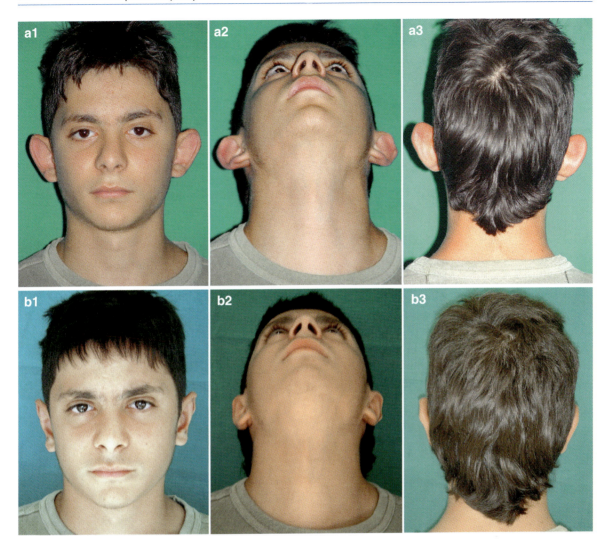

Fig. 54.19 (**a1, a2, a3**) Preoperative 10-year-old boy with prominent ears. (**b1, b2, b3**) One year postoperative

Fig. 54.20 (**a1, a2**) Preoperative 15-year-old boy with mildly asymmetrical prominent ears. (**b1, b2**) One year postoperative.

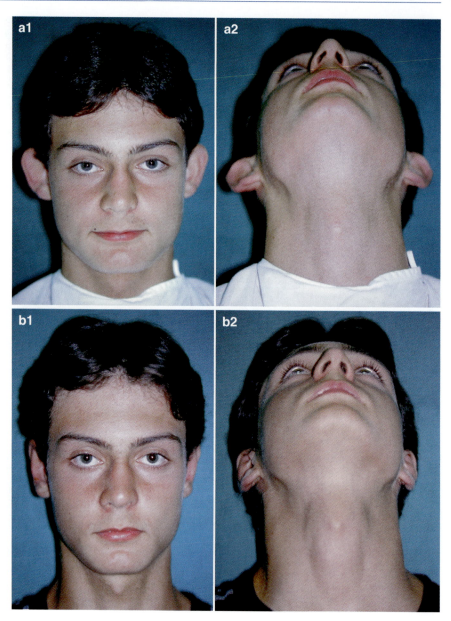

54.5 Conclusions

Otoplasty techniques include a large number of different methods, over 200 techniques, today restricted to the different combination of the elements of few basic techniques. The sunset of full-thickness methods is evident, as well as the current trend of the use of a graduated approach of combining the elements of various techniques.

The author utilizes a combination of techniques that are adapted to the anatomical needs of each deformity which gives natural and pleasant results and few complications. Their basic principles are presented as a graduated approach which is suitable to standardization, thus making this a simple, reliable, versatile, and reproducible method.

References

1. Kompatscher P, Schuler CH, Clemens S, Seifert B, Beer GM. The cartilage-sparing versus the cartilage-cutting technique: a retrospective quality control comparison of the Francesconi and Converse otoplasties. Aesthetic Plast Surg. 2003;27(6):446–53.
2. Janis JE, Rohrich RJ, Gutowsky KA. Otoplasty. Plast Reconstr Surg. 2005;115(4):60e–72e.
3. Matsuo K, Hayashi R, Kiyono M, Hirose T, Netsu Y. Non surgical correction of congenital auricular deformities. Clin Plast Surg. 1990;17(2):383–95.
4. Porter CJW, Tan ST. Congenital auricular anomalies: topographic anatomy, embryology, classification and treatment strategies. Plast Reconstr Surg. 2005;115(6):1701–12.
5. Bennett SPH, Dagash H, McArthur PA. The role of the antitragicus muscle in plical folding of the pinna. Plast Reconstr Surg. 2005;115(5):1266–8.
6. Guyuron B, De Luca L. Ear projection and the posterior auricular muscle insertion. Plast Reconstr Surg. 1997;100(2):457–60.
7. Tan ST, Shibu M, Gault DT. A split for correction of congenital ear. Br J Plast Surg. 1994;47(8):575–8.
8. Tan ST, Abramson DL, MacDonald DM, Mulliken JB. Molding therapy for infants with deformational auricular anomalies. Ann Plast Surg. 1997;38(3):263–8.
9. Matsuo K, Hirose T, Tomoro T, Iwisawa M, Katohda S, Takahashi N, et al. Nonsurgical correction of congenital auricular deformity. Plast Reconstr Surg. 1984;73(1):38–51.
10. Adamson PA, Galli SK. Otoplasty. In: Cummings CW, editor. Otolaryngology – head and neck surgery. 4th ed. Philadelphia: Elsevier Mosby; 2005. p. 853–61.
11. Adamson JE, Horton CE, Crawford HH. The growth pattern of the external ear. Plast Reconstr Surg. 1965;36(4):466–70.
12. Gasques JA, Pereira de Godoy JM, Cruz EM. Psychosocial effects of otoplasty in children with prominent ears. Aesthetic Plast Surg. 2008;32(6):910–4.
13. Gosain AK, Kumar A, Huang G. Prominent ears in children younger than 4 years of age: what is the appropriate timing for otoplasty? Plast Reconstr Surg. 2004;114(5):1042–54.
14. Balogh B, Millesi H. Are growth alterations a consequence of surgery for prominent ears? Plast Reconstr Surg. 1992;89(4):623–30.
15. McDowell AJ. Goals in otoplasty for protruding ears. Plast Reconstr Surg. 1968;41(1):17–27.
16. Richards SD, Jebreel A, Capper R. Otoplasty: a review of the surgical techniques. Clin Otolaryngol. 2005;30(1):2–8.
17. Salgarello M, Gasperoni C, Montagnese A, Farallo E. Otoplasty for prominent ears: a versatile combined technique to master the shape of the ear. Otolaryngol Head Neck Surg. 2007;137(2):224–7.
18. Lavy J, Stearns M. Otoplasty: techniques, results and complications – a review. Clin Otolaryngol Allied Sci. 1997;22(5):390–3.
19. Calder JC, Nassan A. Morbidity of otoplasty: a review of 562 consecutive cases. Br J Plast Surg. 1994;47(3):170–4.
20. Nuara MJ, Mobley SR. Nuances of otoplasty: a comprehensive review of the past 20 years. Facial Plast Surg Clin North Am. 2006;14(2):89–102.
21. Adamson PA, Litner JA. Otoplasty technique. Otolaryngol Clin North Am. 2007;40(2):305–18.
22. Stucker FJ, Vora NM, Lian TS. Otoplasty: an analysis of technique over a 33-year period. Laryngoscope. 2003;113(6):952–6.
23. Kelley P, Hollier L, Stal S. Otoplasty: evaluation, technique, and review. J Craniofac Surg. 2003;14(5):643–53.
24. Petersson RS, Friedman O. Current trends in otoplasty. Facial Plast Surg. 2008;16(4):352–8.
25. Dieffenbach JE. Die Operative Chirurgie. Leipzig: FA Brockhause; 1845.
26. Luckett WH. A new operation for prominent ears based on the anatomy of the deformity. Surg Gynecol Obstet. 1910;10:635.
27. Converse JM, Nigro A, Wilson FA, Johnson N. A technique for surgical correction of lop ears. Plast Reconstr Surg. 1955;15(5):411–8.
28. Chongchet V. A method of antihelix reconstruction. Br J Plast Surg. 1963;16:268–72.
29. Pitanguy I, Rebello C. Ansiform ears. Correction by "island" technique. Acta Chir Plast. 1962;4:267–77.
30. Pitanguy I, Fiazza G, Calixto CA, et al. Prominent ears – Pitanguy's island technique: long-term results. Head Neck Surg. 1985;7:418–26.
31. Gibson T, Davies W. The distortion of autogenous cartilage grafts: its cause and prevention. Br J Plast Surg. 1958;10:257.
32. Stenstroem SJ. A natural technique for correction of congenitally prominent ears. Plast Reconstr Surg. 1963;32:509–18.
33. Bulstrode NW, Huang S, Martin DL. Otoplasty by percutaneous anterior scoring. Another twist to the story: a long term study of 114 patients. Br J Plast Surg. 2003;56(2):145–9.
34. Pilz S, Hintringer T, Bauer M. Otoplasty using a spherical metal head dermabrader to form a retroauricular furrow: five-year results. Aesthetic Plast Surg. 1995;19(1):83–91.
35. Weinzweig N, Chen L, Sullivan WG. Histomorphology of neochondrogenesis after antihelical fold creation: a comparison of three otoplasty techniques in the rabbit. Ann Plast Surg. 1994;33(4):371–6.
36. Mustarde JC. The correction of prominent ears using simple mattress sutures. Br J Plast Surg. 1963;16:170–8.
37. Furnas DW. Correction of prominent ears by concha-mastoid sutures. Plast Reconstr Surg. 1968;42(3):189–93.
38. Scuderi N, Tenna S, Bitonti A, et al. Repositioning of posterior auricular muscle combined with conventional otoplasty: a personal technique. J Plast Reconstr Aesthet Surg. 2007;60:201–4.
39. Wood-Smith D. Otoplasty. In: Rees T, editor. Aesthetic plastic surgery. Philadelphia: W.B. Saunders; 1980. p. 833.
40. Spira M. Otoplasty: what I do now-a 30-year perspective. Plast Reconstr Surg. 1999;104(3):834–40.
41. Farrior RT. A method of otoplasty; normal contour of the antihelix and scaphoid fossa. AMA Arch Otolaryngol. 1959;69(4):400–8.
42. Kaye BL. A simplified method for correcting the prominent ear. Plast Reconstr Surg. 1967;40(1):44–8.
43. Francesconi G, Grassi C, Ciocchetti FC. La nostra esperienza nel trattamento chirurgico dell'orecchio ad ansa. Acta Otorhinolaryngol Ital. 1982;2:163–82.

Rhinoplasty

55

Vladimir Kljajic and Slobodan Savovic

55.1 Introduction

The nose is the most distinctive part of one's face, and its shape and size as well as possible deformities influence its aesthetics and distinction.

The idea of a beautiful nose has changed throughout history, and it is still relative nowadays for beauty is in the eye of the beholder. Unlike the idea of what makes one's nose beautiful, the idea of what makes one's nose symmetrical is easier to define thanks to existence of certain measures and index representing relations between certain anatomic facial structures. Symmetrical nose does not have to indicate a beautiful one, because nasal beauty is defined according to the whole face of an individual; so there are cases when a less symmetrical nose of one person can be more beautiful in relation to a symmetrical nose of another person.

The external nose is most often compared to threefold pyramid which is, by its surface, linked to the other parts of the face and is called the base of the nose. The root of the nose represents its link with the front. Nasal dorsum is the most prominent part of the pyramid. The length of the nose represents the distance from the root to the lower hem of nasal septum. The width of the nose represents the distance between two most distant symmetrical points of nasal wings. The relation between length and width is called nasal index.

In relation to nasal index, there are differences among races; so, white people most often have leptorrhine nose, black people have platyrrhine one, while yellow people have a mesorrhine one [1].

Aesthetically speaking, the nasal profile line is very important and it differs in the nasolabial and profile angles of the nose. The nasolabial angle shows the relation between outer bottom of the nose and frontal part of upper lip. The size of this angle, according to some authors, should be between 80° and 100° in men and 90° and 100° in women. This size influences the position of nasal entrance. Surgical correction of the angle size is often necessary, not only for aesthetic reasons, but also for functional reasons. Profile angle of the nose is formed by facial line and nasal dorsum line. On symmetrical noses this angle is 30°. Noses which have much smaller or much bigger angle than 30° are aesthetically impaired.

Besides these angles, the way nasal profile is linked to facial profile is very important in terms of aesthetics. In symmetrical noses, the size of the nasofrontal angle should be between 127° and 150°. We talk about the Greek nose when nasal profile goes almost directly into frontal profile. When there is greater or lesser recess between nasal root and the front, we can talk about the Roman nose, while the Nordic nose is characterized by a certain convexity degree of the dorsum.

55.2 Types of Nasal Deformity

Nasal deformities can be inborn or gotten throughout a lifetime. Besides thumb sucking, the most common nasal deformities are consequences of nasal injuries or personal massive injury. These injuries can occur during delivery time, in early childhood, or in adulthood. There are more and more injuries that are results of the traffic, industry, and sport development in modern society.

V. Kljajic (✉) and S. Savovic
ENT Clinic, Clinical Center of Vojvodina,
Hajduk Veljkova 1, Novi Sad, Serbia
e-mail: kljaja@eunet.rs; savovics@yahoo.com

Nasal deformities can be isolated or associated with the deformities of surrounding structures (eye, lips, and ear) [2]. Nasal deformities can be limited to bone deformities or deformities of cartilage structures, but they are most often deformities of both cartilage and bone structures.

There are numerous kinds of nasal deformities; although some are really scarce, some others are quite frequent in general population. One of the most frequent deformities is rhinokyphosis (nasal hump), where nasal dorsum is distorted to a greater or a lesser degree. Nasal hump is quite often without septal deviation. It is relatively easy to correct surgically [3].

Rhinoscoliosis is a kind of deformity with greater or lesser medium nasal lines curvatures. The bony pyramid leans to one side. It is asymmetric, with a short, steep slope on the side of the deviation and a long, shallow slope on the opposite side. The cartilaginous pyramid is deformed in a similar way. The triangular cartilages are asymmetric, especially when the trauma occurred in childhood years.

We deal with rhinolordosis in case of dorsum recess. If one's nose is too large (considering length and width) according to a certain face, we deal with macrorhinia, if only the length is too big, we have nasus longus, or if it is too wide, we can talk about the wide nose or pachyrhinia. Platyrrine means that the nose is flat and wide in wings. If the nose is too small in relation to the rest of the face, we have microrhinia. If the nose is too narrow, we deal with stenorhynia.

Isolated deformities of nasal tip are quite common, so we have: nasal tip protrusion (apex nasi prominens), lifted nasal tip (apex nasi excelsus), pointed nose (nasus acutus), obtuse nose (nasus obtusus), lowered nasal tip (ptosis apices nasi), and others.

Nasal wing deformities are quite frequent, the wings being too wide (ala nasi prominens) or too narrow due to weakly developed alar cartilage, so that inhaling can cause nasal wing aspiration (aspiration alarum nasi). Skin part of nasal septum can be lowered (protrusio septi) or widened (hypertonia phyltri). Luxation of lower nasal septum is quite frequent (luxation septi nasi). In case when nasolabial angle is significantly bigger than usual, we deal with nostril declination (declination orificii nasi), and when it is significantly smaller we deal with nostril inclination (inclinatio orificii nasi).

Nasal deformities that can be accurately classified into one of the above deformities are quite scarce. We usually have one leading deformity, while some others follow it and are associated with it.

A special group of deformities are deformities that are the consequences of upper lip fissure, upper jaw, and palate. Some typical disorders can also be manifested by deformities that occur during one's lifetime such as rhinophyma, nose elephantiasis, acromegaly, and others.

Rhinoplasty is a surgical procedure where nasal pyramid is formed according to other facial parts. This is acquired by greater or lesser bone or cartilage structure reduction, by autotransplant implantations or bone or cartilage heterotransplants. Besides these, other materials can also be used. Aesthetic nose surgery is usually combined with functional nose surgery, so nose surgeries for pure aesthetic reasons are quite scarce. Attempting to achieve the best postsurgical result, one cannot forget the main nose function, i.e., breathing. The postsurgical result is not acceptable if the nose is aesthetically beautiful but not functional. If we have a functional postsurgical nose, but not aesthetically beautiful, the result may not be satisfactory either way. It is not always easy to acquire both beautiful and functional noses, but it is a challenge for every surgeon to be knowledgeable, skillful, and experienced and this has to show in each individual case. Every patient and his/her nose represent an isolated case and a new challenge for the surgeon. It is highly important to keep blood circulation of the surgical area. Otherwise, tissue withering can occur or skin malnutrition, which can be manifested by cyanosis, especially in cold weather. In order to have a successful nose surgery both aesthetically and functionally, it is necessary to have a thorough preoperative preparation for every sort of superficiality and negligence can take an enormous toll in reconstructive surgery. Being unsatisfied with the shape of their noses, patients require an aesthetic surgery. Their wish has to be carefully studied and their surgeons should have long and cautious conversations with them prior to the surgery. Sometimes it is necessary to involve a psychologist or a psychiatrist before the surgery in order to make sure that patients' problems won't stay the same after the procedure, because their main problem is not deformity itself but it is their being insecure, scared, and with low self-esteem. Intelligent and well-educated patients are better prepared and better candidates for the surgery than the ones who only listen to what their surgeons have to say. They are expected to have better postsurgical results for they know exactly what they don't like about their looks and what to expect from the surgery. Patients who are less motivated for the surgery, the ones who have a lot of other unsolved issues in their lives, who are less intelligent, who see their surgeon because the members of their families or their friends told them so, are worse candidates for the surgery for they don't really know what they want and expect their surgeons to do wonders for them. Patients who are well motivated for the surgery and who know what to expect after the surgery, are better postoperative patients and in larger numbers show that they are satisfied with postsurgical period [4].

55.3 Preoperative Analysis

When a nose surgery is indicated, it is necessary for the patient to have some blood tests done as well as an internist exam. A thorough presurgical examination of the nose and throat is needed for every catarrh, let alone pustular inflammation, are absolute counter indications for the surgery. There are other factors because of which we cannot perform the surgery such as conjunctivitis, vestibulitis, and herpetic changes in the upper lip area, columella, or nasal wings. These infections can spread onto sinus cavernosus hematogenously by anastomoses between facial vein and ophthalmic vein. All the mentioned infections require a long-term treatment regardless of patients' pressure or patients' friends and family's pressure to perform the surgery as soon as possible [5].

It is necessary to perform a postsurgical nose examination both anterior and posterior, both profiles and the base of the nose as well as the face itself. Afterwards, it is necessary to do nose palpation as well as anterior and posterior rhinoscopy. In case of some vague results, it is necessary to do an endoscopic examination of the nose along with anemisation of nasal mucous membrane, measurements, functional examination of breathing function (rhinomanometry and acoustic rhinometry) [6]. It is necessary to do rhinomanometry and rhinometry before and after nasal mucous membrane anemisation because breathing difficulty can be the consequence of skeletal, mucous, or combined components. These tests can significantly solve the dilemma on the cause of breathing difficulties. Also, it is recommended for every postsurgical patient to undergo an olfactory examination.

Before every rhinoplastic surgery, it is necessary to take at least three photos which would include: profile, base of the face as well as anterior and posterior. Some authors insist on profile photos from the left and from the right, as well as additional photos, but the first three are highly necessary. The photos are necessary to develop the best plan of the surgery, to estimate the process of postsurgical healing having also in mind legal matters in cases of postsurgical lawsuits.

Prior to the surgery itself, it is necessary to explain the procedure to the patient and what can be expected in postsurgical period. A good postsurgical care is very important for it is also a significant factor in surgical results. Thus, with carefully chosen patients, a good presurgical preparation, and an adequate surgical technique that diminishes postsurgical complications, the success of the surgery and patients' satisfaction increase a lot.

Borges et al. [7] have found personality disorders in one-fifth of prospective rhinosurgical patients. There were no significant differences between the genders. Also, their findings state that one-half of surgical patients who underwent rhinoseptoplasty have experienced an increase in self-esteem, notably female patients.

55.4 Surgical Techniques

What we call rhinoplasty is an implementation of different surgical techniques aiming for aesthetic and functional nose change (Figs. 55.1–55.3). Surgical approach covers performing several intranasal or intranasal and extranasal incisions which enable reaching nasal infrastructure.

55.4.1 Incisions in Rhinoplasty

In order to get the easiest approach to nasal pyramid modeling, it is necessary to perform some incisions. The incision location depends on whether the surgery is open or closed. The most frequent nasal septum approach is done through hemitransfixion or transfixion incisions.

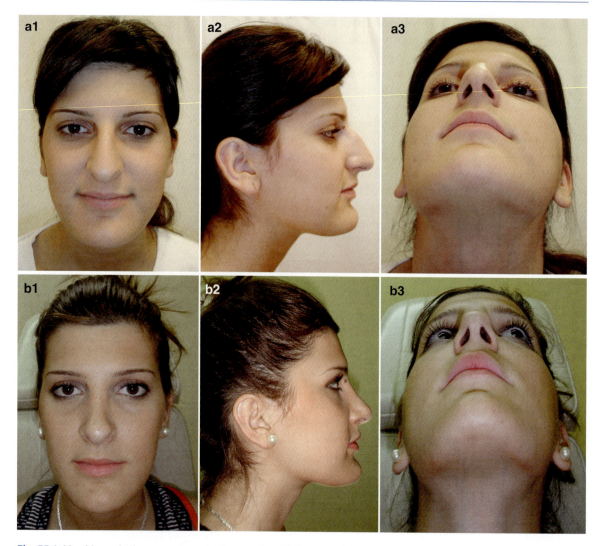

Fig. 55.1 Nasal hump in three proections. (**a**) Preoperative. (**b**) Postoperative

The difference between these two incisions depends on whether the whole thickness of septum in front of caudal edge of septic cartilage is cut or the incision is done only on one side of the septum. The right-handed people perform hemitransfixion incision on the right hand side, while the left-handed do it on the left hand side, although this routine could often be vice versa (Fig. 55.4).

Hemitransfixion incision is done from nasal dorsum toward spini nasalis anterior inferior. If intercartilaginous incision is done (Fig. 55.5), it is necessary to approach nasal dorsum. This incision is done in case of endonasal approach. The incision is performed on the link between alar and triangular cartilage in the area above nasal valvula in the so-called cul de sac so that the incision starts right above the free edge of triangular cartilage laterally and spreads over medially.

When both-sided intercartilaginous incision is done, it is possible to separate suprastructure from infrastructure. This incision enables an easy preparation of cephalic end of alar cartilages. The disadvantage of this incision is that it does not enable the surgeons to work on bifid tip and nasus bullosus.

Approaching alar cartilage is possible through marginal incision (infracartilaginous incision) that is done 1–2 mm in the parallel process with the edge of alar cartilage. This incision is used while decortication of nasal pyramid by widening medial crus of alar cartilage.

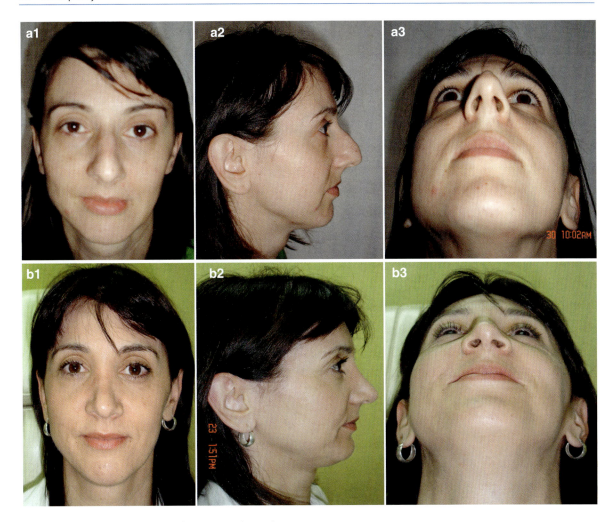

Fig. 55.2 (**a**) Preoperative patient. (**b**) Postoperative patient

Transcartilaginous incision is done through alar cartilage between intercartilaginous and marginal incisions. While performing this incision, a surgeon usually recesses the cephalic part of alar cartilage along with the patient's skin.

Transversal incision of the columella is used in nasal decortication and is often done on the link between lower and medium third of columella.

Vestibular incision is often used by rhino-surgeons who do not separate the complete suprastructure from infrastructure in order to perform lateral osteotomy.

Alar incision is used in cases when it is necessary to make the base of the nose narrow by recessing one part of nasal wing.

55.4.2 Osteotomies in Rhinoplasty

Osteotomy is a procedure in which bones are cut. Chisels and saws can be used. Modern rhinosurgery tends to cut a bone sharply leaving the least possible bone dust. Chisels are recommended for that purpose.

Osteotomies can be transcutaneous when Tardy chisels are used, sublabial when approached through upper vestibulum of the mouth, and endonasal that are most common.

According to the incision location of nasal pyramid, all osteotomies can be divided into: medial, paramedial, lateral, and transverse.

Medial osteotomy is usually performed in cases when the nasal hump is not to be removed. The chisel

Fig. 55.3 Rhinoscoliosis in two proections (**a**) Preoperative. (**b**) Postoperative

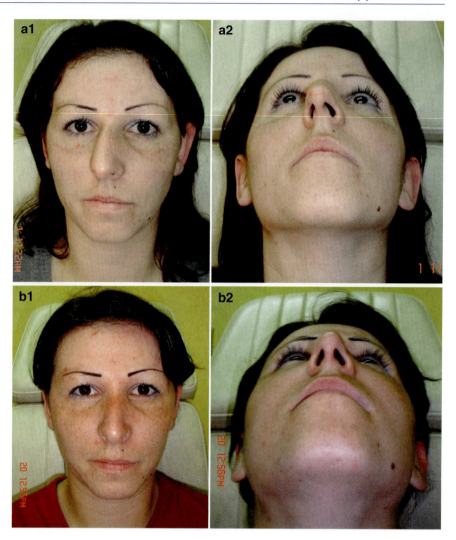

is usually introduced by hemitransfixion incision to the beginning of suture between nasal bones so that the chisel separates nasal bones. The chisel can also be introduced by intercartilaginous incision and it is place at the beginning of the suture of both nasal bones.

Paramedial osteotomy is used in cases when it is necessary to remove the nasal hump or in cases with nasal bone fractures creating the need for the bones to be cut in two levels.

The chisel is usually introduced through intercartilaginous incision or nasal skeleton is reached after lifting of soft tissue in external approach. A wide flat chisel is usually used, with or without guide on both sides. The chisel passes through both nasal bones at a certain level depending on how much is needed to remove the nasal hump or through an old fractural line in case when nasal skeleton is cut in two levels.

Lateral osteotomies serve to close the open nasal roof after removing the hump or in case when nasal dorsum is symmetrical, so it is necessary to correct the height of the nose. Vestibular incision is often used as an approaching way or it is reached through upper vestibulum of mouth cavity, which is extremely rare. They can be low, medium, or high. The line of these osteotomies starts from pyriform aperture, cuts the frontal extension of the upper jaw, passes at about 2–3 mm more dorsal from lacrimal bones, and ends in the area of nasion.

Transversal osteotomies are used in cases when there is no linking between lateral osteotomies and medial or paramedial cuts. The chisel is introduced either through intercartilaginous or vestibular incision.

In transcutaneous osteotomies, the 2 mm skin incision is performed through which a microchisel is introduced

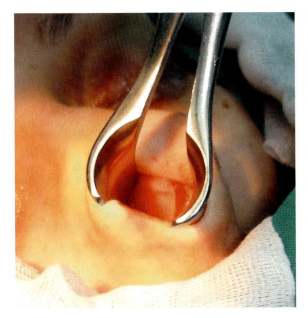

Fig. 55.4 Hemitransfixion incision

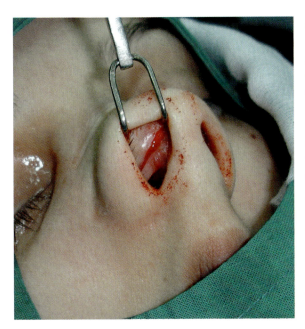

Fig. 55.5 Intercartilaginous incision

making perforation cuts on the frontal extension of the lower jaw and nasal bones following an imaginary line of osteotomies. Afterwards, the fracture is made and roof of nose is closed.

Depending on the kind of the incision, we have two basic surgical techniques, open and closed techniques. The close techniques are also called endonasal while open techniques are called decortications techniques.

Surgeon decides on the technique that is to be implemented during presurgical planning. It should be pointed out that both approaches have their advantages and disadvantages. It is necessary to be knowledgeable about both approaches in order to avoid possible mistakes. Some rhino-surgeons have their own preferences when it comes to choosing a technique.

Decortications or the open technique is characterized by a visible scar on columella. This technique was created by Rethi in the 1920s. Thanks to Padovan, it became popular in the USA. This technique enables surgeons to have a better insight during resection and modeling of the nose tip, and it provides a better overview on the nasal pyramid skeleton. Its drawback lies in the visible scar which is a problem in patients prone to keloid reaction. This technique solves all the deformities of nasal pyramid, although problems can arise in nasal septum. It is indicated in the problem of long noses (nasus longus), big noses (macrorhinia), big nasal tips (nasus bullosus), in nostril asymmetry, in nasal tip augmentation, nasal valve insufficiency, as well as in repeated surgeries.

The surgery begins with a "V" incision or stairway incision of the skin on the link between lower and medium third of columella. This incision is linked to marginal incision (infracartilaginous incision). Skin is carefully lifted until lower edges of medial crus of both lobular cartilages are seen. By following the lobular cartilages, nasal suprastructure is carefully lifted, and triangular cartilages and nasal bones are seen. When a complete insight into nasal pyramid is obtained, surgeons approach nasal septum from the upper and frontal sides. The lobular cartilages are divided and elevated submucosoperichondrial flap on both sides until maxillary spine and crest. All the necessary steps are done regarding correction and reaching the envisaged dimension. If necessary, a scalpel excision of the cartilage part of the hump is done, and then the flat chisel is used to remove the bone part of the hump. Lateral osteotomies on both sides are done. The alar cartilages are modeled. The cartilage grafts are placed, if needed. All nasal cartilages are sutured with Prolene of 5–0 or 6–0 dimensions. Columellar and marginal incisions are closed with interrupted 4–0 or 5–0 chromic gut suture. Nasal packing are placed on both sides and nasal pyramid is immobilized.

Endonasal approach covers incisions on the nasal cavity so that they are invisible. Joseph from Berlin was the first surgeon to solve nasal deformities by endonasal way, which was proven as a revolutionary concept in treating nasal pathologies. He was the first to implement several surgical techniques and introduced several specific instruments in rhino-surgery. His followers in the USA were Aufricht, Safian, and Fomon. Fomon's followers were Cottle and Goldman. Cottle introduced the term of transfixional incision and four tunnel concept in nasal septum preparation. The advantages are shorter postsurgical period, no visible scars, and shorter surgery time. The disadvantages are worse insight in nasal infrastructure and having more difficulty in correcting nasal tip deformity. It is convenient in correcting kyphotic and scoliotic nose.

Endonasal rhinoplasty means incisions to approach nasal septum as well as incisions that enable the approach to nasal suprastructure.

The incision of the authors' choice, in order to approach nasal septum, is hemitransfixion incision, although certain authors prefer transfixion incision. The authors are of the opinion that hemitransfixion incision is better for the better position of the tip of septal cartilage.

It is possible to approach nasal infrastructure through intercartilaginous incision, marginal incision, or transcartilaginous incision. They are usually done with a Bard-Parker 15 blade.

In every rhinoplastic surgery it is highly necessary to solve the nasal septum pathology. Mucoperichondrium is carefully lifted after hemitransfixion incision is done. Septal cartilage is completely prepared (Fig. 55.6).

Nasal septum is modeled to make sure that normal nasal function is obtained. It is necessary to point out that a nasal septum deformity that is not entirely correct can result in further nasal pyramid deformities a couple of months after the surgery. It is necessary to be very careful during nasal septum resection. If nasal septum resection is too big, this can result in nasal tip lowering due to the loss of the support. The best solution is to tend to perform the least possible resection, but not at the expense of the surgery outcome. One of the reasons for postsurgical breathing difficulties is the left deformity of nasal septum. The tip of quadrangular cartilage is shortened if necessary.

After solving nasal septum pathology, one of the nasal suprastructure incisions is performed. The authors prefer intercartilaginous incision. After the incision has been done with fine scissors, nasal suprastructure is carefully lifted (Fig. 55.7).

When the bone part of the pyramid is reached, periosteum is elevated from the bone. When suprastructure is separated from infrastructure in the dorsum area,

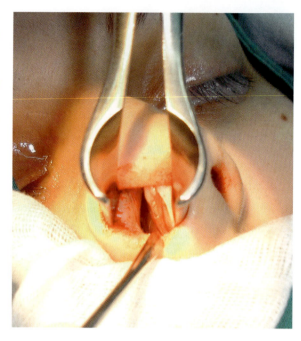

Fig. 55.6 Preparation of caudal part of septum nasi

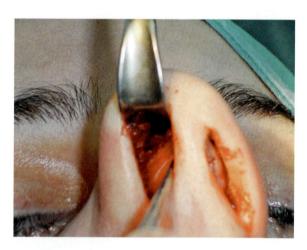

Fig. 55.7 Lifted nasal suprastructure

vestibular incisions are done and the tunnels, through which the chisel will pass during lateral osteotomy, are prepared through them.

In case of dealing with kyphosis scalpels or when scissors are used to remove the cartilage part of the hump, the flat chisel is used to remove the bone part (Fig. 55.8). A file is used to flatten the bone edges. Afterwards, both-sided low osteotomy is performed in order to solve the problem of the open roof. If necessary, it is possible to prepare cephalic end of the lateral crus

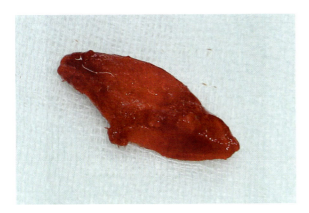

Fig. 55.8 Removed bone–cartilage hump

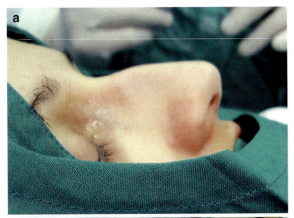

Fig. 55.9 (**a**) The beginning of a nasal surgery. (**b**) The end of a nasal surgery

of the alar cartilage and do necessary corrections on them through transcartilaginous incision.

After finishing the modeling of the nasal pyramid, triangular and quadrangular cartilages are sutured separately. It is preferable to fix caudal end of the septum for the spina nasalis anterior inferior. All the incisions are closed with separate sutures (Fig. 55.9).

It is necessary to put nasal packing in the nasal cavity to prevent hematomas of the nasal septum, and at the same time to stabilize the parts of nasal bones. The nasal pyramid is immobilized.

55.5 Complications

Rettinger [8] states that rhinoplasty is considered a surgery of a high risk, primarily for limited possibilities of influencing its final aesthetic outcome. A good indirect postsurgical result can be a bad one after a year. This is usually the consequence of tissue healing. Several different kinds of tissue heal after a rhinoplastic surgery (bone, cartilage, muscles, skin, fat tissue, etc.) The complications are the consequences of individual reactions and the healing process and surgeons are not responsible for them.

Certain complications occur due to a poor preoperative planning and analysis as well as the selection of the surgical technique [9].

The incidence of complications ranges, according to literature data, from 4% to 18.8%. The percentage of complications is smaller in relation to the occurrence of resurgical procedures undergone by patients [10]. Surgeons are often unaware about the number of procedures their patients undergo due to their discontent with postsurgical results, so they make an appointment and plan another surgery with another surgeon.

The number of resurgical procedures depends on the patients' mental state. Two percent of the patients who undergo aesthetic surgeries have a personality disorder. Borges found a personality disorder in 20% presurgical patients [7]. These patients are prone to exaggerating when it comes to their problems; they are constantly unsatisfied and they need to consult a psychiatrist.

The analysis of clinical material has proven that there were no patients with personality disorders. However, most patients willing to undergo an aesthetic surgery without functional problems do have a disordered idea of whom and what they are and they mostly see themselves as the best at everything.

According to the time of their occurrence, all complications can be divided into:

- Intrasurgical
- Immediate postoperative
- Early postoperative
- Late postoperative

55.5.1 Intrasurgical Complications

Intrasurgical complications cover: excessive bleeding, tearing of mucoperichondrial flaps, nasal dorsum emerging, nasal pyramid bones collapsing, open nasal roof, excessive resection as well as insufficient resection.

Excessive bleeding is quite a rare complication. If hemostatic mechanism disorders are ruled out prior to the surgery, bleeding occurs in less than 1% of the cases. Bleeding occurs due to an *Alvania angularis* injury or injury of some of the bigger branches of *sphenopalatine* artery.

Mucoperichondrial flap tearing occurs in cases of careless nasal suprastructure lifting. This complication needs to be diagnosed and taken care of.

Nasal pyramid bones collapsing usually occur in cases of earlier nasal bone or bone septum parts fracture. However, as this condition is recognized, an adequate bone fragment reposition has not been achieved.

"Open roof" occurs in cases of kyphotic nose correction where both-sided osteotomies is performed. It could occur when a surgeon cannot entirely cover the nose roof, although both-sided lateral osteotomy has been performed. The reason could be inadequate fractured segment adjusting as well as more firmly tamponading. "Open roof" can occur in cases of lesser kyphosis when a surgeon tries to remove the existing deformity by filing without performing lateral osteotomy, most often in female patients for their nose bones are more fragile. A good prevention of the insufficiently covered nose roof with both-sided lateral osteotomy is recovering nose dorsum infrastructure with crashed cartilage.

In cases of "open roof" (Fig. 55.10), nasal mucous membrane grows together with nasal suprastructure in the process of postsurgical healing, causing the change of nose color when the patients have a cold; defect in the bone part of the pyramid can be felt by touching and, can also been seen during examination.

Excessive resections occur due to a poor presurgical planning. They can cause a lordotic nose, stenosis at the level of nose valve, or lowering of the nose tip, when the cartilage part is overly recessed.

Insufficient resections occur due to a poor presurgical planning as well. They are more frequent in inexperienced surgeons who, due to suprastructure nose swelling, cannot estimate the degree of resection. It is usually manifested when the hump is not sufficiently recessed in kyphotic noses or when the hump is to lag in the cartilage part.

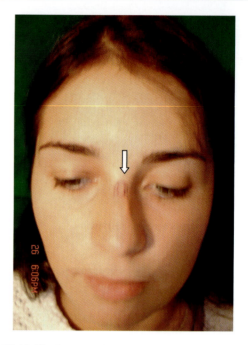

Fig. 55.10 The "open roof"

55.5.2 Immediate Postoperative Complications

These disorders are mainly linked to the use of particular anesthetics. They can occur in the form of anaphylactic reaction, laryngospasm, or visual disturbances.

Anaphylactic reaction is the consequence of the use of local anesthetics or presurgical antibiotic administration in prophylactic purposes.

Respiratory tract obstruction (postextubation laryngospasm) occurs in cases of total anesthesia when laryngospasm occurs after patient extubation and reintubation cannot be implemented because the patient cannot breathe spontaneously. It can be avoided if anesthesia is correctly supervised and when coughing and swallowing reflexes are regained with the help of extubation.

Visual disturbances occur when local anesthetics are administered. They can be transient due to the eye muscle reaction to local anesthetics or permanent that is the consequence of the use of vasoconstrictor leading to eye blood circulation disorders and ischemia [11].

55.5.3 Early Postoperative Complications

Early postoperative complications involve: bleeding, nasal septum hematoma, infections, dehiscence of the wound, toxic shock syndrome, permanent soft tissue edema, skin necrosis, osteomyelitis, cerebrospinal fluid rhinorrhea, olfactory disorder, nose breathing difficulties, contact dermatitis, and the onset of mental disorders.

Bleeding is rare in early postsurgical complications. Nose packing as well as immobilization of nasal bones provides a good pressure that disables bleeding from lesser blood vessels. Bleeding is more frequent after packing. It is necessary to do repacking and protect the patient with antibiotics.

Septal hematoma is the consequence of blood depositing between nasal septum cartilage and mucoperichondrial flaps. As soon as it is noticed, it is necessary to start hematoma draining, repacking, and antibiotics. If not noticed on time, septum abscess can develop along with septal cartilage necrosis which can cause further complications. The worst case scenario is thrombosis of sinus cavernosus or brain abscess.

Infections are quite rare in nasal surgeries. The incidence of the infection of the wound itself, surrounding structures, or septicemia is less than 1%. The operating area is rich in gram-positive bacterial flora with *Staphylococcus aureus* prevailing [12–15].

Toxic shock syndrome is the consequence of the staphylococcus endotoxin effect. It occurs rarely, only in 16 per 1,000 of the total number of surgeries performed [16]. It occurs after nose tamponading. The symptoms occur 2 days after the surgery and tamponading and they include postsurgical fever, vomiting, diarrhea, hypotension and erythematous rash, and the state of shock might occur as well [14, 17–19]. It is necessary to take the tampons out of the nose and give high doses of antibiotics and corticosteroids.

Dehiscence of the wound occurs scarcely. It occurs more frequently in outer approach than in endonasal approach.

Long lasting soft tissue edema occurs rarely. It occurs in patients whose surgeries lasted longer, in more abundant tamponading, in cases of soft tissue infections, but also in people who are prone to more tissue swelling during injuries [20]. Soft tissue swelling lasts longer in cases of open approach and it can last for a couple of months.

Skin necrosis occurs more frequently in cases of careless suprastructure lifting when suprastructure is thinned and consequently necrosis occurs.

Osteomyelitis occurs in cases of infections when smaller bone particles become infected. It is necessary to administer aggressive antibiotic therapy and to perform a revision surgical procedure if needed.

Cerebrospinal fluid rhinorrhea is a rare complication [21]. It occurs most frequently in the area of cribriform plate. It is diagnosed on the basis of finding β2-transferrina or β-trace protein (prostaglandin D-syntethase) in the collected nasal liquid [22]. It can be diagnosed if 5% fluorescein is injected intrathecally. This method is very useful because it is possible to close cerebrospinal fluid rhinorrhea area endoscopically at the same time.

Olfactory disorder is expected in early postsurgical period. It is the consequence of mucous membrane swelling. Anosmia occurs in 1% of the patients in early postsurgical period [23].

Breathing nose difficulties in early postsurgical period can be the consequence of transient nasal mucous membrane swelling. Nasal mucous membrane swelling is the consequence of surgical procedure trauma. Breathing difficulties can also occur in patients who don't have allergic rhinitis.

Contact dermatitis occurs as a reaction to taping material used to immobilize nasal pyramid (Fig. 55.11). This is not a significant complication, although it can

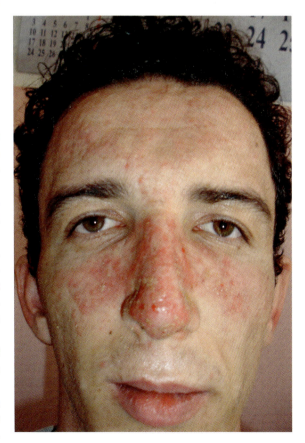

Fig. 55.11 Allergic reaction of the skin to tape

be quite unpleasant. Antihistamines and skin corticosteroids are to be administered.

Early psychological complications are usually manifested as transient periods of tension or depression [24].

55.5.4 Late Postoperative Complications

Late postoperative complications include intranasal synechiae, nasal septum perforations, nasal valvula insufficiency, nasal stenosis, dorsal cyst, nasal pyramid deformities, and persistent mental disorders.

Intranasal synechiae (Fig. 55.12) occur on the spots where mucous membrane of nasal septum and lateral side of the nose are damaged, most frequently lower and medium nasal turbinate. They can lead to nasal septum moving to one side, breathing difficulties, and even nasal pyramid deformation. They are solved by cutting and placing stents to enable reepithelialization of the mucous membrane with no contact.

Nasal septum perforation (Fig. 55.13) is a serious complication that is difficult to solve. It occurs in 3–25% of surgical patients. Perforations are usually asymptomatic. In less serious cases whistling can occur while breathing. If a perforation is bigger due to irregular air flow through nasal cavity, depositing and drying of secretion can occur. Lesser perforations are possible to close with mucosal flaps by placing cartilage grafts while some bigger ones are really difficult to close. There are several techniques for closing perforations of nasal septum [25]. If it persists, it is possible to place a silicone button that would reduce or remove unwanted effects of perforation [26].

Nasal valvula collapse occurs in cases of greater resections of alar cartilage. It is solved by placing spreader cartilage grafts in cases of internal collapse of valvula or alar batten grafts in cases of external valvula collapse.

Nose stenosis is a very serious complication that is difficult to solve. It occurs in the area of nose vestibulum most frequently, in cases when hemi or transfixion incision is linked with intracartilaginous or transcartilaginous during surgery. The patient has breathing difficulties on that side of the nose. It is possible to try "Z" plasty in the area of stenosis. Very good results can be achieved by expanding the stenotic area with long-term dilatation.

Recurrent meningitis occurs in patients with cerebrospinal fluid rhinorrhea. It is necessary to administer antibiotic therapy, diagnose the fistulous area endoscopically with 5% fluorescein, and close the existing defect of duramater cerebri.

Dorsal cyst (Fig. 55.14) occurs in cases when nasal mucosa is transplanted into subcutaneous tissue during surgery. This disorder is quite easy to remove.

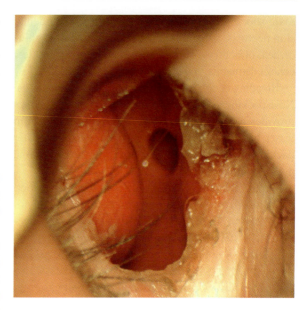

Fig. 55.13 Nasal septal perforation

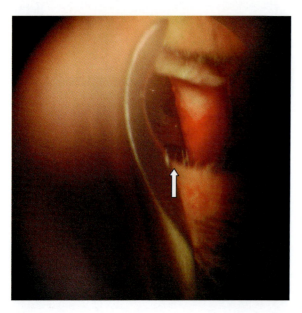

Fig. 55.12 Intranasal synechiae

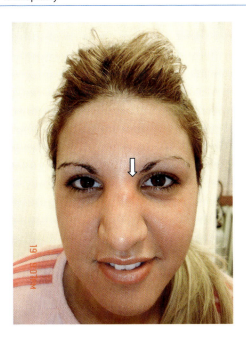

Fig. 55.14 Dorsal cyst

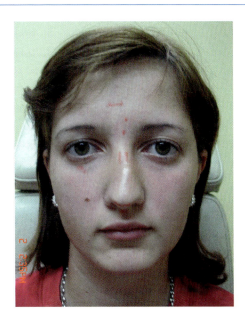

Fig. 55.15 Postsurgical scoliosis

Nasal pyramid deformations usually occur due to a mistake in estimation and presurgical analysis of the patient. It is necessary to highlight that rhinoplasty belongs to the group of surgeries of highest risk when it comes to unfavorable postsurgical results. The occurrence of nasal pyramid deformity after a rhinoplastic surgery can be the consequence of the fact that nasal septum deviation has not been done completely or an error in cartilage and nose bone skeleton deformity. The deformities can be the following:

- Nose scoliosis (Fig. 55.15) – usually occurs due to nose pathology that has not been completely dealt with or in cases when nasal bones have not been equally modeled.
- "Open roof" – occurs when nasal hump is removed without lateral osteotomies, or in cases when nose tamponading has been too firm leading to nasal bones separation.
- Bone or cartilage fragment leftovers after resection – it is manifested with the existence of greater or lesser prominence below skin. They can be spotted only after the withdrawal of nasal soft tissue swelling.
- Excessive nasal resection – this deformity usually leads to lordosis, empty columella (Fig. 55.16), sagging of the cartilaginous dorsum.
- Columella retraction – occurrence of cranial withdrawal of the columella.

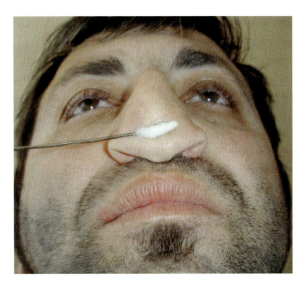

Fig. 55.16 Empty columella

- Cartilage hump (Fig. 55.17) – occurs in cases when a surgeon has not done a complete resection of the bone–cartilage hump causing another cartilage hump in the lower third of the nose (surgical hump).
- Nostril asymmetry – can occur due to a mistake in modeling of alar cartilages or due to uneven nasal bone resection. In the latter case, nasal pyramid is leant on one side.

Persistent psychological disorder occurs only in cases of poor presurgical mental estimation of the patient's

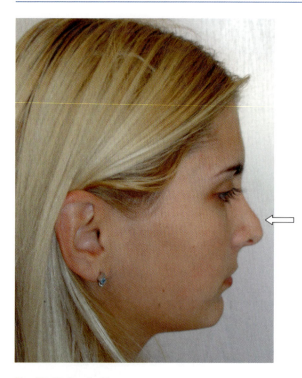

Fig. 55.17 Surgical hump

As for the profile aspect of the face, nose dorsum is the most important being a dimension which cannot be seen by an individual and at the same time the most common reason for undergoing a rhinosurgery.

A kyphotic nose is the most frequent deformity of nasal pyramid, often without nasal septum deviation. It is relatively easy to be operated.

Being knowledgeable about possible complications and solving them is the main condition for a surgeon to be into aesthetic and functional nose surgery.

state. Patients who, along with aesthetic disorder, have a functional one, do not have postsurgical psychological changes as a rule. The change of their looks is linked to the increase of their self-content. The patients who undergo an aesthetic surgery exclusively could be the patients who have underlying mental disorders. Certain authors find more mental disorders in women, while some other in young men [27, 28]. A mental disorder that can have the worst consequences such as suicide or murder of the surgeon is found in patients with dismorphophobia [29].

55.6 Conclusions

While performing a rhinoplastic surgery, it is necessary for the surgeon to think of the function first and aesthetic aspect second.

Presurgical planning is of the highest significance in preventing postsurgical complications.

A psychological profile estimation is extremely important. If a personality disorder is suspected, it is necessary to consult a psychiatrist.

References

1. Šercer A. Otorinolaringologija - Propedeutika 1. Jugoslovenski leksikografski zavod. Zagreb. 1966;77–101.
2. Padovan I. Otorinolaringologija 2. Kirurgija nosa, paranazalnih šupljina i lica. Školska knjiga Zagreb 1984;77–101.
3. Kljajić V, Savović S, Čanji K. Nasal hump – five years analysis. Med Pregl. 2010;63(3–4):159–62.
4. Daniel RK. Rhinoplasty. Boston: Little Brown; 1993. p. 72.
5. Mladina R. Preoperativna priprema. in Deformacije nosnoga septuma i piramide, Školska kinjga Zagreb. 1990; 63–66.
6. Huizing EH, de Groot JA. Functional reconstructive nasal surgery. Stuttgart: Thieme; 2003. p. 103–5.
7. Dinis PB, Dinis M, Gomes A. Psychosocial consequences of nasal aesthetic and functional surgery: a controlled prospective study in an ENT setting. Rhinology. 1998;36(1):32–6.
8. Retinger G. Risks and complications in rhinoplasty. GMS Curr Top Otorhinolaryngol Head Neck Surg. 2007;6: Doc08.
9. Retinger G. Complication or mistake. Facial Plast Surg. 1997;13(1):1.
10. Kljajić V, Savović S, Čanji K. Rhinoplasty – five years retrospective analysis. Med Pregl. 2008;61 Suppl 2:37–40.
11. Gall R, Blakley B, Warrington R, Bell DD. Intraoperative anaphylactic shock from bacitracin nasal packing after septorhinoplasty. Anesthesiology. 1999;91(5):1545–7.
12. Abifadel M, Real JP, Servant JM, Banzet P. Apropos of a case of infection after esthetic rhinoplasty. Ann Chir Plast Esthét. 1990;35(5):415–17.
13. Hetter GP. Infection after rhinoplasty. Plast Reconstr Surg. 1983;71(3):439–40.
14. Silk KL, Ali MB, Cohen BJ, Summersgill JT, Raff MJ. Absence of bacteremia during nasal septoplasty. Arch Otolaryngol Head Neck Surg. 1991;117(1):54–5.
15. Cobouli JL, Guerrissi JO, Mileto A, Cerisola JA. Local infection following aesthetic rhinoplasty. Ann Plast Surg. 1986;17(4):306–9.
16. Jakobson JA, Kasworm EM. Toxic shock syndrome after nasal surgery. Case reports and analysis of risk factors. Arch Otolaryngol Head Neck Surg. 1986;122(3):329–32.
17. Thumfart WT, Volkilein C. Systemic and other complications. Facial Plast Surg. 1997;13:61–9.
18. Holt GR, Garner ET, McLarey D. Postoperative sequelae and complications of rhinoplasty. Otolaryngol Clin North Am. 1987;20(4):853–76.

19. Slavin SA, Rees TD, Guy CL, Goldwyn RM. An investigation of bacteremia during rhinoplasty. Plast Reconstr Surg. 1983;71(2):196–8.
20. Mladina R. Postoperativno razdoblje. in Deformacije nosnoga septuma i piramide, Školska kinjiga. Zagreb. 1990; 107–115.
21. Hallock GG, Trier WC. Cerebrospinal fluid rhinorrhea following rhinoplasty. Plast Reconstr Surg. 1983;17(1): 109–13.
22. Bachmann-Harildstad G. Diagnostic values of beta-2 transferrin and beta-trace protein as markes for cerebrospinal fluid fistula. Rhinology. 2008;46(2):82–5.
23. Kimmelman CP. The risk to olfaction from nasal surgery. Laryngoscope. 1994;104(8 Pt 1):981–8.
24. Sarwer DB, Pertschuk MJ, Wadden TA, Whitaker LA. Psyhological investigations in cosmetic surgery: a look back and a look ahead. Plast Reconstr Surg. 1998;101(4): 1136–42.
25. Huizing EH, de Groot JA. Septal perforation. Functional reconstructive nasal surgery. Stuttgart: Thieme; 2003. p. 180–91.
26. Dosen LK, Haye R. Silicone button in nasal septal perforation. Long term observation. Rhinology. 2008;46(4): 324–7.
27. McKinney P, Cook JQ. A critical evaluation of 200 rhinoplasties. Ann Plast Surg. 1981;7(5):357–61.
28. Guyuron B, Bokhari F. Patient satisfaction following rhinoplasty. Aesthetic Plast Surg. 1981;20:153–7.
29. Hinni ML, Kern EB. Psyhological complications of septorhinoplasty. Facial Plast Surg. 1997;13(1):71–5.

Nonsurgical Rhinoplasty with Radiesse®

George John Bitar, Olalesi Osunsade, and Anuradha Devabhaktuni

56.1 Introduction

Due to its low morbidity and the high patient satisfaction, nonsurgical rhinoplasty (also known as a nonsurgical nosejob) is a viable option for primary nasal augmentation and for correction of nasal deformities. Nonsurgical rhinoplasty, whether performed for primary nasal augmentation or postoperative revision, is increasing in popularity due to advancements in the various soft-tissue fillers. There is no FDA-approved soft-tissue filler specifically directed for nonsurgical rhinoplasty as yet; however, various soft-tissue fillers have been used in off-label protocols with mixed results. Examples of such fillers include injectable silicon (a device banned by the federal government [1]), collagen, non- and crosslinked hyaluronic acid, and calcium hydroxyapatite (CaHA). These alloplasts are regarded as minimally invasive counterparts to cartilage, fat, and other autologous grafts used in surgical nasal augmentation. In recent years, the xenograft Permacol has also been used for nasal augmentation in the UK [2]. With a nonsurgical approach, it is essentially an augmentation rhinoplasty; so it has limitations compared to a surgical rhinoplasty. Various properties of the commercially available calcium hydroxyapatite media (CHM), Radiesse® (BioForm Medical, San Mateo, CA) are discussed with its uses for nonsurgical rhinoplasties and avoidance of pitfalls. Attention is focused on Radiesse® (Fig. 56.1) because of its longevity, ease of administration and molding, as well as its excellent safety profile.

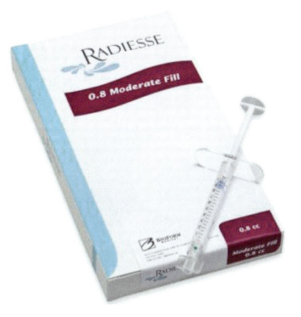

Fig. 56.1 Radiesse® Syringes (Used with permission of Bioform Medical, San Mateo, CA)

G.J. Bitar (✉)
Assistant Clinical Proferssor, George Washington University
Medical Director, Bitar Cosmetic Surgery Institute, 3023 Hamaker Ct, #109 Fairfax, VA 22031, USA
e-mail: georgebitar@drbitar.com

O. Osunsade
George Washington University School of Medicine and Health Sciences, 1121 Arlington Blvd. #702, Arlington, VA 22209, USA
e-mail: olalesi@gwmail.gwu.edu

A. Devabhaktuni
George Washington University School of Medicine and Health Sciences, 1111 25th St NW #509, Washington, DC 20037, USA
e-mail: ardevabh@gwmail.gwu.edu

56.2 Biochemistry

The chemical formula for calcium hydroxyapatite is $Ca_{10}(PO_4)_6(OH)_2$. In the body, hydroxyapatite is a weak base and dissociates into phosphate and hydroxyl ions (Fig. 56.2). Phosphate is capable of accepting up to three protons, but at physiological pH ranges it is only capable of existing as dihydrogen phosphate or hydrogen phosphate ions.

Radiesse® is composed of a sodium carboxymethylcellulose, water, and glycerin suspension (70%) of microspheres (30%; 24–45 μm in diameter) of calcium hydroxyapatite. In Radiesse®, the average microsphere volume is 620 μm³ [3] (Fig. 56.3).

The blend of CaHA with carrier gel is chemically referred to as calcium hydroxyapatite media [4]. Before being mixed with media, sophisticated ceramic processing techniques are utilized to prepare the CaHA particles, which are segregated into a narrow size range, maximizing the volume between the particles [3]. Particles sizes were chosen in order to minimize the possibility of migration and to allow unproblematic injection through a reasonably small needle [3].

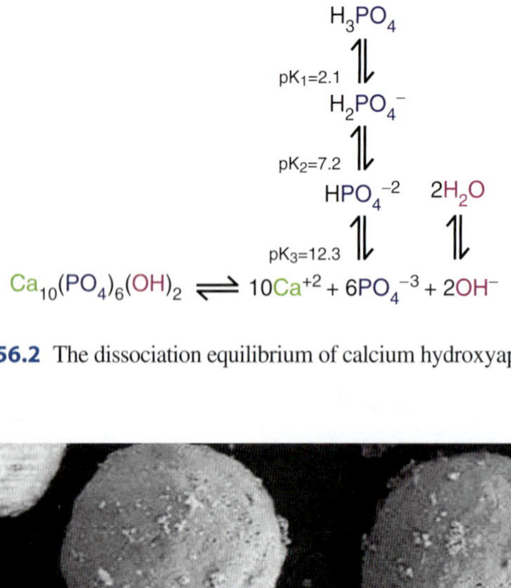

56.3 Storage

Radiesse® comes in 0.3, 0.8, 1.3, and 1.5 ml syringes and can be shipped and stored at room temperature for up to 2 years. It must be injected without any dilutions or alteration, immediately after opening. It should not be reused after initial use for risk of contamination. The current recommendation from the manufacturer is that the Radiesse® that is unused at the first treatment may be stored for up to 3 months for that patient before it must be discarded [5]. It is important that no visible air be present in the capped syringe to prevent premature hardening of the material [5]. The company provides three labels identifying the lot number of the Radiesse syringe in use so that the first and second procedures can be documented in the patient's chart alongside self-adhesive labels.

$$H_3PO_4 \underset{pK_1=2.1}{\rightleftharpoons} H_2PO_4^- \underset{pK_2=7.2}{\rightleftharpoons} HPO_4^{-2} \underset{pK_3=12.3}{\rightleftharpoons} \quad 2H_2O$$

$$Ca_{10}(PO_4)_6(OH)_2 \rightleftharpoons 10Ca^{+2} + 6PO_4^{-3} + 2OH^-$$

Fig. 56.2 The dissociation equilibrium of calcium hydroxyapatite

56.4 Mechanism of Action

Calcium hydroxyapatite media is an injectable soft-tissue filler that is palpable and malleable, allowing the physician to mold it into the appropriate form. Although inorganic, it is found naturally in bones and teeth. After injection into the body, it is eventually absorbed and metabolized into calcium and phosphate ions before being excreted through normal metabolic processes [6].

Positive long-term effects may be explained by the fact that it remains localized at injection sites. While the aqueous gel component is resorbed by 6 months after injection [3], the CaHA microspheres remain as scaffolds for osteoblasts at the periosteum and fibroblasts in the soft tissues for a much longer period of time (Fig. 56.4). Histological evidence shows CaHA microspheres stimulate collagen production (Fig. 56.5), but they do not stimulate bone growth in the periosteum [7]. For this reason, Radiesse® has also been injected with harvested fibroblasts in order to study their combined effects on collagen synthesis [8]. This putative mechanism of action may explain the observation that a smaller volume of Radiesse® is needed for

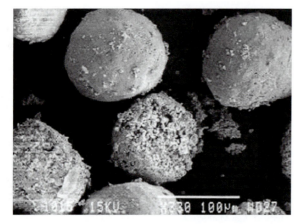

Fig. 56.3 Radiesse® at a microscopic level. CaHA particles after implantation (Image credited to David Goldberg, MD (Used with permission of Bioform Medical, San Mateo, CA)

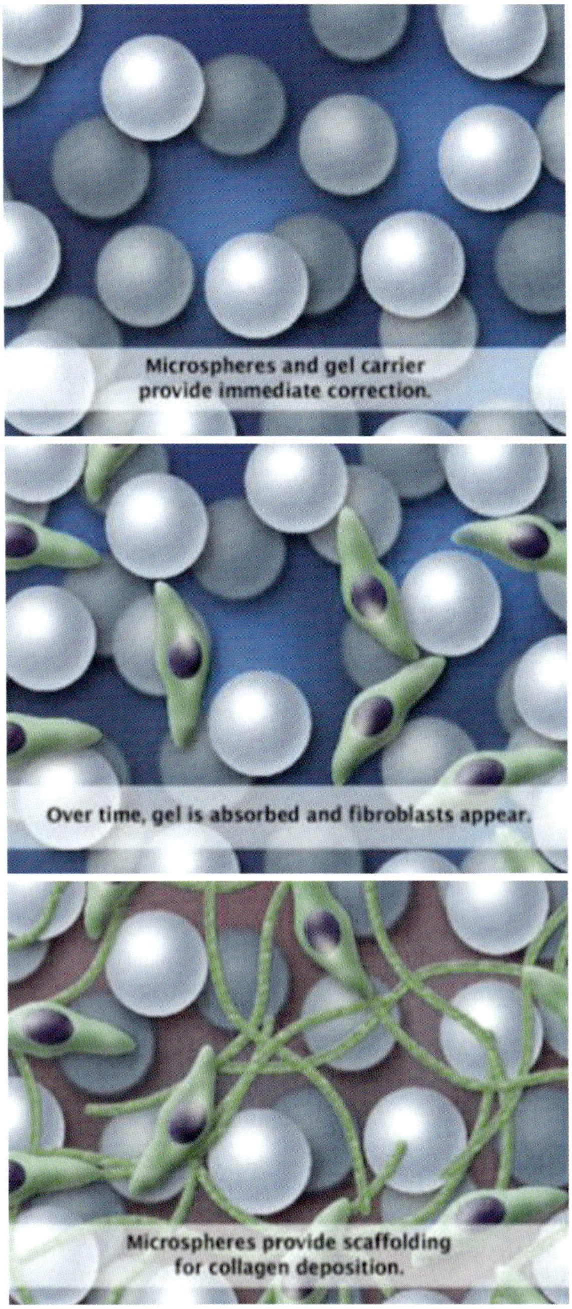

Fig. 56.4 Mechanism of action of Radiesse® (Used with permission of Bioform Medical, San Mateo, CA)

Microspheres and gel carrier provide immediate correction.

Over time, gel is absorbed and fibroblasts appear.

Microspheres provide scaffolding for collagen deposition.

the same degree of correction provided by higher volumes of hyaluronic acid or collagen [7].

Hydroxyapatite cement, which is denser than the granular Radiesse®, has been used for surgical nasal implants for over two decades. This is due to its biocompatibility, which is associated with its osseoconductive and osseoporous properties [9]. It is nonresorpable, however, which leaves risks of infection and extrusion [10].

56.5 Duration of Action

Injectable CaHA lasts longer in areas with less movement, blood supply, and lymphatic drainage because its loss is more limited in these areas [11]. Hence, injecting Radiesse® deep along the periosteum or in facial areas with less movement seems to produce greater longevity than immediately under the skin [11]. In a study involving injection into the neck of the bladder in animals, CaHA lasted for the entire 3 year length of the study [6].

For nonsurgical rhinoplasty, desired results may last 1–2 years [11] (Fig. 56.5) with a single injection (approximately 1.3 ml), although additional touch-up injections may be performed around 6 months after initial treatment to maintain the desired nasal contour. Some patients report longer duration for minor improvements, such as smoothing of irregularities up to 3 years [8]. In one reported case, rhinoplasty revision surgery was performed uneventfully on a patient who received 0.6 ml of Radiesse® 14 months earlier [12]. Interestingly, no residual Radiesse® was noted during that operation [12], which is consistent with the absorption of Radiesse® gradually.

56.6 Clinical Uses

56.6.1 FDA-Approved Uses

Radiesse is approved by the Food and Drug administration (FDA) as a filler to augment vocal cords, for HIV-associated facial lipoatrophy, for nasolabial folds and smile lines, for oral and maxillofacial defects, and a radiopaque marker [13].

56.6.2 Aesthetic Off-Label Uses

The only FDA-approved aesthetic use for Radiesse® is to serve as a soft-tissue filler for correction of moderate to severe facial deficiencies at nasolabial folds and in HIV-associated facial lipoatrophy. The most

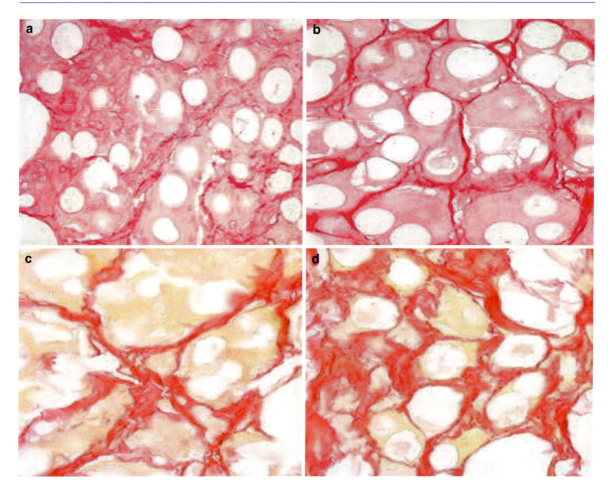

Fig. 56.5 Histological evidence of duration of action. Using picrosirius red staining, increased collagen deposition is seen around the CaHA microspheres at 4 (**a**), 16 (**b**), 32 (**c**), and 78 (**d**) weeks. Note the gradual changes in the appearance of the CaHA microsphere, which can be attributed to their breakdown and resorption through normal metabolic processes. Images credited to David Goldberg, MD (Used with permission of Bioform Medical, San Mateo, CA)

common off-label aesthetic uses of Radiesse® are for nonsurgical facial rejuvenation procedures to smooth wrinkles, fill depressions, and reduce facial asymmetry in lips (where it is sometimes associated with nodule formation [14]), labiomandibular folds, and the prejowl sulcus. It is also a dependable filler for augmenting the facial bony contour, i.e., nose, chin, cheeks, and forehead [5]. Additionally, it has been used in spreader graft injections as a nonsurgical alternative for internal nasal valve collapse patients, minimizing obstruction and improving breathing and snoring [15]. In 2007, Stupak et al. [16] first described the use of Radiesse® for correction of postrhinoplasty contour deficiencies and asymmetries.

Other off-label uses include other facial rejuvenation procedures, bladder dystrophy corrections, nipple projection after failed reconstruction surgery [17], cosmetic correction of enophthalmos [10], and restoration of orbital volume [11]. Radiesse® has received approval for many of these off-label procedures, including nonsurgical rhinoplasty, outside of the USA [13].

56.7 Safety and Efficacy

Due to its inorganic nature Radiesse® is nonimmunogenic, unlike collagen, so no skin testing is needed prior to injection. It has been found to be nontoxic, nonirritating, nonantigenic, and biocompatible through both in vivo and in vitro testing [18, 19]. Should any particles become phagocytized, they are degraded in situ to calcium and phosphate ions like small fragments of bone. Furthermore, it is eventually absorbed by the body, rendering it reversible and preferable to other permanent alloplasts – such as polymethyl methacrylate (PMMA). Because it is semipermeable, it lasts longer than collagen and hyaluronic acid-based fillers, making it more cost effective and reducing frequency of injection.

The major obstacle preventing formal FDA approval of Radiesse® for nonsurgical rhinoplasty and other facial augmentation procedures is the lack of a large, long-term study of its safety and efficacy. There are many studies showing its effectiveness in nasal augmentation on a small scale [8, 12, 16, 19–23] thus warranting further study. A study published in 1996 following more than 200 patients during an 8-year period found the use of porous hydroxyapatite granules – similar to Radiesse® – as favorable means of augmenting the craniofacial skeleton [24]. This study, however, only included a limited number of cases involving nasal augmentation, concluding the method to be investigatory at that time [24]. Similarly, a German study followed 128 augmentations with hydroxylapatite granules filled in a Vicryl-tube in 36 patients from 1986 to 1992 [25]. Implanted in the subperiosteum, these granules proved to be well tolerated and consistently in form in patients with facial deformities [25]. Furthermore, a Chinese study following 50 patients over 8 years found a particulate hydroxyapatite to be aesthetically stable with good long-term results for nasal augmentation [26]; however, this form of hydroxyapatite differs from the granular form found in Radiesse®.

In 2008, a case was reported of a 37-year-old Asian woman who experienced ptosis due to eyelid mass development secondary to receiving CaHA for nasal augmentation 3 days earlier [26]. Symptoms were relieved after surgical excision of the mass 2 months later, but this complication emphasizes the need for proper site selection, meticulous injection techniques, and avoidance of overinjection of CaHA [27].

56.8 Nonsurgical Rhinoplasty

Nonsurgical rhinoplasty with Radiesse® (also known as a Radiesse® rhinoplasty) should be performed by a surgeon with a mastery of nasal anatomy and who is experienced in performing surgical rhinoplasties. Various guidelines have been reported in the literature by clinicians regarding anesthesia, injection, and postoperative care related to Radiesse® rhinoplasty.

56.8.1 Initial Consult

A patient's chief complaint about his or her nose needs to be addressed. The level of nasal deformity as it relates to the magnitude of the patient's concerns should be critically assessed, as well. Past medical history should be reviewed, with an emphasis on drug use, allergies, history of cold sores, presence of autoimmune disorders, history of facial herpes virus, previous facial operations (specifically rhinoplasties or dermal filler treatments), and whether the patient is pregnant or nursing [22]. Patients should also report sinus or nasal congestion, as well as use of decongestants. Due to minor bleeding during injections, patients should not be on any blood thinners including warfarin, NSAIDs, vitamin E (including multivitamin form), certain herbs, and excessive alcohol intake. One recommendation is to cease ingesting anything that can thin the blood for 10 days prior to the procedure [6]. The authors recommend cessation of above products for 2 weeks prior to the procedure with the consent of the patient's primary care physician.

Patients should be informed of the risks and benefits of the procedure in order for them to have realistic expectations toward a satisfactory outcome. They should be informed that the results are not permanent, and may require further revision before acquiring the desired appearance. Moreover, nonsurgical rhinoplasty with Radiesse® does not exclude patients from surgical rhinoplasty in the future. Patients with one or more of the following conditions may also be excluded from the procedure: acute or chronic nasal infection, existing keloid scars, history of systemic collagen diseases, severe bleeding disorders, nasal respiratory impairment, and unrealistic expectations [23].

An essential part of the informed consent is the discussion of a surgical rhinoplasty as a permanent alternative to a nonsurgical rhinoplasty. It is very important for patients to know that both options, the surgical and nonsurgical ones, are viable options if that is the case. Various reasons may sway the patient to have a nonsurgical rhinoplasty such as cost, lower risk, desire for a minimal change, time of recovery, and fear of surgery. Pre and posttreatment photographs should also be taken, and patients should be given the opportunity to speak with previous patients who have undergone nonsurgical rhinoplasty with Radiesse®, if possible.

56.8.2 Physical Examination

Before performing a nonsurgical rhinoplasty with Radiesse®, it is important to examine the nose (Fig. 56.6) thoroughly, including the skin, cartilage, bony pyramid, different relationships of the aesthetic subunits, whether there is septal deviation, enlargement of inferior turbinates, difficulty breathing, prior trauma, as well as identify any possible locations of scar tissue. Also take into consideration that thickness and moisture of skin differs between ethnicities. Treatment should be delayed if any active lesions exist, with initiation of antiviral therapy (e.g., acyclovir) for patients with a history of the facial herpes virus [6].

56.8.3 Nasal Anatomy

For nonsurgical rhinoplasty, good knowledge of the relations of the nasal subunits is essential. Surface anatomy is also of paramount importance. Knowledge of nerve and blood supply will allow the injecting surgeon to avoid complications. For a nonsurgical rhinoplasty, Radiesse® is typically injected into depressions at the fronto-nasal angle, dorsum, nasal tip, columella, and naso-labial angle.

56.8.4 Anesthesia and Prophylaxis

The most common types of anesthesia to injection sites include: lidocaine with epinephrine, topical lidocaine with tetracaine for 30 min [20], anesthetic gel [28], or topical anesthesia with BLT applied for 15–30 min prior to injection. Applying an icepack to the nose decreases sensation and provides good analgesia. A judicious combination of the above may also be used with care not to compromise the blood supply to the nasal tip. Anesthesia can also be used as a means of loosening tissue and cartilage prior to filler injection. For this, a 25 gauge or 27 gauge needle can be used to create a space for the filler from a distal puncture site [21]. For postrhinoplasty contour corrections, injections have been performed without anesthesia (only an alcohol pad), or in the operating room in conjunction with facial procedures [16]. In the latter, it was found that concurrent procedures do not affect injection treatment results [16]. In July 2009, the FDA approved the mixing of Radiesse® with lidocaine. This is another method of anesthesia that has been proven to improve patient comfort and satisfaction with Radiesse® injections [4].

Nerve blocks are helpful mainly when the infiltration of the anesthetic solution may cause undesirable distortion of the surgical site or require an amount of anesthetic that exceeds the maximum recommended dose [21]. For nonsurgical rhinoplasty with Radiesse®, blocking the infraorbital and supratrochlear nerves, which are branches of the trigeminal nerve, has been recommended [21], although neither are used in our institute. An infraorbital nerve block specifically targets the lateral nose [21], but also anesthetizes the lower eyelid area, through the cheeks, and the upper lip [7]. Topical anesthesia may be applied to the oral mucosa prior to anesthetic injection [7]. In our institute, we administer a topical anesthesia of lidocaine 6%, tetracaine 4%, and benzocaine 20% applied for 30–45 min directly to the entire nose, along with ice pack application. That application gives excellent pain control and does not distort the nasal anatomy.

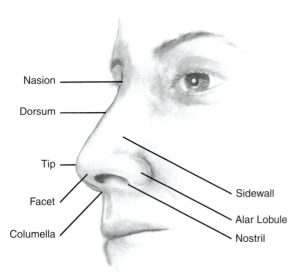

Fig. 56.6 Nasal anatomy

Prophylactic antibiotics are not used for nonsurgical rhinoplasty, but there is anecdotal evidence supporting prophylactic use of Arnica montana, bromelain, and 1% vitamin K1 (phytonadione) cream to reduce bruising [7].

After anesthesia and prophylaxis are administered, patients are marked and then injected subcutaneously or into a subperiosteal plane at the desirable location of the nose. For an experienced surgeon, markings may not be necessary.

56.8.5 Needles

For nonsurgical rhinoplasty, Radiesse® has reportedly been injected in various ways, with any of the following needles: a 23 gauge 1.5-in. straight or angled spreader graft needle [15], a 25 gauge 5/8 in. needle, a 27 gauge 1.75 in. needle [5], a 27 gauge 0.5 in. needle [20], a 30 gauge 1.30 cm needle [16], or a 27 gauge 0.60 cm needle [16]. Our preference is a 27 gauge 0.5 in. needle as it is convenient to inject smoothly but doesn't leave a large needle hole.

56.8.6 Injection Technique

The authors' approach is to address the nose from top to bottom. First, the radix (Fig. 56.7) is assessed. Is it with appropriate height, or does it need to be augmented? Next, the dorsum is injected if necessary. If there is a dorsal hump, injecting cephalad or caudal to it may mask that hump (Fig. 56.7).

If there is a deviated septum, the injections may be done to achieve symmetry by injecting unequal amounts to the left and right side. If there is an isolated depression, it can be addressed with a direct injection to fill it. Caution needs to be exercised if a depression is tethered to the underlying bone or cartilage, since an overly aggressive injection can create a "pin-cushion" effect, with the Radiesse® ending up surrounding the depression rather than filling it.

The nasal tip skin needs to be assessed next (Fig. 56.8). If it is thick and immobile, it may be difficult to change the shape with injections, and may need to be addressed surgically. If the skin is lax, a good outcome can be expected from a nasal tip injection.

The columella can also be injected if it is retracted or deficient. Because it is abundant in sebaceous

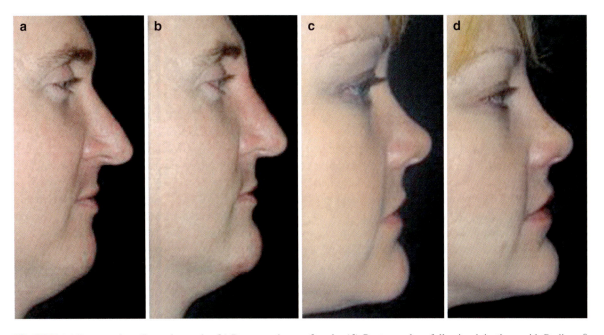

Fig. 56.7 (**a**) Preprocedure Caucasian male. (**b**) Postprocedure following injections with Radiesse® to the dorsum and radix, resulting in increased height. (**c**) Preprocedure Caucasian female. (**d**) Postprocedure following injections with Radiesse® at the dorsum and radix, resulting in increased height

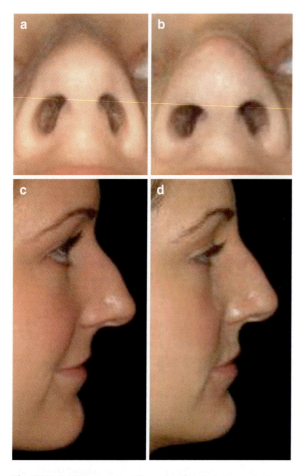

Fig. 56.8 (a) Preprocedure Caucasian female in her early twenties. (b) Postprocedure with injections with Radiesse® to the tip, resulting in a more pointed shape. (c) Preprocedure Caucasian woman in her twenties. (d) Postprocedure after injections with Radiesse® superiorly and inferiorly around a hump on the dorsum, which masked it and resulted in the appearance of a more prominent tip

glands, the nasal tip should be approached preferably from the dorsum to decrease the chance of contamination and infection. Very few times the nasal nares need to be augmented. That should be done with caution as it may narrow the internal nasal valve.

Injection is typically done into the deep dermis in a threaded fashion in doses ranging from 0.1 to 0.3 ml at any given time because higher volumes may create undue tension and cause skin necrosis. Crosshatching, linear, and fanning techniques of injection have been reported [6]. If anesthesia were not used, injections can alternatively be coupled to loosening of subcutaneous tissue as previously described.

Due to its composition, Radiesse® should not be injected into the superficial or middle dermis [5].

Similarly, the thick, white texture of Radiesse® may make it visible under thin skin, which is not aesthetically pleasing. Superficial injections can lead to overcorrection and nodule formation, so it is important to finish injecting before removing the needle. Persistent nodules may be avoided with proper injection of the Radiesse® in the plane immediately deep to the dermis and proper site selection [5]. Areas of extensive scar tissue deposition may be more difficult to treat because of tissue retraction and lack of a bony base for projection. Even so, some correction can often still be achieved in such areas [8]. Care should be taken not to inject into an artery, as this may cause necrosis [20].

56.8.7 Dosage

Doses vary depending on individual patient characteristics, but suggested maximum doses include: 1.5 ml at the fronto-nasal angle, 0.5 ml at the dorsum, 0.5 ml at the tip, and 1.5 ml at the nasolabial angle; as maximum doses to each specific area [21]. We recommend limiting the initial total injection to 1.5 ml to avoid tension on the overlying skin as well as overcorrection. It is better to undercorrect deformities, as they can be filled in or touched up during a follow-up visit in 2 weeks to 3 months.

56.8.8 Postinjection Care

Ice should be applied during breaks between injections and for a period afterwards to reduce edema and ecchymosis. The procedure is typically well tolerated, and no postprocedure pain control is typically required.

Injection is followed by massaging, which molds the desired shape and ensures the absence of palpable lumps. Molding may be enhanced by micropore taping for 24 h after injection [16, 21]. Taping may also help to reduce swelling. Splint placement for a few days after injection may prevent displacement of the filler [6]. At our institute, we do not tape or splint the nose afterwards, but encourage patients to place cold compresses on the nose to decrease the edema for the 24 h following the nonsurgical rhinoplasty. The authors have not seen the filler being displaced by this follow-up care.

The most common adverse effects are local and transient. They include mild pain, erythema, ecchymoses, edema, pruritus, and hematoma [12, 19]. Other adverse effects include soreness, numbness, contour irregularities, tenderness, and irritation. Overall, Radiesse® rhinoplasty is typically well tolerated and patient satisfaction for nonsurgical nasal augmentation is high [8].

Removal of excess Radiesse® with an 18-gauge needle can lead to correction if Radiesse® is injected into the middermis [5] or in excess. Radiesse® has a 1:1 injection-to-augmentation ratio; thus it requires no additional posttreatment augmentation monitoring [29]. Additional touch-ups may be required after 2 weeks to 3 months. Patients are seen 2–3 weeks after injections to ensure that they are satisfied after most of the edema and ecchymosis has subsided.

Radiesse® has also been used to improve postrhinoplasty contour defects, such as dorsal nasal defects (cartilaginous and bony), nasal sidewall depressions, overly deep supratip breaks, and alar asymmetries [16]. Typical candidates include people with ethnic noses: Asians, Middle Easterners, African Americans, and Hispanics. This is because, in general, such people have thicker skin, lower nasal dorsums, and bulbous tips compared to Caucasian patients.

When performing a rhinoplasty on any patient population it is important to take cultural issues into consideration. While such patients seek correction of nasal defects, most patients also cherish subtleties and preservation of their ethnicity. Rhinoplasty should refine facial features while maintaining ethnic identity. When they arise, also recognize language and cultural barriers

56.8.9 Patient Satisfaction

As with any aesthetic procedure, satisfaction depends not only on surgical technique, but realistic expectations from patients, as well as proper prior communication between surgeons and patients. Nonsurgical rhinoplasty with Radiesse® has a high rate of patient satisfaction in the literature [8, 12, 16, 19–23], as well as at our institute. Furthermore, one study found no correlation between patient satisfaction scores and demonstration of improvement by photographic analysis [8].

In the rhinoplasty literature, the standard for measuring patient satisfaction is through patient-reported outcome measures. The most common instruments used to measure patient satisfaction after surgical rhinoplasty are the Rhinoplasty Outcomes Evaluation, the Glasgow Benefit Inventory, and the Facial Appearance Sorting Test [30]. For nonsurgical rhinoplasty with Radiesse®, there is a need for the use of such instruments to assess patient satisfaction.

56.9 Specific Types of Noses

At the nasal radix and dorsum, Radiesse® can be used to augment height, to give a wider appearance, or correct saddle deformities. By correcting retracted columellas, it can give a more prominent nasal tip.

56.9.1 Asian

Augmentation rhinoplasty is a common procedure in the Asian community due to their generally lower and more caudal nasal nasion compared to Caucasian patients. A common misconception is that such rhinoplasty is done to look more "Western," despite the fact that high, narrow bridges are aesthetically pleasing in many Asian cultures [31]. To achieve such results, surgical augmentation is performed with autogenous or alloplastic material placed into the nasal dorsum to make the nasion level higher and more cephalic. Over the years, there has been a debate over the more preferable material. To this end, it has been found that surgeons performing augmentation rhinoplasty on Asian patients have had to recognize that many are unhappy with autogenous implants and prefer alloplasts, particularly silicon, despite long-term side effects [31]. Such surgery, however, may produce conspicuous and unsatisfactory results [32], particularly due to exposure and extrusion of implants. Implant exposure can lead to scarring, which can be difficult to treat with revision surgery [33].

As inhabitants of the largest continent, Asian's noses vary depending on different geographical regions. Northern Asian noses can have dorsal humps and high nasions extending onto the glabella [31]. Filipinos and Polynesians typically have "flat" noses which start off narrow at the bridge and gradually become wide and blunt at the tip [31]. Despite differences, the goal of rhinoplasty in Asian patients can generally be seen as similar to the goal of Occidental rhinoplasty: a strong dorsum with a prominent origin but not competing with the tip as the leading point of the nasal profile [31].

Nonsurgical rhinoplasty with Radiesse® in Asian patients (Fig. 56.9) can increase tip projection, create a higher dorsum, and improve tip contour [34]. Augmentation is also performed at the glabella in response to deficiencies there, and the columella to correct vertical deficiencies. Dorsal augmentation can also be used to create the appearance of a narrow bridge, a procedure also common in African-American noses [35]. In Asian populations, nonsurgical augmentation is also frequently done as part of revision or after removal of an implant.

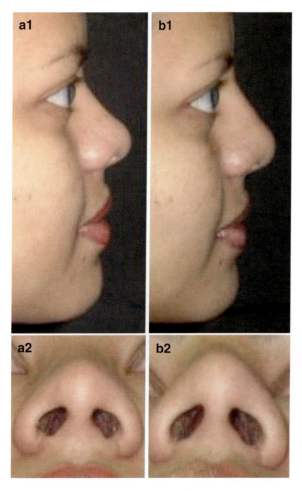
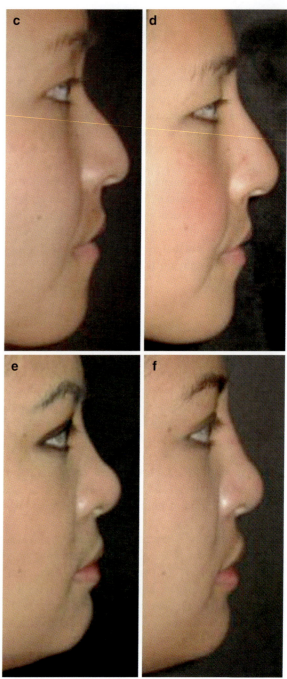

Fig. 56.9 Asian Radiesse® rhinoplasty. (**a1, a2**) pre-injection lateral and worm's eye view respectively. (**b1, b2**) post-injection lateral and worm's eye view respectively (**c**) Preprocedure Chinese woman. (**d**) Postprocedure following injections with Radiesse® to the dorsum and radix. (**e**) Preprocedure 26-year-old Philippino woman. (**f**) Postprocedure after injections with Radiesse® to the radix, bridge, and tip

Fig. 56.9 (continued)

56.9.2 African-American

A frequent complaint of African-American patients is a lack of a projection from the dorsum and the tip. In addition, African-American patients commonly complain of short columella, small nasolabial angle with the upper lip too close to the nasal tip, round nostrils, and excessively broad alae [31].

Augmentation to the dorsum is as routine in African-American patients as hump removal is in Caucasian patients [31]. Approximately 50% of African-Americans are good candidates for augmentation [31]. African-American patients with American Indian heritage frequently also have dorsal humps and high nasions that may extend on the glabella [31]. To this end, nonsurgical rhinoplasty with Radiesse® in African-American patients can increase the height of the dorsum, as well as convert saddle deformities into more linear forms (Fig. 56.10). Dorsal augmentation with Radiesse® is also advantageous because the caudal end of the nose tends to be mobile; therefore rigid implants are not routinely used [31]. In order to address wide-bridge appearances from frontal views, dorsal augmentation alone (without an osteotomy) can create the appearance of a narrower bridge [35].

In African-American patients, tip injections with Radiesse® can also give a more prominent appearance to an otherwise bulbous, flattened tip. The nasal tip in African-American patients has also been described as fleshy, flat, wide, depressed, pendulous, or depressed, while the aim is to create a more sculpted tip [31]. Flared nares cannot be treated with Radiesse® rhinoplasty and need surgical correction.

56.9.3 Hispanic

Nasal surgery is one of the most commonly requested aesthetic surgeries requested by Hispanic Americans. A mestiso nose typically has a narrow and deficient radix that may be augmented with Radiesse® to balance the cephalad aspect with the caudal aspect of the nose. Other common characteristics are insufficient anterior project of the entire nose, wide alar bases, retracted columellas, acute nasolabial angles, and depressed piriformis areas [31].

The dorsum is typically wide, and the goal is to convert it into a straight or slightly concave shape (Fig. 56.11). This is difficult to address with Radiesse®.

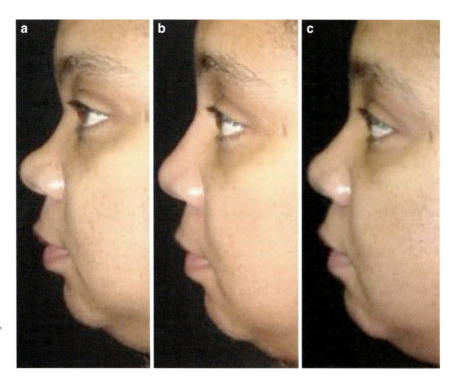

Fig. 56.10 African-American Radiesse® rhinoplasty. (**a**) Pretreatment 42-year-old African-American woman. (**b**) Posttreatment immediately after injections with Radiesse® to the radix, bridge, and tip. (**c**) One month postprocedure after initial swelling subsided

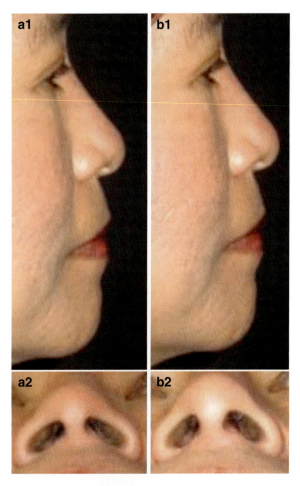

Fig. 56.11 Hispanic Radiesse® rhinoplasty. (**a1, a2**) pre-injection lateral and worm's eye view respectively. (**b1, b2**) post-injection lateral and worm's eye view respectively

The tip is ptotic and Radiesse® can provide a more prominent shape. Another problem site is the columella, which is often weak and found to lie above the alar rim. Radiesse® injection can increase the projection of the columella by adding structure. As with African-Americans, nostril flaring may only be corrected surgically.

56.9.4 Arabic (Middle Eastern)

While generalizations should be avoided, morphologically the Middle Eastern nose falls somewhere between African and Caucasian noses [36]. Some of the most common features of Middle Eastern noses are: wide nasal bones, slight alar flaring, ill-defined bulbous tips, bulky infratip lobules, overprojecting radix, high and wide dorsums, and acute columellar-labial angles [36]. In addition, these patients commonly have thick, sebaceous nasal skin – especially at the tip [36]. Middle Eastern noses can also have dorsal humps and high nasions extending onto the glabella [31]. Correction with Radiesse® should proceed with caution, since this population typically needs a "reduction" rhinoplasty as opposed to an augmentation rhinoplasty. Reduction typically involves a septorhinoplasty in response to a deviated septum, removal of a dorsum hump, correction of a crooked tip, and/or reduction of a broad base [31]. Small improvements can be offered with Radiesse® rhinoplasty such as injections to the radix to augment it if it is deficient, to the tip to offer more definition, as well as to the columella to create a more obtuse columellar-labial angle. In women, this angle should be between 95° and 105°, while in men the angle should be approximately 90° [31]. From a lateral view, the columella should lie 2–3 mm below the alar rim [31].

56.9.5 Aging

Facial aging is a complex process characterized by thinning of the epidermis, atrophy of subcutaneous fat layers, a degree of bone resorption, progressive loss of elastic fibers and collagen organization, and weakening of underlying muscles [7]. In the nose, Radiesse® injection can be used to augment areas affected by the aging processes. For example, augmentation with radiesse to the base of the pyriform aperture can provide the columella with additional support. Nevertheless, it should be noted that Radiesse® can be used to smooth nasal wrinkles and depressions associated with aging in patients (Fig. 56.12). It is already used to improve aesthetic effects of aging on the forehead, cheeks, nasolabial folds, and labiomandibular lines.

56.9.6 Revision Rhinoplasty

Contour irregularities after a rhinoplasty have to be assessed on an individual basis, and may be improved

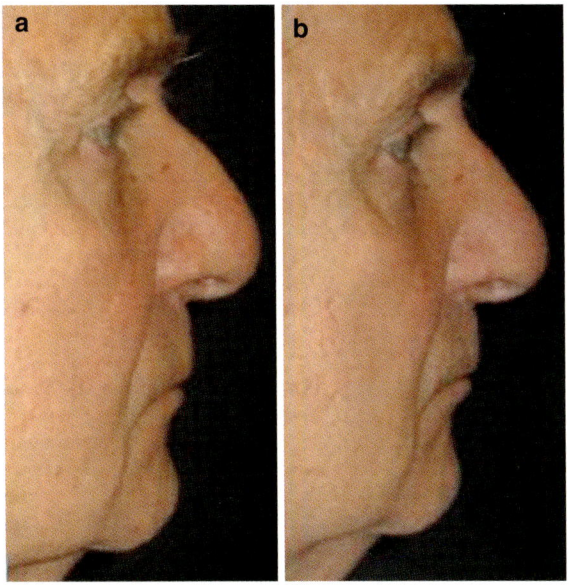

Fig. 56.12 Radiesse® rhinoplasty in response to aging. (**a**) Sixty two-year-old male before treatment. (**b**) Postprocedure after Radiesse® injection above and below a dorsal hump, which masked it

with Radiesse® injections. Because the skin may be compromised or there may be excessive scar tissue, caution needs to be exercised not to compromise the blood supply to the nasal skin with an aggressive injection of Radiesse®. In this category of nonsurgical rhinoplasty correction with Radiesse®, each nasal contour problem is unique and needs to be addressed on an individual basis.

56.10 Discussion

The first report of using an injectable filler for nonsurgical rhinoplasty was by Han et.al [20, 37] in 2006. In that study, hyaluronic acid mixed with autologous human fibroblasts was injected subcutaneously along the nasal dorsum and immediately shaped by hand to correct flat nasal bridges. While hyaluronic acid is known not to be a long-lasting filler, when combined with fibroblasts its aesthetic results last up to approximately 1 year [37]. Drawbacks of this method of nasal augmentation are the significant preparatory time for harvesting fibroblasts and morbidity [20]. With Radiesse®, these drawbacks are negated and results are maintained for an even longer period.

Since the Han et al. study and FDA approval for Radiesse® as a soft-filler for nasolabial folds, which was also in 2006, there have been a plethora of studies where Radiesse® has been used for nonsurgical nasal augmentation. Like other facial rejuvenation procedures, the most important issues for nonsurgical rhinoplasty are longevity, biocompatibility of the soft-tissue filler, low adverse events, and a sound cost-benefit ratio. While rhinoplasty surgery under the correct circumstances can produce astounding results, it is a very costly operation with many consequences. Some patients may prefer to spend $700–$1,000 on Radiesse® rhinoplasty annually or biannually, as opposed to spending $6,000–$13,000 on surgical rhinoplasty.

While complications were previously discussed, another possible risk is internal nasal valve collapse, although no cases have been reported [16]. There is also no evidence of granuloma formation (a problem with injectable silicon) or osteogenesis when CaHA is placed in soft tissue [7]. The problem of nodule of formation seen in the lips has also not been seen in nonsurgical rhinoplasty with Radiesse®. Furthermore, because it is radiopaque there was concern that Radiesse® may interfere with radiological study interpretations, but this theory has been disproved [38].

Because nonsurgical rhinoplasty with Radiesse® is a relatively new procedure, Radiesse® is injected in relatively low doses not only to avoid overcorrection, but due to concerns of safety. In the future, higher doses at more diverse locations may be attempted once longer-term analysis confirms product safety for nonsurgical rhinoplasty [21]. Furthermore, computer-assisted analysis may permit even more objective measurements of nasal symmetry and contour, as seen with surgical rhinoplasty, which may lead to better injection techniques and dosages [21, 39].

Over the last 2 years the authors have performed nonsurgical rhinoplasty with Radiesse® on all ethnic groups discussed previously, with patients ranging from 17 to 62 years old. Nonsurgical rhinoplasty with Radiesse® has also been performed for revision after a primary surgical rhinoplasty. Approximately 30% of patients return for additional touch-ups. Overall, we have experienced no complications or adverse effects, and enjoy an over 95% satisfaction rate. Our high patient satisfaction is a result of good communication and administration of conservative dosages.

56.11 Conclusions

Nonsurgical rhinoplasty with Radiesse® is a feasible alternative for many patients who require nasal augmentation or correction of minor asymmetries, slight depressions, and subtle contour irregularities. A large scale, long-term study of its safety and efficacy in nonsurgical rhinoplasty may lead to Radiesse® being the first FDA-approved soft filler for this procedure, as current indications show Radiesse® is preferable.

Like surgical rhinoplasty, nonsurgical rhinoplasty with Radiesse® requires high-quality consultations, physical examinations, surgical knowledge of nasal anatomy, expert execution of the procedure, and postinjection care. Guidelines have been outlined regarding these steps, including needle specifications, dosages, and use of anesthesia and prophylaxis.

Besides the actual procedural considerations, it is important to identify the potentials and limitations of nonsurgical rhinoplasty with Radiesse®. Typical candidates for the procedure are patients in need of nasal augmentation, particularly patients with ethnic noses, as well as patients with defects related to normal nasal features, aging, or previous surgical rhinoplasty operations. While generalizations can be made regarding how to approach specific ethnic and other nasal features, like surgical rhinoplasty, individual aesthetic subtleties vary between all patients. It is important to approach patients on a case-by-case basis.

With a clear understanding of its background and what it entails, nonsurgical rhinoplasty with Radiesse® is a high satisfaction, comparatively low-cost, and low-risk procedure aesthetic surgeons can easily incorporate into their practices as a cheaper – albeit temporary – alternative to surgical rhinoplasty.

References

1. Kontis TC, Rivkin A. The history of injectable facial fillers. Facial Plast Surg. 2009;25(2):67–72.
2. Pitkin L, Rimmer J, Lo S, Hosni A. Aesthetic augmentation rhinoplasty with Permacol: how we do it. Clin Otolaryngol. 2008;33(6):615–8.
3. Kirwan L: via http://www.cosmeticplasticsurgery.uk.com/skin/radiance-cosmetic-medical-treatment-procedure.php. Last accessed 28 Jul 2009.
4. Busso M, Voigts R. An investigation of changes in physical properties of injectable calcium hydroxylapatite in a carrier gel when mixed with lidocaine and with lidocaine/epinephrine. Dermatol Surg. 2008;34 Suppl 1:S16–23; discussion S24.
5. Godin MS, Majmundar MV, Chrzanowski DS, Dodson KM. Use of Radiesse® in combination with restylane for facial augmentation. Arch Facial Plast Surg. 2006;8(2):92–7.
6. Jones JK. Patient safety considerations regarding dermal filler injections. Plast Surg Nurs. 2006;26:156.
7. Graivier MH, Bass LS, Busso M, Jasin ME, Narins RS, Tzikas TL. Calcium hydroxylapatite (Radiesse®) for correction of the mid-and lower face: consensus recommendations. Plast Reconstr Surg. 2007;120(6 Suppl):55S–66S.
8. Becker H. Nasal augmentation with calcium hydroxylapatite in a carrier-based gel. Plast Reconstr Surg. 2008;121(6): 2142–7.
9. Monhian MCS, Shah SB N. Implants in rhinoplasty. Facial Plast Surg. 1997;13(4):279–90.
10. Renno RZ. Injectable calcium hydroxyapatite filler for minimally invasive delayed treatment of traumatic enophthalmos. Arch Facial Plast Surg. 2007;9(1):62–3.
11. Vagefi MR, McMullan TF, Burroughs JR, White Jr GL, McCann JD, Anderson RL, et al. Injectable calcium hydroxylapatite for orbital volume augmentation. Arch Facial Plast Surg. 2007;9(6):439–42.
12. Dayan SH, Greene RM, Chambers AA. Long-lasting injectable implant for correcting cosmetic nasal deformities. Ear Nose Throat J. 2007;86(1):25–6.
13. Uses and Limitation on Radiesse website, http://www.radiesseusa.com/physicians/uses/. Last accessed 29 Jul 2009.
14. Tzikas T, Mangat D, Mandy S. Radiesse raises the bar in facial augmentation. Aesthetic buyers guide, September/October 2006.
15. Nyte CP. Spreader graft injection with calcium hydroxylapatite: a nonsurgical technique for internal nasal valve collapse. Laryngoscope. 2006;116(7):1291–2.
16. Stupak HD, Moulthrop TH, Wheatley P, Tauman AV, Johnson Jr CM. Calcium hydroxylapatite gel (Radiesse®) injection for the correction of postrhinoplasty contour deficiencies and asymmetries. Arch Facial Plast Surg. 2007;9(2):130–6.
17. Evans KK, Rasko Y, Lenert J, Olding M. The use of calcium hydroxylapatite for nipple projection after failed nipple-areolar reconstruction. Ann Plast Surg. 2005;55(1):25–9.
18. Hubbard W. 36-Month biocompatibility study of calcium hydroxylapatite microspheres in 24 female dogs.
19. Tzikas TL. Evaluation of the Radiance FN soft tissue filler for facial soft tissue augmentation. Arch Facial Plast Surg. 2004;6(4):234–9.
20. Rokhsar C, Ciocon DH. Nonsurgical rhinoplasty: an evaluation of injectable calcium hydroxylapatite filler for nasal contouring. Dermatol Surg. 2008;34(7):944–6.
21. Jacovella PF. Use of calcium hydroxylapatite (Radiesse®) for facial augmentation. Clin Interv Aging. 2008;3(1): 161–74.
22. Siclovan HR, Jomah JA. Injectable calcium hydroxylapatite for correction of nasal bridge deformities. Aesthetic Plast Surg. 2008;33(4):544–8.
23. Jacovella PF. Aesthetic nasal corrections with hydroxylapatite facial filler. Plast Reconstr Surg. 2008;121(5):338e–9e.
24. Gruber R, Kuang A, Kahn D. Asian-American rhinoplasty. Aesthetic Surg J. 2004;24(5):423–30.
25. Röthler G, Waldhart E, Puelacher W, Strobl H. Reconstructive procedures for improving the facial contour [Article in German]. Fortschr Kiefer Gesichtschir. 1994;39:114–6.

26. Guo X, Wu X. Chung-Hua Cheng Hsing Shao Shang Wai Ko Tsa Chih: Augmentation rhinoplasty with particulate hydroxy apatite artificial bone in 50 cases – a follow-up of 8 years [Chinese]. J Plast Surg Burns. 1997;13((3)):185–7.
27. Lee MJ, Sung MS, Kim NJ, Choung HK, Khwarg SI. Eyelid mass secondary to injection of calcium hydroxylapatite facial filler. Ophthal Plast Reconstr Surg. 2008;24(5): 421–3.
28. Braccini F, Dohan ED. Medical rhinoplasty: rationale for atraumatic nasal modelling using botulinum toxin and fillers. Rev Laryngol Otol Rhinol (Bord). 2008;129(4–5): 233–8.
29. Sklar JA, White SM. Radiance FN: a new soft tissue filler. Dermatol Surg. 2004;30(5):764–8.
30. Kosowski TR, McCarthy C, Reavey PL, Scott AM, Wilkins EG, Cano SJ, et al. A systematic review of patient-reported outcome measures after facial cosmetic surgery and/or nonsurgical facial rejuvenation. Plast Reconstr Surg. 2009; 123(6):1819–27.
31. Matory WE. Ethnic considerations in facial aesthetic surgery. Philadelphia: Lippincott-Raven; 1998.
32. Lee CH, Han SK, Kim SB, Kim DW, Kim WK. Augmentation rhinoplasty minimizing nasion level changes: a simple method. Plast Reconstr Surg. 2008;121(5):334e–5e.
33. Hodgkinson DJ. The Eurasian nose: aesthetic principles and techniques for augmentation of the Asian nose with autogenous grafting. Aesthetic Plast Surg. 2007;31(1): 28–31.
34. Toriumi DM, Swartout B. Asian rhinoplasty. Facial Plast Surg Clin North Am. 2007;15(3):293–307.
35. Hubbard TJ. Bridge narrowing in ethnic noses. Ann Plast Surg. 1998;40(3):214–8.
36. Rohrich RJ, Ghavami A. Rhinoplasty for Middle Eastern noses. Plast Reconstr Surg. 2009;123(4):1343–54.
37. Han SK, Shin SH, Kang HJ, Kim WK. Augmentation rhinoplasty using injectable tissue-engineered soft tissue: a pilot study. Ann Plast Surg. 2006;56(3):251–5.
38. Carruthers A, Liebeskind B, Carruthers J, Forster BB. Radiographic and computed tomographic studies of calcium hydroxylapatite for treatment of HIV-associated facial lipoatrophy and correction of nasolabial folds. Dermatol Surg. 2008;34 Suppl 1:S78–84.
39. Coghlan BA, Laitung JK, Pigott RW. A computer-aided method of measuring nasal symmetry in the cleft lip nose. Br J Plast Surg. 1993;46(1):13–7.

Lip Enhancement: Personal Technique

57

Anthony Erian

57.1 Introduction

Cosmetic surgery to the lips is one of the most difficult areas in which to achieve success. As well as the psychological implications compared to other types of surgery, there is a paucity in the literature regarding cosmetic augmentation of the lips. The criteria of beauty for the lips include a fuller look, symmetry, contour definition, and a slightly protruding Cupid's arch. Lips should represent youth, romance, and beauty (Fig. 57.1).

57.2 Anatomical Basics of the Human Lip

The lips (Fig. 57.2) are the shape of a soft M for the upper (Labium superius) and a W for the lower lip (Labium inferius). The lower lip is usually somewhat larger. This should be taken into consideration while injecting. The border between the lips and the surrounding skin is referred to as the vermillion border, or simply the vermilion. The vertical groove on the upper lip is known as the philtrum. The skin of the lip, with 3–5 cellular layers, is very thin compared to typical face skin, which has up to 16 layers. With light skin color, the lip skin contains fewer melanocytes (cells which produce melanin pigment, which give skin its color).

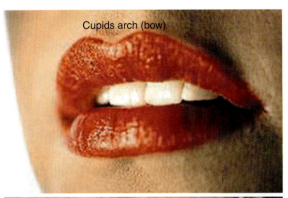
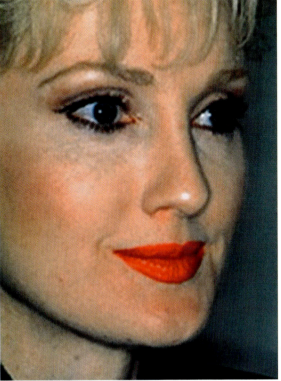

Fig. 57.1 Cupid's arch. Lips should represent youth, romance, and beauty

A. Erian
Pear Tree Cottage, Cambridge Road,
Wimpole 43, SG8 5QD Cambridge, United Kingdom
e-mail: plasticsurgeon@anthonyerian.com

Because of this, the blood vessels appear through the skin of the lips, which leads to their notable red coloring. With darker skin color this effect is less prominent, as in this case the skin of the lips contains more melanin and thus is visually darker. The skin of the lip forms the border between the exterior skin of the face, and the interior mucous membrane of the inside of the mouth. The lip skin is not hairy, and does not have sweat glands or sebaceous glands. Therefore it does not have the usual protection layer of sweat and body oils which keep the skin smooth, inhibit pathogens, and regulate warmth. For these reasons, the lips dry out faster and become chapped more easily [1, 2].

The basic parts of the mouth and lips are:

1. Upper Lip – (labium superfluous entafada) is the strip of smooth skin that borders the upper edge of the mouth. It is usually thinner than the lower lip and can have pronounced peaks to either side of a groove at the center of the mouth.
2. Lower Lip – (labium inferius) is the strip of smooth skin that borders the lower edge of the mouth. It is usually wider and vertically deeper than the upper lip.
3. Vermilion – is the border of the skin of the lips and the surrounding skin of the face. In some individuals this is more pronounced, while in others the two skin types seem to almost blend.
4. Cupid's Bow – is the area in the middle of the upper lip which straightens with age. Carefully placed dermal filler can restore the youthful look of the Cupid's bow.
5. Philtral Columns – is the groove-like indentation often found at the center of the upper lip. It is responsible for the biggest difference in shape between the upper and lower lips and becomes more pronounced when the mouth is puckered. This is an especially important aspect of the lip that requires attention during treatment.
6. Dry Part – is the part under the lip that separates the dry and wet part and is usually used for fullness.
7. Wet Part – adjacent to the dry part and is important for pouting.

The balanced lip size which is the ratio of the height of the upper lip to that of the lower one is ideally 1.4:1.6.

Clinically, the technique is based on the anatomy:

1. For contouring: inject the vermilion border.
2. For fullness: inject the dry part of the inner lip.
3. For pouting: inject the wet part of the inner lip.
4. For philtrum and ridges: inject directly into the subdermal layer.
5. For oral commissure: requires separate injection.

As a person ages, the following changes occur in the lips:

- Loss of lip projection
- Lengthening of white lip
- Flattening of philtrum
- Flattening of Cupid's bow
- Dermal and subcutaneous atrophy
- Atrophy of orbicularis oris

57.3 Injectable Materials

Injectable human-derived collagen comes from a single neonatal human foreskin which was harvested many years ago and which has been shown to be free from known communicable diseases. Examples include CosmoPlast and CosmoDerm. Examples

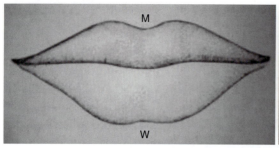
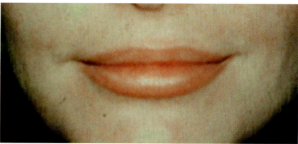

Fig. 57.2 The lips are the shape of a soft M for the upper (Labium superius) and a W for the lower lip (Labium inferius)

ofbovine-derived collagen include Zyplast and Zyderm. The mechanism of action is thought to be due to a direct filling effect. With time, injectable collagen, which is similar to dermal matrix collagen, is metabolized leading to loss of filling effect. Collagen has been in use for over 20 years, and now skin testing for possible allergic reaction is no longer required [3, 4].

Injectable hyaluronic acid (HA) fillers are based on a natural part of the extracellular matrix of bone and cartilage. Examples include Restylane and Juvederm, which are both derived from bacterial fermentation. HA fillers absorb water and form a gel which creates volume. Over approximately 9–12 months this is degraded [5–10]. The author does not recommend the use of nonabsorbable material or Gore-Tex (Fig. 57.3), since long-term complications can occur from these procedures.

57.4 Technique

Emla cream local anesthetic is applied to the lip and skin surrounding the lips approximately 30–60 min before procedure. A complete dental block is performed; this is a vital part of the procedure as lips are very painful and uncomfortable to inject. Good

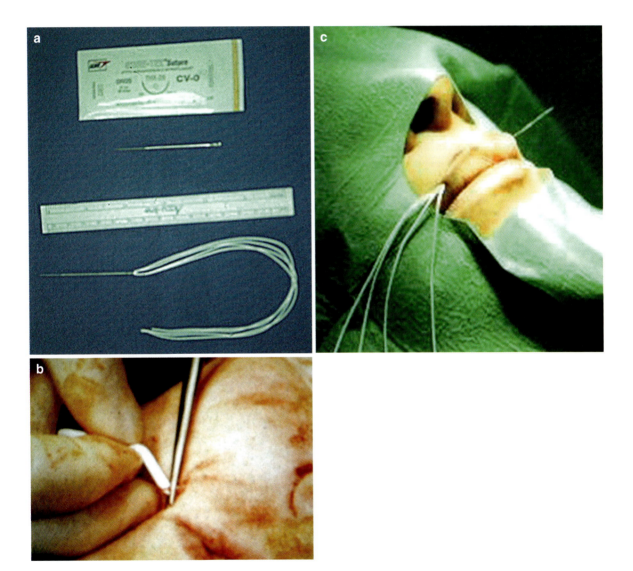

Fig. 57.3 (**a**) Gore-Tex. (**b**) Insertion of Gore-Tex. (**c**) Thicker Gore-Tex being inserted

anatomical knowledge of the nerve supply is vital to the success of the local.

1. The infraorbital nerve is a branch of the maxillary trunk. It supplies not only the upper lip, but much of the skin of the face between the upper lip and the lower eyelid, except for the bridge of the nose (Fig. 57.4).
2. The mental nerve is a branch of the mandibular trunk (via the inferior alveolar nerve). It supplies the skin and mucous membrane of the lower lip and labial gingiva (gum) anteriorly.

Betadine antiseptic solution is used to clean the area. Sterile gloves, a magnifying light, and a mirror are used.

An intramuscular injection using a very fine needle on a Luer-lock syringe is performed. In the upper lip, the needle is inserted into the mucosa and pointed upward on either side of philtrum, in order to fill Cupid's bow and obtain slight eversion. The remaining upper lip is injected through injections at corner of the lips at a 45° angle, progressing slowly toward the midline and philtrum. In the lower lip, the needle is inserted in similar positions to the upper lip. The lip margins are injected superficially to achieve contour definition. This is achieved by injecting parallelly beneath the skin, with slow injection on withdrawal to obtain uniform distribution. Each injection deposits about 0.1 ml of injectable material. This will achieve eversion of the vermilion border, enhance convexity, produce fuller lips, and produce a more youthful appearance due to the improved philtrum and Cupid's bow. Gentle massage to areas after procedure may be performed.

The patient will be able to see the result immediately, which is an additional benefit to this procedure (Fig. 57.5). A touch-up may be considered at anytime. Try to remember the arterial supply in order to avoid bruising as the lips have a very rich blood supply. The facial artery is one of the six nonterminal branches of the external carotid artery. It supplies the lips by its superior and inferior labial branches, each of which bifurcate and anastomose with their companion artery from the other side.

57.5 Postoperative Instructions

Sometimes the lips may swell and be red for 1–2 days; however, when this occurs it is minimal and can be camouflaged with make-up. Clients may continue to work and socialize. No antibiotic or antiviral treatment is required. Ice packs for 24 h may be used to reduce swelling and simple pain medication such as paracetamol may be taken if necessary.

57.6 Complications

Very rarely complications may occur. These include infection, allergic reaction, persistent erythema, lumps, and bleeding. For the best results, do not approach Cupid's bow from superiorly, as this will cause inversion. Fat and collagen do not last long: 3–4 months and 4–6 months respectively, whereas hyaluronic acid lasts 9–12 months. Silicone is no longer available due to possible side effects but may last permanently [11, 12].

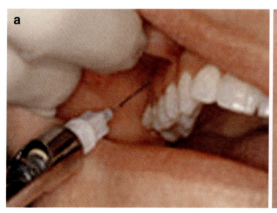
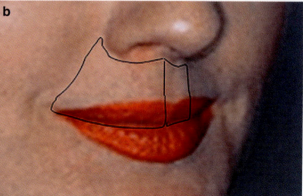

Fig. 57.4 (a) Nerve block. (b) Area numb from maxillary block

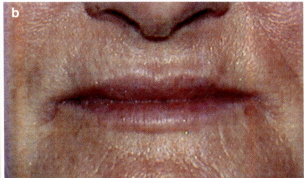

Fig. 57.5 (**a**) Before. (**b**) After injection of hyaluronic acid

More permanent options include Alloderm (homograft of skin) [13, 14] and Polytetrafluoroethylene [15], but these have more complications than the injectable materials. Above all, they may need to be removed due to the client being able to feel the implant, for instance, at the time of eating and kissing.

Other rarer complications for implantable materials include seromas, malposition, infection, extrusion, long-term inflammation, and capsule formation.

57.7 Discussion

In the opinion of the author, the best results for lip enlargement are achieved with injectables, and my advice is to use a filler that is absorbable. The filler is injected superficially (under the dermal layer). When approaching the Cupid's bow or arch, do so from the inferior direction, otherwise it creates inversion of the lip resulting in an unaesthetic appearance. A list of fillers is provided. Most are natural polysaccharides, which are completely biologically degradable. Hyaluronic acid is naturally integrated into the tissues, so nutritive agents pass freely through the implant and cells pass between fragments of gel. Hyaluronic acid exists in the human body and is able to bind water and lubricate movable parts of the body such as muscles. Hyaluronic acid can be extracted from tissues rich in hyaluronan or produced bacterially through fermentation. This can produce hyaluronic acid in unlimited amounts while maintaining high.

Fat transfer techniques have been used to produce aesthetically appealing lips, but there is steep learning curve to this technique. The author prefers the Pearl technique, which injects small aliquots of fat parcels in multiple layers.

A more permanent material is Alloderm which is a homograft of skin, where the soft form is expanded during the procedure. Polytetraflouroethylene is a permanent material but may occasionally require removal. The patients feel these implants during kissing, eating, and other activities. Other complications include seroma, malposition, infection, extrusion, long-term inflammation, and capsule formation. These complications are fortunately rare. Lip augmentation can be performed alone or in combination with facial surgery. In addition to these injectable and implantable procedures, operative procedures may also be considered. This includes operations which involve advancement, lift, and roll techniques. The complications, however, may be significant and hypertrophic scarring, asymmetry, numbness, and lumpiness may be seen [16–23].

References

1. Segall L, Ellis DA. Therapeutic options for lip augmentation. Facial Plast Surg Clin North Am. 2007;15(4):485–90.
2. Wall SJ, Adamson PA. Augmentation, enhancement, and implantation procedures for the lips. Otolaryngol Clin North Am. 2002;35(1):87–102.
3. Kanchwala SK, Holloway L, Bucky LP. Reliable soft tissue augmentation: a clinical comparison of injectable soft-tissue fillers for facial-volume augmentation. Ann Plast Surg. 2005;55(1):30–5.
4. Sclafani AP. Soft tissue fillers for management of the aging perioral complex. Facial Plast Surg. 2005;21(1):74–8.
5. Godin MS, Majmundar MV, Chrzanowski DS, Dodson KM. Use of radiesse in combination with restylane for facial augmentation. Arch Facial Plast Surg. 2006;8(2):92–7.
6. Bagal A, Dahiya R, Tsai V, Adamson PA. Clinical experience with polymethylmethacrylate microspheres (Artecoll)

for soft-tissue augmentation: a retrospective review. Arch Facial Plast Surg. 2007;9(4):275–80.
7. Ersek RA, Beisang III AA. Bioplastique: a new biphasic polymer for minimally invasive injection implantation. Aesthetic Plast Surg. 1992;16(1):59–65.
8. Sarnoff DS, Saini R, Gotkin RH. Comparison of filling agents for lip augmentation. Aesthetic Surg J. 2008;28(5): 556–63.
9. Ali MJ, Ende K, Maas CS. Perioral rejuvenation and lip augmentation. Facial Plast Surg Clin North Am. 2007;15(4): 491–500.
10. Jordan DR. Soft-tissue fillers for wrinkles, folds and volume augmentation. Can J Ophthalmol. 2003;38(4):285–8.
11. Jacinto SS. Ten-year experience using injectable silicone oil for soft tissue augmentation in the Philippines. Dermatol Surg. 2005;31(11 Pt 2):1550–4.
12. Barnett JG, Barnett CR. Silicone augmentation of the lip. Facial Plast Surg Clin North Am. 2007;15(4):501–12.
13. Gryskiewicz JM. Alloderm lip augmentation. Plast Reconstr Surg. 2000;106(4):953–4.
14. Fagien S, Elson ML. Facial soft-tissue augmentation with allogeneic human tissue collagen matrix (Dermalogen and Dermaplant). Clin Plast Surg. 2001;28(1):63–81.
15. Singh S, Baker Jr JL. Use of expanded polytetrafluoroethylene in aesthetic surgery of the face. Clin Plast Surg. 2000; 27(4):579–93.
16. Seymour PE, Leventhal DD, Pribitkin EA. Lip augmentation with porcine small intestinal submucosa. Arch Facial Plast Surg. 2008;10(1):30–3.
17. Trussler AP, Kawamoto HK, Wasson KL, Dickinson BP, Jackson E, Keagle JN, et al. Upper lip augmentation: palmaris longus tendon as an autologous filler. Plast Reconstr Surg. 2008;121(3):1024–32.
18. de Benito J, Fernandez-Sanza I. Galea and subgalea graft for lip augmentation revision. Aesthetic Plast Surg. 1996;20(3): 243–8.
19. Niechajev I. Lip enhancement: surgical alternatives and histologic aspects. Plast Reconstr Surg. 2000;105(3):1173–83; discussion 1184–7.
20. Mutaf M. V-Y in V-Y procedure: new technique for augmentation and protrusion of the upper lip. Ann Plast Surg. 2006;56(6):605–8.
21. Wilkinson TS. Lip enhancement. In: Practical procedures in aesthetic plastic surgery: tips and traps. New York: Springer; 1994, pp. 117–144.
22. Guerrissi JO. Surgical treatment of the senile upper lip. Plast Reconstr Surg. 2000;106(4):938–40.
23. Burres SA. Lip augmentation with preserved fascia lata. Dermatol Surg. 1997;23(6):459–62.

Liposuction of the Neck: Technique and Pitfalls

Anthony Erian

58.1 Introduction

Liposuction of the neck is the removal of unwanted adipose tissue using a tumescent technique, which can restore the jaw line and cervicomental angle. Liposuction of the neck has become a common cosmetic procedure, either on its own or in conjunction with facelifting or other facial procedures. It has many advantages over older techniques. In the author's practice it has improved the results of facial rejuvenation manyfold. The practitioner must be aware of all the pitfalls associated with this procedure. In my opinion most facelifting and facial rejuvenation procedures today require some form of liposculpturing to achieve the best results. Liposuction of the neck achieves excellent results in patients with excess fat along the jowl and in the neck, good skin elasticity, and minimal platysmal banding (Figs. 58.1 and 58.2).

58.2 Advantages

1. Inexpensive.
2. Less traumatic than open procedures.
3. Safe.
4. Small scars.
5. Simple technique.
6. Fat aspirated may be used for lipotransfer [1, 2].

A. Erian
Pear Tree Cottage, Cambridge Road,
Wimpole 43, SG8 5QD Cambridge, United Kingdom
e-mail: plasticsurgeon@anthonyerian.com

58.3 Mechanism of Action

Liposuction of the neck is performed using local anesthesia in the form of a tumescent solution [3, 4]. Fat is aspirated using small cannulas that have been introduced through small incisions below the earlobes and in the submental crease. I use the manual syringe technique to aspirate the fat. Negative pressure formed in the syringe allows adipose tissue to enter the hollow cannula. Back and forth motion of the cannula disrupts fat and creates a series of interlacing tunnels within the fat. Once completed, the patient will wear a compression garment which compresses the tissues and aids in skin contraction. Good knowledge of the anatomy of the neck and musculature of the face is important prior to performing this procedure [5, 6].

58.4 The Tumescent Technique

The tumescent technique was introduced by Klein in 1987 and was the milestone that allowed liposuction to be performed with local anesthesia [7]. Various tumescent solutions have been described, but the author prefers the following:

1. 250 ml of saline
2. Adrenaline 1:1,000
3. Lignocaine 1% 20 ml

This is injected with a 19 gauge needle. The technique of injecting is superficial and in a linear fashion. The nondominant hand, often called the "smart" hand, must be used as a guide for the depth at all times. The linear threading method is the least traumatic.

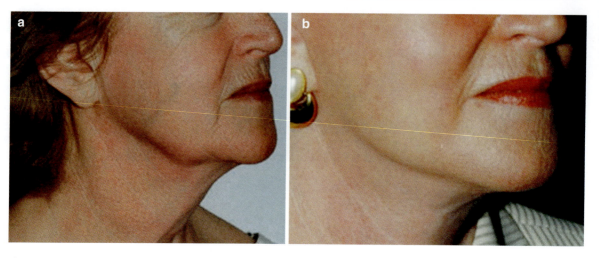

Fig. 58.1 Results in patient with excess fat of jowl and neck. (**a**) Preoperative. (**b**) Following liposuction

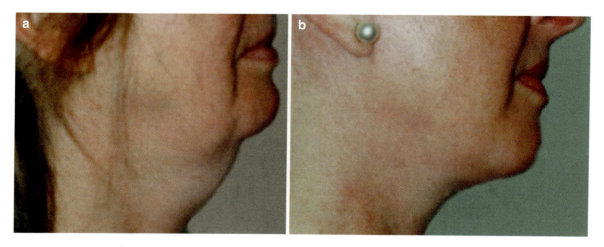

Fig. 58.2 Results in patient with excess fat of jowl and neck. (**a**) Preoperative. (**b**) Following liposuction

58.5 Indications

1. Localized fat deposits in neck and along jawline.
2. Good skin elasticity (Fig. 58.3).
3. Minimal platysmal banding. Patients with banding will require a tightening or excisional procedure of the banding. Patients with minimal neck fat but who have skin wrinkling and banding may best be served with a neck lifting operation [8].
4. Patient is healthy.
5. Discontinued use of aspirin, NSAIDs, and anticoagulation.
6. Patients with a weak chin may require an implant in addition to the liposuction to achieve the best results [9, 10].

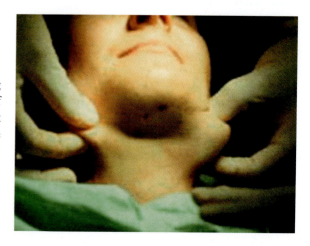

Fig. 58.3 Good skin elasticity

58.6 Contraindications

1. Patients taking anticoagulant or immunosuppressive medication are at a higher risk for complications.
2. History of coagulopathies.
3. History of keloids.
4. History of prior face or neck surgery where the anatomy may be distorted, thus leading to nerve damage.
5. Patients with unrealistic expectations.

58.7 Technique

It is important that the patient lie on a table where the headrest can be dropped to hyperextend the neck. The tumescent solution may be infused manually using a syringe or with the aid of an infusion pump. I prefer handheld aspiration using a 10 ml syringe and a cannula. Approximately 150–300 ml of solution is instilled into the adipose layer of the neck. At least 20 min should be allowed once the solution has been infiltrated. Microcannulas such as the ones the author uses are shown in Fig. 58.4. They come in different designs and each has a special function. For example, the cannula with an opening at the tip is to allow suction close to the skin and the incision site, thus avoiding leaving any thickness in these areas which is very unsightly. Normally 2–3 mm cannulas are used in this technique. It is important to first identify the location of the fat deposits by clinically asking the patient to stick out their tongue. If there is fat above the muscle, the bulging will be larger. It is also vital to leave a thin layer of fat and to not skeletonize the patient's neck. The entirety of neck can be accessed from three incisions. During the procedure, the thickness of the flaps must be assessed constantly and knowing when to stop comes with experience. Finally, while the fat removed is important, it is in fact what remains, which leads to the cosmetic result. As well as the local tumescent solution, many patients will benefit from sedation. Sedation is often best administered by an anesthetist. The patient's face and neck are marked preoperatively in a sitting position to define the base of the neck inferiorly, the anterior border of the sternocleidomastoid muscle laterally, and the jowls superiorly. The stab incision sites may be marked in the submental crease and in the earlobe creases. Above all, the course of the marginal mandibular nerve along the mandible must be noted. Using the stab incisions, the cannula is introduced in a back and forth manner. The cannula is also guided using the "smart" hand in a fan like manner to produce a criss-cross pattern of tunnels within the fat. The cannula openings are generally held face downward, and it is important to avoid rasping the mandible and thus injuring the marginal mandibular nerve. The stab incisions may be sutured, closed with the aid of a steri-strip, or left open. A compression garment is applied to the entire neck. A cervical collar may be used to avoid neck flexion and thus the abnormal creases which may develop. These dressings should be worn for 3 days, after which the patient may shower and apply small bandages to the stab incision sites.

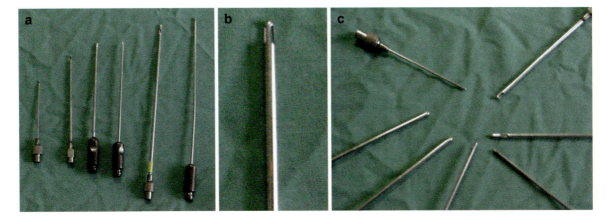

Fig. 58.4 Microcannulas used by the author. (**a**) Microcannulas. (**b**) Cannula with opening at the tip. (**c**) Cannulas with flat inferior opening

58.8 Complications

1. Inadequate result due to poor patient selection
2. Uneven fat removal, skin irregularity, pigmentation
3. Bleeding
4. Hematoma
5. Infection
6. Seroma
7. Scarring
8. Nerve injury
9. Skin perforation
10. Temporary fibrosis and swelling, especially in men (improves with daily massage, monthly steroid injection, and ultrasound therapy) [11, 12]

58.9 Special Considerations

58.9.1 Submandibular Gland Exposure

In some cases, the submandibular gland is ptotic or slightly displaced inferiorly from its anatomic position. Excessive liposuction can aggravate this situation and make the submandibular glands more prominent. In addition, they may then be mistaken for further fat deposits and be injured. Patients must be warned about this prior to surgery.

Correction of submandibular gland ptosis is difficult and many of the described procedures fail. Removal of the glands is unnecessary and can lead to further problems.

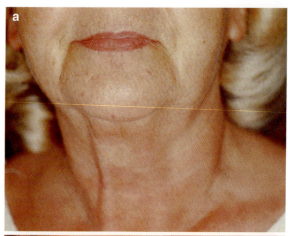
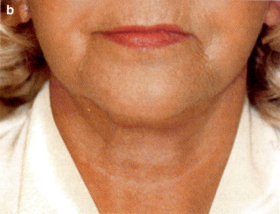

Fig. 58.5 Platysmal band exposed following liposuction of the neck. (**a**) Preoperative. (**b**) Postoperative

58.9.2 Platysmal Band Exposure

Anterior platysmal bands may exist in conjunction with neck and submental fat. Liposuction of the neck can highlight this deformity (Fig. 58.5). Attention must be given to the muscles either simultaneously or on a separate occasion. Many techniques have been described for treating platysmal bands.

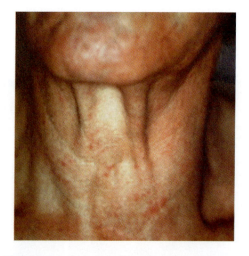

Fig. 58.6 Platysmal band overlying thyroid cartilage

58.9.3 Thyroid Thickness or Band

During the course of my practice, I\the author has come across several cases of a distinct band overlying the thyroid (Fig. 58.6). This band appears to be a thicker layer of adipose tissue which is harder to aspirate. Occasionally an extraincision is required to directly approach this area.

58.9.4 Receding Chin

This is a very common situation which may be associated with a congenital condition, a lack of development, or an undergrowth (Fig. 58.7). It plays a major role toward the shape of the neck especially in profile. During liposuction of the neck, this must be taken into consideration. A chin implant may be required in addition to or instead of liposuction to improve this contour of the neck in profile.

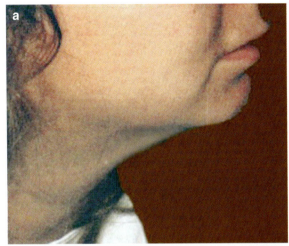

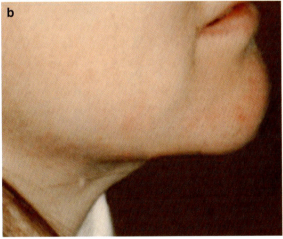

Fig. 58.7 Retrusive jaw. (**a**) Preoperative. (**b**) Postoperative

References

1. Doerr TD. Lipoplasty of the face and neck. Curr Opin Otolaryngol Head Neck Surg. 2007;15(4):228–32.
2. Langdon RC. Liposuction of neck and jowls: five-incision method combining machine-assisted and syringe aspiration. Dermatol Surg. 2000;26(4):388–91.
3. Johnson DS, Cook Jr WR. Advanced techniques in liposuction. Semin Cutan Med Surg. 1999;18(2):139–48.
4. Reznick JB. Cervicofacial liposuction in oral and maxillofacial surgery. J Calif Dent Assoc. 1994;22(5):41–5.
5. Perez MI. An anatomic approach to the rejuvenation of the neck. Dermatol Clin. 2001;19(2):387–96.
6. Goddio AS. Suction lipectomy: the gold triangle at the neck. Aesthetic Plast Surg. 1992;16(1):27–32.
7. Klein JA. The tumescent technique for liposuction surgery. Am J Cosmet Surg. 1987;4:263–7.
8. Ramirez OM. Classification of facial rejuvenation techniques based on the subperiosteal approach and ancillary procedures. Plast Reconstr Surg. 1996;97(1):45–55.
9. Adamson PA, Cormier R, Tropper GJ, McGraw BL. Cervicofacial liposuction: results and controversies. J Otolaryngol. 1990;19(4):267–73.
10. O'Ryan F, Schendel S, Poor D. Submental-submandibular suction lipectomy: indications and surgical technique. Oral Surg Oral Med Oral Pathol. 1989;67(2):117–25.
11. Koehler J. Complications of neck liposuction and submentoplasty. Oral Maxillofac Surg Clin North Am. 2009;21(1):43–52.
12. Bitner JB, Friedman O, Farrior RT, Cook TA. Direct submentoplasty for neck rejuvenation. Arch Facial Plast Surg. 2007;9(3):194–200.

59 Neck Lifting Variations

Harry Mittelman and Joshua D. Rosenberg

59.1 Introduction

The importance of the neck cannot be overstated in the evaluation and treatment of the aging face. Many patients seeking facial rejuvenation report concerns regarding neck skin laxity manifesting as the classic "turkey waddle," platysmal banding, and deep horizontal neck lines as a top priority. In order to achieve an optimal result, both in terms of surgical outcome and patient satisfaction, it is essential to understand the aging process of the neck, properly analyze each individual patient, understand the patient's goals and expectations, and to correctly select the surgical technique with which to correct the patient's pathology.

Over the past century there has been a dramatic evolution of techniques used to correct the aging face and neck. Early teaching and techniques for facial rejuvenation involved simple skin excisions through incisions placed in natural pre and postauricular creases, extensive undermining, and lipectomy [1–3]. The flaps were all subcutaneous in nature and rejuvenation was accomplished through resection of skin. This began to change in the later half of the twentieth century with major innovations in understanding of facial anatomy, its changes with age, and new surgical techniques. A widely heralded achievement was the development of the "Skoog Flap." Zimbler [4] described Skoog's work, published in 1968, where he developed a subplatysmal flap and dissected without detaching the overlying skin. This flap also incorporated the superficial fascia of the lower third of the face which Skoog termed "buccal fascia." The platysma and fascia were undermined anteriorly to the nasolabial and commissure-mandibular grooves and the flap was repositioned posteriorly and affixed to the parotidomasseteric and mastoid fasciae. In 1976, Mitz and Peyronie [5] discovered a fascial layer which invested the mimetic facial musculature and was distinct from the underlying parotidomasseteric fascia. This fascia was called the superficial musculoaponeurotic system (SMAS) and is the basis for SMAS rhytidectomy. Today, approaches to face/neck lifting range from "limited" techniques including multivector face/neck lifts to aggressive, subSMAS procedures.

Coupled with nearly a century of evolution in rhytidoplasty techniques is a long history of evolving techniques addressing the submental region. Bourguet [2] discussed submental lipectomy and transection of platysmal banding. Subsequently, there have been many techniques used to address the aging platysma, such as varieties of midline plication/imbrication, horizontal wedge resection, corset platysmaplasty, interlocking cervicomental suture suspension, and the use of expanded polytetrafluoroethylene (ePTFE) cervical slings [6–8]. Techniques used to address submental adipose tissue initially involved lipectomy while cervicofacial liposuction was a subsequent innovation. The treatment of skin redundancy has involved various approaches such as allowing postoperative adherence and redraping, vertical elliptical skin excision with simple versus Z-plasty, W-plasty, and double advancement flap closure.

H. Mittelman (✉)
Associate Clinical Professor, Stanford University,
Mittelman Plastic Surgery, 810 Altos Oaks Drive,
Los Altos, CA 94024, USA
e-mail: hmittelman@yahoo.com

J.D. Rosenberg
Assistant Professor, Department of Otolaryngology,
Mount Sinai School of Medicine,
Annenberg 10th Floor, One Gustave L. Levy Place,
Box 1189, New York, NY 10029, USA
e-mail: jrosenberg@gmail.com

While great advancements have been made in addressing many aspects of the aging face including the midface and jawline, many of the current techniques fail to completely address the lower half of the neck. This region is easily visible and improvements in this area can be critically important to the overall success of facial rejuvenation surgery. Standard face/neck lift procedures coupled with submentoplasty can effect great improvements in the upper neck and cervicomental angle in the large majority of patients. Nonetheless, in some patients, especially those with pronounced lower neck vertical banding and/or horizontal pleating and deep lines, additional procedures may be beneficial. Standard multivector face/neck lifts as well as deep plane face/neck lifts may incompletely address these pathologies in the lower half of the neck. Two additional neck lifting procedures, the horizontal neck lift and vertical neck lift, may be used, based on individual patient findings. In selected patients, these additional procedures used either concurrently with a face/neck lift or alone in specific situations can be instrumental in the success in of facial rejuvenation surgery.

59.2 Pathophysiology of the Aging Neck

The aging process is dependent upon genetic, anatomic, and environmental factors. The most commonly held theory of cervicofacial aging is one of progressive gravimetric soft tissue descent [9]. With repeated gravitational forces, skin and soft tissue stretch off the bony skeleton, leading to the development of folds, rhytids, and volume loss. However, cervicofacial aging is much more complex and a proper discussion involves dividing the components of facial and neck anatomy into basic categories, including skin, subcutaneous tissue, fascia/muscle, and bone.

59.2.1 Aging Skin

The skin is subject to both extrinsic and intrinsic aging processes. Within the skin, there is thinning of the epidermis, disorganization and reduction in the amount of collagen fibers within the papillary and reticular dermis, including loss of Type I collagen and increased Type III collagen fibers. There is also effacement of rete ridges within the epidermal–papillary dermal junction. Further contributing to the aging appearance is the appearance of dyschromias from accumulation of previous solar damage. This solar elastosis and disorganization leads to thinning of the skin and development of static rhytids. Accumulated exposure to ultraviolet (UV) A and B light leads to direct DNA damage as well as the formation of free radicals which, with the decreased levels of antioxidants with advancing age, are less easily buffered. Furthermore, dehydration of the skin and reduction in sebum production by sebaceous glands leads to further thinning and rhytid formation.

59.2.2 Aging Soft Tissue

Accompanying the changes in the level of the skin are changes in the deeper structures. With advancing age, there is a concomitant decrease in basal metabolic rate, leading to increased adipose tissue. Proportionate fat increases are seen in the face beginning in the fifth decade [9]. Fatty tissue accumulation occurs in depot areas of the body beneath the superficial fascia. In the face and neck, they are located in the periorbital, malar, and submental regions. Progressive fascial and ligamentous laxity leads to decreased support of the adipose tissue resulting in a relative increase in volume of the lower third of the face. While volume loss is a predominant theme in the majority of aging patients, in some, there is increased lyposis, leading to jowl, submental, and lower neck fullness. In these patients, it is important to address the volume accumulation, but also to remain cognizant that adipose tissue may camouflage the aging of other tissues, such as platysmal banding or submandibular gland ptosis.

In many women, as estrogen levels decrease with the onset of menopause, there is a further decrease in superficial fat deposits resulting in thin, poorly supported skin which is easily pulled by the deeper fat. There can also be a loss of subcutaneous adipose tissue resulting in volume depletion and hollowing. There is also increased elasticity of the submuscular aponeurotic system (SMAS) supporting framework leading to vertical descent of the skin-soft tissue envelope of the face and neck. The platysma muscle also loses much of its tone. Repeated contraction, combined with volume loss in the anterior neck, can lead to prominent vertical platysmal bands.

59.2.3 Aging Facial Skeleton

The aging process also affects the skeletal foundation of the face. As the result of hormonal changes, there is an overall decrease in bone density. This decrease is not exclusive to weight-bearing bone, but may also be seen in the facial skeleton. Osteopenia of the zygoma and maxilla leads to a decrease in malar prominence, but also loss of support for the malar fat pads, SMAS, and facial musculature. Osteopenia of the mandible contributes to the formation of the anterior mandibular groove and may accentuate existing microgenia or just a hypoplastic mentum.

59.3 Other Factors

Individual patient factors also play an important role in aging. Perhaps the most important of these factors is tobacco use, which is still quite prevalent and is extremely detrimental to skin quality and blood supply. Model [10] originally coined the term "smoker's face" and attributed to this term the following visual criteria:

1. Lines or wrinkles on the face, typically radiating at right angles from the upper and lower lips or corners of the eyes, deep lines on the cheeks, or numerous shallow lines on the cheeks and lower jaw.
2. A subtle gauntness of the facial features with prominence of the underlying bony contours. Fully developed this change gives the face an "atherosclerotic" look; lesser changes show as slight sinking of the cheeks. In some cases these changes are associated with a leathery, worn, or rugged appearance.
3. An atrophic, slightly pigmented grey appearance of the skin.
4. A plethoric, slightly orange, purple, and red complexion different from the purple blue color of cyanosis or the bloated appearance associated with the pseudo-Cushings's changes of alcoholism.

These qualitative visual criteria reflect physiologic changes occurring beneath the epidermis at the dermal level. Nicotine found in tobacco products leads to increased blood levels of vasopressin, causing peripheral vasoconstriction and a state of dermal ischemia [11–13]. As nicotine blood levels decline, leading to a decrease in vasoconstriction, postischemic reperfusion may lead to the generation of reactive oxygen species which are a major component of UV injury and photoaging [14]. Induction of matrix metalloproteinases within the skin may be yet another mechanism by which tobacco smoke leads to premature skin aging [15].

Other important factors which contribute to the aging of the skin include skin type, history of sun exposure, history of skin irradiation, hyper or hypothyroidism, diabetes, peripheral vascular disease, atherosclerosis, and liver failure. Not only do the aforementioned factors contribute to skin aging, but they may also influence the degree of surgical correction performed by affecting the viability of skin flaps. Ameliorating factors, such as retinoic acid use, routine skin care, and sun protection may serve to retard the aging process.

59.4 Evaluation of the Aging Neck

59.4.1 Analysis and Classification

Previous authors have described visual criteria for the youthful neck which include [16]:

1. Distinct inferior mandibular border from mentum to angle without jowl overhang
2. Subhyoid depression
3. Visible thyroid cartilage bulge
4. Visible anterior border of the sternocleidomastoid muscle distinct in its entire course from the mastoid to sternum
5. Cervicomental angle between 105° and 120°

Another classification system in use is that proposed by Dedo [17]:

> Class I: Minimal deformity: well-defined cervicomental angle, good platysmal tone, no fat accumulation.
> Class II: Early cervical skin elastosis, no fat accumulation, no platysmal weakness.

Class III: Early cervical skin elastosis, fat accumulation, no platysmal weakness.
Class IV: Platysmal muscle accentuation with banding present either in repose or on contraction.
Class V: Congenital or acquired retrognathia/microgenia
Class VI: Low hyoid.

While classification systems serve as useful tools to compare patients and provide goals for rejuvenation, it must be stressed that analysis and treatment should be performed as an individualized approach for each patient, according to his or her personal pathology.

59.4.2 Physical Findings

While patients routinely have a complete facial analysis, this discussion focuses only on findings pertinent to the aging neck. It is important to view the neck as part of the patient's global appearance. To this end we use a comprehensive facial analysis form for all patient consultations (Fig. 59.1). Addressing the neck at the expense of other facial pathology can lead to postoperative imbalance, an unnatural look, and patient dissatisfaction.

Visual inspection begins with assessment of skin quality, which includes dyschromias, static horizontal furrows, and skin lesions such as nevi and skin tags, or acrochordons. Palpation also plays a fundamental role in assessing pathology. Skin elastosis may be visually estimated, but palpation helps confirm the extent of tissue laxity and position of the submandibular glands.

59.5 Jowl/Mandibular Evaluation

Starting in a superior to inferior fashion, evaluation of neck pathology begins with assessment of the chin–mandibular line. On lateral view, the pogonion is the most anterior projection of the chin. The ideal location of the pogonion is tangential to a line perpendicular to the Frankfurt horizontal from the vermilion border of the lower lip [18]. If a patient is in normal Class I occlusion (mesobuccal cusp of the maxillary first molar interdigitates with the buccal groove of the mandibular first molar), and the pogonion is posterior to this line, the mandible is hypoplastic. While a man's ideal pogonion position is tangential to this line, a woman's ideal position may lie 1–2 mm posterior. In addition, the mentolabial sulcus should lie approximately 4 mm posterior to a vertical line from the lower vermilion border to the pogonion [19]. A hypoplastic mentum may be the result of microgenia, a small chin that results from underdevelopment of the mandibular symphysis, or from micrognathia, which is the result of hypoplasia of various parts of the jaw [20]. Alloplastic implantation is indicated for a hypoplastic mentum in patients with normal or near-normal occlusion.

Although the development of a hypoplastic mentum is largely determined by genetic factors, the development of a prejowl sulcus is more the result of aging. However, the prejowl sulcus, or antigonion notch, may also be congenital and be present from childhood [21]. A combination of progressive soft tissue atrophy and gradual bony resorption of the inferior mandibular edge immediately anterior to the jowls (anterior mandibular groove) results in the development of a groove between the chin and the remainder of the body of the mandible [22, 23]. This is known as the prejowl sulcus [24]. With continued aging, the prejowl sulcus may merge with the commissure–mandibular groove, or "Marionette line," further accentuating a classic sign of the aging jawline. Correction of the prejowl sulcus may be accomplished with alloplastic implantation with the Mittelman PreJowl Implant, or submuscular placement of filler substances, such as hyaluronic acid or hydroxylapatite.

Immediately inferior to the mandibular border, lying just anterior to the angle of the mandible, are the submandibular, or submaxillary, glands. With advancing age, glandular ptosis is common and failure to recognize this pathology may compromise the aesthetic cervico-mandibular contour. It is important to point out prominent and ptotic submandibular glands to the patient during the preoperative consultation. While the primary author does not routinely address ptotic glands, a variety of treatment options exist. De Pina and Quinta [25] advocate gland resection at the time of rhytidectomy, through either the rhytidectomy incision or a cervical incision. Singer and Sullivan [26] advocate gland excision through a submental incision while others recommend submental–mastoid suture suspension or imbrication/plication of the periglandular platysma [27].

Fig. 59.1 The author's (HM) standardized patient facial analysis form

Hairline	Low Medium High		Male Pattern Baldness	1 2 3 4 5
Forehead Lines		1 2 3 4 5	Nasoglabellar Lines	1 2 3 4 5
Crow's Feet		1 2 3 4 5	Nasion Lines	1 2 3 4 5
Lower Lid Rhytids		1 2 3 4 5	Diagonal Malar Lines	1 2 3 4 5
Eyebrow Ptosis		R 1 2 3 4 5	L 1 2 3 4 5	

Upper Lids
  Excess Skin   R 1 2 3 4 5   L 1 2 3 4 5
  Fat Protrusion Medial   R 1 2 3 4 5   L 1 2 3 4 5
                       Central   R 1 2 3 4 5   L 1 2 3 4 5
                       Lateral   R 1 2 3 4 5   L 1 2 3 4 5
  Excess Muscle   R 1 2 3 4 5   L 1 2 3 4 5
  Lateral Bony Excess   R 1 2 3 4 5   L 1 2 3 4 5
  Peripheral Visual Loss   R 1 2 3 4 5   L 1 2 3 4 5

Lower Lids
  Excess Skin   R 1 2 3 4 5   L 1 2 3 4 5
  Fat Protrusion R Medial   1 2 3 4 5   L 1 2 3 4 5
                       R Central   1 2 3 4 5   L 1 2 3 4 5
                       R Lateral   1 2 3 4 5   L 1 2 3 4 5
  Excess Muscle   R 1 2 3 4 5   L 1 2 3 4 5
  Laxity   R 1 2 3 4 5   L 1 2 3 4 5
  Scleral Show   R _____ mm   L _____ mm
  Lateral Rounding   R 1 2 3 4 5   L 1 2 3 4 5
  Nasojugal Groove   1 2 3 4 5
  Malar Bags   1 2 3 4 5

Malar Area
  Hypoplastic   1 2 3 4 5   Sub-Malar Cheek Hollow 1 2 3 4 5

Facial Cheek Area
  Cheek Skin Laxity   1 2 3 4 5
  Nasolabial Groove   1 2 3 4 5   Crease 1 2 3 4 5   Fold 1 2 3 4 5

Chin-Mandible Line
  Hypoplastic   1 2 3 4 5   Protruding   1 2 3 4 5
  Pre-Jowl Sulcus   1 2 3 4 5
  J-M Elastosis   1 2 3 4 5
  Jowl Fullness   1 2 3 4 5
  C-M Groove   1 2 3 4 5   Crease 1 2 3 4 5   Fold 1 2 3 4 5
  Depressed COM   R 1 2 3 4 5   L 1 2 3 4 5

Neck Submental
  Skin Elastosis   1 2 3 4 5   Fat 1 2 3 4 5
  Platysmal Banding   C 1 2 3 4 5   R 1 2 3 4 5   L 1 2 3 4 5
  Central Vertical Pleating   1 2 3 4 5

Neck Lower Lateral
  J-M Fullness   1 2 3 4 5   Horizontal Line Depth   1 2 3 4 5

Rhytids
  Perioral   1 2 3 4 5   Upper Lip 1 2 3 4 5   Periorbital 1 2 3 4 5
  Lateral Facial Lines   1 2 3 4 5   Vermilion Loss   1 2 3 4 5

Skin
  Cobblestone   1 2 3 4 5
  Scars _____   Lesions _____   Skin Tone _____

Ears
  Protrusion   1 2 3 4 5

Jowl–mandibular elastosis is estimated by palpating tissue laxity along the mandibular margin, simulating the direction of pull in a rhytidoplasty. Jowl fullness is assessed primarily through visualization of the jowl immediately posterior to the anterior mandibular ligament, and is the result not only of soft tissue descent, but also of accumulation of adipose tissue. Palpation may be used to confirm the presence of adipose tissue.

The commissure–mandibular area is next assessed. This area is commonly referred to as "Marionette lines," but proper clarification of the proper nomenclature is warranted. The commissure–mandibular fold (CMF) refers to the extent of tissue lateral to the actual Marionette line. It is a measure of soft tissue excess and descent. The commissure–mandibular crease refers to the actual depth of etched rhytid formation within the Marionette "Groove." In general, the crease tends to increase in severity with advancing age. The commissure–mandibular groove (CMG) refers to the concavity between the CMF and the lower lip. The distinction in terms is important when discussing the use of fillers and the location of injection. One would never inject the fold as that would accentuate the depth of the groove. However, it is quite appropriate to fill the depth of the crease or to inject the CMG to create a smooth contour and to decrease or eliminate the CMG.

The corner of the mouth, or oral commissure, is next evaluated. With advancing age and loss of soft tissue support, the commissure commonly becomes downturned, creating an "unhappy" appearance. Not only should the degree of the depression be noted, but each side should be compared to document pretreatment asymmetry and to help guide treatment.

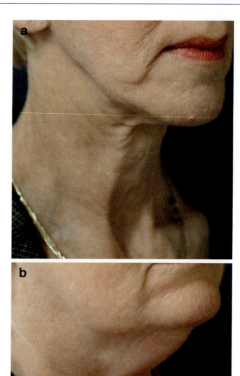

Fig. 59.2 (**a**) Neck with lateral platysmal banding. (**b**) Neck with central platysmal banding

59.6 Submental/Neck Evaluation

The evaluation of the submental area has several components. Skin elastosis is evaluated in a similar manner to that of the jowl–mandibular region using both visual inspection and manual palpation. Medial–lateral as well as superior–inferior movement should be assessed. The amount of adipose tissue, both subcutaneous and subplatysmal, should be estimated by visualization as well as palpation. Accumulation of fat is not universal with age, and skeletonization of subcutaneous muscles should be avoided to preserve a natural appearance. Platysmal banding should be assessed with the patient in repose as well as with animation. A distinction must be made between lateral banding and central banding (Fig. 59.2) as this may dictate treatment. By asking the patient to curl the lower lip or grimace, the anterior edge of the platysma may be brought into relief. Central vertical skin pleating may commonly be found between lateral platysmal banding and represents a medial–lateral skin excess.

Inferiorly in the neck, any lower fullness or adipose tissue should be evaluated. Implications of these findings are further discussed in the surgical technique selection section. The depth of horizontal rhytids should also be assessed.

All of the above findings should be clearly documented on the assessment form. Special description of any unusual pathology should be made. All findings should be demonstrated and explained to the patient, so that surgical recommendations may be better understood and realistic postoperative expectations better achieved.

59.7 Surgical Technique Selection

59.7.1 Nonsurgical Intervention

Prior to discussion of surgical treatment, it is prudent to discuss the concept of noninvasive treatments. In the primary author's practice, this generally includes four different treatment modalities: the use of Botulinum Toxin A, light-based skin tightening procedures, the use of fillers, and resurfacing techniques.

59.7.2 Botulinum Toxin A

Botulinum Toxin A is now a widely used for the nonsurgical treatment of platysmal bands [28, 29]. Originally available only as Botox®, distinct formulations of botulinum toxin A are currently available or will soon be available in the United States. Although possessing similar efficacies, different types of neurotoxins have distinct dosing parameters. For the purpose of this discussion all doses mentioned are appropriate for Botox®.

It appears that the best indication for botulinum toxin A treatment of the aging neck may be for strong, hypertrophic bands that are exaggerated with animation. In the primary author's practice, the technique involves grasping the anterior edge of the platysmal band and injecting 40 units or more along the anterior edges of the right and left platysmal bands. These bands may extend as far inferior as the clavicle. Botulinum toxin A may also be injected intradermally along horizontal rhytids to achieve some degree of effacement, but the results may be inconsistent.

59.7.3 Skin Tightening Procedures

Skin tightening procedures include the use of devices, such as the Affirm Multiplex™, Thermage® or Titan®, to achieve a degree of dermal heating. Thermage® involves the use of radiofrequency energy in order to heat the tissue, while Titan® and the Affirm Multiplex™ use infrared light. These technologies are most appropriately used in patients with skin elastosis, since adipose tissue or muscle banding will not be addressed by superficial dermal heating. Mild to moderate improvement may be seen after two treatments, spaced 1 month apart. These procedures may also have some prophylactic benefit by increasing dermal collagen, while degenerative changes may be delayed or slowed. However, it is extremely important to properly counsel the patient on posttreatment expectations. The best candidates for these treatments may be young adults with Dedo Class II pathology. Again, it must be emphasized that these procedures will not be able to achieve the same degree of improvement in skin laxity as surgery.

59.7.4 Intradermal Fillers

Injectable fillers, such as nonanimal hyaluronic acid (Juvederm™, Restylane®, and Perlane®), or hydroxylapatite (Radiesse®), may be used to fill horizontal neck creases. In the primary author's practice, filling of such creases and grooves is generally limited to nonpermanent fillers, although permanent fillers are available. In terms of mandibular rejuvenation, hyaluronic or hydroxylapatite fillers are ideal for correction of the commissure–mandibular groove and depressed oral commissure when injected intradermally. Temporary correction of the Pre-Jowl groove and microgenia may be achieved with supraperiosteal/submuscular injection of larger volume fillers, such as Perlane® or Radiesse®.

59.7.5 Laser Resurfacing

Resurfacing techniques can be an important adjuvant in many patients seeking facial rejuvenation. Whereas ablative laser resurfacing using traditional carbon dioxide resurfacing had limited utility in the neck, newer fractionated technologies are proving useful [30]. Multiple technologies exist including numerous fractionated carbon dioxide laser systems along with proprietary laser systems such as the Cutera Pearl™ and Affirm Multiplex™. All of these may improve dyschromias, horizontal furrows, and offer some degree of skin tightening. The primary author has recently begun to use a fractionated carbon dioxide laser system coupled with a low powered erbium-YAG laser (Whisper–Erbium YAG Extend Ablation Laser™) for the majority of patients seeking ablative skin resurfacing of the neck.

While noninvasive treatments have merit unto themselves, they may be most appropriate in patients unwilling or unable to undergo surgery. They can also serve as valuable adjuncts to surgical correction. However, there is not currently any noninvasive treatment that can offer the same degree of skin tightening as surgery. Furthermore, only surgery addresses all components of aging: skin elastosis, platysmal laxity and banding, and adipose accumulation.

59.8 Surgical Treatment

The choice of treatment options, especially surgical options, needs to be tailored to the individual and depend on the patient's physical findings. There are also progressive degrees of invasiveness, which usually correspond to progressive degrees of pathology, but may also reflect patient wishes with regard to surgical recovery and postoperative outcome. In the primary author's practice, it is extremely common for patients to preface any discussion of treatment with the phrase: "I want to look natural." While it may be tempting to try to achieve the best possible postoperative result, it is imperative to respect the desires of the patient. However, one must not sacrifice personal standards solely to please the patient. Ideally, if there is a discrepancy between the patient's and surgeon's goals, then a compromise should be reached, or another consultation scheduled for further discussion.

59.8.1 Liposculpting

Liposculpting of the jowl–mandibular and submental regions offers the least invasive means of surgical improvement. An ideal candidate is generally someone younger with mild adipose accumulation in the jowl, submandibular, and submental regions without severe skin elastosis or platysmal laxity or banding.

The jowl–mandibular region can be reached using a 2 mm punch biopsy or stab incision postauricularly at the level of the lobule (Fig. 59.3). The primary author prefers to use microliposuction cannulas for this region in order to avoid skeletonization and also to achieve a gradual transition, or "feathering" into untreated areas. The degree of adipose tissue in the submental region dictates the type of incision and cannula to be used. With minimal subcutaneous fat, a small stab incision in the submental crease allows introduction of a microliposuction cannula. The use of standard 3 mm liposuction cannulas can be used in the submental region to remove subcutaneous fat. While adequate negative pressure may be achieved in many

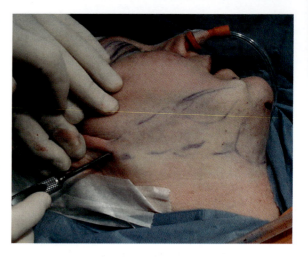

Fig. 59.3 A patient undergoing jowl–mandibular liposculpture. In this situation a standard number 3 spatula open liposuction cannula is being used. However, a multifenestrated microliposuction cannula is more commonly used for "closed" liposculpturing in this area

cases with standard wall suction, it is frequently necessary to employ a liposuction machine to generate sufficient negative pressure.

In patients with a greater degree of submental adipose tissue, a standard submentoplasty incision, 2.5–3.0 cm in length posterior to the submental crease may be optimal. It is important to detach the membranous raphe beneath the submental crease from the overlying skin to diminish the depth of the submental crease. Improved visualization and access allows for more accurate liposuction as well as visualization of the platysma muscle and decussation.

In some patients with more fibrous adipose tissue, the results of cannula liposuction are limited. Lipectomy, under direct vision, may be performed with care taken to remain above the level of the platysma. However, due to the risk of skeletonization, a conservative approach should be taken and feathering with a microliposuction cannula should be performed lateral to the region of direct lipectomy in order to achieve a gradual transition.

If the patient has obvious subplatysmal fat, it may be addressed in a judicious manner. Small perforations in the platysmal decussation may be made to allow prolapse of the adipose tissue. A standard spatula liposuction cannula will then remove the prolapsed fat and will not violate the platysmal muscle or decussation. This conservative approach will avoid complications involved with subplatysmal dissection under limited visualization and offers a substantial improvement in the heavy neck.

While liposuction coupled with direct lipectomy when appropriate remain effective and widely used, alternative techniques in liposculpture of the jawline and neck continue to evolve. Becker et al. [31] and Schaeffer [32] have reported on their use of endoscopic liposhaving for liposculpture of the jawline and submental region. The technique involves the creation of approximately 2 cm postauricular incisions with or without a small submental incision. Using traditional sharp dissection skin flaps are raised over the areas requiring contouring. The subcutaneous fat is then shaved using a microdebrider visualized via a 30° endoscope. Adjunctive techniques including platysmal resection and corset platysmaplasty are used as needed.

Liposculpture alone, without addressing the platysma or skin elastosis, will affect a modest improvement in the submental and jowl–mandibular regions. Postoperatively, the primary author has all patients wear a supportive headband so that adhesion of the skin to the underlying soft tissue occurs in a superior fashion.

It bears mentioning that a patient with a large degree of submental adiposity has relatively less skin than a neck with a smaller degree of adipose tissue. This paradoxical finding is demonstrated in Fig. 59.4. It is important to keep this relative skin paucity in mind when reapproximating the submental incision. If excess skin is excised, there may be too much skin tension on the final closure leading to a widened scar or incisional dehiscence.

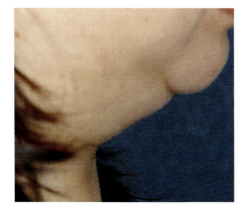

Fig. 59.4 A patient with abundant submental adipose tissue

59.8.2 Platysmaplasty

If the patient has a Dedo Class IV neck with platysmal banding or laxity, then this must be addressed to optimally improve the cervicomental angle. Pre and intraoperative analysis is essential in selecting the proper surgical technique to correct the patient's pathology but avoid an unnatural, "operated" appearance. As mentioned in the previous section, platysmal banding is classified as central versus right and left. Central platysmal banding often occurs secondary to subplatysmal fat accumulation with weakening of the platysmal decussation. In one cadaveric study three different forms of platysmal decussation were found [33]. The first type, seen most commonly, involved decussation from the mandibular margin for 1–2 cm below the mentum with separation in the suprahyoid region. The second type, seen less often, involved decussation from the mentum to the thyroid cartilage. The third type, seen least commonly, involved a complete absence of decussation. In general, the degree of decussation correlates with the amount of soft tissue support given to the subplatysmal structures in the midline and will affect the type of platysmal banding found in patients.

Central banding may be found primarily in patients with a Type II decussation. With a complete decussation of muscle fibers, there will be no anterior edge of the platysma muscle to form lateral banding. With a Type I decussation, central banding may be seen in the suprahyoid neck in the region of the intact decussation. Conversely, lateral banding may be observed primarily in patients with a Type III, or absent, decussation. Due to the lack of platysmal fiber interdigitation, there is no central support for the subplatysmal soft tissue and lateral banding may be found at the anterior edge of the platysma on either side. Lateral banding may also be seen in Type I decussation in the region of the neck below the intact decussation, especially in the infrahyoid region. Lateral banding may extend as far inferiorly as the clavicle, in which case, it is very difficult to improve.

If central banding is due to subcutaneous adipose tissue, then liposuction or lipectomy may be adequate. However, if there is significant platysmal decussation laxity, two therapeutic options exist. If direct lipectomy has been performed, then often some degree of central platysmal resection may concurrently occur. If that is the case, the cut edges of the platysma may be imbricated together with a 3–0 Prolene suture in an interrupted or continuous fashion. This will afford some central tightening and reinforcement of cervicomental fascial support. An alternate option is not to disrupt the weakened decussation, but to tighten the platysmal sling posteriorly with plication or imbrication as part of a rhytidoplasty, or face–neck lift.

The treatment of lateral banding depends on the severity, extent, and location of the bands. Rohrich [27] categorizes lateral platysmal banding into wide (greater than 2 cm) and narrow (less than 2 cm). While the primary author does not use the exact interband distance to determine treatment options, the interband distance relative to the size of the entire neck helps dictate treatment. For those bands that are sufficiently close together, a vertical resection of muscle along both bands is performed to the level of the hyoid. Prolene sutures (3–0), in an interrupted or continuous fashion, are then used to approximate the edges of the muscle in a corset fashion. If the bands are pronounced below the hyoid, then a horizontal wedge is resected on either side at the cervicomental angle. This horizontal section allows the inferior portion of the band to fall posteriorly and inferiorly when platysmal plication/imbrication is performed subsequently during rhytidoplasty. For extreme inferior banding (Fig. 59.5) to the level of the sternum/clavicle, a vertical neck lift may be helpful, which is subsequently described in greater detail.

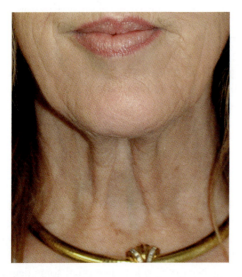

Fig. 59.5 A patient with extreme inferior platysmal banding. This degree of inferior banding is difficult to correct with a classic face/neck lift and submentoplasty. A vertical neck lift will help correct this pathology

If the interband distance is sufficiently wide so that reapproximation of the bands would result in excess tension, the bands are not reapproximated and the incision is left open until after the rhytidoplasty. With posterior platysmal plication or imbrication, the bands may be pulled even further apart. If they have been previously reapproximated, then the posterior pull will be limited and this may limit the improvement in lateral neck laxity. After the rhytidoplasty has been completed, the submental region may be reevaluated and, if able to be done without excess tension, the platysmal bands may be reapproximated at this time.

A number of techniques have been described as adjuncts or alternatives to platysmal section, imbrication, and plication. Although the primary author does not typically use them of particular note is Giampapa's interlocking mattress suture technique [7]. Coupled with liposculpture of the jawline and submental region interlocking sutures are placed subcutaneously running from the right platysma to the left mastoid and left platysma to right mastoid. The sutures are placed so they run obliquely from just off midline inferiorly toward the mastoid superiorly. The desired effect is to pull the platysma muscles together in the midline and pull the anterior neck upward defining the jawline and cervicomental angle. Variations on this technique using endoscopy can also be employed [34].

After the adipose tissue and platysma has been addressed, the skin may be evaluated. In the large majority of patients in the primary author's practice, no submental skin excision is performed during primary submentoplasty. In cases of severe skin excess, or in select revision cases, a vertical ellipse of skin may be excised, creating a "T"-shaped scar. Meticulous closure of the vertical portion of the "T" with intradermal sutures and long-term use of Steri-Strips™ helps to avoid postoperative scar widening. Alternative techniques in the treatment of skin redundancy include vertical elliptical skin excision coupled with Z-plasty, W-plasty, and double advancement flap closure [35]. If there is significant inferior skin redundancy, then a horizontal neck lift may be required for optimal correction. This procedure is discussed later in the chapter.

Isolated submentoplasty may be performed for patients with excess submental adipose tissue and minimal skin elastosis. With younger patients having good skin elasticity, one can expect a significant degree of postoperative skin retraction and redraping. Another indication is for patients with mild platysmal banding and adipose tissue. These patients tend to be in the fourth and fifth decades of life without significant skin excess. As mentioned previously, it is important to have the patient wear a support sling postoperatively to ensure optimal skin envelope adherence. Figure 59.6 demonstrates an ideal candidate for isolated submentoplasty, jowl–mandibular liposculpturing, and alloplastic mandibular augmentation.

59.8.3 Rhytidoplasty

The preceding paragraphs all addressed surgical correction of the submental area. However, unless there is minimal skin laxity, improvement of the cervicomental angle cannot be adequately improved without some form of rhytidoplasty. In the primary author's practice, the term "face/neck lift" is used in patient discussion

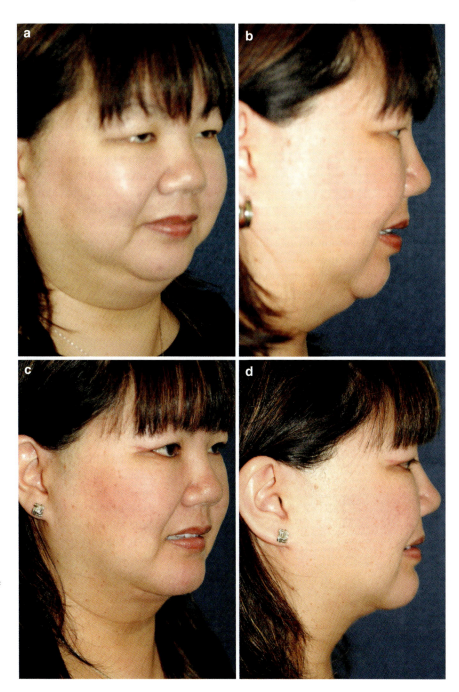

Fig. 59.6 (**a, b**) Preoperative patient with microgenia, significant submental and jowl–mandibular adipose tissue. (**c, d**) Postoperative after submentoplasty, and placement of an alloplastic chin–jowl implant

as it better confers the principle that a rhytidoplasty, although offering some improvement in the lower and midface, is especially efficacious in addressing jowl–mandibular elastosis and the upper third of the neck. Although detailed discussion of rhytidoplasty techniques are beyond the scope of this chapter, the different ranges of rhytidoplasty employed by the primary author and others reflect different degrees of subcutaneous undermining, the length and location of skin incisions, and the degree to which the SMAS/Platysma complex and thus the upper third of the neck can be addressed.

The primary author employs a multivector SMAS/Platysma suspension technique with variations depending on the needs of a particular patient. Extensive sub-SMAS/Platysmal undermining is not performed. It is felt that this does not offer a significant advantage in lifting the SMAS/Platysma complex, but does increase the risk of facial nerve branch injury. In fact, when resuspending the SMAS/Platysma complex, the lift of the inferior portion of the SMAS/Platysma is only along the nonundermined portion. A more complete, uniform lift is achieved without any undermining. With the multivector suspension, the direction of vector pull is determined by the tissue pathology. Figure 59.7 shows the various vector directions for the SMAS/platysma imbrication or plication. In general, the most inferior SMAS suture vector focuses on improvement of the submental area, cervico-mental angle, and upper neck with a primarily vertical direction of suspension superiorly at the angle of the mandible. For many patients seeking improvement in the neck selection of appropriate face/neck lifting techniques are of utmost importance.

59.9 Special Neck Lifting

Although the upper neck and cervicomental angle can be greatly improved in the large majority of patients through face/neck lifting, submentoplasty and liposculpture, additional procedures may be beneficial. Standard multivector face/neck lifts as well as deep plane face/neck lifts may incompletely address the lower half of the neck. Two additional neck lifting procedures, the horizontal neck lift and vertical neck lift, may be used, based on individual patient findings. Both of the procedures may be performed concurrently with a face/neck lift, subsequent to a face/neck lift in a patient who desires further improvement, or as the sole surgical procedure in patients without a prior history of surgery.

59.9.1 Vertical Neck Lift

While the classic face/neck lift provides generally adequate results when combined with a submentoplasty/platysmaplasty, the lower half of the neck may have insufficient improvement in a certain percentage of patients. Most patients presenting for face/neck lift/submentoplasty display most of the aging in the upper half of the neck. As much as 30% of the face/neck lift population display considerable aging in the lower half of the neck, most commonly characterized by vertical platysmal bands extending to the clavicle. This type of patient can sometimes display inadequate improvement in the vertical bands in the lower half of the neck postoperatively. Until recently, we have provided very little in the way of a solution to this dilemma.

In the past few years, the author (HM) has utilized an extension of the classic face/neck lift along the hairline to create massive undermining in the lower half of the neck, extending almost to the midline. In doing this, one is able to affect a posterior pull on the platysma onto the firm and less mobile sternocleidomastoid fascia. In doing this, one can achieve a more dramatic improvement of the vertical bands in the lower half of the neck. This procedure has been coined

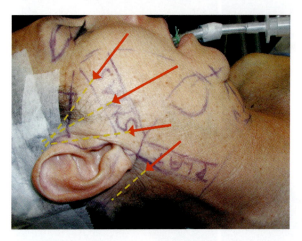

Fig. 59.7 Demonstrating the different vectors of pull in the multivector SMAS plication

"The Vertical Neck Lift." While not perfect, it is the best, in our experience, in improving the platysmal bands of the lower half of the neck. This also seems to help lower and midneck central vertical skin pleating.

The candidates for this type of procedure are limited. If a woman wants to wear pulled straight back, this scar is visible and may not be desirable. Vertical neck scars do not heal as well as horizontal neck scars and are more prone to hypertrophic scarring. Another limitation is a patient with a high posterior hairline. In a patient with a high posterior hairline, the incision cannot be carried far enough inferiorly to effect the desired improvement in the vertical bands of the lower half of the neck. The ideal patient has a very low posterior hairline and does not wear their hair straight back.

The vertical neck lift addresses platysmal banding of the inferior neck as well as vertical skin pleating (Fig. 59.5). Commonly, this procedure is done in conjunction with the face/neck lift. The skin incision is carried inferiorly from the postauricular aspect of the face/neck lift along the hairline (Fig. 59.8). It is extremely important to preoperatively evaluate the patient's hairline and inquire about hairstyle preference. The inferior aspect of the incision is the inferior border of the hairline, and the ideal patient is one with a low posterior hairline. Patients with a high posterior hairline are poor candidates for the vertical neck lift as the access provided by limited incision will be inadequate to reach the posterior platysmal border and improve inferior platysmal banding and skin pleating. In addition, patients who prefer to wear their hair in a pulled-back fashion should be advised that this may lead to scar visibility and a postoperative hairstyle change may be advisable.

The skin flap is undermined and elevated well past the posterior border of the platysma (Fig. 59.8) about 2–3 cm from the midline. This extensive undermining allows the inferior platysma to be resuspended posteriorly and superiorly to the fascia of the sternocleidomastoid where it is more stable (Fig. 59.8). This resuspension allows for improvement of the inferior portion of the platysmal bands which would be inaccessible in a traditional face/neck lift.

In addition to improved platysmal suspension, another important advantage of the vertical neck lift is the improvement in redraping of the lower neck skin flap. A significant amount of posterior neck skin may be removed which permits a smoother contour with a more subtle transition to the nonundermined neck skin (Fig. 59.8).

One might be surprised at how much additional skin can be removed in the neck when combined with the classic face/neck lift. Certainly, such a large amount of skin removal must contribute to a more dramatic change to the lower half of the neck in the short and long term.

It is very important for surgeons to realize that the vertical neck lift can be done as an additional procedure long after a classic face/neck lift. For example, the surgeon and patient may see a lack of satisfactory improvement in the lower half of the neck after 1 year and can easily perform this procedure under local anesthesia. It is possible that an adequate face/neck lift with good results at 50 years of age can persist in the upper half of the neck while the lower half of the neck shows undesirable results again at 55 years of age. One can then do an isolated vertical neck lift bilaterally and, even at times, unilaterally. In the senior author's experience, the classic limited neck lift for the upper half of the neck is not effective as an isolated procedure; however, the vertical neck lift is effective as an isolated procedure for the lower half of the neck.

The most significant disadvantage of the vertical neck lift is the resultant scar. It is essential that the skin closure be performed in a tension-free manner with long-term absorbable or permanent dermal sutures. If there are early signs of scar hypertrophy or keloid formation, then this should be promptly addressed. Other disadvantages include a longer surgical time, potential for more neck ecchymosis, and the creation of a long, narrow postauricular skin flap. It is generally agreed that long, narrow skin flaps are more prone to epidermolysis, less optimal wound healing, and even regional necrosis. Although skin flap necrosis may be possible, the primary author has not yet experienced this. Figure 59.8 demonstrates the degree of improvement that may be achieved with the vertical neck lift. Patients have uniformly recognized the value of the vertical neck lift as the improvement is substantial and not subtle.

59.9.2 Horizontal Neck Lift

There is a group of patients where a significant aging process occurs in a horizontal direction rather than the vertical direction described above. Certainly the vertical platysmal banding is more common than what is

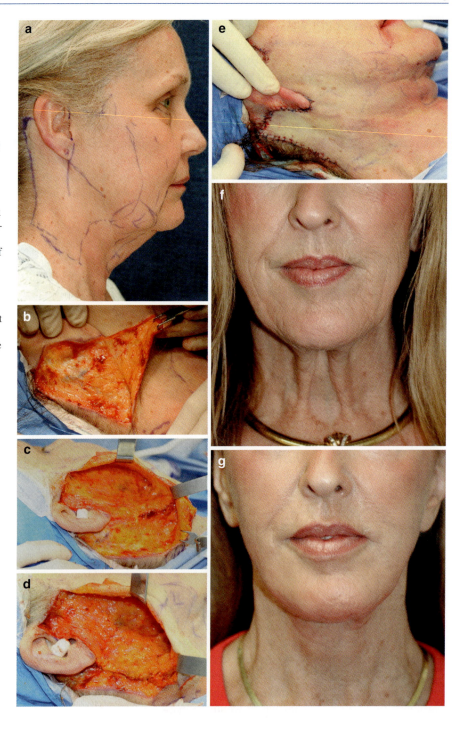

Fig. 59.8 (**a**) Preoperative markings for the vertical neck lift. The preauricular portion is the same as the classic face/neck lift while the postauricular incision extends inferiorly along the postauricular hairline. (**b**) Intraoperative showing elevation of the postauricular skin flap achieved with the extended vertical neck lift incision. (**c**) Intraoperative demonstrating the access to the SMAS/platysma complex after subcutaneous undermining. (**d**) Intraoperative showing the inferior extent of the platysmal plication achieved with the vertical neck lift. (**e**) Intraoperative demonstrating the postauricular skin redraping without any bunching or contour irregularities. (**f**) Preoperative patient with extreme inferior platysmal banding. (**g**) Postoperative after a vertical neck lift demonstrating virtual elimination of the platysmal banding

described relating to the horizontal neck aging. This group of patients demonstrates deep, long, multiple horizontal neck lines as well as redundant horizontal neck skin between these "etched-in" lines. A posterior pull on the neck, in this type of patient, will not provide the desired result. The senior author has seen this group of patients in the past without daring to perform an excision of skin and sometimes fat by creating a visible scar line across the lower, central neck. With some trepidation, this procedure is carried out with the idea that a meticulously approximated 12–17 cm scar is less conspicuous than the more conspicuous deep horizontal "etched-in" neck lines already present in this group of patients. The vertical height of the elliptical excision in the horizontal neck lift may range from 2–4 cm. The senior author has never found the resulting scars to be a detriment to doing this procedure because the improvement is so much more rewarding.

The horizontal neck lift is used primarily to improve lower neck horizontal pleating or excess skin and to improve the number of deep horizontal skin furrows, as demonstrated by the patient in Fig. 59.9a. In the primary author's practice, the horizontal neck lift is commonly performed as a sole procedure in a patient with horizontal neck laxity after a prior face/neck lift. However, in certain circumstances, it may be performed concurrently with a face/neck lift and submentoplasty. A central neck vertical excess of skin and/or fat will not be adequately addressed with a posterior–superior vector of pull achieved with a traditional face/neck lift or even the vertical neck lift. However, the horizontal neck lift is an excellent means by which this difficult problem may be improved.

The technique involves an elliptical excision of the horizontal neck redundancy. Determination of the amount of skin to be resected is done using a pinch technique. The ellipse is centered on an existing horizontal neck furrow. The height of the ellipse is determined by grasping the excess skin until the neck is taut with the head in a slightly extended position (Fig. 59.9). The resulting amount of skin to be removed is at least 2 cm and, much more commonly, around 4 cm. The resulting scar from the elliptical excision will replace a preoperative existing horizontal neck furrow. Excision of the skin is then performed along with a thin layer of subcutaneous adipose tissue.

Depending on the individual patient findings, open subcutaneous liposuction may be performed in the exposed area, as needed, with a #3 spatula cannula. Further closed liposuction in surrounding areas can be accomplished, if needed. A microliposuction cannula may be used to feather the periphery of the ellipse or the area of closed liposuction to create a smooth transition zone. Additionally, if vertical platysmal bands are encountered,

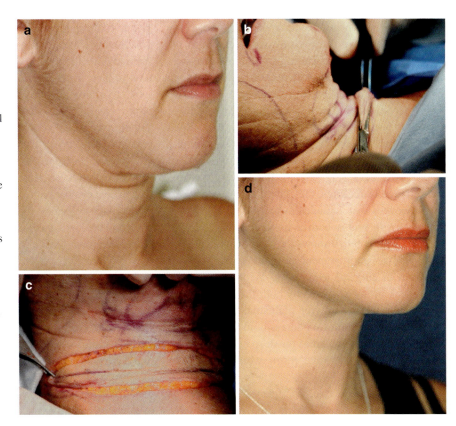

Fig. 59.9 (**a**) Preoperative patient with deep horizontal neck furrows and a horizontal excess of lower neck skin. (**b**) Preoperative marking of the ellipse in the horizontal neck lift. The extent of vertical skin excision is in the surgeon's judgment but should be aggressive. The neck is extended and the excess horizontal neck skin is grasped with a forceps or Allis clamp until the skin contour is smooth. (**c**) Intraoperative just after incision of the ellipse demonstrating the amount of skin that can be safely removed. (**d**) Postoperative demonstrating a dramatic improvement in the depth of horizontal neck furrows as well as elimination of the horizontal excess neck skin

they may be addressed through vertical or horizontal resection and imbrications/plication as described previously in the discussion of submentoplasty.

The advantages of the horizontal neck lift include the ability to use local anesthetic if done as a sole surgical procedure, the ability to reduce lower neck horizontal pleating and excess skin, the ability to reduce the severity and decrease the number of deep transverse neck furrows, and the fact that, if properly closed, the scar is generally not as deep or visible as the original horizontal furrow it replaces. It is extremely important that the incision be closed meticulously with numerous dermal sutures and the skin edges everted with vertical mattress sutures. Steri-Strips™ should be used for several weeks after the sutures have been removed. The patient should also be instructed to avoid extreme neck extension during the recovery period.

The disadvantages of the horizontal neck lift include restricted neck extension if the height of the excised ellipse is too much, a horizontal neck scar, and the possible need for repeat excision of skin if the initial excision is too conservative. This additional horizontal excision is not uncommon, as the surgeon tends to be conservative in his initial horizontal neck lift (Fig. 59.9).

The patients on whom the author (HM) has performed horizontal neck lifts, have uniformly been very satisfied and realize the obvious improvement in the lower half of the neck. These procedures have most commonly been done under local anesthesia when they are not combined with other procedures.

A special circumstance is one in which a patient may have both extreme vertical neck skin excess and vertical platysmal banding combined excess skin in a horizontal direction with horizontal rolls of excess fat in the lower neck (Fig. 59.10). If a patient has this combination of findings, they can undergo one surgical procedure that includes submentoplasty, classic face/neck lift, and a both a horizontal and vertical neck lift. Figure 59.10 shows the significant degree of postoperative improvement possible using the full spectrum of surgical techniques. Without the additional neck lifting provided by both the vertical neck lift (to improve the inferior platysmal banding) and the horizontal neck lift (to address both the horizontal skin and fat excess as well as the deep horizontal neck creases), the postoperative result would have been suboptimal.

These two simple, easily performed procedures of the vertical neck lift and horizontal neck lift have added enormously to the results one can achieve in a limited group of aging neck patients, more specifically the lower half of the neck. These are easily added to any surgeon's armamentarium and can be provided to patients with problems in the lower half of the neck.

59.10 Clinical Pearls and Pitfalls

The importance of an individual patient approach to the aging neck cannot be overemphasized. There is not a "one size fits all" approach to rejuvenation. In order to optimally treat each patient, all aspects of patient aging must be understood and addressed.

The patient consultation is the first impression of you practice and will set the stage for future expectations. Besides instilling a sense of professionalism and comfort in the prospective patient, the consultation provides the surgeon with the opportunity to educate his patient on his or her specific pathology. A better understanding of pathology will help the patient understand the surgeon's recommendations and will also increase the likelihood that the surgeon's treatment recommendations will be followed. Patient wishes must be respected and no unrealistic promises be given. If the patient stresses a natural, conservative postoperative appearance, this should be clearly documented in the patient medical record. It is not uncommon to have a patient, previously espousing a natural look, to return wanting a more extreme degree of improvement. Documentation during the initial consultation can help remind both the surgeon and the patient of any earlier discussions.

A systematic approach to facial analysis is essential in rejuvenation treatment. In this endeavor, a standardized patient evaluation form is extremely valuable. Such an approach helps develop a complete pattern of evaluation and creates a qualitative analysis and quantitative record of patient features and the degree of aging which serves to individualize patient analysis and records. The evaluation form not only provides a valuable intraoperative reference, but greatly facilitates a review of patient findings long after the initial consultation.

Any preoperative asymmetry or unusual findings must be documented and discussed with the patient. Standardized photographs help to provide a record of the preoperative appearance. Patients frequently forget their "old face" and these photos can help remind them of previous pathology. It is common for lines and skin lesions on the face and neck to move to a different

Fig. 59.10 (**a, b**) Preoperative patient with extreme horizontal neck skin excess with many deep horizontal furrow and inferior platysmal banding. This degree of neck pathology is not fully addressed with a classic multivector SMAS face/neck rhytidoplasty and submentoplasty. (**c, d**) Postoperative after a submentoplasty, classic face/neck lift, and both vertical neck lift and horizontal neck left. There is virtually complete elimination of the horizontal neck skin excess, effacement of the horizontal skin furrows, and great improvement in the inferior platysmal banding

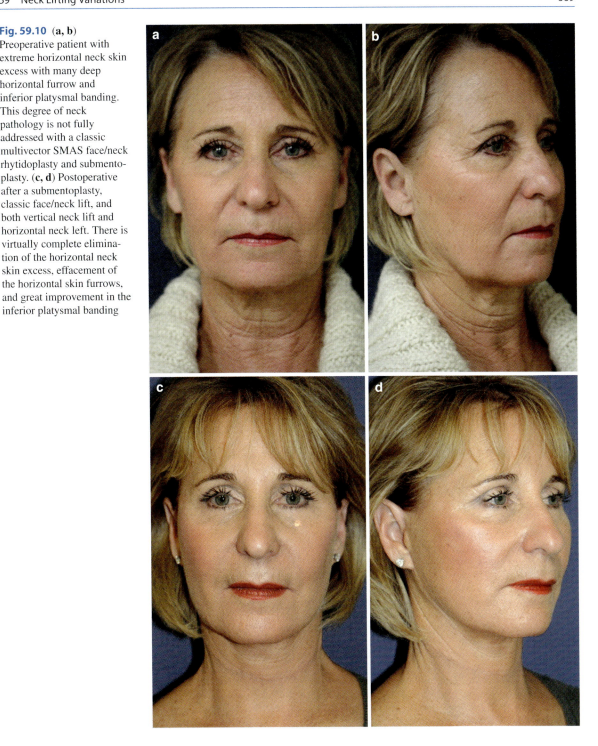

position postoperatively and reviewing the preoperative photos with the patient can help remind him or her that this is not a surgical complication.

Remember the Horizontal Neck Lift for improving the supraclavicular redundant neck skin. A long horizontal scar in a previous horizontal neck crease is far more aesthetic than horizontal pleats of supraclavicular or midneck skin.

Do not promise great results in the aging lower half of the neck. Do not forget that the Vertical Neck Lift is the path toward your best lower neck skin redundancy and supraclavicular platysmal banding.

It is important to avoid the temptation to overcorrect any patient pathology. This can lead to excess wound tension with scar widening as well as an unnatural, "pulled" appearance. It is far better to be conservative and to do a small secondary procedure in the future than to have a complication from trying to be too aggressive initially. Any early signs of complications, such as scar hypertrophy or keloid formation, or skin flap compromise, must be quickly diagnosed and treated. Frequent postoperative patient appointments help not only follow the surgical recovery, but also to convey a sense of patient importance. A solid surgeon–patient relationship will help carry the patient through any postoperative setbacks and ensure a successful postoperative result with a satisfied, happy patient that will be a positive reflection to the practice.

References

1. Adamson PA, Litner JA. Evolution of rhytidectomy techniques. Facial Plast Surg Clin North Am. 2005;13(3): 383–91.
2. Bourguet J. La disparition chiurgicale des rides et plis du visave. Bull Acad Med (Paris). 1919;82:183.
3. Bettman A. Plastic and cosmetic surgery of the face. Northwest Med. 1920;19:205.
4. Zimbler MS. Tord skoog: facelift innovator. Arch Facial Plast Surg. 2001;3(1):63.
5. Mitz V, Peyronie M. The superficial musculo-aponeurotic system (SMAS) in the parotid and cheek area. Plast Reconstr Surg. 1976;58(1):80–8.
6. Feldman JJ. Corset platysmaplasty. Plast Reconstr Surg. 1990;85(3):333–43.
7. Giampapa VC, Di Bernardo BE. Neck recontouring with suture suspension and liposuction: an alternative for the early rhytidectomy candidate. Aesthetic Plast Surg. 1995; 19(3):217–23.
8. Prabhat A, Dyer II WK. Improving surgery on the aging neck with an adjustable expanded polytetrafluoroethylene cervical sling. Arch Facial Plast Surg. 2003;5(6):491–501.
9. LaTrenta GS. Atlas of aesthetic face and neck surgery. Philadelphia: Saunders; 2001.
10. Model D. Smoker's face: an underrated clinical sign? Br Med J (Clin Res Ed). 1985;291(6511):160–76.
11. Reus WF, Robson MC, Zachary K, Heffers JP. Acute effects of tobacco smoking on blood flow in the cutaneous microcirculation. Br J Plast Surg. 1984;37(2):213–5.
12. Richardson D. Effects of tobacco smoke inhalation on capillary blood flow in human skin. Arch Environ Health. 1987;42(1):19–25.
13. Tur E, Yosipovitch G, Oren-Vulfs S. Chronic and acute effects of cigarette smoking on skin blood flow. Angiology. 1992;43(4):328–35.
14. Fisher GJ, Wang ZQ, Datta SC, Varani J, Kang S, Voorhees JJ. Pathophysiology of premature skin aging induced by ultraviolet light. N Engl J Med. 1997;337(20):1419–28.
15. Lahmann C, Bergemann J, Harrison G, Young AR. Matrix metalloproteinase-1 and skin aging in smokers. Lancet. 2001;357(9260):935–6.
16. Ellenbogen R, Karlin JV. Visual criteria for success in restoring the youthful neck. Plast Reconstr Surg. 1980;66(6): 826–37.
17. Dedo DD. "How I do it" –plastic surgery. Practical suggestions on facial plastic surgery. A preoperative classification of the neck for cervicofacial rhytidectomy. Laryngoscope. 1980;90(11 Pt 1):1894–6.
18. Gonzalez-Ulloa M. A quantum method for the appreciation of the morphology of the face. Plast Reconstr Surg. 1964;34: 241–6.
19. McGraw-Wall B. Facial analysis. In: Bailey B, editor. Head and neck surgery–otolaryngology. Philadelphia: Lippincott Williams & Wilkins; 2001. p. 2183–8.
20. Mittelman H, Jen A. Aesthetic mandibular implants. In: Papel I, editor. Facial plastic and reconstructive surgery. New York: Thieme; 2009.
21. Hollinshead WH. Anatomy for surgeons: the head and neck. Philadelphia: Harper & Row; 1982.
22. Shire JR. The importance of the prejowl notch in face lifting: the prejowl implant. Facial Plast Surg Clin North Am. 2008;16(1):87–97.
23. Anderson JE. Grant's atlas of anatomy. Baltimore: Williams & Wilkins; 1983.
24. Mittelman H. The anatomy of the aging mandible and its importance to facelift surgery. Facial Plast Surg Clin North Am. 1994;2:301–11.
25. de Pina DP, Quinta WC. Aesthetic resection of the submandibular salivary gland. Plast Reconstr Surg. 1991;88(5): 645–52.
26. Singer DP, Sullivan PK. Submandibular gland I: an anatomic evaluation and surgical approach to submandibular gland resection for facial rejuvenation. Plast Reconstr Surg. 2003; 112(4):1150–4.
27. Rohrich RJ, Rios JL, Smith PD, Gutowski KA. Neck rejuvenation revisited. Plast Reconstr Surg. 2006;118(5): 1251–63.
28. Kane MA. Nonsurgical treatment of platysma bands with injection of botulinum toxin a revisited. Plast Reconstr Surg. 2003;112(5 Suppl):125S–6S.
29. Matarasso A, Matarasso SL. Botulinum A exotoxin for the management of platysma bands. Plast Reconstr Surg. 2003;112 Suppl 5:138S–40S.
30. Tierney EP, Hanke CW. Ablative fractionated CO_2, laser resurfacing for the neck: prospective study and review of the literature. J Drugs Dermatol. 2009;8(8):723–31.
31. Becker DG, Cook TA, Wang TD, Park SS, Kreit JD, Tardy Jr ME. Gross CW: a 3 year multi-institutional experience with the liposhaver. Arch Facial Plast Surg. 1999;1(3):171–6.
32. Schaeffer BT. Endoscopic liposhaving for neck recontouring. Arch Facial Plast Surg. 2000;2(4):264–8.
33. De Castro CC. The anatomy of the platysma muscle. Plast Reconstr Surg. 1980;66(5):680–3.
34. Keller GS, Hutcherson R. Percutaneous videoendoscopic neck lift with suture suspension. Facial Plast Surg Clin North Am. 1997;5:179–84.
35. Bitner JB, Friedman O, Farrior RT, Cook TA. Direct submentoplasty for neck rejuvenation. Arch Facial Plast Surg. 2007;9(3):194–200.

Exodermlift: Nonsurgical Facial Rejuvenation

Clara Santos

60.1 Introduction

As the face is the most exposed area, it shows initially when the signs of aging appear. Aging skin signs like wrinkles and flaccidity are usually present in the elderly population. Sunlight exposure abbreviates skin aging and causes worsening of wrinkles, laxity, and changes in skin pigmentation like freckles, solar lentigo, and melasma. Also neoplastic growth as solar keratosis, basal cell carcinoma, or epidermoid carcinoma are present mostly in skin exposed areas. All these together, skin laxity, wrinkles, pigment disorders, and leather texture contribute to the loss of beauty and attractiveness and can cause aesthetic and psychological problems.

Among several rejuvenating technologies Exoderm buffered deep peel has shown to be a fantastic tool for dermatologists as well as for plastic and cosmetic surgeons. This peel was developed 25 years ago by Fintsi. Exoderm is the result of medical research over many years and is composed of 12 components, including phenol, resorcin, citric acid, and a variety of natural oils. More than a decade of experience in more than 20,000 patients and 35 countries has shown that this method is safe and minimizes any systemic side effects or permanent damage. The results are impressive and cause a high degree of patient satisfaction and long-lasting results (Fig. 60.1). It is not a substitute for surgery, but in several cases, it can be done instead of surgery or it can be complementary after facial surgery has been performed.

C. Santos
Dermatology in Private Practice, Department of Dermatology, Avenida Brasil, 583 Jardim Europa,
CEP 01431-000 São Paulo, Brazil
e-mail: clara_santos@terra.com.br

60.2 Technique

It is interesting to have skin preparation as it is in any other chemical peel. This is especially important if skin is thicker, in darker skin type, and when hyperpigmentation disorder is present.

When the patient decides to have Exoderm done, basic blood analysis and cardiac evaluation should be done as the procedure is under intravenous (IV) sedation.

The procedure is easy to perform. Patients feel comfortable as IV sedation prevents pain. A point to be taken into careful attention is related to postpeeling edema. Facial swelling is a normal and expected reaction, but as it is important, patients and family must know about it in advance in order to avoid misunderstandings. Also temporary (from 8 to 12 weeks) postpeeling redness has to be fully understood and accepted as it is normal in post peel evolution (Fig. 60.2). Patients must know they are allowed to make up to blend this erythema after the eighth day.

60.3 Instructions

60.3.1 Day of Treatment

1. Patients must wash the face completely with water and a neutral soap.
2. The anesthetist must see the patient in advance and make the prescription of the preoperative medication as well as take care of the monitoring and IV sedation during the procedure. Scrub carefully the entire face with 100% acetone to degrease the skin thoroughly. To achieve a proper scrub, use two 4×4 gauzes and apply it with little pressure. Be sure to

Fig. 60.1 (**a1, a2**) Pretreatment. (**b1, b2**) Post-treatment

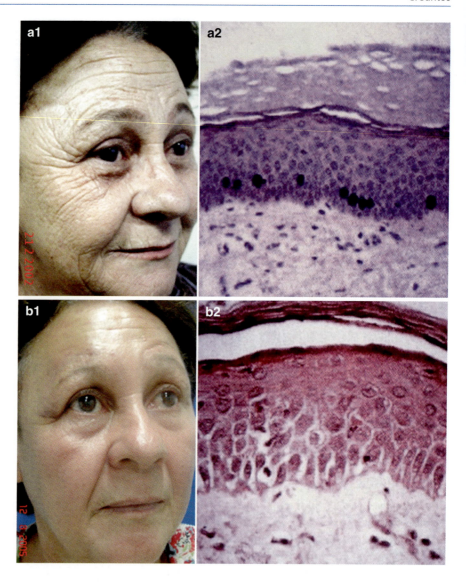

go to the eye lids only when the gauzes are dry, but over the lids no pressure is necessary. If correctly done, the facial skin will present a homogeneous erythematic aspect. Ask the patient to sit down and then mark a line 1–2 cm below the mandible ridges as the endpoint for application.
3. Tie the hair behind and use a plastic cap to cover it.
4. Stir (shake) the bottle well before using it. Soak a cotton Q-tip (Fig. 60.3) with the Exoderm solution and squeeze the Q-tip against the bottleneck several times to remove excess solution.
5. Start by applying with a rolling motion with slight pressure into the frontal hairline and forehead until you get an even frosting (Fig. 60.3). Have a dry cotton ball and clean the Exoderm solution excess right after the frost appears. Apply solution a few millimeters into the hairline in all areas. Gradually cover the entire forehead and then continue on to the temples, eyebrows, eyelids, cheeks, nose, chin, perioral region, etc.
6. Apply the Exoderm solution with a longer Q-tip. Use a cotton ball to clean the Exoderm solution excess right after the frost appears. Gradually cover the entire forehead and then continue working following the anatomical units.
7. Apply 1 mm to the lower vermilion border on the lips (Fig. 60.4). A little more pressure may be used in deep perioral lines. After having done this area, a tiny

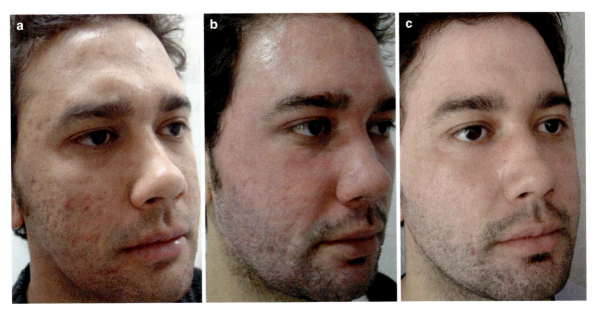

Fig. 60.2 (**a**) Pretreatment male with severe acne scars. (**b**) Two weeks posttreatment with erythema. (**c**) Two months posttreatment without erythema

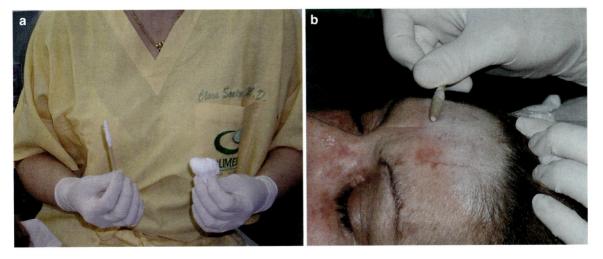

Fig. 60.3 (**a**) Apply the Exoderm using a long Q-tip and use a cotton ball to remove the excess solution. (**b**) Start by applying with a rolling motion with slight pressure into the frontal hairline and forehead until you get an even frosting

wood stick should be applied into each wrinkle line over the lips. This is useful because peribuccal wrinkles are hard to treat. There will be some cases where next day abrasion may be necessary. But it is useful to comment to patient that applying the Exoderm solution and abrading the lips may have a potential risk of hypochromia. Most patients avoid this possibility and understand that most heavy peribuccal wrinkles will clear but maybe there will still be some lines. Patients understand this easily and they do not get disappointed if they know it in advance. We always work going into the vermilion border and this does not cause any special discomfort to patients at all. It is imperative to know if patient has a positive past history for simplex herpes. In this case, antiviral drugs should be started 2 days in advance.

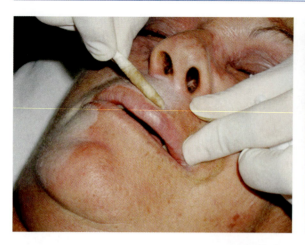

Fig. 60.4 Apply 1 mm Exoderm to the lower vermilion border on the lips

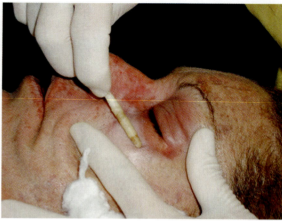

Fig. 60.5 No pressure is necessary to apply the Exoderm solution on eyelids

8. The eyelids will be the most sensitive area for application and should be treated in the moment the patient is sleeping deeper. No pressure is necessary to apply the Exoderm solution on eyelids (Fig. 60.5).
9. On the eyebrows, the application should be in the opposite direction of the hair growth to be certain all the skin is treated.
10. On the eyelids make sure that the Q-tip is nearly dry and apply right to the eyelash margin on the upper and lower lids. When applying to the eyelids, the application should be in the direction away from the eyelid margin. Always have a dry gauze ready to absorb any tears prior to or during the application of the solution.
11. The first application should take about 50–55 min. After the full face is done, start a second coat. This time you can do faster. A third application will be done only over the more damaged area (s) as on wrinkles and scars using little more pressure.
12. Be sure to treat into the hairline all around and in the sideburns and upper preauricular area.
13. Dry the skin before applying the tape. Use medium size Micropore tape to cover the entire face except the upper eyelids and eyebrows in an overlapping manner. Several layers will be necessary in order to get a perfect occlusion. You must apply the tape overlapping many times, that you won't be able to see the skin through its transparency. The Micropore mask will be completed when a white color like "snow" is achieved. Stretch the wrinkles and crow's feet before applying the white color tape to reduce the chances of air pockets developing.
14. Tape the shower cap down to the frontal scalp and along the temporal hairline.
15. Feather the edges of the tape like a stepladder below the mandible. Leave 0.5–1 cm free at the bottom.
16. Once the tape mask is in place, press firmly down on the face to eliminate any possible air pockets and secure it on the face.

60.3.2 Second Day: Micropore Tape Mask Removal and Application of Subgalatic Mask

17. A complete set of pictures of all Exoderm steps, (Fig. 60.6).
18. Remove the tape mask after 24 h. Start releasing it kindly, from the top at the hairline pulling downward.
19. The old skin mostly presents liquefied. Clean off all the liquefied skin with a Q-tip soaked in normal saline.
20. If there is crusting present in any areas, apply saline-soaked gauze to help their removal. It may

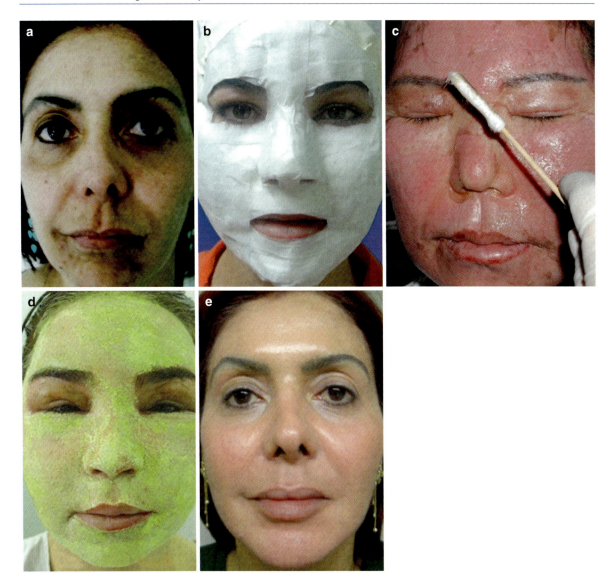

Fig. 60.6 Typical case Exoderm evolution. (**a**) Pretreatment. (**b**) End of the procedure, patient with Micropore mask. (**c**) One day after treatment with Micropore mask removal and cleaning skin liquefaction. (**d**) Subgalatic bismuth mask (7 days). (**e**) Eight months posttreatment

be necessary to use mild gauze soaked in normal saline for a light abrasion in these areas. But do it kindly. If it is difficult to remove, leave it. These darker areas represent dead skin and will peel off anyhow together with the bismuth subgalatic mask.

21. Apply Exoderm to the areas of the deepest wrinkles, pigmented area, and scars once more using your pretreatment drawing. If you are treating acne scarring, use gauze abrasion over the edges of the scars or the Exoderm Chemo Abrasion, according to the proper technique.
22. Apply the bismuth subgalatic powder evenly with a rolling motion of a Q-tip to the entire face except the upper eyelids. If the powder does not stick in an area, use mild gauze abrasion and sterile saline and then try to reapply the powder.

60.3.3 Eighth Day: Bismuth Subgalatic Mask Removal

On the eighth day, the patient will apply Vaseline to remove the powder mask at home. The Vaseline is applied continually for several hours (usually 3–5 h). After the fourth time of Vaseline massage the patient can shower using normal temperature water, never hot water. It is totally forbidden to use hot water. This shower will help the mask removal, but it is not obligatory. At first, small pieces will come off followed progressively by larger pieces. Make sure that the patient does not pull off the mask.

The use of the prescribed sun protection and topical agents are necessary to prevent unwanted pigment changes and the sunscreen as well. It is important that the patient follows this regimen carefully.

60.4 Patient Instructions

60.4.1 Shopping List

1. Vaseline. Organize to have liquid foods like different types of juices and teas, soups, etc., as you will have liquid diet for the first days.
2. Medicines and topical agents according to your prescription.
3. Q tips.
4. Mouth wash (cleaning your teeth is difficult in the rigid powder mask).
5. "Big Straws" and semisolid foods/drinks.
6. Sunscreen (SPF 30+, preferably with titanium dioxide).

60.4.2 Night Before Procedure

1. Remove all makeup and eyeliner.
2. Wash your hair.

60.4.3 The Procedure (Day 1)

Remember for the previous 8 hours before the procedure you are not allowed to eat or drink. You should have nothing leading up to the procedure, except for taking regular medications, with a minimum sip of water. Before coming for treatment, wash the face thoroughly with soap and water.

A few minutes before the procedure, you will be given prepeeling prescription to relax you and prevent the procedure from being painful. Two coats of solution are applied, and then a tape mask is put in place and firmly pressed onto the face and will remain for approximately 24 h. You need to return to have this first mask removed. Make sure to have the time to return as scheduled. Anytime if you have any doubts feel free to contact us.

60.4.4 Day 2

The tape mask is peeled off and the liquified skin cleaned away. A further coat of solution is applied to problem areas with the deeper wrinkles and then the powder mask is applied.

60.4.5 Day 3

The latter part of day 2 and day 3 is the most uncomfortable time, and you may feel a little "low." It is possible to be feverish and paracetamol is adequate for this.

There may be swelling of the face, neck, and even the upper chest. This also produces itching as the nerve endings in the remaining skin are stretched. You must sleep semirecline, rather than lying flat, as this reduces the swelling (e.g., "Lazy Boy Chair").

At this stage, there may also be some fluid oozing through the mask or slight cracking, and it is good to apply a little more powder in these areas yourself with a Q tip.

Swelling of the eyelids tends to force the eyes to close, and they should be opened regularly with two Q tips. Your may wish to irrigate them with the sterile solution to remove any powder or exudate.

60.4.6 Days Four (4) to Seven (7)

The swelling rapidly reduces, and you become much more comfortable. The main thing is to avoid cracking your mask by chewing or other facial expressions like laughing. This is where the "Big Straws" and semisolid food is essential. High-calorie drinks can also be very useful.

60.4.7 Mask Removal on Day Eight (8)

Vaseline should be massaged firmly into the mask hourly five to six times, until it can be peeled off piece by piece. This can be done safely at home as you are not peeling off skin, only the mask. The skin was removed by liquefaction in the first 24 h. This whole procedure takes 6–7 h.

At first there will be many new lines on the skin… "Don't Panic!" These are not wrinkles, but just indentations from the rigid mask and will resolve completely over the next few days.

The new skin is red initially, but this will pass over the next 8–10 weeks. However, it is a good idea to use plenty of your aqueous cream and consult your beauty therapist immediately for makeup to cover the redness until it resolves. This allows you to get back to a normal life as soon as possible.

Also you should apply the prescription your physician gave to you to prevent unwanted pigment changes and the sunscreen as well. It is important to follow this regime carefully.

60.5 Remember

If you have any questions or problems after the procedure or at any time, please contact me or one of our staff.
   Dr. _____
   Dr. Assistant_____
   Nurse:_____

60.6 Complications

Apart from the excellent and impressive results, the best on Exoderm is the safety. The buffered solution does not penetrate any further than the middermis, so dermatologic side effect reactions like scars or achromia is avoided when the technique is correctly performed. Systemic complications like arrhythmias and organ damage (especially kidneys) are equally not seen here.

In close to 2,000 patients treated over 15 years, we had delayed healing with posterior hyperthrophic scar formation only in two patients. It is interesting to remark technical mistakes that might have contributed to these two complications. Both patients were female. They had past history of previous face-lift. In both there were skin healing problem around the mandible area. In these patients, tumescent solution was infiltrated. This solution is well known by its marvellous effect to promote local anesthesia especially for liposuction. I tried this solution on the face as I thought it could be helpful to avoid local sedation and to reduce the need for postpeeling pain killers. The author feels that the tumescent solution changes local microcirculation and favors deeper absorption with this dangerous consequence. The second conclusion here was to be very careful on patients past facial surgery history as this area around the mandible may be covered by neck skin as the facial surgery lifts and brings up the surround skin. This solution has been used in another case that coincidently had previous mini face-lift, but have had no healing complication by the time of the surgery. This third patient is the only patient who has had discoloration and the skin became much lighter than it was expected.

60.7 Discussion

Several techniques are available to treat facial aging.

Ablative lasers do promote beautiful physical resurfacing, but in our experience, postop is longer and potential complication like bacterial infection or viral infection is more prone to happen. Ablative laser therapies require antibiotic and antiviral drugs while Exoderm only requires pain killers. The only situation to prescribe antiviral for Exoderm is in case when patient has positive past history for simplex herpes eruption.

Other rejuvenate techniques like botulinum toxin and fillers have a special role in the battle against aging. They can bring patient expressive results but neither of them treats the problem literally speaking, as patients keep inside the same aged tissue.

Exoderm represents an optimal solution to the aging phenomenon. Exoderm is performed ambulatory, under IV sedation. After the eighth day, patient recovery is completed and patient can return to normal activities.

60.8 Conclusions

Exoderm represents the best deep peel solution. The little phenol amount in the formula is not a problem due to the buffer system that autoblocks Exoderm in the medium dermis. This auto blockage mechanism is responsible for Exoderm security.

Patient satisfaction and long-standing effect have proved the Exoderms goals to be true: preserve long-lasting clinical and histological results (Figs. 60.7–60.9).

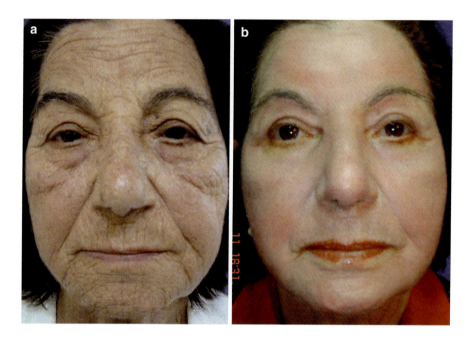

Fig. 60.7 (**a**) Pretreatment. (**b**) Posttreatment

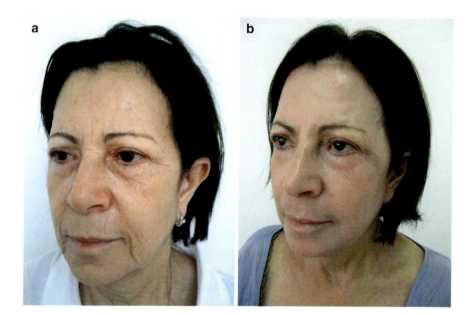

Fig. 60.8 (**a**) Pretreatment. (**b**) Posttreatment

Fig. 60.9 (**a**) Pretreatment. (**b**) Posttreatment

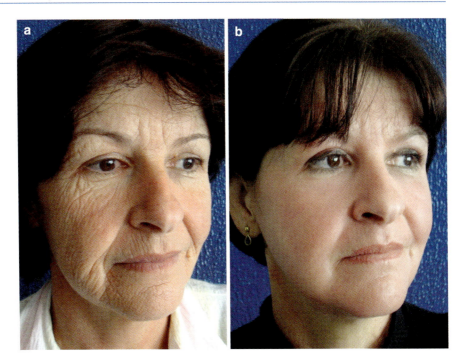

New Concepts of Makeup and Tattooing After Facial Rejuvenation Surgery

Karen Betts

61.1 Applications of Permanent Cosmetics

Permanent cosmetics can be used to complement a range of facial rejuvenation procedures. Using modern techniques, equipment and pigments, a broad spectrum of end results are achievable. These range from skin camouflage procedures to natural-looking enhancements, to the imitation of more youthful facial features, and finally to the replication of traditional makeup.

In terms of facial procedures, the most significant changes in appearance can be achieved through permanent cosmetics for eyebrows and lips. Eyebrows can be enhanced and reshaped, or imitated entirely where there are none. These procedures are particularly useful after brow-lifts, whereby new eyebrows can be designed and pigmented to complement the outcomes of the surgical procedure.

Permanent cosmetics can also provide an excellent complement to lip augmentation surgery. In the first instance, permanent cosmetics can be used to improve the definition of the lip line and also enhance the intensity of color within the lips. Should a significant change to the shape of the lip be required, permanent cosmetics can be used to redesign the lip contour.

Procedures around the eyes also have a role to play. After blepharoplasty surgery, patients can benefit from enhancements designed to add extra definition to the eyelids. These can take the form of subtle lash enhancements through to eyeliner procedures in imitation of traditional makeup. As with traditional makeup techniques for the eyes, permanent cosmetics can also be selectively utilized to improve the illusion of balance, size, and symmetry.

61.2 Preprocedure Preparation

Following a general consultation during which requirements and medical health are assessed, all clients should undertake a sensitivity patch test for pigments and topical anesthetics. Reactions to permanent cosmetic pigments are relatively rare. Topical anesthetics are required to aid the patient and to minimize any flinch responses, thus helping to maximize control and accuracy of depth when implanting pigment.

61.3 Pigment Blends

Best results are achieved if pigments are individually blended to suit the requirements of each patient (Fig. 61.1). At this point, the base tone of the pigment blend must be compared to the natural skin tone of the client to minimize the risk of an unnatural-looking color fade in future years.

61.4 Eyebrows

The eyebrow enhancement should be custom-designed and sketched onto the skin using a cosmetic pencil (Fig. 61.2). The general flow and direction of any natural hairs should be imitated for a realistic-looking result (Fig. 61.3). The procedure begins with a light first pass to provide a general indication of the guidelines. The design is quickly sketched in with the needles using light pressure and minimal depth (Fig. 61.4a).

K. Betts
Nouveau Beauty Group, Nouveau House, Barnsley Rd.,
South Elmsall, Pontefract, West Yorkshire, WF9 2HR, UK
e-mail: info@karenbetts.co.uk

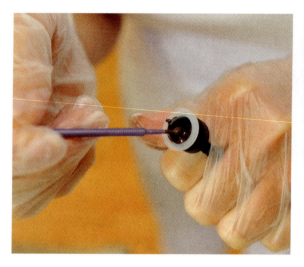

Fig. 61.1 Pigments are individually blended to suit the requirements of each client

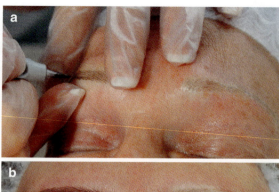

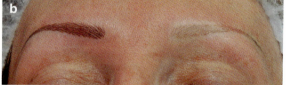

Fig. 61.4 (**a**) The first pass is extremely light and is intended to provide a general indication of the new eyebrow design. (**b**) More pressure is applied in the second pass to implant pigment to the required depth. Note the difference between the first and second passes

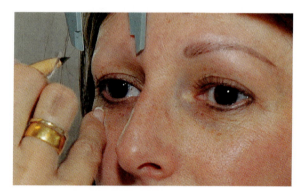

Fig. 61.2 Eyebrow enhancements should be custom-designed, using callipers to assess symmetry and estimate general guidelines

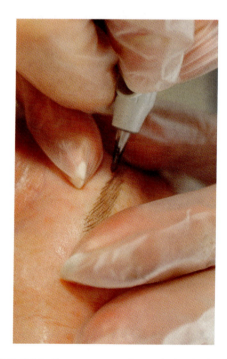

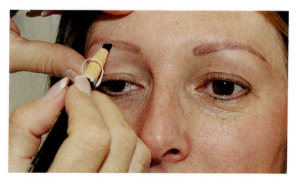

Fig. 61.3 The general flow and direction of any natural hairs should be imitated for a realistic looking result

More pressure is applied in the second pass to implant pigment to the required depth (Fig. 61.4b).

Depth is ascertained by tightly stretching around the work area and monitoring the vibrations in the skin (Fig. 61.4a).

Fig. 61.5 Subtle line curvature and a gradual reduction in line thickness can make the difference between a line that looks like an eyebrow hair and a line that looks like a tattooed line

Subtle line curvature and a gradual reduction in line thickness can make the difference between a line that looks like an eyebrow hair and a line that looks like a tattooed line (Fig. 61.5). Changes to line thickness are achieved by varying the depth into which the needles are implanted into the skin.

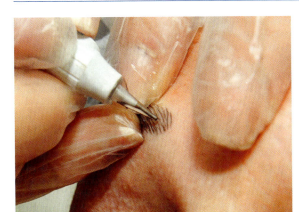

Fig. 61.6 Careful imitation of the finer features of natural brow hairs, particularly at the bulb and tail, are then added to maintain the visual illusion of real eyebrows

Careful imitation of the finer features of natural brow hairs, particularly at the bulb and tail, are then added to maintain the visual illusion of real eyebrows (Fig. 61.6).

Final healed results can be seen in Figs. 61.7 and 61.8.

61.5 Lips

Decisions regarding lip shape must be considered alongside the pigment color to be used. This is because increased depth of color and use of shading will add to the visual illusion of size and plumpness (Fig. 61.9).

A gentle first pass is used to delineate the new lip line, using light pressure and minimal depth (Fig. 61.10). The second pass is used to fully define the lip line (Fig. 61.11). A fine needle grouping is used to enhance color intensity and provide a crisp outline.

Permanent cosmetic pigments are translucent. It is therefore necessary to compensate for differences in the underlying skin tone when applying them. In Fig. 61.12, the areas of skin outside of the natural vermilion border have been intensely pigmented with a relatively small needle grouping. A larger needle grouping and slightly modified pigment blend is used to shade within the vermillion border (Fig. 61.13). This provides less intensity of color, which helps to compensate for differences in skin tone between the new lip contour and the natural lip.

Shading techniques allow for subtle visual illusions, enabling flatter areas of the lip to be highlighted, thus giving the impression of more rounded and plump lips (Figs. 61.14 and 61.15).

Subtle modifications to the pigment blend and the use of different needle groupings and shading techniques are essential elements in producing natural-looking outcomes (Figs. 61.16 and 61.17).

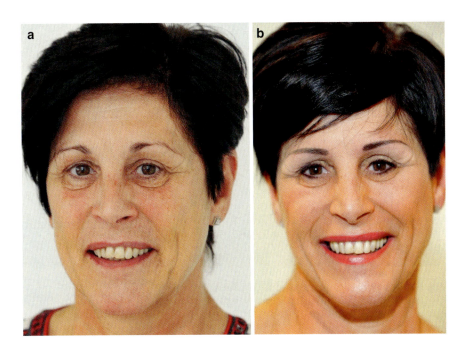

Fig. 61.7 (**a**) Before treatment. (**b**) After permanent makeup of eyebrows (healed result)

Fig. 61.8 (**a**) Before treatment. (**b**) After permanent makeup of eyebrows and lips (healed result)

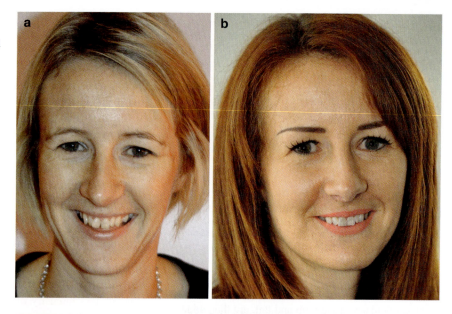

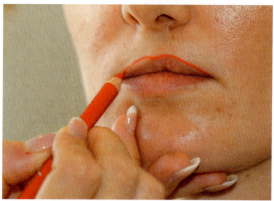

Fig. 61.9 Increased depth of color and use of shading will add to the visual illusion of size and plumpness, these factors need to be considered at the design stage

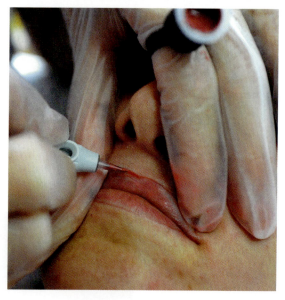

Fig. 61.11 The second pass is used to fully define the lip line

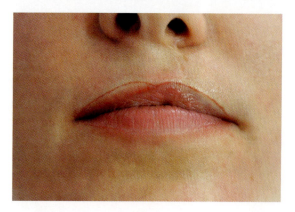

Fig. 61.10 A gentle first pass is used to delineate the new lip line, using light pressure and minimal depth. Note the significant change to the upper lip contour

61.6 Postprocedure Considerations

The final healed result color will be 30–60% lighter than it appears directly after the procedure. Skin healing balms can be beneficial in reducing pigment loss due to scabbing.

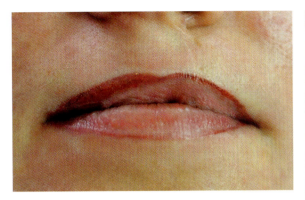

Fig. 61.12 The areas of skin outside of the natural vermilion border have been intensely pigmented with a smaller needle configuration

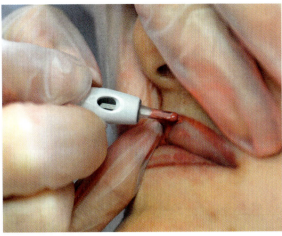

Fig. 61.14 Shading techniques allow for subtle visual illusions, enabling flatter areas of the lip to be highlighted, thus giving the impression of more rounded and plump lips

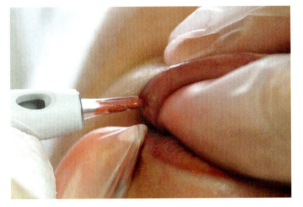

Fig. 61.13 A larger needle grouping and slightly modified pigment blend is used to shade within the vermillion border

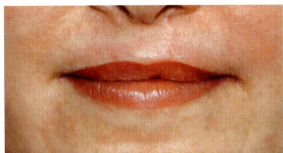

Fig. 61.15 Final healed result

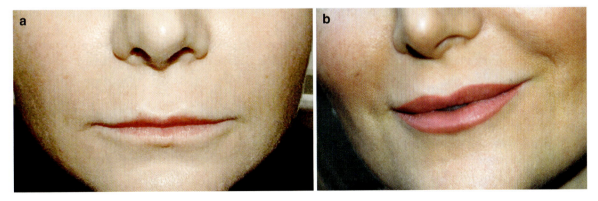

Fig. 61.16 (**a**) Before treatment. (**b**) After permanent makeup of the lips (healed result)

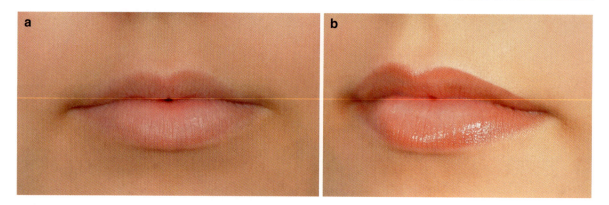

Fig. 61.17 (a) Before treatment. (b) After permanent makeup of the lips (healed result)

61.6.1 Longevity

After 30–45 days an assessment should be carried out to assess the healed result. A touchup may be required to ensure evenness of color tones. The client may benefit from a color boost 12–18 months after the initial procedure, particularly if they chose subtle pigment colors. After 18–24 months, fading and degrading of the color is likely to commence.

61.6.2 Risks

In the majority of instances, permanent cosmetics should be applied after surgical procedures. If changes to the facial structure are made following permanent cosmetics, there is a risk that the symmetries and placement will alter and become problematic. This is particularly relevant for eyebrow procedures. Removal of some pigment may be required, plus correctional work.

By contrast, it is advisable that permanent cosmetics are applied prior to lip augmentation procedures. This allows the lip shape to be accurately assessed and contoured prior to any changes effected by the surgical procedure.

The color-fade associated with permanent cosmetics is often seen as a benefit because it enables the pigment to be refreshed or the design amended to suit the needs of the client in future years. If the pigment is implanted too deeply, it will not fade sufficiently. Instead, the pigment will be subjected to the typical aging process of traditional tattoos, which are more susceptible to pigment migration and often undesirable changes in color tones. Removal of the pigment is usually required in these instances.

During the fading stage, some clients can experience a type of color fade that causes the base colors to be accentuated – most commonly reddish or grey hues. Color correction techniques can be used to neutralize these colors and restore the desired color.

Other risks associated with permanent cosmetics are similar to those of traditional tattoos and include infections, allergic reactions to pigments, scarring, and ink migration. Client dissatisfaction regarding the shape, placement, and color of the procedure outcome is also a potential risk.

61.7 Conclusions

Permanent cosmetics can be used alone, or in conjunction with a range of facial rejuvenation procedures. The range of achievable outcomes is extremely broad, ranging from subtle camouflage to more dramatic recontouring and recoloring. In the hands of professionals, permanent cosmetics can form a beneficial final step in the treatment of many clients.

Recommended Reading

Armstrong ML, Saunders JC, Roberts AE. Older women and cosmetic tattooing experiences. J Women Aging. 2009; 21(3):186–97.
De Cuyper C. Permanent makeup: indications and complications. Clin Dermatol. 2008;26(1):30–4.

Hoffman H, Gisbert M, Ortega A. Micropigmentation: technology, methodology and practice. Madrid Videocinco. 2008.

Mazza Jr JF, Rager C. Advances in cosmetic micropigmentation. Plast Reconstr Surg. 1993;92(4):750–1.

Traquina AC. Micropigmentation as an adjuvant in cosmetic surgery of the scalp. Dermatol Surg. 2001;27(2):123–8.

Vassileva S, Hristakieva E. Medical applications of tattooing. Clin Dermatol. 2007;25(4):367–74.

Part VI

HIV Facial Lipodystrophy

Poly-L-Lactic Acid for the Treatment of HIV-Associated Facial Lipoatrophy

Douglas R. Mest and Gail M. Humble

62.1 Introduction

Since the introduction of highly active antiretroviral therapy (HAART) in 1996, the mortality of patients with human immunodeficiency virus (HIV) has decreased greatly making HIV infection a more manageable chronic disease [1]. However, there has been an increase in metabolic and morphological changes known collectively as HIV-associated lipodystrophy. This syndrome, with a reported prevalence in 50% of patients on HAART for more than 12 months [2], is of increasing significance to patients and their physicians.

Lipodystrophy syndrome, first reported in 1998 [3] is now believed to be comprised of two main components: lipodystrophy and lipoatrophy. Lipodystrophy is manifested by serum lipid abnormalities, insulin resistance, and increased fatty deposits (especially around the viscera and in the dorsal cervical region), while lipoatrophy is manifested by loss of subcutaneous fat in the periphery, buttocks, and face. This subcutaneous fat loss is distinct from the HIV-associated wasting seen in patients before the advent of HAART, which is secondary to loss of lean body mass. Loss of facial fat is perhaps the most stigmatizing aspect of HIV-associated lipoatrophy because it cannot be disguised [4]. As a result, treatment options tend to focus on this aspect of the syndrome.

Despite years of in-depth research, both on a clinical and cellular level, the exact mechanism of HIV-associated facial lipoatrophy is unknown.

Indeed, current research suggests the cause is multifactorial [5, 6]. No specific antiretroviral agent has been shown to be causative. However, a strong association exists with thymidine nucleoside reverse transcriptase inhibitors (tNRTIs), most likely through inhibition of mitochondrial DNA polymerase γ, leading to depleted mitochondrial DNA in the adipose tissue and consequent cellular dysfunction. More important than specific antiretroviral agents is the influence of patient factors such as age (>40 years), gender (men more than women), and race (whites than nonwhites) [5]. The strongest predictor of lipoatrophy development appears to be low CD4 count (<100 cells/mm^3), especially in patients whose counts remained unimproved with treatment [5]. Thus prolonged delay in treatment, often requested by patients to avoid lipoatrophy, may be counterproductive to this goal.

Many methods have been used to diagnose HIV-associated lipoatrophy, including dual-energy x-ray absorptiometry (DEXA), magnetic resonance imaging, computed tomography, ultrasound, and anthropometric calipers. Although useful for research, these methods unfortunately have high costs, problematic access issues, and/or high patient-to-patient variability. A promising new technique for measuring treatment effectiveness for facial lipoatrophy is advanced photographic three-dimensional microtopography imaging. Because of these testing limitations, a clinical diagnosis is most commonly performed. James et al. [7] proposed a clinical grading scale (from 1–4) 1 = mild to 4 = severe for facial lipoatrophy (Table 62.1) based on buccal-area fat loss and visualization of underlying facial musculature. Although not validated, this scale is useful for documentation. A validated, reliable clinical scale that considers other facial areas was published by Ascher et al. [9] in 2006 but has not been widely adopted.

D.R. Mest (✉) and G.M. Humble
Blue Pacific Aesthetic Medical Group, Inc,
2301 Rosecrans Ave., #1135, El Segundo, CA 90245, USA
e-mail: drmest@aol.com; gailhum@aol.com

Table 62.1 James facial lipoatrophy severity scale

	Description
Grade 1	Mild and localized facial lipoatrophy
Grade 2	Deeper and longer atrophy, with the facial muscles beginning to show through
Grade 3	Atrophic area is even deeper and wider, with the muscles clearly showing
Grade 4	Lipoatrophy covers a wide area, extending up toward the eye sockets, and the facial skin lies directly on the muscles

Reproduced with permission from Burgess and Quiroga [8]

The psychosocial effects of facial lipoatrophy are well known. Facial lipoatrophy is the most visible and perhaps the most stigmatizing manifestation of HIV-associated lipoatrophy [4, 10]. Patients often perceive facial lipoatrophy as the "Kaposi sarcoma of the twenty-first century" with resultant anxiety over the inadvertent disclosure of HIV status [11]. Gradual fat loss and resulting disfigurement of HIV-associated facial lipoatrophy have caused depression and lowered self-esteem in patients, leading to poor social functioning and increased social isolation [10, 11]. In addition, the reduced libido sometimes seen with the condition may create quality-of-life issues [12]. Perceived or genuine employment discrimination has been reported [11].

The fear of treatment-related facial lipoatrophy has been cited as a reason to postpone treatment [13]. More important, this fear has been reported to help reduce patient adherence to treatment [10]. The unsupervised cessation of treatment poses the risk for increasing the prevalence of drug-resistant strains of HIV [14]. Fortunately, physicians now recognize the psychosocial effects of facial lipoatrophy and the need for treatment [11]. Further education is needed, however, for governmental agencies and the health insurance industry.

There are many options available for treatment of this disorder, including autologous fat transfer, surgical implants as well as a number of injectable devices. Of the injectable products, only two are FDA approved at this time in the United States. For the purpose of this chapter the remaining discussion are dedicated to the history, efficacy, mechanism of action, injection technique, duration of action, and complications associated with the use of Poly-L-Lactic Acid (PLLA) in the treatment of HIV-associated lipoatrophy.

62.2 History of Poly-L-Lactic Acid (PLLA)

PLLA was first synthesized by a French chemist in 1956. It is produced by carbohydrate fermentation of corn dextrose. Because PLLA is of a synthetic origin, no animal sensitivity testing is needed. This means no allergy testing is required. PLLA is biocompatible, biodegradable, and immunologically inert. Polylactic acid has been used since the early 1960s in the human body. When this synthetic polymer is implanted in the body, hydrolysis of the polymer backbone reduces the weight of the polymer and their degraded products are then metabolized by the body. Because of this the polymer has been used extensively in drug delivery systems and tissue engineering applications. There is at least a 45-year safety history of polylactic acid in the human body. It has been used since the early 1960s in absorbable sutures such as Vicryl™ and Dexon™. It has also been used as fixation devices in orthopedic surgery, in urethral and tracheal stents, and in dental implants. There have been over 7,000 published articles on uses of polylactic acid in humans. As previously stated the polylactides have been shown histologically to break down to the lactic acid monomer. This process takes 12–18 months, depending on the size and shape of the polylactic acid.

Injectable PLLA, which is FDA approved in the United States under the trade name Sculptra™, consists of microparticles of the L isomer of polylactic acid which are 40–60 μm in diameter and of an irregular shape. Each particle has a molecular weight up to 140,000 Da. These microparticles come in the form of a freeze-dried powder combined with apyrogenic mannitol and sodium carboxymethylcellulose. It is thought that the irregular product shape as well as the heavy molecular weight of the microparticles contributes to the slow degradation kinetics (up to 18 months) of the product (Fig. 62.1). Each vial of Sculptra™ contains 150 mg of PLLA, Sodium Carboxymethylcellulose 90 mg, and 127.5 mg Mannitol. The lyophilizate needs to be reconstituted with sterile water prior to injection.

Metabolism involves bioabsorption and gradual degradation. Polylactic acid is gradually hydrolyzed by nonenzymatic hydrolysis into mono or oligomers ($C_3H_6O_3$) of lactic acid. These fragments are then phagocytized by macrophages before being eliminated in the form of CO_2 and water or glucose and lactate (Fig. 62.2).

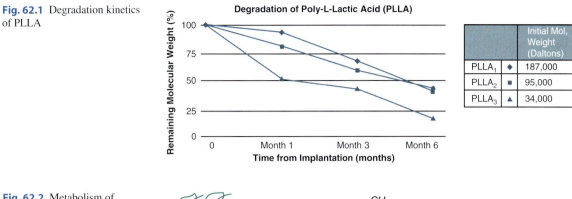

Fig. 62.1 Degradation kinetics of PLLA

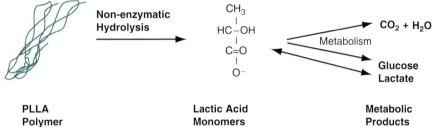

Fig. 62.2 Metabolism of PLLA

Poly-L-Lactic Acid was first marketed as a cosmetic line filler, with minimal dilution amount (1 ml) and dilution time, in Europe under the name of New Fill™. It has been used as an injectable filler since 1999 in more than 30 different countries. At that time, it was manufactured by Biotech Industries S.A. in Luxembourg. It achieved CME mark certification in Europe first as a line filler and then later as a volumizer. It is now owned and distributed by Dermik Aesthetics which is a subsidiary of Sanofi-Aventis (Bridgewater, New Jersey, USA).

The first data related to the use of PLLA in HIV-associated lipoatrophy was presented in abstract form by Amard and Saint Marc in Sept of 2000 [15]. Twenty-six HIV+lipoatrophy patients were treated with PLLA. Ultrasound measurement was used to measure dermal thickness. A 151% increase in dermal thickness was found at 3 months, 196% at 6 months, and 131% at 54 weeks.

A 96 week study was presented at the 10th Conference for Retroviral and Opportunistic Infection in Boston in February of 2003 and subsequently published in the journal AIDS in 2003 [16]. Researchers from the VEGA study presented the results of 50 HIV-positive patients after receiving PLLA for correction of facial lipoatrophy using a 3 ml dilution and a 2 week treatment interval. Change in dermal thickness was evaluated using ultrasound and color Doppler preformed by the same trained radiologists. They found a threefold increase in dermal thickness that was sustained at 72 and 96 weeks.

An early study performed by Lafaurie et al. [17], involved treating 40 patients with facial lipoatrophy. In this study, the product was diluted with 3 ccs of sterile water and 1 ml Lidocaine and the patients were treated with 150 mg (1 Vial) per cheek every 15 days. Efficacy was evaluated at 2 months and after 6 months utilizing 3D photos analyzed by digital surface photogeometry software. Results showed a mean increase of dermal thickness of 2.3 mm at the end of treatment. Results were maintained at 2 and 6 months.

Moyle et al. [18] performed the first randomized clinical trial using PLLA as a treatment for HIV-Associated lipoatrophy. Thirty patients were randomized to either immediate or delayed treatments, using three fixed treatments at 2 week intervals. Efficacy was measured by ultrasound measurement of skin thickness. Mean increases in skin thickness of 4–5 mm were observed in the treated but not in the untreated group. After delayed treatment, no inter group differences were observed. Of note, ultrasound measurements in nearby, but untreated areas, did not show any increase in skin thickness.

In 2002 in the United States when PLLA was still under the name of New Fill™, PLLA was first obtained to treat individual patients with facial lipoatrophy using the personal use importation (PUI) process regulated by the Food and Drug Administration (FDA). The PUI requires that the foreign drug or device be distributed noncommercially in volumes not considered excessive. (i.e., a 3 month period supply or less). The FDA stipulated the intended use of the drug or device be appropriately identified and affirmation had to be made in writing by the patient that the treatment was for personal use [19].

The data of two US studies, the APEX002 [20] and the Blue Pacific Study [21], were used when PLLA was submitted to the United States FDA for approval of the treatment of HIV-associated lipoatrophy, which was granted in August, 2004. Both were open-labeled single-center Investigational Device Exemption (IDE) studies meant to assess the efficacy and safety of PLLA in HIV-associated lipoatrophy.

The APEX002 trial involved 99 patients who were given one to six treatment sessions, 4–6 weeks apart, with PLLA. The average treatment sessions ranged from three to four. Patients and physicians rated the degree of lipoatrophy on a scale of 1–5 before, immediately after treatment, at 6 months and at 12 months. Patients were followed with serial photography. Seventy-seven patients considered both their cheeks and temples to be affected by lipoatrophy and 22 patients at baseline considered only their cheeks to be affected. On a scale of 1–5 (1=mild, 5=most severe), mean lipoatrophy at baseline was 3.58 in the cheek area, compared with 2.36 in the temples, decreasing to 1.51 and 1.32, respectively, prior to final treatment. Six months and 12 months after treatment cheek lipoatrophy was rated at 0.97 and 0.79, respectively: and at these time points the temples were rated 1.01– 0.47, respectively. On a satisfaction scale of 1–5, with 1 being unsatisfied and 5 very satisfied, at the end of treatment satisfaction was 4.71, at 6 months 4.83, and at 12 months 4.69.

In the Blue Pacific study patients received deep dermal/subdermal injections of PLLA into targeted treatment areas using 1–6 ml of PLLA, reconstituted with 3 ml of sterile water for injection per vial (50 mg of PLLA per milliliter), per session. Volume of PLLA injected at each treatment session was subjective and individualized to produce the desired filling effect for that patient based on the investigators previous experience. A typical treatment session involved injecting 6 ml of the product. No more than 6 ml of reconstituted PLLA (two vials) were used at any one treatment session. Sessions were scheduled 3 weeks apart with an allowed variability of 10 days. In order to assess the desired correction during the study period and for 6 and 12 months following the last treatment session, buccal skin thickness was measured by skin calipers. A total of 99 patients (97 males, 2 females) consented for participation in the study.

Of the 97 patients who completed the treatment series, 75 patients physically returned to the study site for their 12-month follow-up visit. Of these 75 patients, all patients experienced an increase in skin thickness as measured by skin calipers. Compared with baseline skin thickness, patients at the end of the treatment had an average 65.1% increase, which increased to 68.8% at 6 months and was maintained at 73% at the 12-month follow-up period. The increases in skin thickness were statistically significant at all time points.

On a scale of 1–5 with 1 being Dissatisfied and 5 being Very Satisfied, 97 patients reported a mean satisfaction score of 4.6 at the end of treatment, 77 patients reported a mean of 4.6 at 6 months, and 75 patients reported a mean of 4.8 at the 12 month follow-up visit. Mean Physician Satisfaction with overall correction was 4.5 at the end of treatment, 4.7 at 6-month follow-up, and 4.8 at 12-month follow-up. Initial facial lipoatrophy severity, as graded by the published James Scale [7] (Table 62.1) ranged from 1 (mild) to 4 (severe). The mean was 2.8. Table 62.2 displays the median number of treatments required for full correction, as it relates to initial degree of facial lipoatrophy. Most patients required between three and six treatments. Four patients (4.1%), with the most severe lipoatrophy, clinically could have used more than six treatments but were limited by the study design. There were no

Table 62.2 Distribution of patients by James Scale Class and median number of treatments required for full correction

James Scale	No. of patients	Median number of treatments by James Scale Class
1 = Mild	10	3
2	23	4
3[a]	43	5
4 = Severe	22	6
Total	98[a]	

Reproduced with permission from Mest and Humble [21]
[a]One patient found to be HIV and was removed from study after one treatment

clinically significant changes seen in serum venous lactate levels throughout the study.

The last study that should be briefly mentioned for completion of the history of this product is the cosmetic trial that was completed in 2006 (Table 62.3) [29]. The study was a 13 month, multicenter trial involving 233 subjects. The study was randomized and the evaluators were blinded. A split-face subjective evaluation was used as one side of the patients face at the nasolabial crease was injected with Cosmoplast™ (human collagen) and the other with Sculptra™. The objective of the study was to determine longevity and satisfaction with correction compared with the gold standard at the time which was Cosmoplast™. The Cosmoplast™ side demonstrated satisfactory improvement until 3 months and the Sculptra™ side up to end of the clinical trial

Table 62.3 Summary of studies of PLLA treatment and HIV lipoatrophy

	N	Injection method	Needle size	Reconstitution volume	Treatment interval	Nodule/papule rate (%)
Studies using cross-fanning injection technique						
Mest and Humble [21] (Blue Pacific study)	99	Cross-fanning	25 gauge 1.5 in.	3 ml SWFI	3 weeks (±10 days)	13
Mest et al. [22] (Blue Pacific study)	65	Cross-fanning	25 gauge 1.5 in.	3 ml SWFI	5 weeks (±10 days)	8
Hanke and Redbord [23]	65 (27 HIV+; 38 HIV−)	Cross-fanning	25 gauge 1 in.	3 ml SWFI 2 ml lidocaine	4–6 weeks	6
Burgess and Quiroga [8]	61	Cross-fanning	25 gauge 1.5 in.	4–6 cc bacteriostatic water	3–6 weeks	3
Woerle et al. [24]	300	Cross-fanning	26 gauge	3 ml SWFI 2 ml lidocaine	4–6 weeks	<1
Studies using other injection techniques						
Valantin et al. [16] (VEGA study)	50	NR	NR	3–4 ml SWFI	2 weeks	44
Moyle et al. [18] and (Chelsea and Westminster study) 18	30	NR	NR	2 ml SWFI 1 ml lidocaine	2 weeks	31
Onesti et al. [25]	4	NR	25 gauge	3–4 cc SWFI	2–3 weeks	25
Guaraldi et al. [26]	59	NR	26 gauge	4 ml SWFI	4 weeks	23
Lafaurie et al. [17]	94	NR	26 gauge 0.5 in.	3 ml SWFI 1 ml lidocaine	2 weeks	13
Engelhard and Knies [20] (Apex 002 study) (Data on file, sanofi-aventis U.S. LLC)	99	NR	NR	3 ml SWFI	4–6 weeks (±10 days)	6
Cattelan et al. [27]	50	Multiple parallel or crisscross passes	NR	3–4 ml SWFI 6–8 ml SWFI (for thinner skin)	2–4 weeks	0
Borelli et al. [28]	14	Tunneling (Crisscross and fan shape)	26 guage	4–5 ml SWFI 1 ml lidocaine	4–6 weeks	0

HIV− human immunodeficiency virus negative, *HIV+* human immunodeficiency virus positive, *NR* not reported, *SWFI* sterile water for injection

period which was 13 months. Evaluation of safety data showed a similar incidence of nodule production and papule rate (6.9% vs. 6.0% and 8.6% vs. 3.4%) between products.

62.3 Efficacy

Direct comparison of PLLA studies for efficacy is difficult secondary to the variability in study design. Treatment numbers vary significantly depending on whether the study used a fixed number of treatments [16, 18, 30] or adjusted number of treatment vials to obtain maximal patient correction of the underlying lipoatrophy [8, 20, 21, 28]. Variability in facial lipoatrophy severity and heterogeneity of study subjects add to the difficulty. The most common objective measure of efficacy has been ultrasound of skin thickness, ideally performed by a single radiologist [16, 18, 26, 28]. Recently, Carey has called into question the validity and reproducibility of ultrasound as a measure of facial lipoatrophy [31]. Other measures include 3D photography, Visual Analog Scale (VAS), skin calipers, and CT scans for linear measurement at fixed points. Regardless of the instrument used, the range of improvement that is documented is in the millimeters of improvement. What is more noticeable is the marked visual improvement in patients after treatment with PLLA (Figs. 62.3–62.5).

In general, the number of treatments needed for full correction of normal contours is directly related to the degree of facial lipoatrophy present. This was reinforced with the findings of the original Blue Pacific study [21]. There is a natural variability to patient response to PLLA as it is 100% dependent on the patient's reaction to the PLLA and reported subsequent stimulation of endogenous collagen. In the author's experience, darker skin types respond very well to PLLA as do younger patients and patients with thicker skin. This individual patient response to treatment was documented in the VEGA study [16]. In this study, although individual variability in ultrasound thickness with treatment was noted, all patients did statistically significantly respond to treatment at all time points measured.

As a secondary measure of efficacy, patient and physician satisfaction has been measured after treatment with PLLA. Again, use of various scales and end points make direct comparisons between studies impossible. However, despite the differing measurement tools utilized, the persistent overlying finding is one of significant patient satisfaction that persists through the follow-up period (Table 62.4). This consistent degree of patient satisfaction supports the efficacy of PLLA treatment of facial lipoatrophy. In the longest study to date (36 months) Mest and Humble [33] showed a continued high degree of patient satisfaction (4.9 on a scale of 1–5) at 36 months. Of note, in a study by Orlando et al. [32], it is stated that the presence of "lumps" did not alter patient satisfaction, reflecting the importance of the return of normal contours to this patient population.

An additional secondary efficacy measure that has been studied is the effect of PLLA treatment on the Quality of Life (QoL) of patients with HIV-associated lipoatrophy. These results are at first very confusing and mixed with some studies showing a significant improvement in the QoL of patients [16, 26], others not showing any improvement, and several studies showing a mixed pattern [18, 30]. The earliest studies, such as the one by Lafaurie et al. [17] used QoL questionnaires

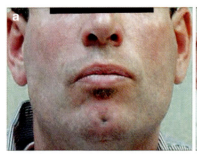
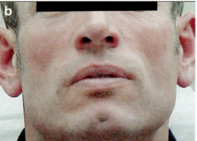
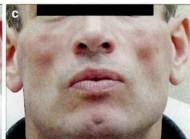

Fig. 62.3 (**a**) Before treatment. (**b**) After treatment. (**c**) One year after treatment

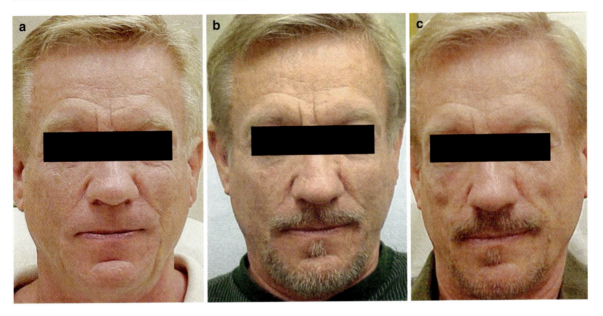

Fig. 62.4 (a) Before treatment. (b) Three months after treatment. (c) One year after treatment

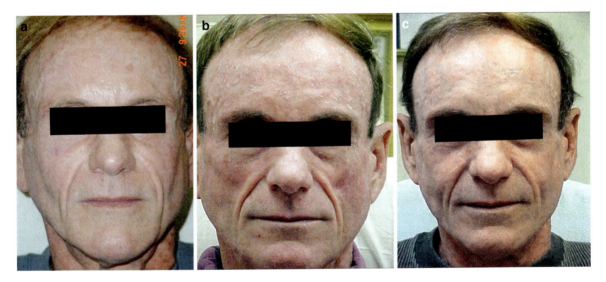

Fig. 62.5 (a) Before treatment. (b) Three months after treatment. (c) One year after treatment

that were developed for HIV patients prior to the use of HAART therapy and its resultant body changes. Use of updated QoL questionnaires such as the Short Form 36v2 Health Survey [34] showed statistically significant improvement in components of the mental health portion but not the physical health summary [30]. Using newly developed scales (Multidimensional Body-Self Relations questionnaire-Appearance Scales) Carey [30] was able to show improvement between randomized patients undergoing immediate versus delayed treatment with PLLA. Perhaps the best developed and studied tool is the AIDS Clinical Treatment Group (ACTG) Assessment of Body Change and Distress (ABCD) scale. Several studies [26, 32] have confirmed the importance of PLLA treatment for facial lipoatrophy using the ABCD scale.

Table 62.4 PLLA patient satisfaction

Study	N	Scale			
Guaraldi et al. [26]	20	Aesthetic facial satisfaction score (scale not specified), mean ± SD			
		Baseline	Week 24	Change	
		20 ± 20	83 ± 17	51 ± 32	
Orlando et al. [32]	91	Aesthetic facial satisfaction score (0=poor, 10=best), mean ± SD			
		Baseline	Week 48	p-value	
		3.3 ± 2.1	6.2 ± 2.0	<0.0001	
Lafaurie et al. [17]	94	Satisfaction about the aspect of your face in relation to the lipoatrophy (0 = dissatisfied, 10 = total satisfaction), median score (min:max)			
		Baseline	End of treatment	12 mo FU	p-value
		3.4 (0:9.3)	6.8 (1.7:9.9)	7 (1.8:9.5)	<0.0001
Mest and Humble [21]	98	Satisfaction score (1=dissatisfied, 5=very satisfied) mean rating			
		End of treatment	6 month FU	12 month FU	
		4.6	4.6	4.8	

62.4 Mechanism of Action/Histology

PLLA differs from other fillers in that it is dependent on the host response to accomplish filling. Clinically, this is represented by an initial volume effect, due to the volume of hydrogel (diluent water plus PLLA microparticles) injected. This effect lasts up to 1 week. The secondary, long lasting clinical effect is believed to involve collagen synthesis, which by definition is a delayed mechanism of action. PLLA is one of the few soft tissue fillers which can be termed a true biocatalyst or biostimulant [35–37]. Since the host immune response is involved in fibroblast behavior to some degree, and fibroblasts are responsible for collagen synthesis, potential differences to treatment with PLLA in patients with an intact immune system have been proposed as possible. In terms of response to treatment, in the authors over 8 years of experience with both cosmetic and HIV patients, this has not been the case. Cosmetic patients in general require fewer treatments in that the volume loss due to the lipoatrophy of aging is much less than HIV-associated lipoatrophy. The slightly greater potential for delayed complications in nonimmune suppressed individuals is discussed in more detail in the complication section of this chapter.

This delayed mechanism of action is important to remember when treating patients with HIV-associated lipoatrophy with PLLA. The current recommendation is to wait 4–6 weeks after treatment to access the need for additional treatment. This treatment interval can be lengthened as patients approach full correction to maximize time for the correction to occur and minimize the chance of overcorrection. In the original Blue Pacific study, patients appeared to improve clinically in their correction up to 6 months after their last treatment [21].

Well-controlled, sequential, multipatient clinical histology documenting the exact mechanism of action in humans is lacking for PLLA. In the mouse model, Gogolewski et al. [3] showed, at 1 month after PLLA implantation, a microparticle polylactide surrounded by a 100 mm thick capsulation with an increase in vascularity. Histology at 3 months revealed a decrease in cell numbers and capsule thickness of 80 mm. At 6 months capsule thickness had decreased and the surrounding areas were composed entirely of collagen fibers. At 18 months the microparticles were shown to still exist with collagen neogenesis and no signs of inflammation. Lemperle [38] studied the histologic reaction in his own forearm to poly-L-lactic acid. At 1 month there was a fine capsule around the implant. At 3 months the PLLA microspheres were intact, and surrounded by macrophages and lymphocytes. At 6 months the PLLA microspheres were degraded and deformed, and surrounded by macrophages and giant cells. At 9 months the PLLA microparticles completely degraded and there was no detectable scar tissue. This differs somewhat

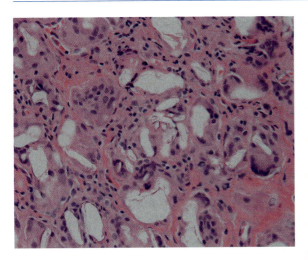

Fig. 62.6 Biopsy of papule (×100), with H&E stain, showing birefringent particles surrounded by giant cells

from the accepted clinical duration of PLLA in HIV-associated lipoatrophy of 18 months [16, 33] or longer in cosmetic patients [39, 40].

Histology in clinical patients has been confined to biopsies of nodules and papules. These biopsies are rare in that most patients are not clinically bothered by these events in that the vast majority of nodules and papules are palpable, but nonvisible. Therefore, patients rarely opt to have them excised for microscopic examination. In the Blue Pacific study [21], one patient developed an infraorbital papule that the patient elected to have surgically removed at a scheduled blepharoplasty. Histology showed birefringent particles surrounded by giant cells (Fig. 62.6). Beljaards et al. [41] reported similar histologic findings in their report of complications with early, cosmetic use of PLLA. It is unknown, but assumed that nodule/papule formation is related in some way to the generalized, underlying mechanism of action of PLLA.

62.5 Technique

A brief review of facial anatomy or more specifically facial fat anatomy is relevant to understand the changes that occur on the anatomic level with HIV-associated lipoatrophy. An understanding of this anatomy is helpful in planning how and where to place the PLLA for optimum results.

The facial fat can be divided into two layers. The first layer is superficial, between the skin and the superficialis fascia. Its function is essentially protective and has a fairly even distribution. The thickness of this layer is dependent on total body fat, as well as genetics and nationality. The other layer is deep, under the superficialis fascia. Its principal function is mechanical. This layer is made up of several fat pads, including the intraorbital fat pad, the suborbicularis oculi fat pad (SOOF), the retro-orbicularis oculi fat pad (ROOF), the galeal fat pad, the temporal fat pad, the malar fat pad, and the buccal fat pad. Of these, the temporal, malar, and buccal fat pads are the most commonly affected by HIV facial wasting. However, the pattern is quite variable from patient to patient.

Fat is a well-vascularized tissue with high metabolic activity. In addition to its structural role, fat tissue serves as a reservoir for energy storage. The number of fat cells generally is assumed to be stable after the completion of adolescent growth. Changes in the volume of fatty tissue relate to the size of the cells and their overall lipid content. Cells removed by liposuction or other surgical procedures do not regenerate. In healthy patients, cells shrink with overall weight loss and in fact, may dedifferentiate. However, subsequent weight gain causes redifferentiation of the cells with an increase in volume.

Fat tissue consists of fat cells, which have thin cell membranes enmeshed in a fibrous network. Without the supporting fibers, the cells tend to collapse. An additional supporting network of connective tissue structure creates lobules of fat.

As a side effect of HAART, HIV-associated lipoatrophy may result and can progress toward near complete subdermal facial fat loss in some patients. There is also an associated reduction in the size of the deeper fat pads. This fat loss causes changes in the other soft tissues of the face, leaving atrophic regions of generalized tissue ptosis and loss of the convex contour of the face that represents normal health and youth.

An individual, regional anatomic assessment of the face and the associated underlying fat structures affected by the lipoatrophy better guide the treatment for the optimum benefit from soft tissue fillers. With soft tissue fillers, one is essentially remaking the underlying fatty support to correct the flattening and hollowing that is present and replacing it with the normal contours of the face. Although not replacing fat with fat, correct placement of soft tissue fillers can dramatically reshape the face (Figs. 62.3–62.5).

The technique used to administer PLLA has evolved considerably since its introduction in Europe in 1999. Originally considered a dermal line filler, and not fully appreciating the mechanism of action led to its dilution with the minimal amount of water (1 mL) and placement higher in the dermis. This led to too robust of collagen synthesis with resulting surface irregularities and relatively poor outcomes [41]. Subsequent initial studies [16, 18, 20, 21] of PLLA in HIV lipoatrophy involved dilution to 3 ml with excellent efficacy but still somewhat high rates of adverse events. Further refinement of technique has evolved to greater dilution volumes (6+ ml total diluent), greater dilution times (>24 h), longer treatment intervals (4–6 weeks), and post procedure massage as standards of care when using PLLA. The overlying concept is that as a particulate suspension that stimulates collagen formation gradually, it is important to deliver the PLLA particles in as uniform of a manner as possible.

Factors such as age and the area for correction should be taken into account when planning a treatment regimen [42]. In general, the number of injections per session and total volume of correction is determined by the size of the area to be corrected. For example, if lipoatrophy is particularly severe, a cheek may require as many as 20 injections of 0.1–0.2 ml each [42]. Small marks can be made with a water-soluble surgical pen around the area to be injected. Marks should be made with the patient in the sitting position to better assess facial laxity.

There are two types of injection techniques recommended for PLLA, which are known as threading/tunneling and depot. Threading or tunneling is the most appropriate technique for the mid and lower face (cheek, preauricular and malar regions) and should be administered in a cross-hatching type pattern to more evenly cover the desired treatment area and avoid any skip areas [28]. In this area, the needle should be inserted past the deep dermis to the junction with the upper subcutaneous layer at a 30°–40° angle, followed by lowering of the needle to inject parallel to the skin [43]. A change in tissue resistance should be felt as the needle traverses the dermal–subcutaneous junction [24]. Poly-L-lactic acid is injected as the needle is withdrawn in a retrograde fashion, stopping short of the dermis. A recent refinement of technique is the additional placement of PLLA in the supraperiosteal plane where available, such as the midface. The benefit of this being improved efficacy secondary to the subsequent volume enhancement being only able to move in an anterior or forward direction.

The depot technique is recommended for other areas, such as the temples or upper zygoma. Specifically for the infraorbital area, PLLA injection should be reduced to small boluses of 0.05 ml per injection. The needle should be placed below the orbicularis oculi muscle, depositing the product just above the periosteum [24]. When treating the temples, the needle should be inserted at a 45° angle, with the final product placed below the level of the temporalis muscle fascia. When injecting, it is important to use a reflux maneuver before depositing PLLA to ensure that a blood vessel has not been entered [28].

As a biostimulant, PLLA is dependent on the patient's own stimulation of fibroblasts to lay down new collagen. Areas of active muscle, such as the orbicularis oculi and facial muscles around the mouth area, cause an increase in fibroblast stimulation. As such, these areas tend to require less product per square centimeter as well as fewer treatment sessions. In general, to avoid overcorrection, a minimal amount of product should be used for each injection (0.1–0.2 ml) and each injection site should be spaced at 0.5–1 cm intervals apart [42]. Of note, deeper, more atrophic areas are corrected with additional treatment sessions rather than additional product at the initial treatment, to avoid an overabundant formation of collagen in that area. Injections are carried out with a 25- or 26-gauge needle and the treated area should be massaged following every two to three injections [42]. Patients should also be advised to massage the treatment area periodically for several days after treatment. Lidocaine may be added to the product immediately prior to use to increase patient comfort.

62.6 Longevity

When discussing longevity with any reconstructive treatment, it is important to clarify between absolute duration of action and more importantly, clinical duration of action. That is, specifically, the time to clinical retreatment. This is especially important in patients with HIV facial lipoatrophy as the psychological meaning to patients of even a mild decrease in correction of the normal facial contours is significant. Naturally, this threshold will vary from patient to patient.

This concept becomes important when analyzing various long-term studies using PLLA in facial lipoatrophy. In the VEGA study [16], patients were not allowed interval treatments for 96 weeks. At the end of the study, patients were still visually improved compared to baseline. Since this was one of the pivotal studies used as part of the US FDA approval of PLLA, the product labeling for duration of PLLA effect is that the product "persists" for up to 2 years. In the other pivotal study evaluated by the US FDA, Moyle et al. [18] found that 14 of 27 patients had received additional PLLA treatments between the end of the initial study (6 months) and the long-term follow up visit at 18 months. It should be noted that in 10 of these patients, treatment was in areas not previously treated, which highlights the fact that clinically, physicians treating patients with facial lipoatrophy are dealing with possible continued fat loss. Patients should be counseled as such when undergoing treatment with any substance. In addition, this study used a fixed dosing scheme and therefore some patients may not have been fully corrected after the initial treatment series. Lafaurie et al. [17] in a 2005 study found that statistically, the probability of reinjection 15 months after the end of treatment was 45% as assessed by the Kaplan–Meier method. Of the 61 patients reported by Burgess [8], following fixed three treatments, significant improvement and dermal thickening was retained in 37 patients for 6 months, 1 year for 10 patients, 18 months for 9 patients, and 2 or more years for 5 patients.

In the longest-term follow-up study (36 months) to date on PLLA and HIV facial lipoatrophy, the extension study of the original Blue Pacific study examined the 75 patients who returned for measurement at month 12 [33]. PLLA was reconstituted with 5 ml of sterile water 2 h prior to injection and was injected into target treatment areas in the deep dermal/subcutaneous layer. A total of 1–10 ml of PLLA was given via a cross-fanning injection technique; utilizing a 25-gauge 1.5-in. needle, 0.1–0.2 ml threads of PLLA were placed per injection in a retrograde manner. Similar injections were then placed at approximately 90° to the original injections in the treatment areas. No more than 10 ml of reconstituted PLLA was injected at any single treatment session. Patients were treated at 5-week intervals (maximum deviation of 10 days) until full correction was obtained. Patients could receive a maximum of 12 treatment sessions over the 24-month study period if need was mutually agreed on by the treating physician and the patient. Caliper skin thickness was measured, and serial digital photographs were taken before each subsequent treatment session to assess the continued efficacy of PLLA.

Of 75 patients, 65 (63 male and 2 female) required retreatment during the study period and consented to participate in the retreatment study. Of the ten eligible patients who did not enter the retreatment study, nine continued to have persistent correction after 36 months and did not require retreatment during the extension phase, and one patient was treated at 30 months by his local physician.

Table 62.5 demonstrates the study results according to severity of original (presenting) facial lipoatrophy by the James scale: 1 ($n=8$), 2 ($n=11$), 3 ($n=32$), and 4 ($n=14$). The time to first retreatment varied by the original James scale score: 1 (21.4 months), 2 (15.7 months), 3 (14.0 months), and 4 (13.0 months). Patients with mild (James scale score 1) facial lipoatrophy had a mean of 1.9 retreatments, whereas those with moderate to severe facial lipoatrophy required more retreatments: for James scale score 2, 3, and 4 the mean number of retreatments were 3.4, 4.4, and 4.8, respectively. Approximately 50% of patients ($n=34$) required

Table 62.5 Distribution of treatments and retreatments by original James Scale

Original James Scale classification	1($n=8$)	2($n=11$)	3($n=32$)	4($n=14$)
Mean number of treatments in original Blue Pacific study	3.3	4.3	5.2	5.5
Mean skin thickness change[a] before first retreatment (mm)	+0.2	0	−0.3	+0.3[b]
Mean time to first retreatment (months)	21.4	15.7	14.0	13.0
Mean number of retreatments over the 24-month study	1.9	3.4	4.4	4.8

Reproduced with permission from Mest and Humble [33]

[a]Change from end of treatment in the Blue Pacific study to time of first retreatment

[b]Includes one patient who presented for initial retreatment with areas of overcorrection/irregular growth. Exclusion of this patient yields −0.2 mm

≤3 retreatment sessions to maintain satisfactory correction as determined by both patient and physician.

The mean skin thickness change before first retreatment generally varied by presenting James scale score: 1 (+0.2 mm), 2 (0), and 3 (−0.3). It should be noted that the mean increase (+0.3) in skin thickness observed in patients with severe facial lipoatrophy (James scale score 4) was solely attributed to areas of overgrowth in 1 patient that skewed the results. Mean change for all other patients with James scale scores of 4, excluding this patient, was −0.2 mm.

This study design was limited by the absence of a predetermined threshold to determine the need for retreatment. This may have contributed to the large number of patients (36 of 75) who opted to have their first retreatment at the time of their 12-month, on site, follow-up from the original Blue Pacific study [21]. These patients were already at the study site, eligible for retreatment and may have elected to undergo retreatment with the goal of maintaining correction rather than wait for a decrease in correction. In addition, this study did not limit treatment to areas already treated. It was noted by the study authors that a few patients actually had an increase in skin caliper measurement in their originally treated (and measured) areas but requested treatment in other areas not previously treated. Consequently, the study authors concluded that an exact answer to the rate of loss of correction over time was not possible from their study. The study also concluded that, in general, PLLA was a safe and effective long-term treatment option for HIV-associated facial lipoatrophy. Patients with milder facial lipoatrophy required fewer injections and had more sustained correction than those with severe facial lipoatrophy. Twelve percent of patients had greater than 36 months of sustained correction. All patients receiving treatment of facial lipoatrophy with PLLA were highly satisfied with the results of the therapy.

The conclusion as to the longevity of the product is therefore somewhat variable. Whether it is 6 months or 36 months and beyond depends on a number of factors including individual response to treatment, possible ongoing fat loss, treatment technique variability, and treatment quantities utilized. Clinically, the average time to re-retreatment in the chapter authors experience is approximately 18 months. As such, it is at least reasonable to consider PLLA a semipermanent filler. Of note, there appears to be a difference in longevity when comparing the use of PLLA in HIV-Associated facial lipoatrophy and the lipoatrophy of aging. Published reports out of Europe [39, 40, 42] have documented a cosmetic indication duration of effect of 3–4 years and beyond.

62.7 Complications

Possible adverse events common to all injectable products may include tissue response to the injection procedure itself, such as bruising and swelling. Adverse events may relate to the properties of the product used or the technique of administration [44]. In regards to PLLA, the most common adverse event that is prominently discussed is the possibility of small (<5 mm) subcutaneous papules. In key studies for PLLA, subcutaneous papules were found in 44% [16], 31% [18], 6.1% [20], and 13.1% [21] of the patients. A more complete papule/nodule rate of various studies on PLLA in HIV facial lipoatrophy is found in Table 62.2. Rates as low as 0.139% have been reported in a long-term mixed population of cosmetic and HIV+ patients [39].

These subcutaneous papules tend to be nonvisible and asymptomatic (noninflammatory). These papules are rarely biopsied as they are not usually bothersome to patients. Therefore the exact histopathology is lacking. Isolated biopsies have shown birefringent particles surrounded by giant cells (Fig. 62.6). In general, the common clinical belief is that they represent a localized, excessive, collection of PLLA particles, reactive cells, and resultant collagen bundles.

The risk of adverse events associated with PLLA is minimized if appropriate preinjection and injection procedures are employed. The area selected for treatment should be appropriate; injections to the periorbital area should be reserved for experienced injectors and injections should be avoided in areas such as the lips, neck, or glabella. Based on initial studies, a minimum of 2 weeks is recommended in the product insert, between each treatment. However, clinical experience has shown it is best to wait 4–6 weeks between treatment sessions as this allows the physician to properly assess the needs of the patient and the effects of the treatment.

It is also important that PLLA is reconstituted properly, as nonhomogeneous reconstitution of PLLA or injection less than 2 h after reconstitution have both been associated with an increased risk of side effects.

It has been found that papule/nodule formation may be associated with high concentrations of localized PLLA (i.e., dilution of the contents of one vial with 3 ml sterile water for injection [SWFI]). Published information also suggests that additional dilution time (24 h) beyond the 2 h minimum may further decrease the risk of papule/nodule formation [24, 28]. Therefore, a recommended technique is to dilute PLLA with 6 ml SWFI and to reconstitute for at least 2 h prior to use. Again, additional dilution time (>24 h) may be beneficial. Of note, in cosmetic patients the dilution amount is usually higher in an attempt to further minimize papule/nodule formation in this patient population that tends to be risk averse. Administration should be by superficial subcutaneous injection. Finally, to ensure that the product is evenly dispersed throughout the tissues the injection area should always be massaged posttreatment. Patients are also encouraged to massage the treated areas postprocedure for several days. By avoiding a localized accumulation of PLLA, the risk of papule/nodule formation will be minimized.

A clearer picture is evolving regarding the long-term natural course of resolution of these subcutaneous papules. The 24-month VEGA study [16] reported that 6 of 22 papules resolved spontaneously. In the 36-month Blue Pacific follow-up study [33], the authors reported that all but one (12 of 13) of the small (<5 mm) papules that formed during the original study had resolved by the end of the retreatment study. In addition, in 5 (7.7%) of the 65 patients, a total of five new, small (<5 mm), nonvisible papules were reported all occurring within 2 and 7 months after retreatment. Four resolved spontaneously; one patient elected surgical excision of an infraorbital papule that was resistant to conservative treatment measures (including needle desiccation and dilution and treatment with intralesional 5-fluorouracil (5FU)/steroid injection). Another patient presented at retreatment with areas of relative overcorrection, but no discrete papules. This patient had severe lipoatrophy (James scale score of 4) in the original study; the overgrowth was believed to be secondary to an overaggressive original treatment dosage per area. The patient responded to treatment that was administered in adjacent areas of the face to minimize the contour irregularities.

The majority of the studies on PLLA and HIV facial lipoatrophy have been heavily weighted to White males. As part of the US FDA approval of PLLA, a post-marketing study looking at PLLA to treat people of color and women with lipoatrophy was required. Enrollment started in November 2005 on a 5 year, multi-center phase four registry study. The 1-year, interim analysis abstract [22] showed that there were numerically fewer adverse events (nodules/papules) in darker skin types. There were also no reports of hypertrophic scars or keloids in darker skin types. In addition, there was no difference in clinical response between genders.

As it appears that most of these papules are self limited, the treatment of them should therefore be conservative. The ideal one is to avoid them by following the above procedures. The formation of a papule, if it is to occur, is somewhat delayed, usually in the range of 2–7 months. Initial treatment consists of physically attempting to break up the accumulation of PLLA particles. This can be accomplished by an injection of the papule and surrounding area with local anesthetic containing epinephrine and subsequent needle desiccation/subcision with a small caliber needle (25 or 26 gauge). The goal of treatment is not to completely rid the patient of the papule but to make it smaller and therefore more prone to the natural degradation process. This treatment can be done weekly as necessary. If the physician or patient requires a more aggressive treatment, low dose Triamcinolone-10 (0.2 ml) with 5FU 50 mg/ml (0.8 ml) can be used to slow the mitotic activity of the fibroblasts stimulated by the PLLA. Of note, high-dose, nondilute triamcinolone is not recommended as the majority of the papules are self limited and the subsequent skin depression possible after use of high-dose triamcinolone may become apparent after the papule resolves (Fig. 62.7).

There have been isolated reports of rare (<0.1%) inflammatory papules occurring late after PLLA usage [45]. This inflammatory reaction is very robust and routinely occurs no sooner than 12 months after PLLA treatment. It is felt to be a T cell-mediated delayed sensitivity response and therefore has been reported more in patients with an intact immune system, but the chapter authors are aware of at least two cases in patients who were HIV positive (personal communication). In both of these cases, the reactions occurred after a spike in the patients T cells. Treatment of these nodules involves short-course, high-dose, systemic steroid treatment, as well as localized steroid injection to the papules to blunt the inflammatory response in addition to several months of daily Doxycycline. Treatment of these extremely rare inflammatory papules is usually very successful (Fig. 62.7).

```
                        ┌─────────────┐
                        │   NODULE    │
                        └──────┬──────┘
              ┌────────────────┴────────────────┐
┌─────────────────────────────┐    ┌─────────────────────────────────┐
│         INACTIVE            │    │            ACTIVE               │
│ Usually occur <6 months     │    │ Very rare                       │
│ post treatment              │    │ Usually late onset >12 months   │
│ Hard                        │    │ post treatment                  │
│ Non-inflammatory            │    │ Inflamed                        │
│ Confined to treatment area  │    │ May appear beyond treatment area│
│ Evidence of histiocytes     │    │ Evidence of inflammatory cells  │
└─────────────────────────────┘    └─────────────────────────────────┘
```

TREATMENT

```
┌─────────────────────────────────────┐   ┌────────────────────────────────────────┐
│ Subcision with 25 G needle          │   │ Every 1–2 weeks:                       │
│ Inject sterile water to dilute      │   │ Intralesional injection of triamcinolone│
│ poly-L-lactic acid at site          │   │ or methylprednisolone + 5–fluorouracil*.│
│ Massage following injection         │   │ Precision delivery with 27 G needle     │
│              OR                     │   │                 PLUS                    │
│ Heat treatment, ultrasound,         │   │ Systemic therapy with prednisolone or   │
│ mechanical vibration                │   │ doxycycline*                            │
│              OR                     │   │                                         │
│ Excision of nodule (last resort)    │   │                                         │
└─────────────────────────────────────┘   └────────────────────────────────────────┘
```

* See individual summaries of product characteristics for dosing recommendations

Fig. 62.7 Papule/nodule treatment algorithm

62.8 Conclusions

HIV-associated facial lipoatrophy is a long-term issue with no simple solution. The hope of finding a single cure is doubtful because the cause appears multifactorial. Therefore, long-term, multidisciplinary solutions need to be sought. The advantages of treating this condition can be neither underestimated nor undervalued. PLLA provides a safe and effective treatment option for this condition (Table 62.5). It is important that the correct overall injection technique is employed when using PLLA, including proper reconstitution and injection, massage, and enough time between treatments to evaluate the effects. This will allow the physician to achieve the most natural-looking result with minimal adverse events.

References

1. Palella Jr FJ, Delaney KM, Moorman AC, Loveless MO, Fuhrer J, Salten GA, et al. Declining morbidity and mortality among patients with advanced human immunodeficiency virus infection. HIV outpatient study investigators. N Engl J Med. 1998;338(13):853–60.
2. Miller J, Carr A, Emery S, Low M, Mallal S, Baker D, et al. HIV lipodystrophy: prevalence, severity and correlates of risk in Australia. HIV Med. 2003;4:293–301.
3. Carr A, Samaras K, Burton S. A syndrome of peripheral lipodystrophy, hyperlipidaemia and insulin resistance in patients receiving HIV protease inhibitors. AIDS. 1999;12(7):F51–8.
4. Carrieri P, Cailleton V, Le Mong V. The dynamic of adherence to highly active antiretroviral therapy: results from the French National APROCO cohort. J Acquir Immune Defic Syndr. 2001;28:232–9.
5. Lichtenstein KA, Delaney KM, Armon C, Ward D, Moorman A, Wood K, et al. Incidence of and risk factor for lipoatrophy (abnormal fat loss) in ambulatory HIV-1 infected patients. J Acquir Immune Defic Syndr. 2003;32:48–56.
6. Mallon P, Miller J, Cooper D, Carr A. Prospective evaluation of the effects of antiretroviral therapy on body composition in HIV-1 infected men starting therapy. AIDS. 2003;17: 971–9.
7. James J, Carruthers A, Carruthers J. HIV-associated facial lipoatrophy. Dermatol Surg. 2002;28(11):979–86.
8. Burgess CM, Quiroga RM. Assessment of the safety and efficacy of poly-L-lactic acid for the treatment of HIV-associated facial lipoatrophy. J Am Acad Dermatol. 2005; 52:233–9.
9. Ascher B, Coleman S, Alster T. Full scope of effect of facial lipoatrophy: a framework of disease understanding. Dermatol Surg. 2006;32:1058–69.

10. Martinez E, Garcia-Viejo MA, Blanch L, Gotell JM. Lipodystrophy syndrome in patients with HIV disease: quality of life issues. Drug Saf. 2001;24(3):157–66.
11. Power P, Tate HL, McGill SM, Taylor C. A qualitative study of the psychological implications of lipodystrophy syndrome on HIV positive individuals. Sex Transm Infect. 2003;79: 137–41.
12. Dukers NH, Stolte IG, Albrecht N, Coutinho RA, de Witt JB. The impact of experiencing liodystrophy on the sexual behaviour and well-being among HIV-infected homosexual men. AIDS. 2001;15:812–3.
13. Duran S, Saves M, Spire B, Cailleton V, Sobel A, Carrieri P, et al. Failure to maintain long-term adherence to highly active antiretroviral therapy: the role of lipodystrophy. AIDS. 2001;15(18):2441–4.
14. Miller V, Sabin C, Hertogs K, Bloor S, Martinez-Picado J, D'Aquila R, et al. Virological and immunological effects of treatment interruptions in HIV-1 infected patients with treatment failure. AIDS. 2000;14(18):2857–67.
15. Amard P, Saint Marc T. Polylactic acid in the treatment of HIV-associated lipoatrophy. Second lipodystrophy workshop, Toronto, Sep 2000.
16. Valantin MA, Aubron-Olivier C, Ghosn J, Laglenne E, Parchard M, Schoen H, et al. Polylactic acid implants (new-fill®) to correct facial lipoatrophy in HIV-infected patients: results of the open-label study VEGA. AIDS. 2003;17: 2471–7.
17. Lafaurie M, Dolivo M, Porcher R, Rudant J, Pharm IM, Molina JM. Treatment of facial lipoatrophy with intradermal injections of polylactic acid in HIV-infected patients. J Acquir Immune Defic Syndr. 2005;38(4):393–8.
18. Moyle GJ, Lysakova L, Brown S, Sibtain N, Healy J, Priest C, et al. A randomized open-label study of immediate versus delayed polylactic acid injections for the cosmetic management of facial lipoatrophy in persons with HIV infection. HIV Med. 2004;5:82–7.
19. Administration USFDA. Policy on importing unapproved AIDS drugs, vol. 2004; 1998.
20. Engelhard P, Knies M. Safety and efficacy of new-fill™ (Poly-L-lactic acid) in the treatment of HIV-associated lipoatrophy of the face (HALF). XIV International AIDS conference, Barcelona, Jul 2002.
21. Mest DR, Humble G. Safety and efficacy of poly-L-lactic acid injections in persons with HIV-associated lipoatrophy: the US experience. Dermatol Surg. 2006;32(11):1336–45.
22. Mest D, Humble G, Pierone, G. Interim results of a 5-year open-label study for the correction of HIV-related facial lipoatrophy with injectable PLLA. summer AAD, Boston; Jul 2009.
23. Hanke CW, Redbord KP. Safety and efficacy of poly-L-lactic acid in HIV lipoatrophy and lipoatrophy of aging. J Drugs Dermatol. 2007;6:123–8.
24. Woerle B, Hanke CW, Sattler G. Poly-L-lactic acid: a temporary filler for soft tissue augmentation. J Drugs Dermatol. 2004;3(4):385–9.
25. Onesti MG, Renzi LF, Paoletti F, Scuderi N. Use of polylactic acid in face lipodystrophy in HIV positive patients undergoing treatment with antiretroviral drugs (HAART). Acta Chir Plast. 2004;46:12–5.
26. Guaraldi G, Orlando G, De Fazio D, De Lorenzi I, Rottino A, De Santis G. Comparison of three different interventions for the correction of HIV-associated facial lipoatrophy: a prospective study. Antivir Ther. 2005;10(6):756–9.
27. Cattelan AM, Bauer U, Trevenzoli M. Use of polylactic acid implants to correct facial lipoatrophy in human immunodeficiency virus 1 positive individuals receiving combination antiretroviral therapy. Arch Dermatol. 2006;142:329–34.
28. Borelli C, Kunte C, Weisenseel P, Thoma-Gerber E, Korting HC, Konz B. Deep subcutaneous application of poly-L-lactic acid as a filler for facial lipoatrophy in HIV-infected patients. Skin Pharmacol Physiol. 2005;18:273–8.
29. Narins R. Abstract ASDS, Oct 2006.
30. Carey DL, Baker D, Rogers GD, Petoumenos K, Chuah J, Easey N. A randomized, mulitcentre, open-lable study of poly-L-lactic acid for HIV-1 facial lipoatrophy. J Acquir Immune Defic Syndr. 2007;46(5):581–9.
31. Carey D, Wand H, Martin A. Evaluation of ultrasound for assessing facial lipoatrophy in a randomized, placebo-controlled trial. AIDS. 2005;19:1321–7.
32. Orlando G, Guaraldi G, De Fazio D, Rottino A, Grisotti A, Blini M. Long-term psychometric outcomes of facial lipoatrophy therapy: forty-eight week observational, nonrandomized study. AIDS Patient Care STDs. 2007;21(11):833–41.
33. Mest DR, Humble GM. Retreatment with injectable poly-L-lactic acid for HIV-associated facial lipoatrophy: 24-month extension of the Blue Pacific study. Dermatol Surg. 2009;35: 350–9.
34. Ware Jr JE, Sherbourne CD. The MOS-36 item short-form health survey (SF-36) conceptual framework and item selection. Med Care. 1992;30:473–83.
35. Gogolewski S, Jovanovic M, Perren SM, Dillon JG, Hughes MK. Tissue response and in vivo degradation of selected polyhydroxyacids: polylactides (PLA), poly (3-hydroxybutyrate) (PHB) and poly (3-hydroxybutyrate-co-3-hydroxyvalerate) (PHB/VA). J Biomed Mater Res. 1993; 27:1135–48.
36. Brady JM, Cutright DE, Miller RS, Barristone GC. Resorption rate, route, route of elimination and ultrastructure of the implant site of polylactic acid in the abdominal wall of the rat. J Biomed Mater Res. 1973;7(2):155–66.
37. Pietrzak WS, Sarver DR, Verstynen ML. Bioabsorbable polymer science for the practicing surgeon. J Craniofac Surg. 1997;8:87–91.
38. Lemperle G, Morhenn V, Charrier U. Human histology and persistence of various injectable filler substances for soft tissue augmentation. Aesthetic Plast Surg. 2003;27(5): 354–66.
39. Bauer U. Correction of facial deformities with poly-L-lactic acid: 40-month follow-up. J Eur Acad Dermatol Venereol. 2004;18:193–57.
40. Vleggaar D. Facial volumetric correction with injectable poly-L-lactic acid. Dermatol Surg. 2005;31(11 Pt2):1511–7.
41. Beljaards R, de Roos K, Bruins F. NewFill for skin augmentation. A new filler or failure? Dermatol Surg. 2005;31: 772–7.
42. Vleggaar D. Poly-L-lactic acid: consultation on the injection techniques. J Eur Acad Dermatol Venereol. 2006;20 (Supple 1):17–21.
43. Dermik Laboratories, Sculptra™ Product Information. Available at http://www.sculptra.com/US/resources/SculptraPI.pdf, 2006.
44. Lowe NJ, Maxwell CA, Patnaik R. Adverse reactions to dermal fillers. J Dermatol Surg. 2005;31:1616–25.
45. Vleggaar D. Soft tissue augmentation and the role of poly-L-lactic acid. Plast Reconstr Surg. 2006;118:46S–54.

Autologous Fat Transfer for HIV-Associated Facial Lipodystrophy

Lisa Nelson and Kenneth J. Stewart

63.1 HIV-Associated Lipodystrophy Syndrome

Although the survival of HIV-infected patients has improved dramatically due to highly active antiretroviral therapy (HAART), prolonged HAART is associated with side effects including HIV-associated lipodystrophy. This is a syndrome consisting of morphological changes (central fat accumulation and peripheral fat atrophy) and metabolic changes (hyperlipidemia and insulin resistance) which has been increasingly reported in patients since 1998 [1]. The consequence of body fat changes is social stigmatisation that may negatively affect the quality of life of patients with HIV disease and may pose a barrier to treatment and reduce medical adherence.

63.2 Prevalence

From the era of HAART (Highly Active Antiretroviral Therapy), a spectrum of changes in body fat has been reported to occur in 20–80% of subjects receiving these therapies [2–6]. Variations in the reported prevalence rates are related to a variety of many factors, including age, genetics, HIV medications and case definition.

63.3 Clinical Features

63.3.1 Morphological Changes

Changes in body fat distribution are characteristic of HIV-associated lipodystrophy. The most prominent clinical sign is a loss of subcutaneous fat in the face and extremities. Facial lipoatrophy has been attributed to the loss of buccal, parotid and pre-auricular fat pads [7], and may be accentuated by parotid hypertrophy in some patients. Adipose tissue loss from the peripheral regions occasionally leads to prominent veins resembling varicosities. Some patients have concomitant deposition of excess adipose tissue around the neck (Fig. 63.1), over the dorso-cervical spine (Fig. 63.2),

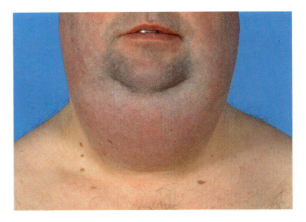

Fig. 63.1 Deposition of excess adipose tissue around the neck

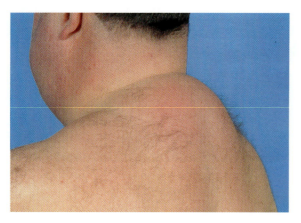

Fig. 63.2 Excess deposition of fat over the dorso-cervical spine

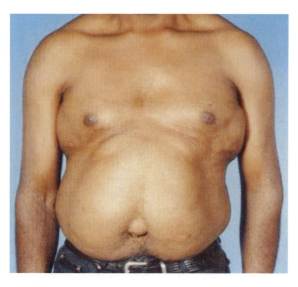

Fig. 63.3 Excess deposition of fat of the upper torso and intra-abdominal region

upper torso and intra-abdominal region (Fig. 63.3) [8, 9]. Dorso-cervical fat accumulation can be disfiguring and is associated with the development of neck pain and sleep apnea [10]. This can also be associated with fat accumulation around the occipital region. Breast enlargement has been reported in both sexes, although it is unclear whether this is due to excess subcutaneous fat, glandular hypertrophy, or both [11, 12].

On body shape changes alone, three different patterns of lipodystrophy have been described: some patients have only lipohypertrophy, some have only lipoatrophy and some patients exhibit a mixed clinical presentation. Because no uniform morphologic changes occur with HIV lipodystrophy, there is now accumulating evidence that lipoatrophy, central adiposity and the combination of both are considered distinct entities with different risk factors and metabolic processes underlying their development [13].

Several techniques are suitable for measuring regional fat distribution including dual energy x-ray absorptometry (DEXA), computer tomography (CT), magnetic resonance imaging (MRI) and ultrasound. Anthropometric measurements, including waist circumference, sagittal diameter and skin fold thickness are cheaper and easier to perform than imaging techniques but are operator dependant [13]. Three-dimensional laser scans have been used for measurement of facial volumes [14–16] and may provide an objective tool for monitoring changes in facial lipoatrophy [17].

63.3.2 Metabolic Changes

Frequently, complex metabolic alterations are associated with the described body shape alterations. These include peripheral and hepatic insulin resistance, impaired glucose tolerance, type 2 diabetes, hypertriglyceridemia, hypercholesterolemia, increased free fatty acids and reduced high-density lipoproteins [18]. The prevalence of insulin resistance and glucose tolerance is reported in the literature at 20–50% depending on study design and measurement methods [19, 20].

63.3.3 Pathogenesis

The reasons for fat depletion and accumulation in HIV-infected patients receiving antiretroviral therapy remain unclear. The pathogenesis of HIV lipodystrophy is complex and the aetiology is likely to be multifactorial. Studies published provide evidence for two assumptions: first, lipoatrophy and lipoaccumulation result from divergent mechanisms. Second, the various classes of antiretroviral drugs contribute to the lipodystrophy syndrome by different and probably overlapping mechanisms.

63.3.4 Protease Inhibitors

Many studies have suggested a link between the use of protease inhibitors and the development of lipodystrophy. Protease-inhibitor (PI) binding of cytoplasmic retinoic-acid binding protein type 1 may prevent a cascade of molecular events leading to peripheral adipocyte differentiation and apoptosis. An alternative suggested mechanism is that PI therapy inhibits adipogenesis by a process involving sterol regulatory element binding proteins (SREBPs), which play a central role in cellular lipid homeostasis [21]. Differences in the metabolic activity of central, dorso-cervical and peripheral adipocytes have been proposed. Thus, the impaired fat storage and hyperlipidemia associated with protease inhibitor treatment may lead to preferential central accumulation of fat. A link between PI therapy and altered apolipoprotein (B and C-III) synthesis has also been postulated [22].

63.3.5 Non-Nucleoside Reverse Transcription Inhibitors

Mitochondrial toxicity associated with nonnucleoside reverse transcription inhibitors (NRTIs) has also been well established and is thought to contribute to the fat redistribution syndrome seen in patients with HIV infection [23, 24]. It has been suggested that the pattern of lipodystrophy varies with drug therapy: NRTIs are associated with lipoatrophy alone, while NRTI combined with PI therapy is associated with lipoatrophy and lipohypertrophy. However, the wide variety of drug combinations used make it difficult to identify risk associated with particular drugs.

63.4 HIV Infection

The development of HIV lipodystrophy has been positively associated with the duration of HIV infection, negatively associated with previous HIV viral load and both positively and negatively associated with blood CD4 lymphocyte counts in various studies [16].

63.5 Nutritional Status, Age, and Adiposity

Body adiposity before receiving antiretroviral therapy may also affect features of lipodystrophy. In one cross-sectional study, patients with BMI greater than 28 kg/m^2 had higher prevalence of buffalo hump and breast enlargement, but a lower prevalence of facial and gluteal fat loss compared with underweight patients (BMI < 20 kg/m^2) [25]. Older people tend to have greater body fat mass, particularly intra-abdominal fat, which may contribute to the body fat changes seen in HIV-associated lipodystrophy [26].

63.6 Female Sex

Trunk obesity rather than subcutaneous fat wasting appears to be more common in women than in men [27], although prospective studies are required to evaluate whether there are true differences between the sexes.

63.7 Cytokines

There is an association between lipodystrophy and levels of serum inflammatory factors. One study analysed the mRNA expression of adipocytokines and transcriptional factors in fat samples from 26 patients with peripheral lipoatrophy [28]. The patients' fat showed higher values of apoptosis, fibrosis, vessel density and macrophage infiltration than controls, together with lower adiponectin and leptin mRNA levels and higher interleukin (IL)-6 and tumour necrosis factor (TNF) alpha mRNA levels. Elevated levels of the soluble type 2 tumour necrosis factor-alpha receptor has been linked with insulin resistance associated with lipodystrophy.

C-peptide has been shown to be the strongest metabolic predictor of future lipodystrophy severity in patients receiving combined NRTI and protease inhibitor therapy [29].

63.8 Management

63.8.1 Nonsurgical Treatment of HIV Facial Lipoatrophy

No specific medical treatment exists for HIV-associated lipodystrophy. The use of recombinant growth hormone can be beneficial in patients with visceral abdominal fat or dorso-cervical fat pad; however, it is not recommended for the treatment of patients with features of lipoatrophy as it may lead to a reduction in peripheral fat. In general, dietary modification, exercise and switching antiretrovirals that are implicated in the lipodystrophy syndrome may improve metabolic abnormalities but the impact on body fat is very small [30].

63.8.2 Surgical Treatment of HIV-Associated Facial Lipoatrophy

The most common site for lipoatrophy is the face, and is often the most distressing for the patient as it identifies them as being affected by HIV. Anatomically, facial fat lies in three planes: subcutaneous fat, fat within the SMAS layer and the deep fat pads. The deep fat of the cheek constitutes the Bichat fat sack, which has three branches: temporal, buccinator and retromandibular [31]. In the literature, facial atrophy has been attributed to either atrophy of the deep facial fat pads, or atrophy of all layers of facial fat [31]. However, one recent study which evaluated the anatomy of the buccal fat pad of Bichat in HIV-related facial atrophy reported normal position and caliber of the fat pad and suggests that the cache tic appearance of the face is likely secondary to profound atrophy of the subcutaneous tissues in these areas [8].

Surgical options for HIV-associated facial lipoatrophy include: autologous fat transfer, dermis-fat graft, flaps, rhytidectomy, malar implants and soft-tissue fillers. Autologous tissue is the ideal tissue filler for physiological reasons. The potential advantages include biocompatibility, versatility, stability and natural appearance [29].

and emphasised the importance of small grafts for more predictable results [32]. This was followed by reports of free fat autographs to fill soft-tissue defects by Czerny [33], Lexer [34] and Rehn [35]. In 1911, Bruning was the first to inject autologous fat into the subcutaneous tissue for the purpose of soft-tissue augmentation [36]. In 1912, Hollander published photographs showing the results of fat infiltration into two patients with lipoatrophy of the face [37]. In 1926, Miller wrote about his experiences with infiltration of fatty tissue through cannulas [38]. Early optimism was tempered by Peer in 1950, who demonstrated histologically that fat grafts lost approximately 45% of their weight and mass 1 year or more after transplantation [39].

Interest in autologous fat transfer diminished until the advent of liposuction surgery in the 1980s which provided plastic surgeons with semiliquid fat which could be grafted with relative ease. In the 1980s, Illouz and Fournier [40, 41] developed an approach to fat transfer by syringe harvesting called 'microlipoinjection'. Initial experimentation with this new technique yielded variable results. In the early 1990s, Ersek reported disappointing results, with fat loss ranging from 20% to 90%, which generated a widespread negative perception of the technique [42]. Since the mid-1990s, Coleman has confirmed the efficacy and permanence of grafted fat, but stresses that this is dependent on the harvesting and grafting technique adopted [43]. Indeed, ongoing variability in results has been reported depending on choice of technique, the area treated, patient factors and surgical experience. In recent years, many different techniques have evolved and a standard procedure that is adopted by all practitioners has not yet been developed.

63.9 Autologous Fat Transfer

63.9.1 History of Autologous Fat Transfer

Autologous transplantation of adipose tissue is a practice that has gained increasing popularity over the past two decades. However, the concept of fat transfer is not new. The earliest recorded human free fat transfer was by Neuber in 1893, who reported using upper extremity fat to recontour soft-tissue facial defects,

63.10 Theories of Fat Graft Survival

There have been two major theories proposed for the survival of fat grafts. The 'host cell replacement theory' was based on the work of Neuhof and Hirshfeld in 1923. It postulated that transplanted fat undergoes complete cell death and that histiocytes would scavenge lipid material and eventually replace all the host tissue [44]. The more popular theory in recent years is the cell survival theory, which states that some of the graft adipose tissue survives after the host reaction subsides and is based on the work of Peer [45].

The graft of adipose tissue goes through an initial period of ischemia and obtains nutrition through plasmatic imbibition [46]. Circulation is restored to the grafted fat cells in a manner similar to the revascularisation of a skin graft. In the first 4 days, host cells, such as polymorphonuclear leukocytes (PMNs), plasma cells, lymphocytes and eosinophils, infiltrate the graft. On or about the fourth day, neovascularisation is evident. Histiocytes act only to remove fat from disrupted cells.

More recently, the role of adipose-derived stem cells and pre-adipocytes in transplanted fat has been investigated. These cells appear to be more resistant to trauma than mature adipocytes due to lower oxygen consumption requirements. Some researchers have proposed that survival of adipose-derived stem cells in the stromal cell fraction of transplanted fat is a major factor and may account for the variability in survival of fat grafts between individuals [43].

63.11 Histological Evaluation of Transplanted Fat

Multiple animal models have been proposed to study the technique of autologous fat transfer. Recent histologic evaluation of transplanted fat grafts to the lips of rabbits has demonstrated an early inflammatory response to the injected fat followed by sequestration of nonviable tissue. The transplanted fat remained viable at 1 year, with good overall survivability and minimal fibrosis [47]. However, there are few studies to evaluate the histologic fate of reinjected fat in humans. Niechajev et al. obtained biopsies of transplanted fat to the cheeks of 9 patients with subcutaneous fat atrophy, 7–36 months after transplantation. Histologic analysis showed an organised lobular structure of transplanted fat at 7 months with more pronounced fibrosis between lobules in the specimens obtained at 36 months [48].

Carpaneda studied collagen alterations in adipose tissue transplanted to abdominal subcutaneous fat prior to abdominoplasty [49]. He found a type 1 collagen capsule around the grafted fat and several alterations to type 1 and type 3 collagen synthesis, degradation and remodelling. A shift in the inflammatory process from the peripheral viable region to the central unviable region was also demonstrated, where pseudocysts were present. Chajchir et al. [50] performed biopsies on the sites of grafted fat at intervals. Three months after transfer, zones of cystosteatonecrosis, lipophagic granulomas, lymphocytes, adipocytes, giant multinucleated cells and new vessels were found. At 6–8 months, the specimens were infiltrated heavily by PMNs in a fibrotic matrix, and, at 1 year, a large amount of connective tissue and fibrotic reaction was present. Some fat was still present, but the authors felt that the inflammatory reaction may contribute more to the long-term result. There is some disagreement about the role of fibrosis. Some authors believe that fibroblasts cause contraction, while others believe that they can provide augmentation. A fibrous host reaction may be all that occurs in some patients although it may be argued that it ultimately fulfilled the role of soft-tissue augmentation.

63.12 Technique

63.12.1 Assessment of Patients with HIV-Associated Lipodystrophy

Autologous fat transfer for the treatment of HIV-associated lipodystrophy may be performed under local or general anaesthesia depending on patient preference and anaesthetic risk. Assessment of anaesthetic risk in HIV-infected patients requires knowledge of the potential effects of HIV infection on each organ system combined with a full history, examination and appropriate investigations.

To ensure optimal safety for both the patient and the operating team, it is recommended that the HIV-1 RNA viral load should be maximally suppressed at the time of surgery (HIV-1 RNA < 50 copies/ml) [51]. Recommendations on preoperative CD4 count are lacking, although a CD4 count less than 200 cells/µl is considered suboptimal for elective procedures by some surgeons.

Surgical assessment of patients with HIV facial lipoatrophy involves quantification of the severity of facial wasting, and generalised clinical examination to identify other morphological features of HIV lipodystrophy and potential donor sites for fat harvest.

A classification of facial lipoatrophy has been proposed by James et al. to assist in treatment decisions [29]. Grade 1 is mild and localised, and the appearance is almost normal. Grade 2 has longer and deeper central cheek atrophy, with the facial muscles (especially zygomaticus major) beginning to show through. In grade 3, the atrophic area is even deeper and wider with the muscles clearly showing and in grade 4 atrophy covers a wide area and extends up towards the orbit (Fig. 63.4).

63.13 Surgical Technique

A greater understanding of how to maintain viable fat has led to modifications in technique that are believed to improve clinical results. These modifications are

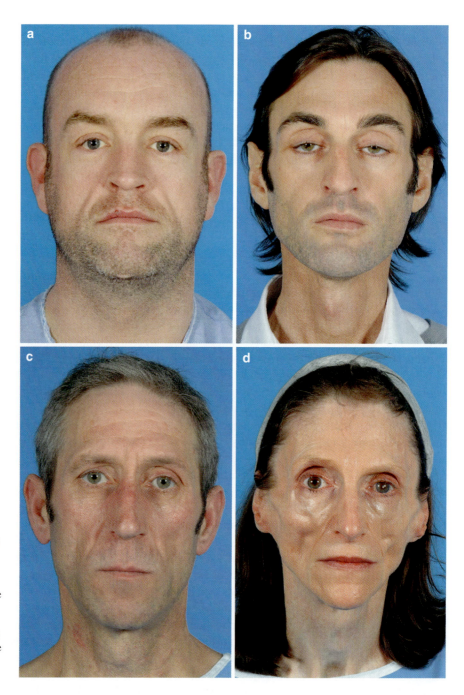

Fig. 63.4 (**a**) Grade 1 with mild and localised fat that appears almost normal. (**b**) Grade 2 with longer and deeper central cheek atrophy and with the facial muscles (especially zygomaticus major) beginning to show through. (**c**) Grade 3 with the atrophic area even deeper and wider with the muscles clearly showing. (**d**) Grade 4 with atrophy covering a wide area and extending up towards the orbit

intended to preserve the delicate structure of adipocytes and provide a robust blood supply on which fat cells are extremely dependant. However, there is little objective scientific evidence and studies are difficult to compare as authors use different harvesting techniques, reinjection techniques and means of evaluating the outcome.

63.13.1 Anaesthesia of the Donor Site

The use of local anaesthesia at the harvest site has been debated. While some practitioners argue that vasoconstriction by local application of epinephrine may have a detrimental effect on the graft, others believe that reduced bleeding helps to maintain viability [52]. Some studies have also shown that lidocaine may potentially inhibit adipocyte metabolism in culture, but this effect persists only as long as the lidocaine is present and has not been demonstrated in vivo [53].

According to a recent survey of American plastic surgeons, the majority of practitioners use a wetting solution, with a mixture of lidocaine and epinephrine (e.g. 50 ml 1% lidocaine plus 1 ml of epinephrine 1:1,000 plus 1 l of normal saline) [54].

63.13.2 Choice of Donor Site

The most common sites for fat harvest include the abdomen (Fig. 63.5), thigh, flank, gluteal region and knee. In patients with HIV-associated lipodystrophy, sites of lipohypertrophy such as the dorso-cervical fat pad may also be utilised for fat harvest. When assessing central adiposity, it is important to evaluate whether the fat accumulation lies within the subcutaneous tissue or peritoneum. Abdominal computed tomography scans have shown that the increase in girth in patients with HIV lipodystrophy is largely due to fat accumulation in the perivisceral region, which is less accessible for harvesting of fat grafts.

Some authors have suggested that adipocytes from the gluteal–femoral region are larger and have greater lipogenic activity, making them the ideal choice for donor fat [55]. However, other studies have shown no difference between choice of donor site following assessment of histological parameters [56] or adipocyte

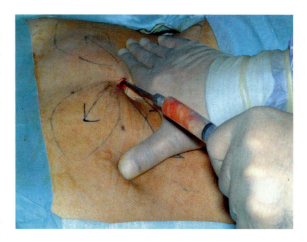

Fig. 63.5 The most common sites for fat harvest includes the abdomen

viability using cell proliferation techniques [57]. Thus, the donor site may be chosen based on surgeon or patient preference. The solutions are infiltrated in a ratio of roughly 1 cc of solution per cubic centimetre of fat to be harvested.

63.13.3 Harvesting Method

Common harvesting techniques used for fat isolation include syringe aspiration and lipoaspiration. It has been hypothesised that liposuction may be more detrimental to the fat fells than syringe aspiration. However, laboratory studies comparing the techniques have reported contradictory results. Various studies have shown no difference in fat cell viability, as assessed by cell proliferation, graft weight maintenance, or histological evaluations [58, 59]. Some investigators argue that adipose aspirates from conventional liposuction have suboptimal levels of cellular function despite maintenance of normal structure and numbers of viable fat cells, and therefore may not survive well after transplantation [59, 60].

The negative pressure applied using either technique appears to determine the extent of cell damage. A number of authors recommend using half the normal suction pressure to avoid mechanical injury to adipocytes during aspiration [48]. Nguyen et al. showed 90% adipocyte injury at −760 mmHg on histological sections compared to 5% injury after gentle syringe aspiration [61]. It is estimated that the pressure when a syringe plunger is pulled is 40% of liposuction pressures. However, it has been demonstrated that negative pressures can reach 100% of liposuction pressures when a 10-cc syringe plunger is pulled maximally [58].

The Coleman technique is now the most popular method of autologous fat transfer. It was first described in 1994 using a syringe, cannula and centrifuge and later refined with the use of Coleman instruments [62]. For harvesting fat, Coleman recommends a 3 mm diameter, 2-hole Coleman harvesting cannula attached to a 10-ml Luer-Lok syringe. Via a small stab incision, the blunt cannula is advanced and retracted through the harvest site using digital manipulation of the plunger to create gentle negative pressure. Parcels of fat are delivered to the cannula and once full, the syringe and plunger are disconnected and a plug is attached before placement in the centrifuge.

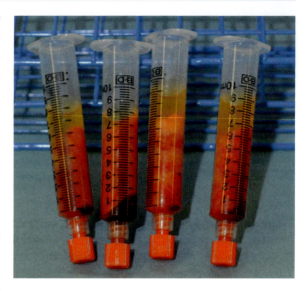

Fig. 63.6 Centrifuging syringes of fat at 3,000 rpm for 3 min separates the harvested material into three layers

63.14 Method of Refinement

There are various methods of fat refinement advocated to improve the long-term take of fat grafts. These include centrifugation, washing, rolling and treatment with other substances ranging from growth factors to growth medium [63, 64].

Washing liposuction aspirate with saline, Ringer's lactate or sterile water is felt by some authors to obtain the highest proportion of viable cells [65]. However, Coleman argues that washing of harvested tissue may disrupt the fragile fatty tissue architecture and also remove fibrin, thus hampering anchorage of fat to the surrounding tissues [66].

Centrifugation, popularised by the Coleman technique remains the most widely practised method of fat purification. The rationale for centrifugation is to remove excess blood, oil and local infiltration fluid. Thus a purified, predictable volume of fat may be re-injected. Prevention of inflammatory reaction to debris by centrifugation or washing is also an intuitive argument. Studies to evaluate adipocyte viability between centrifuged and non-centrifuged fat samples are also conflicting. One study investigating cell proliferation has shown no difference between groups although the authors acknowledge that evaluation of long-term cell viability requires an in vivo animal model [57]. Further scientific studies are required to determine the best method of cell isolation whether by centrifugation or other means.

The Coleman protocol for centrifugation involves centrifuging syringes of fat at 3,000 rpm for 3 min, which separates the harvested material into 3 layers (Fig. 63.6). The upper layer is composed of oil from ruptured adipocytes and should be decanted. Absorbent material can be used to wick off any remaining oil. The bottom layer is composed of blood, water and local anaesthesia, and is allowed to drain by gravity after the plug is removed. The middle layer is composed of refined fat, which is transferred to 1 ml Luer-Lok syringes for infiltration. During the transfer process, most authors favour a closed technique. Advantages include maintenance of sterility and avoidance of exposure to air, which may lead to desiccation of adipocytes.

63.15 Placement

Infiltration cannulas devised by Coleman are commonly used for placement of fat grafts. For the treatment of facial lipoatrophy, a blunt 17-gauge cannula is recommended. The cannula is inserted to the recipient tissues via 2 mm incisions and fat is injected on withdrawal of

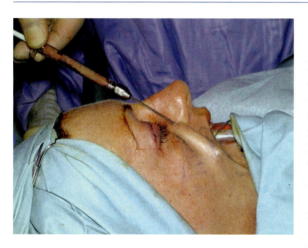

Fig. 63.7 Fat is injected on withdrawal of the cannula in multiple planes

the cannula in multiple planes (Fig. 63.7). In the face, the maximum amount of fat deposited with each withdrawal should be 1/10th ml. Placement of small parcels of fat is recommended to maximise the surface area of contact between the harvested fat and recipient site. Studies have shown that only 40% of grafted fat tissue is viable 1 mm from the edge of the graft at 60 days [66]. Therefore, decreasing the diameter of the grafted fat parcels ensures adequate blood supply to central adipocytes for nutrition and respiration. Ideally, the threads of fat should not exceed 3 mm diameter. An additional benefit of maximising the surface area of grafted fat is increased stability and fat anchorage via host fibrin [66].

Although some authors believe that injection of fat graft into muscle is associated with increased viability due to improved vascularity, clinical evidence shows good survival in scarred tissue despite reduced vascularity in these conditions [67].

Because of the tendency for fat resorption, many surgeons believe it is necessary to overcorrect the soft-tissue defect. For surgeons who follow this practise, the amount of overcorrection thought to be required varies between 10% and 50% [54].

63.16 Post-operative Care

To minimise oedema some authors suggest the use of elevation, cold therapy and external pressure with elastic tape. Compression to the grafted area should be avoided to prevent migration of fat.

63.17 Complications

Fat grafting is considered to be a relatively safe procedure with few serious complications. The most common complications are aesthetic. Undercorrection may result from insufficient volume correction intra-operatively or resorption of grafted fat over time. Overcorrection can lead to several problems and is generally more difficult to resolve than undercorrection. Placement of excess adipose tissue in a particular area can lead to graft necrosis through failure of revascularisation. Fat migration may also be related to overcorrection of an area as pressure and insufficient blood supply force the graft into an undesirable site.

Contour irregularities may develop as a consequence of graft necrosis, surgical technique or migration of grafted fat. Clumping can be corrected to some extent by scar massage.

Fat graft hypertrophy has been documented by several authors [68, 69], and is a problem particularly noted in patients with HIV-associated lipodystrophy.

Damage to underlying structures such as nerves, muscles, glands and blood vessels is rare although can result from this technique. In particular, intra-arterial injection is a potentially devastating complication. Reports of unilateral blindness following treatment of glabellar frown lines have been documented as a result of intra-vascular emboli [48]. The use of a blunt cannula is recommended to avoid these complications. Donor site contour irregularities can result from overly aggressive harvesting in a small area. Another problem relating to patients with HIV lipodystrophy is insufficient subcutaneous fat reserves in some patients secondary to generalised lipoatrophy. In patients with HIV lipodystrophy, fat is often harvested from areas of dystrophic fat (e.g. the dorso-cervical fat pad) which is extremely fibrous and often requires multiple aspirations.

Variable degrees of oedema can result from the procedure depending on the amount and location of grafted fat. Oedema is usually evident for 2 weeks after the procedure; however, it be prolonged and troubling to the patient. Bleeding complications and bruising may also occur but are usually associated with the use of sharp needles for fat graft placement. Although rare, infections can occur wherever the skin envelope is violated. The most common source of infection is the oral mucosa.

63.18 Discussion

The degree of resorption of autologous fat grafts remains a topic of debate and is mainly based on subjective observation of surgically treated areas over time. Indeed, studies are difficult to compare due to the wide variability in technique, experience of the surgeon and means of evaluating outcome. Compared to other non-permanent fillers, the longevity of autologous fat is not as easily predictable. For patients with HIV lipodsytrophy, the unpredictable nature of the technique is even more apparent due to the underlying systemic lipodystrophic process. Quantification of surgical outcome in HIV-infected patients undergoing autologous fat transfer for facial lipoatrophy is lacking, and studies are limited by small numbers, subjective assessment and lack of long-term data.

In one study, 38 patients received autologous fat injections using the Coleman technique for HIV facial lipoatrophy [31]. The cosmetic result was evaluated at 6 months, after which 12 patients required a new injection of fat to improve symmetry and resorption. At 1 year, the cosmetic result was rated as good to excellent by the patient, the clinic nurse and the surgeon. Less resorption was reported in cases where the fat was not centrifuged and the authors suggest that this may be due to decreased trauma to the fat. In another study, the outcome of the Coleman technique was evaluated in 33 HIV-infected patients by clinical examination, biochemical data, patient satisfaction and standardised photographs at baseline and 1 year following lipostructure [70]. Improvement was found in 12 patients by 3 independent evaluators at 12 months and 93% of patients were satisfied with the results. The authors also report that quantity of fat injected and low serum triglyceride level before surgery were significantly associated with improvement of facial lipoatrophy.

Similar outcome measures were evaluated in two further studies to demonstrate the efficacy of lipostructure in HIV-infected patients using the Coleman technique for facial lipoatrophy. Levan et al. reported 93% patient satisfaction and 'acceptable', 'good' or 'very good' results in 13 out of 14 patients evaluated by a 5-member jury 6 months following the procedure [71]. Caye et al. evaluated 29 HIV-infected patients treated using the Coleman technique and reports durability of fat grafts at 6 months based on serial photography [72]. The results were deemed good in 72.4%, acceptable in 13.8% and poor in 13.8%. Davison et al. have utilised lipoaspirate in patients undergoing suction-assisted liposuction for buffalo hump deformities to correct associated facial wasting [73]. In these cases, the fat grafts were not centrifuged to avoid aerosolisation of the virus. The authors report graft take of approximately 40–50% based on subjective assessment, and postulate that fat harvested from dystrophic sites possesses different biochemical properties from non-hypertrophic fat and may lead to more sustained results in these patients.

However, Talmor et al. feel that the quality of fat rendered from dystrophic sites makes it unsuitable for transfer due to its extremely fibrous nature [8]. Also, the potential for fat graft hypertrophy when utilised from dystrophic sites should be considered. Since HIV lipodystrophy is a systemic, metabolic disease, the effect of transferring dystrophic fat can be unpredictable. In one study of 41 patients who received autologous fat injections for HIV-associated lipoatrophy, 4 patients developed disfiguring facial lipohypertrophy at the injection site [74]. The fat source was the dorso-cervical fat pad in three of these patients. The pathogenic mechanism for this is unknown. The authors hypothesise that the mechanism may be related to adipocyte receptors and mitochondrial toxicity: receptor expression could be transferred from the harvest site and remain sensitive to lipohypertrophy determinants. Another hypothesis is that lipohypertrophy of the cheeks may be the result of expansion of brown fat that is transferred with the intervention. Histological examination of hypertrophied fat graft to the nasogenian area was carried out following surgical resection in one patient. Fibroadipose tissue and dystrophic adipocytes of various sizes were demonstrated. The authors postulate that a non-adaptive response could be partly related to dysfunction of adipocyte receptor expression and a mutated DNA toxicity-related mechanism.

The perceived success of autologous fat transfer depends on whether one considers long-term resorption disappointing or potentially superior to the anticipated longevity of other non-permanent fillers. Multiple treatments with autologous fat transfer may be required in patients with severe facial lipoatrophy to achieve volume augmentation (Fig. 63.8). Paucity of subcutaneous donor fat is another limitation of the technique in patients with generalised lipoatrophy and synthetic injectable fillers may be an alternative treatment option. The use of various facial fillers has been reported in the treatment of HIV facial lipoatrophy. Eviatar et al. have evaluated the safety and efficacy of calcium hydroxyapatite (Radiesse®) in 100 patients

Fig. 63.8 Multiple treatments with autologous fat transfer may be required in patients with severe facial lipoatrophy to achieve volume augmentation. (**a**) Pre-operative. (**b**) Post-operative 4 months following first fat transfer. (**c**) Ten months following second fat transfer

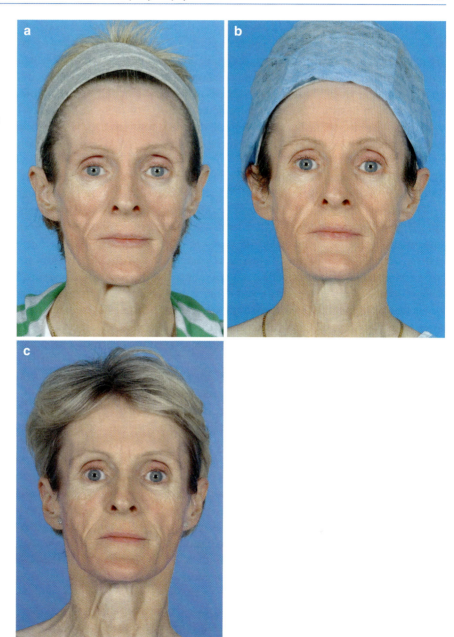

with HIV-associated facial lipoatrophy [75]. Eighty-five percent of patients received touch-up injections at 1 month following initial treatment. The study demonstrated that all patients had improved aesthetic outcomes at 6 months as scored on a facial global aesthetic improvement rating scale. The use of hyaluronic acid has been evaluated for soft-tissue augmentation of HIV-associated facial lipodystrophy in five patients [76]. Each patient received approximately 5–6 ml in total of hyaluronic acid in the malar area via intradermal injection. The technique was found to provide a good cosmetic result for at least 6 months, with high patient satisfaction and no adverse events. Another study of seven patients with HIV-associated facial lipodystrophy treated with hyaluronic acid revealed high patient satisfaction with regard to cosmetic improvement, and no side effects of treatment [77].

The VEGA study evaluated the safety and efficacy of Poly-L-lactic acid injections (New-fill) in 50 patients with HIV-associated lipoatrophy by means of an open-label, single-arm, pilot study [78]. The authors report a significant increase in dermal thickness from baseline, as assessed by facial ultrasound, for a duration of 96 weeks post treatment. There were no serious adverse events although in 44% of patients, palpable but non-visible subcutaneous nodules developed. Similar results were found by Moyle et al. who report a mean increase in dermal thickness of 4–5 mm within 12 weeks of treatment with effects persisting at least 18 weeks beyond the last injection [79].

There have been reports on the use of liquid injectable silicone in patients with HIV-associated facial lipoatrophy including a case report of 1 patient [80] and larger study of 77 patients [81]. Facial contours were restored and significant patient satisfaction was achieved with no adverse events noted. Both papers conclude that silicone oil is a safe and effective treatment for HIV-associated facial lipoatrophy. However, longer-term safety and efficacy in HIV patients remains unproven.

Several studies have reported stability, tolerance and safety of Bio-Alcamid® with permanent, satisfactory improvement in appearance for patients with lipodystrophy [82–84]. In one study, 90% of the 73 patients required a second injection of Bio-Alcamid® (4 weeks after the first injection) to improve implant appearance [84]. The aesthetic results were deemed excellent by both physicians and patients at follow-up of 3 years. However, the long-term results of Bio-Alcamid® are uncertain and complications such as infection, capsular contraction and migration have been reported, necessitating removal of the product [85].

Thus, the less predicable long-term volume augmentation achievable with autologous fat must be balanced against the risks of allergic responses and other complications relating to synthetic injectable fillers. The simplicity and safety of autologous fat transfer also makes it an attractive option compared to other surgical options for HIV facial lipoatrophy including the use of dermis-fat grafts, flaps and implants.

Peer advocated the use of free fat grafts with overlying dermis for patients with soft-tissue defects in 1956. The results of dermis-fat graft transfer to the malar area in patients with HIV-associated lipodystrophy have been variable. Strauch et al. evaluated this technique in five patients (four female and one male) with HIV-associated facial lipodystrophy [86]. Dermis-fat grafts were transferred from the abdominal wall to malar pockets through a trans-oral approach. Patients were overcorrected to twice the expected final volume and they reached final volume (50% of initial augmentation) in 3–5 months. The aesthetic results were maintained during the follow-up period of 14–30 months. However, others reporting on the use of a dermis-fat graft to treat HIV-associated lipodystrophy have been sceptical about the technique as a consequence of patient dissatisfaction and surgical complications [87]. The donor site scars may also be unacceptable. Breast tissue from gynaecomastia resection has also been reported in HIV patients and has minimal donor site scar although the small risk of potential carcinomatous change is a drawback.

With the advent of microvascular surgery and free flap transfer, numerous flaps have been used to treat patients with lipodystrophy including a double paddle dermis-fat forearm free flap [88], adipofascial free radial forearm flap [89] and a temporalis muscle rotation flap [90]. However, potential disadvantages with free tissue transfer include multiple procedures, lengthy operation, flap failure, hematoma and donor site defects [89, 91].

The use of submalar silicone implants has been evaluated in patients with HIV-associated lipodystrophy. In one study, three patients with facial lipoatrophy underwent reconstruction with submalar silicone implants via an intra-oral approach [8]. No infection or extrusion was encountered, although one patient required implant repositioning on one side. At 15 months follow-up, both patients and surgeons were satisfied with the results. However, the decreased immunity inherent to the HIV-positive surgical patient and the risk of peri-implant infection represents a significant concern. Indeed, reports of infection and erosion of the implant through the anterior maxilla have been published [92, 93].

63.19 Conclusions

The treatment of HIV-associated lipodystrophy remains a challenging problem for physicians. The wide choice of treatment options and problems inherent to HIV-infected individuals can make management decisions difficult. In general, autologous fat transfer is an effective treatment due to the biocompatibility, safety and satisfactory aesthetic results of this technique. However, paucity of donor and unpredictable resorption rates are the main drawbacks in the treatment of patients with HIV-associated lipodystrophy, and the use of synthetic fillers or alternative surgical techniques may be considered. Further studies using objective measures are required to quantify the long-term outcome of autologous fat grafting, particularly in patients with HIV-associated lipodystrophy, who may respond differently from non-lipodystrophic patients.

References

1. Carr A, Samaras K, Burton S, Law M, Freund J, Chisholm DJ, et al. A syndrome of peripheral dystrophy, hyperlipidaemia, and insulin resistance in patients receiving HIV protease inhibitors. AIDS. 1998;12(7):F51–8.
2. Miller J, Carr A, Emery S, Law M, Mallal S, Baker D, et al. HIV lipodystrophy: prevalence severity and correlates of risk in Australia. HIV Med. 2003;4(3):293–301.
3. Sanchez Torres AM, Munoz Muniz R, Madero R, Borque C, Garcia-Miguel MJ, De Jose Gomez MI. Prevalence of fat redistribution and metabolic disorders in human immunodeficiency virus-infected children. Eur J Paediatr. 2005;164(5):271–6.
4. Puttawong S, Prasithsirikul W, Vadcharavivad S. Prevalence of lipodystrophy in Thai-HIV infected patients. J Med Assoc Thai. 2004;87(6):605–11.
5. Sattler F. Body habitus changes relating to lipodystrophy. Clin Infect Dis. 2003;36 Suppl 2:S84–90.
6. Carr A, Emery S, Law M, Puls R, Lundgren JD, et al. An objective case definition of lipodystrophy in HIV-infected adults: a case-control study. Lancet. 2003;361(9359):726–35.
7. Chen D, Misra A, Garg A. Lipodystrophy in human immunodeficiency virus-infected patients. J Clin Endocrinol Metab. 2002;87(11):4845–56.
8. Talmor M, Hoffman L, LaTrenta GS. Facial atrophy in HIV-related fat redistribution syndrome: anatomic evaluation and surgical reconstruction. Ann Plast Surg. 2002;49(1):11–8.
9. Carr A, Cooper DA. Adverse effects of antiretroviral therapy. Lancet. 2000;356(9239):1423–30.
10. Piliero PJ, Hubbard M, King J, Faragon JJ. Use of ultrasonography-assisted liposuction for the treatment of human immunodeficiency virus-associated enlargement of the dorsocervical fat pad. Clin Infect Dis. 2003;37(10):1374–7.
11. Paech V, Lorenzen T, von Krosigk A, Graefe K, Stoehr A, Plettenberg A. Gynaecomastia in HIV-infected men: association with effects of antiretroviral therapy. AIDS. 2002;16(8):1193–5.
12. Qazi NA, Morlese JF, King DM, Ahmad RS, Gazzard BG, Nelson MR. Gynaecomastia without lipodystrophy in HIV-1-seropositive patients on efavirenz: an alternative hypothesis. AIDS. 2002;16(3):506–7.
13. Behrens GM, Schmidt RE. The lipodystrophy syndrome. In: Hoffmann C, Rockstroh J, Kamps BS, editors. HIV medicine 2003. www.HIVMedicine.com; 2003. pp. 263–283.
14. Ras F, Habets LL, van Ginkel FC, Prahl-Anderson B. Quantification of facial morphology using stereophotography – a demonstration of a new concept. J Dent. 1996;24(5):369–74.
15. Bourne CO, Kerr WJ, Ayoub AF. Development of a three-dimensional imaging system for analysis of facial change. Clin Orthod Res. 2001;4(2):105–11.
16. Hajeer MY, Ayoub AF, Millet DT, Bock M, Siebert JP. Three-dimensional imaging in orthognathic surgery: the clinical application of a new method. Int J Orthod Orthognath Surg. 2002;17(4):1–5.
17. Benn P, Ruff C, Cartledge J, Sauret V, Copas A, Linney A, et al. Overcoming subjectivity in assessing facial lipoatrophy: is there a role for three dimensional laser scans? HIV Med. 2003;4(4):325–31.
18. Sekhar RV, Jahoor F, White AC, Pownall HJ, Visnegarwala F, et al. Metabolic basis of HIV-lipodystrophy. Am J Physiol Endocrinol Metab. 2002;283(2):332–7.
19. van der Valk M, Casula M, Weverlingz GJ, van Kuijik K, van Eck-Smit B, et al. Prevalence of lipoatrophy and mitochondrial DNA content of blood and subcutaneous fat in HIV-1-infected patients randomly allocated to zidovudine- or stavudine-based therapy. Antivir Ther. 2004;9(3):385–93.
20. Carr A, Samaras K, Thorisdottir A, Kaufman GR, Chisholm DJ, Cooper DA. Diagnosis, prediction, and natural course of HIV-protease-inhibitor-associated lipodystrophy, hyperlipidaemia, and diabetes mellitus: a cohort study. Lancet. 1999;353(9170):2093–9.
21. Tershakovee AM, Frank I, Rader D. HIV-related lipodystrophy and related factors. Atherosclerosis. 2004;174(1):1–10.
22. Carr A. Pathogenesis of HIV-1-protease inhibitor-associated peripheral lipodystrophy, hyperlipidaemia, and insulin resistance. Lancet. 1998;351(9119):1881–3.
23. Shevitz A, Wanke CA, Falutz J, Kotler DP. Clinical perspectives on HIV-associated lipodystrophy syndrome: an update. AIDS. 2001;15(15):1917–30.
24. McComsey GA, Walker UA. Role of mitochondria in HIV lipoatrophy: insight into pathogenesis and potential therapies. Mitochondrion. 2004;4(2–3):111–8.
25. Pettit R, Kotler D, Falutz J, et al. Abnormalities in HIV-associated lipodystrophy syndrome that vary by weight status. [Abstract 63]. 1st International workshop on adverse drug reactions and lipodystrophy in HIV, San Diego, 1999, p. 53.
26. Mercie P, Tchamgoue S, Dabis F. Lipodystrophy in HIV-1-infected patients. Lancet. 1999;354(9181):867–8.
27. Hadigan C, Miller K, Corcoran C, Anderson E, Basgoz N, Grinspoon S. Fasting hyperinsulinaemia and changes in regional body composition in HIV-infected women. J Clin Endocrinol Metab. 1999;84(6):1932–7.
28. Jan V, Cervera P, Maachi M, Baudrimont M, Kim M, et al. Altered fat differentiation and adipocytokine expression are inter-related and linked to morphological changes and insulin resistance in HIV-1-infected lipodystrophic patients. Antivir Ther. 2004;9(4):555–64.
29. James J, Carruthers A, Carruthers J. HIV-associated facial lipoatrophy. Dermatol Surg. 2002;28(11):979–86.
30. Milinkovic A, Martinez E. Current perspectives on HIV-associated lipodystrophy syndrome. J Antimicrobial Chemother. 2005;56(1):6–9.

31. Serra-Renom JM, Fontdevila J. Treatment of facial fat atrophy related to treatment with protease inhibitors by autologous fat injection in patients with Human Immunodeficiency Virus infection. Plast Reconstr Surg. 2004;114(2):551–5.
32. Neuber G. Fettransplantation. Verh Dtsch Ges Chir. 1893;22:66.
33. Czerny A. Plastischer Ersatzder Brustdruse durch ein Lipoma. Chir Kongr Verhandl. 1895;216:2.
34. Lexer E. Freie fettgewebstransplantation. Dtsch Med Wochenschr. 1910;36:46.
35. Rehn E. Die fetttransplantation. Arch Klin Chir. 1912;98:1.
36. Bruning P. Contribution a l'etude des greffes adipeuses. Bull Acad R Méd Belg. 1919;28:263.
37. Joseph M. Handbuch der kosmetik. Leipzig: Veit & Co; 1912. p. 690–1.
38. Miller C. Cannula implants and review of implantation techniques in esthetic surgery. Chicago: The Oak Press; 1926.
39. Peer LA. Loss of weight and volume in human fat grafts. Plast Reconstr Surg. 1950;5:217.
40. Illouz YG. The fat cell "graft". A new technique to fill depressions. Plast Reconstr Surg. 1986;78(1):122–3.
41. Fournier PF. Microlipoextraction et microlipoinjection. Rev Chir Esthet Lang Franc. 1985;10:36–40.
42. Ersek RA. Transplantation of purified autologous fat: a 3-year follow-up is disappointing. Plast Reconstr Surg. 1991;87(2):219–27.
43. Coleman SR. Structural fat grafting: more than a permanent filler. Plast Reconstr Surg. 2006;118 Suppl 3:108S–20.
44. Neuhof H, Hirshfeld S. The transplantation of tissues. New York: D. Appleton; 1923.
45. Peer LA. Cell survival theory versus replacement theory. Plast Reconstr Surg. 1955;16(3):161–8.
46. Billings Jr E, May Jr JW. Historical review and present status of free fat graft autotransplantation in plastic and reconstructive surgery. Plast Reconstr Surg. 1998;83(2):368–81.
47. Brucker M, Sati S, Spangenberger A, Weinzweig J. Long-term fate of transplanted autologous fat in a novel rabbit facial model. Plast Reconstr Surg. 2008;122(3):749–54.
48. Niechajev I, Sevcuk O. Long-term results of fat transplantation: clinical and histologic studies. Plast Reconstr Surg. 1994;94(3):496–506.
49. Carpaneda CA. Collagen alterations in adipose autografts. Aesthetic Plast Surg. 1994;18(1):11–5.
50. Chajchir J, Benzaquen I, Wexler E, Arellano A. Fat injection. Aesthetic Plast Surg. 1990;14(2):127–36.
51. Quinn TC, Wawer MJ, Sewankambo N, Serwadda D, Li C, et al. Viral load and heterosexual transmission of human immunodeficiency virus type 1. N Engl J Med. 2000;342(13):921–9.
52. Sommer B, Sattler G. Current concepts of fat graft survival: histology of aspirated adipose tissue and review of the literature. Dermatol Surg. 2000;26(12):1159–66.
53. Moore Jr JH, Kolaczynski JW, Morales LM, Considine RV, Pietrzkowski Z, Noto PF, et al. Viability of fat obtained by syringe suction lipectomy: effects of local anaesthesia with lidocaine. Aesthetic Plast Surg. 1995;19(4):335–9.
54. Kaufman MR, Bradley JP, Dickinson B. Autologous fat transfer national consensus survey: trends in techniques for harvest, preparation, and application, and perception of short- and long-term results. Plast Reconstr Surg. 2007;119(1):323–31.
55. Hudson D, Lambert EV, Bloch CE. Site selection for autotransplantation: some observations. Aesthetic Plast Surg. 1990;14(3):195–7.
56. Ullmann Y, Shoshani O, Fodor A. Searching for the favorable donor site for fat injection: in vivo study using the nude mice model. Dermatol Surg. 2005;31(10):1304–7.
57. Rohrich R, Sorokin E, Brown S. In search of improved fat transfer viability: a quantitative analysis of the role of centrifugation and harvest site. Plast Reconstr Surg. 2004;113(1):391–5.
58. Smith P, Adams W, Lipschitz A, Chau B, Sorokin E, Rohrich RJ, et al. Autologous human fat grafting: effect of harvesting and preparation on adipocyte graft survival. Plast Reconstr Surg. 2006;117(6):1836–44.
59. Pu LL, Coleman SR, Cui X, Ferguson RE, Vasconez HC. Autologous fat grafts harvested and refined by the Coleman technique: a comparative study. Plast Reconstr Surg. 2008;122(3):932–7.
60. Pu LL, Cui X, Fink BF, Cibull ML, Gao D. The viability of fatty tissues within adipose aspirates after conventional liposuction: a comprehensive study. Ann Plast Surg. 2005;54(3):288–92.
61. Nguyen A, Pasyk KA, Bouvier TN, Hassett CA, Argenta LC. Comparative study of survival of autologous adipose tissue taken and transplanted by different techniques. Plast Reconstr Surg. 1990;85(3):378–86.
62. Coleman SR. Facial recontouring with lipostructure. Clin Plast Surg. 1997;24(2):347–67.
63. Yuksel E, Weinfeld AB, Cleek R, Wamsley S, Jensen J, et al. Increased free fat-graft survival with the long-term, local delivery of insulin, insulin-like growth factor-1, and basic fibroblast growth factor by PLGA/PEG microspheres. Plast Reconstr Surg. 2000;105(5):1712–20.
64. Eppley BL, Sidner RA, Platis JM, Sadove AM. Bioactivation of free-fat transfers: a potential new approach to improving graft survival. Plast Reconstr Surg. 1992;90(6):1022–30.
65. Rubin A, Hoefflin S. Fat purification: survival of the fittest. Plast Reconstr Surg. 2002;109(4):1463–4.
66. Coleman SR. Hand rejuvenation with structural fat grafting. Plast Reconstr Surg. 2002;110(7):1731–44.
67. Rigotti G, Marchi A, Galie M, Baroni G, Benati D, Krampera M, et al. Clinical treatment of radiotherapy tissue damages by lipoaspirates transplant: a healing process mediated by adipose derived stem cells. Plast Reconstr Surg. 2007;19(5):1409–22.
68. Miller JJ. Fat hypertrophy after autologous fat transfer. Ophthal Plast Reconstr Surg. 2002;18(3):228–31.
69. Latoni JD, Marshall DM, Wolfe S. Overgrowth of fat autotransplanted for correction of localized steroid-induced atrophy. Plast Reconstr Surg. 2000;106(7):1566–9.
70. Burnouf M, Buffet M, Schwarzinger M, Roman P, Bui P, et al. Evaluation of Coleman lipostructure for the treatment of facial lipoatrophy in patients with human immunodeficiency virus and parameters associated with the efficiency of this technique. Arch Dermatol. 2005;141(10):1220–4.
71. Levan P, Nguyen T, Lallemand F, Mazetier L, Mimoun M, Rozenbaum W, et al. Correction of facial lipoatrophy in HIV-infected patients on highly active antiretroviral therapy by injection of autologous fatty tissue. AIDS. 2002;16(14):1985–7.

72. Caye N, Le Fourn B, Pannier M. Surgical treatment of facial lipoatrophy. Ann Chir Plast Esthét. 2003;48(1):2–12.
73. Davidson SP, Timpone Jr J. Hannan CM: surgical algorithm for the management of HIV lipodsytrophy. Plast Reconstr Surg. 2007;120(7):1843–58.
74. Guaraldi G, De Fazio D, Orlando G, Murri R, Wu A, Guaraldi P, et al. Facial lipohypertrophy in HIV-infected subjects who underwent autologous fat tissue transplantation. Clin Infect Dis. 2005;40(2):e13–5.
75. Eviatar JA, Silvers SL, Echavez MI. Restorative treatment of HIV-associated facial lipoatrophy. Plast Reconstr Surg. 2005;116(3):29–30.
76. Gooderham M, Solish N. Use of hyaluronic acid for soft tissue augmentation of HIV-associated facial lipodystrophy. Dermatol Surg. 2005;31(1):104–8.
77. Ritt MJ, Hillebrand-Haverkort ME, Veen JH. Local treatment of facial lipodystrophy in patients receiving HIV protease inhibitor therapy. Acta Chir Plast. 2001;43(2):54–6.
78. Valantin MC, Aubron-Olivier C, Ghosn J, Laglenne E, Pauchard M, et al. Polylactic acid implants (Newfill)® to correct facial lipoatrophy in HIV-infected patients: results of the open-label study VEGA. AIDS. 2003;17(17):2471–7.
79. Moyle GJ, Lysakova L, Brown S, Sibtain N, Healy J, Priest C, et al. A randomized open-label study of immediate versus delayed polylactic acid injections for the cosmetic management of facial lipoatrophy in persons with HIV infection. HIV Med. 2004;5(2):82–7.
80. Orentreich D, Leone AS. A case of HIV-associated facial lipoatrophy treated with 1000-cs liquid injectable silicone. Dermatol Surg. 2004;30(4 Pt 1):548–51.
81. Jones DH, Carruthers A, Orentreich D, Brody HJ, Lai MY, Azen S, et al. Highly purified 100-csSt silicone oil for the treatment of human immunodeficiency virus-associated facial lipoatrophy: an open pilot trial. Dermatol Surg. 2004; 30(10):1279–86.
82. Protopapa C, Sito G, Caporale D, Cammarota N. Bio-alcamid in drug-induced lipodystrophy. J Cosmet Laser Ther. 2003;5(3–4):226–30.
83. Formigli L, Zecchi S, Protopapa C, Caporale D, Cammarota N, Lotti TM. Bio-alcamid: an electron microscopic study after skin implantation. Plast Reconstr Surg. 2004; 113(3):1104–6.
84. Pacini S, Ruggiero M, Cammarota N, Protopapa C, Gulisano M. Bio-alcamid, a novel prosthetic polymer, does not interfere with morphological and functional characteristics of human skin fibroblasts. Plast Reconstr Surg. 2003;111(1): 489–91.
85. Karim RB, Hage JJ, van Rozelaar L, et al. Complications of polyalkylimide 4% injections (Bio-alcamid™): a report of 18 cases. J Plast Reconstr Aesthet Surg. 2006;59(12): 1409–14.
86. Strauch B, Baum T, Robbins N. Treatment of human immunodeficiency virus-associated lipodystrophy with dermafat graft transfer to the malar area. Plast Reconstr Surg. 2004;113(1):363–70.
87. Wechselberger G, Sarcletti M, Meirer R, Bauer T, Schoeller T. Dermis-fat graft for facial lipodystrophy in HIV-positive patients: is it worthwhile? Ann Plast Surg. 2001;47(1): 99–100.
88. Endo T, Nakayama Y, Matsuura E, Natsui H, Soeda S. Facial contour reconstruction in lipodystrophy using a double paddle dermis-fat radial forearm free flap. Ann Plast Surg. 1994;32(1):93–6.
89. Koshy CE, Evans J. Facial contour reconstruction in localized lipodystrophy using free radial forearm adipofascial flaps. Br J Plast Surg. 1998;51(7):499–502.
90. van der Wal KG, Mulder JW. Facial contour reconstruction in partial lipodystrophy using two temporalis muscle flaps. A case report. Int J Oral Maxillofac Surg. 1998;27(1): 14–6.
91. Longaker M, Flynn A, Siebert J. Microsurgical correction of bilateral facial contour deformities. Plast Reconstr Surg. 1996;98(5):951–7.
92. Adams JR, Kawamoto HK. Late infection following aesthetic malar augmentation with proplast implants. Plast Reconstr Surg. 1995;95(2):382–4.
93. Williams CW. Malar implant infections resulting from recurrent infections of adjacent dental pathology. Plast Reconstr Surg. 1994;93(7):1533–4.

Comparison of Three Different Methods for Correction of HIV-Associated Facial Lipodystrophy

Giovanni Guaraldi, Pier Luigi Bonucci, and Domenico De Fazio

64.1 Introduction

Lipodystrophy (LD), referring to morphologic changes and metabolic alterations, affecting HIV-1-infected patients, was first described in 1998 [1–5]. The main clinical features are peripheral fat loss or lipoatrophy of the face, limbs, and buttocks and central fat accumulation within the abdomen, breast, and the dorsocervical spine both of which may be present in the same individual [6, 7].

Facial lipoatrophy, in particular, includes loss of the buccal fat and temporal fat pads and leads to facial skeletonization with concave cheeks, prominent nasolabial folds, periorbital hollowing, and visible facial musculature [8–10]. This volume deficit alters the contour of the face from youthful, healthy, convex curves to aged, pathologic, concave contours [11–14]. The net aesthetic result is of an accelerated aging process of the face appearance.

It is intuitive that facial lipoatrophy is the most stigmatizing feature of HIV-related LD, as face cannot be masked by clothes and usually it is perceived as the manifestation of our health. Many studies have demonstrated that LD causes negative psychosocial impact and an impairment of quality of life because of erosion of self-image and self-esteem, demoralization and depression, problems in social and sexual relations, and threats to locus of control. Often LD forces HIV disclosure [15].

Surgical treatments for facial lipoatrophy include autologous fat transplant (AFT) from a subcutaneous abdominal graft or injections of biodegradable or nonbiodegradable fillers into the lipoatrophic areas of the face.

64.2 Comparative Studies

It is surprising how very few studies have assessed safety, efficacy, and durability of these interventions and only two partially randomized studies have compared different surgical approaches [16, 17].

The first partially randomized study was conducted at the Metabolic Clinic of the University of Modena and Reggio Emilia, where an extensive surgery experience for HIV-related facial lipoatrophy has been gathered from 2001. Eligible individuals with enough residual subcutaneous fat were offered to receive AFT; the others were blindly assigned to two different surgical teams who administered a set of PLA or PAAG injections every 4 weeks. The primary endpoint was the measurement of Bichat's fat pad region determined by the result of dermal plus subcutaneous thickness. Secondary endpoints included body image evaluation (ABCD questionnaire), facial aesthetic satisfaction (Visual Analogue Scale), and aesthetic pre and

G. Guaraldi (✉)
Department of Medicine and Medicine Specialities,
Infectious Diseases Clinic, University of Modena
and Reggio Emilia School of Medicine,
Via del Pozzo 71, 41100, Modena, Italy
e-mail: giovanni.guaraldi@unimore.it

P.L. Bonucci
Chirurgia plastica, Salus Hospital, Reggio Emilia,
Italy and Hesperia Hospital Modena, Modena, Italy
e-mail: pierluigibonucci@virgilio.it

D. De Fazio
Chirurgia plastica, Salus Hospital, Reggio Emilia,
Italy and casa di cura: S. Pio X, Milano, Italy
e-mail: dododefazio@libero.it

postpicture comparisons by independent reviewers. All variables were measured at baseline and week 24.

Twenty-four individuals received AFT and 35 were selectively randomized to PLA [18] or PAAG [15] infiltrations. PLA and PAAG groups received a mean of five to six injections, respectively ($p=ns$). The mean change in fat thickness was respectively 3.3 ± 4.1; 3.5 ± 4.0; 2.1 ± 3.0 mm ($p = .687$). The mean change in ABCD score result was poorer in the AFT arm but there were no other differences in other measured parameters. Four serious adverse events were documented in the AFT arm represented by facial fat graft hypertrophy, which occurred at the beginning of the authors' clinical experience when areas of fat hypertrophy (mainly buffalo hump) were used for graft site. These subjects developed facial fat hypertrophy at the same time of recurrence of fat hypertrophy in the harvest site. Patients described themselves as "hamster" because of the swollen cheeks, and this clinical picture has been published as "Hamster syndrome" [16]. This phenomenon is no more observed since the use of fat hypertrophy for harvest site is avoided. All three interventional techniques were highly effective in improving the aesthetic satisfaction of the patients. Figure 64.1 represents three cases from this series in which an equal satisfactory aesthetic result was obtained. Physical examination does not allow the identification of which surgical procedure was performed in each case.

The second study by Negredo et al., evaluated the clinical efficacy of facial infiltrations with autologous fat, polylactic acid, and polyacrylamide gel using clinical inspection and facial photographs as well as patient satisfaction, emotional status, and quality of life. Evaluations were made at 48-week follow-up. Analysis included 138 patients: 8, 25, and 105 in the fat, polylactic acid, and polyacrylamide gel groups, respectively. At baseline, almost 50% of the patients (67/138) presented grades 3 and 4 lipoatrophy, but at week 48 only 7.5% (7/93) remained in these advanced grades (no patients from the polyacrylamide group). A new round of infiltrations at week 48 was necessary in 35% (33/93) of patients (88%, 84%, and 8% in the fat, polylactic, and polyacrylamide groups, respectively). No serious adverse events were detected with any of the substances. Patient satisfaction and quality of life improved significantly in all three groups. Infiltrations with autologous fat, polylactic acid, or polyacrylamide gel have appeared to be an effective and safe alternative to repair facial lipoatrophy, at least up to 48 weeks, significantly improving patient quality of life. Similar results were observed for all degrees of severity and between genders. Polyacrylamide gel provided the longest-lasting benefits.

Establishing endpoints is challenging for comparative studies of facial fillers that work by different mechanisms. Assessment by photographs may not lead to reproducible results and is operator-dependent, and the continuation of specific antiretroviral therapies may also influence outcomes. Fortunately, some attempts at comparison have been made, and funding for additional comparative data is being sought.

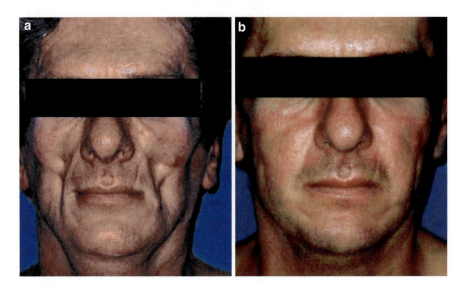

Fig. 64.1 (**a**) Preoperative. (**b**) Following 10 ml of autologous fat injected into each cheek

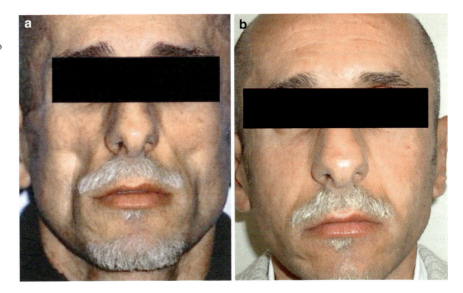

Fig. 64.2 (a) Preoperative. (b) Following 12 ml of PLA (polylactic acid) injected into each cheek

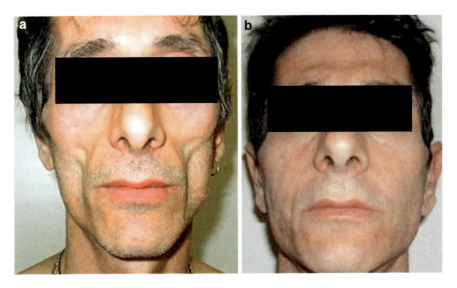

Fig. 64.3 (a) Preoperative. (b) After injection of 12 ml of PAAG (polyacrylamide gel) injected into each cheek

Some studies have utilized pictures comparisons and ultrasound assessment of cheek thickness as aesthetic outcomes. As previously said, it is necessary to consider PRO such as the assessment of BI, aesthetic perception, depression, and QoL. Long-term psychometric outcomes of plastic surgery for treatment of facial lipoatrophy have been described by Orlando et al. [19] in an observational, prospective, nonrandomized study of 299 participants (70.8% male). Fifty-four (18.1%) have undergone lipofilling (Fig. 64.1), 24 (8%) after an initial lipofilling have needed polylactic acid injections to correct cheek asymmetry, 91 (30.4%) have received only polylactic acid infiltrations (Fig. 64.2), 130 (43.5%) only polyacrylamide infiltrations (Fig. 64.3). At 48 weeks after end of surgery participants have shown an improvement of face satisfaction (by a Visual Analogue Scale from 2.9 ± 2.1 to 6.2 ± 2.1 ($p<.0001$), of body image satisfaction (ABCD question 7 from 3.8 ± 1 to 3.1 ± 1 $p<.0001$ and ABCD question 8 from 70.7 ± 16.7 to 77.2 ± 17.2 $p<.0001$), as well as improvement of objective outcome as the augmentation of both cheeks thickness (right cheek from 4.3 ± 1.9 to 9.5 ± 3 mm $p<.0001$, left cheek from 4.4 ± 2 to 9.6 ± 3.1 mm, $p<.0001$). Notwithstanding surgery has been limited to the face; all patients have reported body image improvement even though the ABCD questionnaire had no specific questions or items referring to facial lipoatrophy. Apparently facial surgery has resulted in an improvement of whole body aesthetic satisfaction and psycho-social life (social and sexual life, health perception, habits, affections, relationships). This positive effect was evident in the overall sample and in the polylactic acid and polyacrylamide groups, while it has reached no statistical significance in the lipofilling group. One of the most striking impacts of surgery was on depression as assessed by the Beck depression inventory (BDI) [20]. This is a self-administered 21 item scale measuring supposed manifestations of depression. It includes factors reflecting negative attitudes towards self, performance impairment and somatic disturbances, as well as a general factor of depression [18]. The BDI takes approximately 10 min to complete. The higher the score, the greater the state of depression. Total possible score ranges from 0 to 63. Mild depression was defined as a value between 9 and 17, a moderate depression between 18 and 29, and a severe depression for values greater than 30. At follow-up, the change in BDI revealed a significant improvement in the depression score for the overall cohort from 11.4 ± 8.3 (corresponding to mild depression) to 9.4 ± 7.8 (almost absence of depression), $p = 0.001$. Nevertheless, analyzing the score by single surgery group the change was significant in the polylactic acid and polyacrylamide groups only (lipofilling score changed from 10 ± 8.3 to 10.4 ± 8.7, $p = ns$; lipofilling + polylactic acid score changed from $15.6 + 10.5$ to 12.7 ± 12.1, $p = ns$; polylactic acid score changed from 10.7 ± 7.4 to 8 ± 6.5, $p = 0.001$; polyacrylamide score changed from 11.8 ± 8.5 to 9.6 ± 8.1, $p = 0.014$).

Table 64.1 summarizes the studies that have assessed safety, efficacy, and durability of different surgical interventions for treatment of facial lipoatropy.

64.3 How to Choose Different Surgical Procedures to Treat HIV-Related Facial Lipoatrophy

The most important prerequisite to the choice is the expertise of the health care worker; thus plastic reconstructive surgeons should always be the preferred ones, and are needed to perform autologous fat transplant. Given the excellent aesthetic result of lipofilling and both biodegradable and nonbiodegradable fillers the choice of the best surgical procedure is not a matter of aesthetic issues. Generally speaking biodegradable fillers should be the first choice in younger people in order to allow a better adaptation of the filler with the physiological aging process, unless grade 4 facial lipoatrophy where high volume injection is needed. This result, indeed, can be obtained mainly with autologous fat transplant, when feasible, or with nonbiodegradable fillers. In case of patients often suffering from sinusitis or dental granuloma or undergoing odonto-stomatologic procedure, nonbiodegradable fillers should be avoided because of the risk of local infection or granuloma that may potentially occur years after the filling procedure as long-term complications. Short-term complications, mainly represented by local edema, infection, and bleeding are few when filler are injected with small-gauge needle, and always self-limiting, but

Table 64.1 Studies that have assessed safety, efficacy, and durability of different surgical interventions for treatment of facial lipoatropy

Author, journal, year	Material	Number of pts	Efficacy objectively assessed (method)	Efficacy subjectively assessed (QoL domains)	Safety (AES, %)	Durability (weeks of f-u)
Negredo, *AIDS Patient Care STDS*, 2006 [17]	Polylactic acid	$N=25$	NA	+	+	48
	Polyacrylamide gel	$N=105$				
	Autologous fat transplant	$N=8$				
Guaraldi, *Antivir Ther*, 2005 [16]	Polylactic acid	$N=20$	+	+	+	24
	Polyacrylamide gel	$N=15$	(US)		+	
	Autologous fat transplant	$N=24$			(SAE, 18%)	

QoL quality of life, *AE* adverse event, *f-u* follow up, *US* ultrasound, *NA* not available, + effective or save, *SAE* serious adverse events

Table 64.2 Clinical considerations for various fillers

	Autologous fat transplant	Biodegradable fillers	Nonbiodegradable fillers
Expertise of the health care worker	Highly required	Highly required	Highly required
Safety	Potential short-term complications as local edema, infection, and bleeding	Potential subcutaneous skin nodules after injecting polylactic acid	Potential long-term complications as local infection or granuloma
Severity	Preferable when there is need of high-volume injection	Preferable when there is no need of high-volume injection	Preferable when there is need of high-volume injection
Costs	Presumably most costly	Potentially costly when many retouches needed	Costly but definite
Age	Preferable in all ages	Preferable in younger people	Preferable in older people
Reimbursement	Depends on country policy	Depends on country policy	Depends on country policy

they may occur hypothetically with all fillers. Different countries' policies about reimbursement of these procedures underpin all the comments on the different costs. In general it can be assumed that lipofilling procedure is very expensive, but given its permanent result, it costs less in comparison to the cost of biodegradable filler that needs yearly retouch procedures.

Reimbursement of surgical treatment for HIV-related lipoatrophy is possible in UK and France and to some extent in Spain and Italy. We encourage public health authority to recognize facial lipoatrophy as a common clinical picture associated to HIV infection and guarantee access to surgical treatment for the quality-of-life implication of its results.

Table 64.2 summarizes these clinical considerations.

Acknowledgement We thank G. Orlando, M.D. and C. Stentarelli, M.D. for their assistance in the project.

References

1. Carr A, Samaras K, Burton S, Law M, Freund J, Chisholm DJ, et al. A syndrome of peripheral lipodystrophy, hyperlipidaemia and insulin resistance in patients receiving HIV protease inhibitors. AIDS. 1998;12(7):F51–8.
2. Lo JC, Mulligan K, Tai VW, Algren H, Schambelan M. "Buffalo hump" in men with HIV-1 infection. Lancet. 1998;351(9106):867–70.
3. Stricker RB, Goldberg B. Fat accumulation and HIV-1 protease inhibitors. Lancet. 1998;352(9137):1392.
4. Saint-Marc T, Partisani M, Poizot-Martin I, Bruno F, Rouviere O, Lang JM. A syndrome of peripheral fat wasting (lipodystrophy) in patients receiving long-term nucleoside analogue therapy. AIDS. 1999;13(13):1659–67.
5. Miller KD, Jones E, Yanovski JA, Shankar R, Feuerstein I, Falloon J. Visceral abdominal-fat accumulation associated with use of indinavir. Lancet. 1998;351(9106):871–5.
6. Carr A, Miller J, Law M, Cooper DA. A syndrome of lipoatrophy, lactic acidaemia and liver dysfunction associated with HIV nucleoside analogue therapy: contribution to protease inhibitor-related lipodystrophy syndrome. AIDS. 2000;14(3):F25–32.
7. Saint-Marc T, Partisani M, Poizot-Martin I, Rouviere O, Bruno F, Avellaneda R, et al. Fat distribution evaluated by computed tomography and metabolic abnormalities in patients undergoing antiretroviral therapy: preliminary results of the LIPOCO study. AIDS. 2000;14(1):37–49.
8. Carr A, Law M. An objective lipodystrophy severity grading scale derived from the lipodystrophy case definition score. J Acquir Immune Defic Syndr. 2003;33(5):571–6.
9. Garg A. Acquired and inherited lipodystrophies. N Engl J Med. 2004;350(12):1220–34.
10. James J, Carruthers A, Carruthers J. HIV-associated facial lipoatrophy. Dermatol Surg. 2002;28(11):979–86.
11. Fenske NA, Lober CW. Structural and functional changes of normal aging skin. J Am Acad Dermatol. 1986;15(4 Pt 1):571–85.
12. Gonzalez-Ulloa MSF, Flores E. The anatomy of the aging face. In: Hueston JT, editor. Transactions of the fifth international congress of plastic and reconstructive surgery. London: Butterworth; 1971. p. 1059–66.
13. Hall DA, Blackett AD, Zajac AR, Switala S, Airey CM. Changes in skinfold thickness with increasing age. Age Ageing. 1981;10(1):19–23.
14. Tan CY, Statham B, Marks R, Payne PA. Skin thickness measurement by pulsed ultrasound: its reproducibility, validation and variability. Br J Dermatol. 1982;106(6):657–67.
15. Collins E, Wagner C, Walmsley S. Psychosocial impact of the lipodystrophy syndrome in HIV infection. AIDS Read. 2000;10(9):546–50.
16. Guaraldi G, Orlando G, De Fazio D, De Lorenzi I, Rottino A, De Santis G, et al. Comparison of three different interventions for the correction of HIV-associated facial lipoatrophy: a prospective study. Antivir Ther. 2005;10(6):753–9.
17. Negredo E, Higueras C, Adell X, Martinez JC, Martinez E, Puig J, et al. Reconstructive treatment for antiretroviral-

associated facial lipoatrophy: a prospective study comparing autologous fat and synthetic substances. AIDS Patient Care STDs. 2006;20(12):829–37.
18. Brown C, Schulberg HC. Diagnosis and treatment of depression in primary medical care practice: the application of research findings to clinical practice. J Clin Psychol. 1998; 54(3):303–14.
19. Orlando G, Guaraldi G, De Fazio D, Rottino A, Grisotti A, Blini M, et al. Long term psychometric outcomes of facial lipoatrophy therapy. AIDS Patient Care STDs. 2007; 21(11):833–42.
20. Beck AT, Steer RA. Internal consistencies of the original and revised Beck Depression Inventory. J Clin Psychol. 1984; 40(6):1365–7.

Part VII
Medical Legal

Medical Malpractice Lawsuits: What Causes Them, How to Prevent Them, and How to Deal with Them When You Are the Defendant

Ronald A. Fragen

65.1 Introduction

In 45 years of medical practice and 30 years as an expert witness, the author has seen angry patients and incompetent lawyers devastate physicians' psyche. Except for the outlying percent of physicians who are impaired or have serious psychological problems, every other physician wants no part of a lawsuit and will, if instructed properly, avoid them at considerable cost of time, money, and effort. Unfortunately in the years of training and teaching in medical school and residency programs there was no instruction on avoiding lawsuits. It was assumed that if you, as a physician, made no mistake then a lawsuit would never happen. We all know this is a fallacy, especially in the cosmetic aspects of surgery. Since we can never truly know what will make the patient happy or what offhand remark by a third party may change a satisfied patient to an unhappy patient, we must arm ourselves with the information to help prevent lawsuits.

Where do we get this information on how to prevent lawsuits? We talk to colleagues who are usually far too upset to discuss their experiences and only see the complaint rather than the whole picture. We take risk management courses provided by insurance companies and we listen to discussion by attorneys at national or regional medical meetings. The thing that all these courses have in common is they are presented by lawyers or educators who have never experienced the total patient contact from first phone calls to the office to 2 months postoperation. These courses discuss the technical aspects of lawsuits but rarely the personal and emotional aspects. The success ratio of countersuing plaintiffs and their lawyers is next to zero. So forget about getting even.

As a physician, not a lawyer, is how the author views medical malpractice, nothing in this article should be construed as legal advice. The following is a synopsis of the main points discussed by others in regard to risk management assuming a cosmetic practice where patients seek you rather than involvement as part of the trauma team.

65.2 Four Elements of Medical Malpractice: Duty, Breach of Duty, Causation, and Damages

65.2.1 Duty

Do we have an obligation to treat everyone? No, but there are subtle legalities that create a doctor–patient relationship. If you find a patient or a complex problem you do not wish to begin or continue treating, make it clear in your chart and refer the patient.

Suppose a patient with a body dysmorphia comes for consultation for her fifth rhinoplasty. Display understanding of the patient's point of view; explain that the

R.A. Fragen
Assistant Professor of Surgery, Division of Otolaryngology,
University Medical School, 1900 E. Tahquitz Canton Way,
Suite A2, Palm Springs, CA 92262-7060, USA
e-mail: ron@thefragens.com

problem is not one you feel comfortable handling and document to who you refer the patient.

65.2.2 Breach of Duty (Negligence)

Implies the physician failed to render the required standard of care, a level of care a reasonably prudent physician would provide under the same or similar circumstances.

Describe in your chart note, and to the patient verbally, the patient's complaint, by restating their reason for consultation. Also state your findings, diagnoses, treatment plan and why, the risks, and alternatives.

65.2.3 Causation

The plaintiff must prove that your breach of duty (negligence) caused the injury. As we all know in the current atmosphere of turf wars the plaintiff's attorney can usually pay for, and find, an adversarial physician to support their contention of malpractice.

In one case, a board-certified physician testified that injection of more than 10 mg of triamcinolone at any one time was below that standard of care and caused damage. The defendant physician was severely penalized over this absolute falsehood.

65.2.4 Damages

Compensation for the breach can be economic (loss of wages), noneconomic (pain and suffering), or punitive, usually the result of acts such as being impaired, sexual assault, changing the record, or extreme gross negligence. Of course, the lawyers, courts, and plaintiffs twist the facts so the outcome of the suit is often a turkey shoot with the defendant doctor being the turkey.

Other areas frequently discussed in risk management are advertising, consent forms, and chart notes. Review your website do not advertise that you are the best or credentials that you do not have. This is a frequent part of the complaint, especially if one of your turf war colleagues is the opposing expert.

Medical records are the first place lawyers look to trip you. Risk management will tell you the notes should be legible, accurate, and complete. We know our notes rarely meet their standard. We write contemporaneously and are often never going to see the patient seeking consultation again. However, your notes should tell a story and substantiate your reasoning. Document a reasoned history, chief complaint, physical examination of pertinent areas, diagnosis, and treatment options. Document informed consent and include pertinent positives as sun damaged skin and pertinent negatives such as no evidence of infection. Document informed refusal. An example may be a patient who has slight neck skin laxity 6 months post facelift. You offer a tuck up to correct the problem and the patient refuses, put this in a chart note – it starts the statue of limitations and lets the patient know you are their advocate.

Part of your chart is your informed consent. An informed consent is more than a signed piece of paper. It should include what a reasonable person would want to know as a beginning. Also include pages of as many risks as you can collect from any source; do not be afraid to copy from your colleagues. In addition, document as a separate chart note that the patient has read, understood, and (after reading and signing the consent) agrees to surgery. If you do not personally go over all of your forms, have the person who does, enter a note and sign and date it. Especially in cosmetic surgery, not only document in the chart but explain to the patient what you see, what you plan, what you expect the result to be, and whether you anticipate more than one surgery or treatment session and who would be financially responsible for subsequent treatment. Examples would include facial filler, secondary surgery for a difficult nose, and deep resurfacing post-facelift in a patient with deep etched rhytids. Learn to prevent lapses in record keeping and communication that cause malpractice suits over unwanted results that are clearly not negligence.

Another trap is the area of vicarious liability. You are held responsible for errors of those you have a duty to supervise. Your staff and what they say is an obvious trap. You should at least discuss patient confidentiality and demeanor in the office and over the phone. Have your staff inform you when patients are unhappy. The patient will often discuss with the staff what they will not tell you. This applies even before they meet you for the first consultation.

"Res ipsa loquiter" – It speaks for itself, i.e., a sponge left in an operative site.

Ideally the physician on call for you and covering your practice should have the same certification and privileges as you.

When you are only a consultant, remember you have an independent duty to the patient and a duty to have knowledge of pertinent lab, x-ray, and history, i.e., review records or document the patient is supposed to bring records.

65.3 Avoiding Lawsuits

Lawsuits come from angry, frustrated patients looking for a result or answer to a problem and are left feeling their doctor has either deceived or abandoned them. Patients sue because of greed, lawyers, unrealistic expectations, poor outcomes, perception of poor care, failure to keep the patient and family informed, and poor communication.

Your medical team's relationships, doctors, nurses, technicians, and front office personnel are also responsible for patient relationships. Thirty percent of suits are urged by another health care professional. Remember patients do not sue doctors they like and trust because they do not want to damage the relationship. In this age of the computer, email, and text messages, almost everyone hungers for interaction with a person they admire and respect.

We have all known physicians who have frequent complications but rarely get sued. Why is this? Rapport is defined as a close relationship with agreement and harmony. Make people feel comfortable with you. Let them know you care about them not just one or more of their body parts. Stop treating patients as conditions and treat them as people. Interact with patients like they are a most valued friend. Listen and show it, look at them, touch them, call them by name, and do not interrupt them. Sit and actively listen to you patient. Use body language, eye contact, leaning in, facial expression, and touching to show your interest. Paraphrase the patient's story and requests using your own words to show you care. This may help clear up any misunderstanding of their requests and concerns.

Avoiding lawsuits begins with the first office contact. Your office must be courteous, friendly, and respectful to patients at all times. Do not put them on hold for long periods, if you are a little late explain why and apologize. You and your staff should engage the patient like they are the most important person in the world and that you are happy they called your office. When the patient arrives for consultation be efficient and helpful. However, train yourself and your staff to look out for the patient from Hell! The body dysmorphic, overly flirtatious, the patient who has called and cancelled repeatedly, and the patient spending their last dime all should raise a caution flag. When you, the physician, meet the patient, look at them, not your computer, know their name and ask, "What can I do for you?" Take enough time, listen, and ask, "Is there anything else?"

Listen first, then write or dictate and excuse yourself from the close contact to look away to write and organize the information. Then return to patient contact and become your patient's guide and counselor, be chatty about their job, family, or other personal areas.

Carefully explain your expectations and what their expectations should be. If your expectations differ from the patients original expectations, resolve the differences before moving forward. Explain how the patient can help or diminish the result. Discuss alternatives and likelihood of secondary and/or revision surgeries and if there will be additional charges. Common examples are additional fat grafts or fillers with face-lifts, possible skin excision, or touch-ups after liposuction. Ask if there are any questions. When the consultation is over thank the patient by name for coming to consult with you.

Patients will sue if angry. They will get angry if you or your staff are rude, insulting, or if you abandon them.

When it comes to surgery, be rigorous in your charting, planning, photographs, lab work, history, and physical exam. Try to operate with the same team; make sure the patient is positioned properly and that you have the medicines, implants, and equipment that you need. Try to do things in a regular and repetitive way to avoid mistakes. Concentrate on the task at hand and avoid interruptions that break your concentration. Get your helpers to concentrate on the patient, not the phone or computer.

When you have a problem with a result, stay on top of it, call consultants and see the patient often. Explain what is going on, how you plan to handle it, and how long you expect until resolution. Keep the patient on your side, support them, and do not deny the problem. Always make them feel you will be there for them. It is often a good idea to enlist a family member or friend in the care of the patient.

We have all run across physicians who have many complications and never seem to get sued. Why is this?

People will sue an expert technician who does not perform to their expectations. People rarely sue their friend and counselor.

How well we handle problems often significantly affects whether a suit will follow. When dealing with an angry patient, listen and do not respond to each complaint. Wait until the patient is done, actively listen, and ask if there is anything else. Paraphrase the complaint and ask for confirmation. Above all: Do not get defensive. Attempt to explain the cause of the problem, i.e., thick skin and a fibrous supratip poly beak. Explain a proposed treatment and a time frame. Explain how the patient can help. Do not promise anything! Follow up with a phone call. Communicate bad news or a significant problem forthrightly and in private. Notify patients of lab results and do not make them wait since waiting creates angst and then anger if something pertinent is late in being discussed or if a normal is not delivered timely.

What can we do with the noncompliant patient? Educate the patient and ask them to repeat so you and they understand. Ask in what other areas they have been noncompliant. If the patient does not follow through in one area maybe there are others they are not letting you know about. Get the patient and a family member or friend involved with the treatment. Often ask what part of compliance will be most difficult for the patient and if they will agree to change behavior. How many patients either overclean or do not clean postauricular incisions?

Confidentiality is especially important in a cosmetic practice. Get permission to use and show photos. Make sure your staff is aware what happens in the office stays there. Have them sign a confidentiality agreement and make sure they do not gossip about patients in the office because they may be overheard. When a patient asks to speak to another person who has had the same procedure, protect identities by using only first name and ask the former patient to contact the future patient so nuisance phone calls come only if the former patient gives out their phone number.

65.4 What to Do When a Lawsuit Is Threatened or Filed

When a case does not go well and you get a request for a chart to be sent elsewhere or a lawsuit is either threatened or filed, review the chart. *Do Not Alter* the chart. Write contemporaneous notes about the case, not in the chart. Ask your staff to do the same since often they are privy to information you do not have. Patients are often bumped in the nose postrhinoplasty and tell only your receptionist. One of my patients was socked in the face by a boyfriend 2 days post cheek implant and the patient did not tell me when displacement occurred. However, she sobbingly related the incident to our patient counselor. The patient went on to file a lawsuit which was stopped when we informed her lawyer of the assault by the boyfriend. These personal notes should be in the form of a letter to your attorney so they can protect you.

Always review a chart before copying as this is often the first sign of an impending lawsuit. Never allow staff or anyone to copy a chart you have not reviewed.

Always be involved with your insurance company and defense attorney. No one else knows the case better than you. Review your notes and other information supplied by the patient, your diagnosis, treatment plan, what happened, and why. Look up literature just as if you were to be the expert on the case. Remember, lawsuits take 2–5 years (or more) to come to trial. The notes you make will help you remember later.

What happens when we are served notice of a lawsuit? It ruins your day but do not let it ruin you. A lawsuit usually demeans your professional competence and your integrity. This usually gets you angry and creates great stress. Remember, lawsuits are about money and are a part of doing business. They are the reason we have insurance companies and why we pay those premiums. Clear some time and take a deep breath. Notify your insurance carrier.

Unfortunately, malpractice lawsuits are about us and are personal. If the suit were about a fence one foot over the property line we would not take it personally. Try to put the suit and the accompanying angst in that category of the fence rather than a personal attack. Do not be afraid to contact a friend or mentor in this field. There is probably no mature physician in the field of cosmetic surgery who has not been sued. Try to compartmentalize the stress, remembering the process will usually take years. We are all compulsive perfectionist personalities and our tendency is to review the incident and make sure we do not commit the error again. We obsess about it. This leads to sleepless nights and continued stress and the likelihood of making additional errors because of fatigue. Control your working hours and maintain a balance of work, rest, recreation, and sex. Work on your personal relationships and emphasize people skills. Do not get into a depressive funk. Especially monitor your use of medication and alcohol. Post lawsuit stress is real. Lawsuits can take months and years for resolution. Be reasonable and go back to work. Statistically, we are twice as prone to be sued a second time in the 12 months after being notified of a first lawsuit.

The author is a big proponent of arbitration; it takes less time, costs less, and presentation is in front of a person or panel educated enough to recognize the nuances of scientific and technical matters. The physician does not need to be present during testimony. There is little to no grandstanding by the attorneys. The emotional defendant is blunted. As an expert witness for many years the author feels that the defendant physician gets a better deal. There is usually no problem with getting patients to sign arbitration agreements.

What can you do about an opposing expert witness who lies under oath? The American College of Legal Medicine (ACLM) has produced legal guidelines for the ethical conduct of physician expert witnesses. The testimony is considered the practice of medicine and as such this testimony (in the trial records) can be sent to the American Medical Association (AMA), the physician's specialty board, and the physician's state medical board. Experts are given wide discretion by courts who do not know medical facts, but the ACLM's guidelines state that the expert must not be an advocate or partisan for either party, the expert should have recent experience in the area of testimony, the expert should testify honestly without excluding relevant information, there should be no conflict of interest with the clients or attorneys, and testimony should be based on literature or stated that it is opinion. The author would encourage plaintiffs or defendants who feel wronged by testimony to complain to the appropriate agencies and boards.

The author realizes this is a different approach than you are used to. Most risk management courses involve how you advertise, your chart notes, history, and physical, reports, consent forms, and other documentation. You all should know these are important.

It is the art of being your patient's advocate, friend, and counselor that keeps the lawsuits away. It is the documentation that helps you win, not prevent, the suit and the author's experience, as a malpractice expert witness, is that most suits involve technical issues. It is easier for a good expert witness to explain, document, and footnote your defense before an arbitration judge or panel. Most juries do not understand even the simplest technical points and tend to write off both the plaintiff and defendant experts as a balance. Juries look to the emotional distress and is it justified given the less than desired result. The more convinced the jury is that the result of surgery led to significant and justifiable distress to the plaintiff, the more likely is the plaintiff's verdict or settlement even though your treatment was within the standard of care.

If you have problems call and ask for advice. If you are sued, participate in your own defense. "RON'S Rules" state almost all patients lie either by omission or commission and when the patient decides to sue, everyone lies: The patient, the family, their experts, and their lawyer.

There are many subtle aspects of avoiding suits and winning those you are unable to avoid. Of all the things you wear, your expression is the most important. Be kinder than necessary because everyone you meet is fighting some kind of battle.

Index

A
Abdelkader, M., 18
Abscess, 619
Advanced cardiac life support (ACLS), 50
Allergic reactions, 217
Alopecia, 129, 334, 475, 515, 531
Aly, A.S., 467
American Society of Anesthesiologists (ASA), 49, 51, 77
American Society of Plastic and Reconstructive Surgery (ASPRS), 232
American Society of Plastic Surgeons (ASPS), 211, 463
Arlt's method, 578–580
ASA classification, 51
Ascher, B., 691
ASPRS. *See* American Society of Plastic and Reconstructive Surgery
ASPS. *See* American Society of Plastic Surgeons
Asymmetry, 308, 449, 471, 480, 515, 538, 575, 645, 668, 686
Aufricht, G., 241, 459
Autologous fat, 212, 235–239, 346
    grafting, 532, 552, 564, 592
    transfer, 465, 710, 711, 724

B
Baker, D.C., 247
Baker, T.J., 193
Basal metabolic index (BMI), 463
Basic life support (BLS), 50
Baum ratio, 17, 18
Beck depression inventory (BDI), 726
Becker, D.G., 661
Beeson, W.H., 193
Bell's phenomenon, 557
Berg, D., 137, 149, 151
Bettman, A.G., 449, 459
Bichat's fat pad, 447, 451
Biller, J.A., 18
Bircoll, M., 232
Blair's method, 580, 582
Bleeding, 157, 217, 259, 261–262, 308, 442, 471, 538, 618, 619, 650, 715
Blepharochalasis, 549
Blindness, 218, 553, 566, 592, 715
BMI. *See* Basal metabolic index
Boulogne, G.B., 31
Bourguet, J., 449, 459

Bourguet, J., 241, 558
Brow ptosis, 227
Bruning, P., 710
Buccal fat pad, 39
Buck, D.W., 216
Bukkewitz, H., 288
Bulstrode, N.W., 602, 603
Burgess, C.M., 701
Burrow's triangle, 364

C
Carboxytherapy, 112, 113
Carey, D.L., 697
Carpaneda, C.A., 711
Carruthers, J., 177
Castañares, S., 519, 524
Certified Registered Nurse Anesthetist (CRNA), 49, 50, 62
Cervicomental angle, 655
Chajchir, A., 476
Chajchir, J., 711
Chemical peel, 109–111, 113, 181, 182, 184, 186–189, 193–199, 559, 560, 567, 671, 672, 674, 675
Cheney, M.L., 482
Christie, J.L., 57
Coiffman, F., 512
Coleman, S.R., 232, 710, 714
Coleman technique, 716
Connelly, B.F., 241
Converse, J.M., 580
Converse's method, 581
Cook, T.A., 560
Core, G.B., 495
Courtiss, E., 241
CRNA. *See* Certified Registered Nurse Anesthetist
Crow's feet, 227, 497, 500, 534, 550, 556
Crumley, R.J., 17
Cytochrome P450, 248
Czerny, A., 710
Czerny, V., 231, 233

D
Davis, R.A., 403
de Castro, C.C., 246
Dedo, D.D., 245, 655
Dehiscence, 158, 471, 520, 554, 567, 618, 619
Del Campo method, 582

Dermatochalasis, 571
Diabetes mellitus, 54
Dieffenbach, J.E., 601
Dingman, R.O., 247, 403
Dog ear, 471
Douse-Dean, T., 592
Duchenne, D.E., 31
Dzubow, L.M., 316

E
Ecchymosis, 227, 308
Ectropion, 201, 557, 565
Edema, 157, 260, 308, 449, 472, 575, 619, 715
Edwars, 511
Entropion, 557
Epiphora, 553, 566
Erol, Ö.O., 289
Ersek, R.A., 710
Erythema, 189, 195, 589, 644
Eviatar, J.A., 716
Eyebrow ptosis, 479, 486, 491, 506, 512, 516, 519, 524, 527–529
Eyelid ptosis, 227, 549

F
Facial
    arteries, 13, 40, 234
    fat, 4, 5, 9, 10
    ligaments, 234
    mimetic muscles, 7–9, 406–407
    muscles, 31–33, 477, 478, 528
    nerves, 11–13, 23–28, 39, 40, 44, 198, 219, 234, 235, 247, 260, 331, 355, 397–398, 403, 407, 476, 485, 488, 498, 499, 644
    retaining ligaments, 6, 7, 336–337, 339–346, 349, 407–408
    skeleton, 3, 4
Faivre, J., 461
Farrior technique, 603
Fat graft hypertrophy, 716
Fat hypertrophy, 715, 724
Fat transfer, 233
Feldman, J.J., 241
Fernandez-Cossío, S., 592
Fibrosis, 316
Fillers, 468, 469, 552, 563, 587, 588, 591, 625, 626, 630–638, 642–644, 659, 692, 693, 695, 696, 698, 700–703, 718
Fischer, G., 231
Fitzpatrick classification, 170
Fitzpatrick skin types, 183, 196, 261, 365
Flowers' method, 582
Follicular unit, 131, 132, 144–149, 151, 152
Fomon, S., 511
Fournier, P.F., 710
Francesconi, G., 602, 603
Frankfurt horizontal line, 656
Frankfurt's horizontal plane, 243–244, 251
Frankfurt horizontal plane, 17, 19
Furnas, D.W., 408, 409, 602
Furnas ligaments, 42

G
Giampapa, V.C., 662
Gibson, T., 602
Glogau classification of photoaging, 183
Gogolewski, S., 698
Golden ratio, 19, 20
Goldman, L., 51
Gonzalez Ulloa, M., 476
Gosain, A.K., 403
Granulomas, 554, 637, 711
Granulomatous reactions, 217
Greenberg, R., 408
Gryskiewicz, J., 242
Gunter, J.P., 450

H
Hamra, S.T., 379, 425, 450, 460, 461
Har-Shaip, Y., 405
Hematoma, 259, 261–262, 333, 403, 448, 449, 472, 482, 515, 521, 552–554, 565–566, 600, 618, 619, 650
Hernandez-Perez, E., 289, 290
Hester, T.R., 450
Hiraga's method, 579
Hoeffin states, 118
Holdaway, R., 21
Hollander, E., 459
Hume, 117
Hunt, H.L., 475, 511
Hyperpigmentation, 173, 175, 177, 187, 188, 195, 197, 201, 202, 261, 473
Hypertension, 53, 54
Hypopigmentation, 175, 558

I
Illouz, Y.G., 234, 710
Implants, 206–209, 251–252, 468
Infection, 157, 173, 177, 188, 189, 195, 202, 217, 237, 261, 308, 333, 442, 448, 472, 492, 515, 521, 538, 600, 611, 618, 619, 650, 686
Intense pulsed light (IPL), 175–178, 321, 322
Isse, N.G., 476

J
James, J., 711
Jessner's peel, 186
Johnson, G.W., 232
Joseph, J., 459, 511

K
Kamer, F.M., 460, 461
Kaye, B.L., 476, 602
Kelley, P., 602
Klein, J.A., 241, 247, 248
Knize, D.M., 522
Krulig, E., 232

L
Lafaurie, M., 693, 696
Lagophthalmus, 549, 550, 553
Lambros, V.S., 592

Lazor, J.B., 482
LD. See Lipodystrophy
Leach, J., 17
Lemmon, M.L., 460
Lemperle, G., 698
Levan, P., 716
Lexer, E., 231, 459, 511, 710
Lipodystrophy (LD), 707, 708, 715, 716, 723
Lipodystrophy syndrome, 691
Lipohypertrophy, 708
Little, J.W., 243
Local anesthetic toxicity, 57, 58, 248
Lorenz, 118
Lowe, N.J., 468
Ludwig, E., 130
Ludwig classification, 131
Lyand, M., 495

M
MAC. See Monitored Anesthesia Care
Malignant hyperthermia, 56
Marchand, F., 233
Marino, H., 476, 511
Marquardt, S.R., 20
Matsuo, K., 595
McDowell, A.J., 596
McGregor's patch, 7, 42, 408–409
Mendelson, B.C., 409, 415
Mest, D.R., 696, 701
Microdermabrasion, 111, 113, 320
Microgenia, 207
Midfacial fat atrophy, 467
Milia, 195, 553, 566
Miller, C.C., 459, 495, 710
Mitz, V., 6, 450, 460
Moelleken, B., 450
Monitored Anesthesia Care (MAC), 77, 78
Moyle, G.J., 693, 718
Mueller's muscle, 548
Mustarde, J.C., 602
Mustarde's method, 581, 582

N
Nasal septum perforation, 620
Nasal stenosis, 620
Necrosis, 218, 276, 333, 472, 492, 515, 600, 619
Negredo, E., 724
Nerve block, 630
Neuber, F., 211, 212, 231, 468, 532
Neuber, G., 710
Neuhof, H., 234, 710
Newman, J., 232
Niechajev, I., 711
Noël, A., 459, 511
Nordstrom, R.E., 131
Norwood classification, 130

O
Obesity, 52, 463
Olsen, E.A., 130
Orlando, G., 696

Ostad, A., 57
Osteomyelitis, 619

P
Papules, 703
Park's method, 580, 581
Passot, R., 459, 475, 476
Peck, H., 20, 21
Peer, L.A., 231, 234, 710
Peyronie, M., 460
Pitanguy, I., 403
Pitman, G.H., 57
Platelet-rich plasma (PRP), 469
Platysmal banding, 459, 654, 658, 661, 662
Polyacrylamide gel filler, 724, 725
Powell, N., 17, 20
PRP. See Platelet-rich plasma
Psillakis, J.M., 446, 450, 461
Pulmonary embolism, 65

R
Ramirez, J., 479, 482, 484–492
Ramirez, O.M., 446, 450, 460
Rehn, E., 710
Res ipsa loquitur, 732
Retaining ligament, 408–418
Retro-orbicularis oculi fat (ROOF), 699
Rettinger, G., 617
Richards, S.D., 596
Ricketts, R.M., 20
Rogman's method, 579
Roizen, M.F., 51
ROOF. See Retro-orbicularis oculi fat
Ruff, G., 286

S
Santana, P.M., 446
Sasaki, G.H., 290
Scar, 158, 173, 177, 188, 195, 333, 334, 340, 341, 373, 374,
    448, 449, 467, 473, 475, 476, 482–484, 486, 491, 492,
    508, 515, 521, 523, 531, 558, 567, 584, 600, 645, 649,
    650, 666, 675, 677, 686, 703, 715
Schaeffer, B.T., 661
Serdev, N.P., 291
Seroma, 260, 449, 473, 650
Simons ratio, 17, 18
Skoog, K., 460
Skoog, T., 450
Sleep apnea, 55
SMAS. See Subcutaneous musculoaponeurotic system;
    Superficial musculoaponeurotic system
Smoking, 55, 316, 329
SOOF. See Suborbicularis oculi fat
Stenstrom, S.J., 602
Stenström otoabraders, 598
Straatsma, C.R., 231
Stuzin, J.M., 403, 415
Subcutaneous musculoaponeurotic system (SMAS), 207, 405,
    406, 414, 416–418, 437, 445, 447, 450, 478
Suborbicularis oculi fat (SOOF), 447, 448, 461, 557, 564, 669
Sulamanidze, M.A., 282, 286, 290

Superficial musculoaponeurotic system (SMAS), 6, 7, 24, 25, 35, 37, 39, 234, 247, 279, 293–295, 298, 299, 301, 318, 331, 332, 335, 336, 339–347, 349, 358–360, 373–382, 384–386, 388–391, 393, 394, 397–402, 404, 460, 461, 466, 467, 653, 654, 664
Superficial peels, 185
Swelling, 200, 237, 515, 534, 589

T
Talmor, M., 716
Telangiectasias, 567
Telephone ear deformity, 600
Tessier, P., 446, 451
Thromboembolism, 65
Tosti, A., 133
Toxic shock syndrome, 189, 619
Tubercle of Whitnall, 556
Tuffier, T., 231

U
Uchida, J.I., 511
Uchida method, 582, 583
Unna, P.G., 181

V
Vanluchene, A.L., 79
Vasconez. L.O., 476
Verderame, P., 233
Vermillion border, 15
Viñas, J.C., 476, 512, 519, 523, 524
Von Ammon's method, 578, 583, 584

W
Watanabe's method, 579
Webster, R.C., 460
Weinzweig, N., 602
Wilson sedation scale, 78
Wu, W., 285

Y
Yousif, N.J., 290

Printing and Binding: Stürtz GmbH, Würzburg